IMMUNOFLUORESCENCE TECHNOLOGY
Selected theoretical and clinical aspects

IMMUNOFLUORESCENCE TECHNOLOGY

Selected theoretical and clinical aspects

Editors:
G. WICK
K.N. TRAILL
K. SCHAUENSTEIN

Institute for General and Experimental Pathology, University of Innsbruck Medical School, Fritz-Pregl-Strasse 3, A-6020 Innsbruck, Austria

1982
ELSEVIER BIOMEDICAL PRESS
AMSTERDAM · NEW YORK · OXFORD

ISBN 0444 80398 X

Published by:
Elsevier Biomedical Press B.V.
1 Molenwerf, 1014 AG. P.O. Box 211
Amsterdam, The Netherlands

Sole distributors for the USA and Canada:
Elsevier Science Publishing Company Inc.
52 Vanderbilt Avenue
New York, N.Y. 10017

Library of Congress Cataloging in Publication Data
Main entry under title:

Immunofluorescence technology

Bibliography: p.
Includes index.
I. Immunofluorescence. I. Wick, G. (Georg)
II. Traill, K.N. III. Schauenstein, K.
QR187.I48I44 1982 616.9'780756 82-13776
ISBN 0-444-80398-X

Printed in The Netherlands

Foreword

More than ten years ago, with the initial sponsorship of W.H.O., we held the first of what has since become an annual postgraduate course in immunofluorescence. Due to the continuing interest in immunohistological techniques we are currently organizing the 11th course of this type. A booklet describing the basic principles of immunofluorescence with emphasis on problems of standardization was published to serve as a manual for this purpose.

The programme of these events includes both practical exercises and lectures on theoretical aspects. Each year, as one of the highlights of the course, we invite a distinguished immunologist to give a talk on a selected topic of immunofluorescence. These guest lectures always deal with some advanced aspects of the technique and its application such as pattern recognition, ways of standardization, flow cytometry, immunofluorescence as a tool for the study of local immunity, etc. Since they were always met with great interest we considered asking some of these speakers and also some additional authors to help us compile a second volume dealing with these more specialized aspects of immunofluorescence and putting the use of this technique into a broader context. All of our colleagues whom we asked for contributions reacted positively and this volume is the result of that endeavour. We would like to take this opportunity to thank all the authors for their cooperation as well as the publishing house for its patience in preparing this book and bringing it to its present form. The aim of this publication cannot, of course, be to cover all aspects of new developments in immunofluorescence, but rather to provide detailed technical data in some selected areas which are of interest to workers in the theoretical field as well as to clinicians. It is intended as a reference book giving practical details and we hope that it will be useful both for students of the postgraduate courses and for those using this technique for the first time in the laboratory. Since labelled antibody technology, and in particular immunofluorescence, is a rapidly expanding field, it was a great pleasure for the editors both to receive these papers from the contributors and to discuss the work described in the manuscripts with them.

We do hope that the readers will enjoy this book as much as we did preparing it.

G. Wick
K.N. Traill
K. Schauenstein

Innsbruck, Austria

List of contributors

B. ALBINI, Department of Microbiology, State University of New York at Buffalo School of Medicine, 240B Cary Hall, Buffalo, NY 14214, U.S.A.

P. BERGER, Institute for General and Experimental Pathology, University of Innsbruck Medical School, Fritz-Pregl-Strasse 3, A-6020 Innsbruck, Austria

G. BÖCK, Institute for General and Experimental Pathology, University of Innsbruck Medical School, Fritz-Pregl-Strasse 3, A-6020 Innsbruck, Austria

P. BRANDTZAEG, Histochemical Laboratory, Institute of Pathology, The National Hospital, Rikshospitalet, Oslo, Norway

S. CHANTLER, Bone and Joint Research Unit, London Hospital Medical College, London, U.K.

H. DENK, Division of Gastroenterologic Pathology and Hepatopathology (Hans Popper Laboratory), Department of Pathology, University of Vienna School of Medicine, A-1090 Vienna, Austria

G.J. Van den ENGH, Department of Radiobiology, Erasmus University, 151 Lange Kleiweg, 2288 GJ Rijswijk, The Netherlands

J.J. HAAIJMAN, Institute for Experimental Gerontology TNO, P.O.Box 5815, 2280 HV Rijswijk, The Netherlands

E.J. HOLBOROW, Bone and Joint Research Unit, London Hospital Medical College, London, U.K.

G.D. JOHNSON, Bone and Joint Research Unit, London Hospital Medical College, London, U.K.

D. KERJASCHKI, Department of Cell Biology, Yale University, New Haven, CT, U.S.A.

W. KNAPP, Institute for Immunology, University of Vienna, A-1090 Vienna, Austria

R. KOFLER, Institute for General and Experimental Pathology, University of Innsbruck Medical School, Fritz-Pregl-Strasse 3, A-6020 Innsbruck, Austria

B. NOBLE, Department of Microbiology, 2403 Cary Hall, State University of New York at Buffalo, Buffalo, New York 14214, U.S.A.

E. PENNER, Department of Gastroenterology and Computer Science, II. Universitäts Klinik für Gastroenterologie und Hepatologie, Allgemeines Krankenhaus Wien, Garnisongasse 13, A-1090 Vienna, Austria

B. PLATZER, Division of Gastroenterologic Pathology and Hepatopathology (Hans Popper Laboratory), Department of Pathology, University of Vienna School of Medicine, A-1090 Vienna, Austria

J.S. PLOEM, Department of Histochemistry and Cytochemistry, Sylvius Laboratories, University of Leiden, Wassenaarseweg 72, 2333 AL Leiden, The Netherlands

T. RADASZKIEWICZ, Division of Gastroenterologic Pathology and Hepatopathology (Hans Popper Laboratory), Department of Pathology, University of Vienna School of Medicine, A-1090 Vienna, Austria

K. SCHAUENSTEIN, Institute for General and Experimental Pathology, University of Innsbruck Medical School, Fritz-Pregl-Strasse 3, A-6020 Innsbruck, Austria

J.W.M. VISSER, Radiobiology Institute TNO, 151 Lange Kleiweg, 2288 GJ Rijswijk, The Netherlands

G. WICK, Institute for General and Experimental Pathology, University of Innsbruck Medical School, Fritz-Pregl-Strasse 3, A-6020 Innsbruck, Austria

H. WOLF, Institute for General and Experimental Pathology, University of Innsbruck Medical School, Fritz-Pregl-Strasse 3, A-6020 Innsbruck, Austria

Contents list

List of abbreviations

AAb, autoantibodies
ABC, antigen-binding cells
ABM, alveolar basement membrane
AC, alternating current
ADCC, antibody-dependent cellular cytotoxicity
ADM, aperture-defined microvolume
AFP, alpha-1-fetoprotein
ANA, antinuclear antibody
ANF, antinuclear factor
ARS, arsinilic acid
BCGP, breast carcinoma glycoprotein
BG, blood group
BMD, basement membrane dense deposit disease
BSA, bovine serum albumin
BUN, blood urea nitrogen
CEA, carcinoembryonic antigen
CEX, CEA-associated antigen
CGN, chronic glomerulonephritis
CNBr, cyanogen bromide
Con A, concanavalin A
CSS, chronic serum sickness
DC, direct current
DEG, diffuse extracapillary (crescentic) glomerulonephritis
DEPG, diffuse endocapillary proliferative glomerulonephritis
DMG, diffuse mesangiocapillary glomerulonephritis
DMSO, dimethyl sulphoxide
DNA, deoxyribonucleic acid
DASS, defined antigenic substrate spheres (system)
DNP, dinitrophenol
DSG, diffuse (chronic) sclerosis glomerulonephritis
ELISA, enzyme-linked immunosorbent assay
FAA, fibrin-associated antigen
FACS, fluorescence-activated cell sorter
FDA, fluorescein diacetate
FG, focal glomerulonephritis
FIF, formaldehyde-induced fluorescence
FIAPS, fluorescence immunoassay with plain surface
FICA, fluoro-immuno-cytoadherence
FITC, fluorescein isothiocyanate
FPR, fluorescence-photobleaching recovery

FSA, fetal sulphoglycoprotein antigen
FSH, follicle-stimulating hormone
FSHS, focal and segmental hyalinosis and sclerosis
GBM, glomerular basement membrane
GFR, glomerular filtration rate
GN, glomerulonephritides
HAT, hypoxanthine–aminopterin–thymidine (medium)
hCG, human chorionic gonadotropin
HLTAA, human lung tumor-associated antigen
IC, immune complexes
ICA, islet cell antibodies
IF, immunofluorescence
IFM, immunofluorescence microscopy
IIF, indirect immunofluorescence
IN, interstitial nephrotides
ITP, idiopathic thrombocytopenic purpura
IUIS, International Union on Immunological Societies
LH, luteinizing hormone
MAb, monoclonal antibodies
MeIF, membrane immunofluorescence
MGL, minimal glomerular lesion
MGN, membranous glomerulonephritides
MHC, major histocompatibility complex
MMF, semiautomated microassay
MPG, mesangial proliferative glomerulonephritis
MUF, 4-methylumbelliferone
NA, numerical aperture
NCA, normal cross-reacting antigen
NCS, normal chicken serum
NGP, normal glycoprotein
NMS, normal mouse serum
NSN, nephrotoxic serum nephritis
OS, Obese strain
PAS, periodic acid–Schiff
PAP, peroxidase–antiperoxidase
PBV, packed bead volume
PI, propidium iodide
PM, photomultiplier
PSGN, post-streptococcal glomerulonephritis
RBC, red blood cells
RFC, rosette-forming cells
RIA, radioimmunoassay
RIg, rabbit immunoglobulin
SAT, spontaneous autoimmune thyroiditis
SBM, single bead measurement

SITS, 4-acetamido-4-isothiocyanostilbene-2,2′-disulphonic acid
SLE, systemic lupus erythematosis
Tg-BC, thyroglobulin-binding cells
TI, tubulointerstitial
TMB, tubular basement membrane
TRITC, tetramethylrhodamine isothiocyanate
TSH, thyroid-stimulating hormone
XRITC, tetra-*N*-cyclopropylrhodamine

Wick et al. (eds) Immunofluorescence Technology. Selected Theoretical and Clinical Aspects © Elsevier Biomedical Press, 1982

CHAPTER 1

Use of international reference preparations for immunofluorescence

E.J. HOLBOROW, G.D. JOHNSON and SHIREEN CHANTLER

Bone and Joint Research Unit, London Hospital, Medical College, London (U.K.)

1.1. HISTORICAL ASPECTS

The increased use of immunofluorescence (IF) techniques in routine laboratories during the 1960s focussed attention on the problems encountered in different laboratories using reagents from a variety of sources. Variation in results was seen not only between laboratories using a similar procedure but also within individual laboratories performing tests on different occasions. Recognition of the need for standardisation in diagnostic immunofluorescence in the field of autoimmune serology led to the acquisition and evaluation of a pool of serum with autoantibody activity of defined specificity, "antinuclear antibody", by the Division of Biological Standards, London, working closely with the World Health Organisation (WHO) [1]. As described below, this was subsequently accepted as an International Reference Preparation for antinuclear factor (ANF).

It was also apparent that the conjugate is of crucial importance in determining both the performance and reproducibility of autoantibody assays and several workers emphasised the need for improving the quality of commercially available conjugates [3, 4, 7–9, 13]. This stimulated interest in the U.K. in the process of standardisation and culminated in the publication by a Medical Research Council (MRC) Working Party (1971) of recommendations for conjugate preparation.

There was also considerable international interest in the field of standardisation in its widest context. This resulted in the formal establishment of the International Union of Immunological Societies' (IUIS) Standardisation Committee in 1971 with Professor Raynaud as Chairman and Mrs. Irene Batty as Secretary. The objectives of this group were to encourage international representation of scientific and professional bodies with a common interest in standardisation, to minimise any duplication of effort, to identify priorities in the field of immunological standardisation, and finally to ensure that specifications for potential international standard and reference preparations were compiled by informed specialists in the relevant areas. Members of this committee felt that the objectives outlined above would be best achieved by means of sub-committees comprised of experts in those fields of immunology in which the need for standardisation was greatest.

Since the activities of IUIS in respect of standardisation were complementary to those of WHO, formal liaison between the two organisations was desirable to ensure agreement on acceptable standards. In 1972, Irene Batty was given the task of setting up a secretariat within the division of immunology at WHO, Geneva, which would be responsible for coordinating the activities of different WHO/IUIS sub-committees and administering government grants from Canada, Germany, Holland, Israel, Norway, Sweden, Switzerland, United Kingdom and U.S.A. channelled via WHO for IUIS/WHO standardisation efforts.

The first IUIS immunofluorescence committee chaired by Professor Astrid Fagraeus was established in 1971 and as a result of the efforts of this group, two WHO/IUIS International Standard conjugate preparations and Reference serum containing antinuclear antibody (ANA) of IgM class (HL) were adopted by WHO. These preparations, FITC-labelled sheep anti-human Ig (480010), FITC-labelled sheep anti-human IgM (anti-μ chain) and IgM class ANA (HL) are available from the WHO Immunology Unit, Geneva. The current WHO/IUIS sub-committee are in the final stages of evaluating a candidate FITC-labelled anti-human IgG (anti-γ chain) conjugate prior to its submission to the WHO expert committee.

1.2. PURPOSES OF STANDARDISATION

Immunological reagents are for the most part biological materials which cannot be characterised adequately by chemical and/or physical means alone. Common reference materials (standards) are therefore required to provide results which are "quantitatively consistent and which can be reliably related from one laboratory to another and from one time to another" [2]. Standards should ideally be qualitatively identical to test materials; plots of their respective dose responses should be parallel and show linearity, and they should have long-term stability. If these conditions are met the ratio of the potency of the test material to that of the standard is independent of the method used and should remain constant. The assignment of an arbitrary unitage to the standard or reference material and the expression of results in relative units minimised interlaboratory differences due to technical variation. Unfortunately, biological materials rarely satisfy all of these requirements. Their performance is affected by qualitative and quantitative differences related to antibody avidity and specificity and, in the case of fluorochrome-labelled reagents, additional factors related to the method of preparation. Many of these diverse factors affecting performance are well documented so that their adverse effects can be minimised by careful preparation, characterisation and selection of materials which satisfy defined minimal requirements. However, although the suitability of labelled reagents for use as standards can be predicted from a knowledge of selected physico-chemical characteristics, their practical adequacy can only be established by their performance in a definitive system. The prime function of international immunofluorescence standards and reference preparations is thus to enable reactions detectable by immunofluorescence to be quantified in uniform terms throughout the world and also to provide a check on specificity. The WHO nomenclature used for immunological comparison materials of this sort is given in Table 1.I.

TABLE 1.I

NOMENCLATURE FOR IMMUNOLOGICAL COMPARISON MATERIALS

Material	Potency assigned	Intended use	Available for immunofluorescence
WHO Internat. Standards	Assigned Internat. Unitage (I.U.)	Calibration of local materials for control of quality and for potency	FITC anti-human Ig conjugates: sheep anti-human Ig sheep anti-human IgM (anti-μ chain) sheep anti-human IgG (anti-γ chain)
WHO Internat. Reference Preparations	May or may not be assigned I.U.	Provided as a service reagent; also suitable for calibrating local material	antinuclear factor (homogeneous) 66/233 (100 I.U./ampoule) IgM class antinuclear antibody HL
WHO Internat. Reference Reagents	—	Qualitative use in identification (high specificity)	—

1.3. THE ROLE OF INTERNATIONAL COLLABORATIVE ASSAYS

The suitability of immunofluorescence standards has been assessed by a sequence of collaborative assays carried out on an international basis with the aim of answering the question "Are the proposed materials useful to ensure uniformity of results?" "Results", here, means attempts to measure the amount or activity of reagents in various immunofluorescent reactions. It might be thought that uniformity of results would be best achieved by specifying a standard technique to be used in each laboratory routinely performing a given test. However, the variables in immunofluorescence methodology are numerous and it would not be practicable to impose technical restrictions on them all. They include i) the optical features and illumination systems used in the microscopy, ii) the properties of the fluorochrome conjugated antibody, iii) in indirect IF the quality and quantity of antibody in the patient's serum, iv) the antigen-containing substrate, and v) the observer. Thus, the accepted approach to promoting uniformity of reporting immunofluorescence test results is to use collaborative studies in order to establish a standard material of uniform and stable potency suitable for monitoring local reference preparations for potency and specificity. This approach is exemplified by the studies leading to the provision of antinuclear antibody reference preparations.

1.4. ANTINUCLEAR ANTIBODY (ANA) REFERENCE PREPARATIONS

The IF test for antinuclear antibodies is among the most frequently performed autoantibody tests. The reason for this is that, although we still have no clear understanding of why ANA appear in disease, we know that the highest titres cluster in patients with systemic lupus erythematosus, that a negative result virtually excludes this diagnosis, and that published results of innumerable studies of the incidence of ANA in human disease appear increasingly open to the interpretation that a positive ANA test reflects a degree of disturbance of the control mechanisms by which the immune system regulates its own responses. For several reasons, therefore, rheumatologists, haematologists, hepatologists and other physicians need not only to know whether ANA is present, but to be able to monitor its serum levels. In turn, the laboratories to which they are sending their blood specimens need to define the level of sensitivity which in each laboratory determines a negative report.

As mentioned above, the first reference preparation to be presented to the WHO expert committee on Biological Standardisation was a freeze-dried batch of ANA-positive serum pooled from six British and Dutch patients with systemic lupus erythematosus, which was originally proposed as a British Research Standard. With this preparation, known as 66/233, an international collaborative assay involving eleven laboratories was undertaken, each participating laboratory using its own technique for testing and, in addition, a suggested common technique. Five other ANA positive sera were provided for assay in comparison with the proposed standard. Geometric mean titres were calculated for each preparation and for each technique, local or common. At the same time the potencies of each preparation in relation to the standard 66/233 were estimated and expressed as percentages.

The results of this study led to two general conclusions. Firstly, the variability of estimates of potency of the five ANA-positive sera was reduced if potencies relative to the reference material were compared, rather than mean titres. Secondly – and this was an important conclusion for its influence on the planning of future studies of proposed standards and reference preparations in IF – it was shown that estimates of potency are not more uniform, i.e. less variable, when a common technique rather than a local technique is used in a collaborative study. The study thus clearly demonstrated that the real value of a reference preparation of this sort is to permit different workers in different laboratories usefully to compare their results *without altering or modifying their methods*, although the results of such comparisons may, of course, lead some workers to consider changing their techniques to improve specificity or sensitivity. As a consequence of this study the preparation was accepted as a WHO International Reference Preparation.

1.4.1. Method of use of the international reference preparation for antinuclear factor 66/233

The principle of how a reference preparation such as antinuclear factor 66/233 should be used is well known, but since this one appears rarely to be put to proper use even now, ten years after its introduction, it may be set out again here.

The ampoule provided contains an arbitrary 100 units of ANA activity as lyophilised serum. The material is dissolved in the diluent used routinely so as to contain, say, 100 units/ml, and doubling dilutions are titrated on nuclear substrate, e.g. cryostat sections of liver as employed in the local method under precisely the conditions employed for routine tests. The end-point is the highest dilution showing weak nuclear fluorescence, i.e. giving minimal nuclear staining distinguishable from a negative reaction. If, for example, the end-point defined in this way is 1 : 160, then under routine conditions of test for this observer, the end-point dilution contains $1/160 \times 100$ International Units per ml = 0.625 I.U/ml. For another observer, with another system, the end-point might represent less or more I.U. per ml of ANA activity. Such differences between systems are nullified by expressing results of test sera in I.U. per ml, calculated by multiplying the reciprocals of their dilutions at their titration end-points by the number of units of activity present in the reference preparation at its titration end-point in the laboratory concerned.

This, then, is how the ANA reference preparation (and any other such preparations forthcoming) should be used, and we strongly urge that clinical immunology laboratories take note of the Report of the Second Joint IUIS/

WHO Consultation, 1976, and report antinuclear antibody levels in I.U. per ml.

Abuses of the ANF reference preparation mostly arise from failure to take account of the complex nature of the active material in it. The antibody activity is directed against nuclear antigens which impart a diffuse nuclear fluorescence; these are probably nucleoproteins, although this specificity has not been formally shown for the reference preparation. Thus, serum 66/233 is an inappropriate reference for speckled and other patterns of nuclear fluorescence. Further, sera giving selective nuclear staining in some tissues and not others (e.g. staining renal tubular cell nuclei but not hepatocyte nuclei) are unsuitable for comparison with serum 66/233, which contains antibodies reactive with cell nuclei in widely different tissues. Secondly, as with other antibody titrations, the end-point is the resultant of total antibody content and antibody avidity, and sera containing the same total amounts of less or more avid antinuclear antibodies may give different end-points. Thirdly, the reference preparation 66/233 has its antinuclear antibody activity preponderantly in the IgG fraction. Its best use, therefore, is as a comparison material for test sera in which the ANA activity is also of the IgG class; and used in this way it provides an invaluable yardstick against which to assess not only the potency of unknown test sera, but also the overall sensitivity of the immunofluorescence methodology for detection of ANA in use in any given laboratory.

1.4.2. IgM class-specific antinuclear antibody

As a yardstick of IgM antibody specificity, a WHO/IUIS reference preparation of IgM ANA (monoclonal in nature) designated "IgM class antinuclear antibody HL" is also available, but in limited supply. It is reactive with speckled nuclear antigen and is best demonstrated on tissue sections fixed with paraformaldehyde.

1.5. INTERNATIONAL STANDARD FITC-LABELLED ANTI-HUMAN Ig CONJUGATES

IUIS/WHO International standard conjugates with activity against human Ig and human IgM respectively are already available, and a third against human IgG is being submitted for acceptance. All three have been prepared from antisera raised in sheep injected with appropriate immunoglobulin antigens and checked for specificity by accepted methods. The total protein, the antibody protein and the fluorescein : protein weight and molar ratios of the conjugates determined by accepted methods were measured, and the freeze-dried conjugates were then distributed to expert laboratories for collaborative study* as to their suitability as reference standards. At this

* These collaborative studies have been organised by the Immunofluorescence Sub-Committee of the IUIS Standardisation Committee.

point, it may be useful to recapitulate why IUIS/WHO thought (and still thinks) it is desirable to provide standard conjugates, and also the criteria on which the suitability of candidate conjugates is judged.

Conjugated antibodies to human immunoglobulins are used in immunofluorescence for diagnostic and other purposes in clinical and research laboratories, both specialised and unspecialised, throughout the world. As emphasised above, the quality of the conjugate has a profound effect upon the results obtained. The primary need of the laboratory worker is thus for reassurance about the quality of conjugates (usually supplied commercially) in routine use at the bench, and it is this need that the standards are designed to meet. Apart from deficiencies due to gross over- or under-labelling, the performances of conjugates differ for reasons of potency and immunological specificity.

The time-honoured, and indeed still the most satisfactory method of assessing the potency of conjugates in indirect immunofluorescence is by their performance in a chessboard titration of dilutions of conjugate against dilutions of the same middle layer serum known to contain antibody such as ANA. The first requirement of a satisfactory conjugate is that it should give a constant titre for the middle layer serum over a wide range of conjugate dilutions, the middle layer titre thereafter dropping significantly. The constant end-point dilution of the middle layer is the "plateau titre", and the highest conjugate dilution at which the plateau titre is maintained is the "plateau end-point" of the conjugate. The working dilution of a conjugate for a given test system should be at least twice the concentration at the plateau end-point.

The plateau titre (perhaps "plateau height" is a better term) is an expression of the resultant of antibody content and antibody avidity for a given middle layer serum. Its height, however, is also significantly affected by the fluorochrome : protein ratio of the conjugate used to measure it. The plateau end-point, on the other hand, expresses the antibody potency of a conjugate, and it is well recognised that conjugates giving plateau end-points at high dilution, and hence used at high working dilutions, are more efficient because at such dilutions they give less background staining.

A comparison of plateau titres (heights) and plateau end-points between standard and local conjugates therefore gives a useful measure of the performance of the latter. It may be noted, moreover, that this comparison can be made without knowledge on the part of the user of the protein content, antibody content or fluorescein : protein ratio of either conjugate. Although these measurements will have been determined for each standard conjugate and the results confirm that the conjugated material is likely to be satisfactory as a standard for the purposes described, its suitability is ultimately decided by its behaviour by block titration in collaborative studies. Unless they have special reasons for doing so, laboratory users of conjugates thus do not usually need to measure their immunochemical and biochemical characteristics, since comparative chessboard titrations can tell them what they need to know about the relative potency and specificity. On this count, we disagree with the view expressed by Beutner et al. [6] that standard reference conjugates are contraindicated, and that IUIS/WHO is in "inappropriate competition with industry" in providing them. It is apparent that, far from attempting to compete, IUIS/WHO offers international standard anti-immunoglobulin conjugates as yardsticks of performance for both potency and specificity, vouched for by the results of collaborative assay by experts world-wide. Like laboratory workers, manufacturers may, if they so wish, use such standards as comparison materials.

To define the specificity of a conjugate in indirect immunofluorescence, it is necessary to test it under conditions where the middle layer is varied to contain antibodies of different immunoglobulin classes, taking separate account of at least IgG, IgA and IgM antibodies. A comparison of class specificities is in fact a difficult one for the user to make, for middle layer reagents with antibody specificity exclusively of a single defined class, especially other than IgG, are not readily available. Another difficulty confronting the user wishing to compare the performances of conjugates is that special processing of the substrate tissue may have been used in the original assays of the standard conjugate; for example, as described above, the standard anti-IgM conjugate has been collaboratively assayed on rat liver sections prefixed in 4% paraformaldehyde in order to retain otherwise soluble nuclear antigens reactive with the monoclonal IgM antinuclear antibody reference preparation HL used in the middle layer.

The specificity of anti-immunoglobulin conjugates in direct testing is a different question, which has to take into account the uses to which they are to be put. Thus, it appears (Dr. W. Hijmans, personal communication) that anti-Ig conjugates that are satisfactorily class-specific on monoclonal bone marrow cells or on artificial substrates comprised of antigens coupled to Sepharose beads, may not be so when tested under double-staining conditions on polyclonal bone marrow. Likewise, the appropriateness for direct staining of lymphocyte membrane Ig of conjugates which are Ig class-specific under indirect conditions has to be separately established.

1.5.1. Limitations of use of standard anti-Ig conjugates

WHO International Standard Conjugates are supplied in ampoules which contain 100 I.U. It should therefore be possible to define the relative potency of other conjugates in terms of I.U. by comparison of their respective titres obtained by block titration on the lines described above for the use of the antinuclear factor reference preparation. In practice, however, the following reservations must apply.

1. Valid comparisons of titre can only be made between reagents of identical immunological specificity.

2. The results of block titration reflect two independent variables in the case of the conjugate: fluorochrome : protein ratio as a function of plateau

height and antibody potency which determines the plateau end-point titre of the conjugate.

Thus only in a given test system employing conjugate of the same specificity as the standard and having a similar fluorochrome : protein ratio is it possible to express the activity of the conjugate under test in terms of International Units. This is clearly important when considering the potential use of WHO conjugates for standardisation of commercial reagents.

1.6. CONCLUSIONS

Thirty years after the definitive description of the immunofluorescence procedure [10] its adoption in routine diagnostic laboratories continues to expand and new applications of its versatility as a research tool are being reported. Although the influence on sensitivity of the diverse variables inherent in the procedure is understood, technical restrictions on the methodology employed have not been established. This has undoubtedly been responsible for many new observations and such technical diversity should continue to be encouraged.

Essential for this policy, however, are the means of ensuring consistency within the laboratory and comparability between different laboratories, particularly in the field of clinical immunology and microbiology. The progress already made by WHO/IUIS in meeting this need by provision of the standard materials described above and their general adoption should go a long way towards improving the quality of immunofluorescent testing. It is to be hoped that the panel of materials available will be expanded to include standards for other fluorescent conjugates and for other antibodies of clinical importance – including autoantibodies and antibodies to microorganisms – for which immunofluorescence continues to be the screening method of choice.

REFERENCES

1 Anderson, S.G., Addison, I.E. and Dixon, H.G. (1971) Antinuclear factor serum (homogeneous): an international collaborative study of the proposed research standard 66/233. Ann. N.Y. Acad. Sci. *77,* 337–345.

2 Bangham, D.R. and Cotes, P.M. (1974) Standardisation and standards. Br. Med. Bull. *30,* 12–17.

3 Beutner, E.H., Holborow, E.J. and Johnson, G.D. (1967) Quantitative studies of immunofluorescent staining I. Immunology *12,* 327–337.

4 Beutner, E.H., Sepulveda, M.R. and Barnett, E.V. (1968) Quantitative studies of immunofluorescent staining. II. Bull. W.H.O. *39,* 587–606.

5 Beutner, E.H., Monin, K. and Wypych, J.I. (1971) Field trials by ten laboratories of six commercial conjugates prepared from antisera to human IgG. Ann. N.Y. Acad. Sci. *177,* 361–404.

6 Beutner, E.H., Kumar, V and Binder, W.L. (1980) State of the art of immunofluorescence techniques in tissues. *In:* Kertges, P.W. and Nakamura, R.M. (eds.), Diagnostic Immunology:

Current and Future Trends (College of American Pathologists, Illinois) pp. 88–99 (in press).
7 Brighton, W.D. and Hayhoe, J. (1970) Comparison of the activity of commercial conjugates in different antigen-antibody systems. *In* Holborow, E.J. (ed.), Standardisation in Immunofluorescence (Blackwell Scientific Publications, Oxford), pp. 205–208.
8 Brighton, W.D., Taylor, C.E.D., Tomlinson, A.H. and Wilkinson, A.E. (1967) A provisional specification for fluorescein labelled antibody against human globulin (IgG). Mon. Bull. Minist. Health Public Health Lab. Serv. *26,* 179–181.
9 Cherry, W.B. and Reimer, C.B. (1973) Diagnostic immunofluorescence. Bull. W.H.O. *43,* 737–746.
10 Coons, A.H. and Kaplan, M.H. (1950) Localisation of antigen in tissue cells II: improvements in a method for the detection of antigen by means of fluorescent antibody. J. Exp. Med. *91,* 1–13.
11 Johnson, G.D., Chantler, S., Batty, I and Holborow, E.J. (1979) Use and abuse of international reference preparations in immunofluorescence. *In* Dumonde, D.C. and Stewart, M.W. (eds.), Laboratory Tests in the Rheumatic Diseases (MIP Press Ltd.) pp. 81–91.
12 MRC Working Party (1971) Recommendations on the characterisation of antisera as reagents. Immunology *20,* 1–10.
13 Nairn, R.C. (1968) Standardisation in immunofluorescence. Clin. Exp. Immunol. *3,* 465–476.
14 Report of Second Joint IUIS/WHO Consultation (1976) Standardisation of immunological reagents for diagnostic purposes.

Wick et al. (eds) Immunofluorescence Technology. Selected Theoretical and Clinical Aspects © *Elsevier Biomedical Press, 1982*

CHAPTER 2

Preparation and use of defined antigenic substrates for standardized immunofluorescence

W. KNAPP

Institute for Immunology, University of Vienna, Austria

2.1. INTRODUCTION

During the last 16 years several attempts have been made to use antigens coupled to inert matrices or polymerized antigen itself as an artificial substrate in immunofluorescence [2, 3, 5, 6, 31, 41, 46, 47].

The main advantages of artificial substrates over biological substrates such as tissue sections or cells are 1) better defined antigenic composition of artificial substrates in qualitative as well as quantitative terms, 2) the homogeneous fluorescence pattern of most artificial substrates necessary for reliable quantitation, and 3) the usually significantly better storing stability.

During the last several years the most frequently used defined antigenic substrate is the so-called defined antigenic substrate spheres (DASS) system [4, 7–14, 16, 18, 20, 21, 25–27, 29, 36, 47]. This chapter will primarily emphasize the DASS system.

2.2. PREPARATION OF DEFINED ANTIGENIC SUBSTRATES

2.2.1. Carrier material

We are using agarose beads (Sepharose 4B from Pharmacia, Uppsala, Sweden) as relatively inert carriers to which protein antigens can easily be covalently coupled by the Bromcyan method [35]. Raybould and Chantler [36] recently proposed the use of cross-linked Sepharose 4B (Sepharose CL4B, Pharmacia) instead of Sepharose 4B, since a lower staining variation of individual beads was observed when using Sepharose CL4B. We have also tried other materials such as cross-linked dextran particles, but the best contrast in fluorescence between negative and positive reactions was obtained with agarose material.

2.2.2. Cyanogen bromide (CNBr) activation of Sepharose 4B beads

All manipulations of the CNBr activation procedure are performed in a fume cupboard. Sepharose 4B is first washed exhaustively with distilled water in order to remove the preservative added by the manufacturer.

One volume of washed Sepharose consisting of equal volumes of packed beads and water (= 50% v/v) is added to one volume of 2 M sodium carbonate. The mixture is then placed into an ice bath and slowly stirred in order not to break the beaded material. During stirring 0.05 volume of a solution of CNBr (Fluka Ag, Buchs, Switzerland) in acetonitrile (Sigma, St. Louis, MO) (2 g CNBr/ml acetonitrile) is added. The CNBr solution in acetonitrile is usable for several months when stored at –20°C. Stirring is continued for 1–2 min and then the gel is quickly washed on a coarse-sintered glass funnel (Type D3, Schott, F.R.G.) with 5–10 volumes of the following ice-cold solutions: a) 0.1 M sodium bicarbonate, pH 9.5; b) distilled water; and c) 0.2 M bicarbonate, pH 9.5.

2.2.3. Coupling procedure

Immediately following this washing procedure the gel is sucked almost dry and transferred to a tube containing one volume of 0.2 M sodium bicarbonate, pH 9.5, and one volume of protein (usually dissolved in phosphate-buffered saline, pH 7.2; PBS*) to be coupled. Antigen preparations should be dialysed against PBS before coupling in order to remove substances like NaN_3, glycine, Tris, etc. which interfere with the coupling. This suspension is then gently mixed and incubated for 8–12 h on a rollerbank at 4°C.

* 0.15 M NaCl, 0.01 M sodium phosphate, pH 7.2.

2.2.4. *Deactivation of residual active groups*

The residual active groups are subsequently deactivated by overnight incubation with 2 volumes of 0.5 M ethanolamine (Sigma, St. Louis, MO) adjusted to a pH of 9.0. After deactivation with ethanolamine the beads are washed again on a coarse-sintered glass funnel (Schott, Type D3) with 20 volumes of the following solutions: a) 0.1 M sodium acetate, pH 4.0, with 0.65 M NaCl; b) 2 M urea with 0.65 M NaCl; c) 0.1 M sodium bicarbonate, pH 9.5, with 0.65 M NaCl; and d) PBS, pH 7.2.

Beads are usually stored as a 5–20% suspension at 4°C (volume packed beads after 5 min centrifugation at 400 g/ total volume suspension). When only small volumes of bead suspensions are available the estimation of the bead suspension density can be performed in microhaematocrit tubes and the results read with a microhaematocrit reader (e.g. from Hawksley, U.K.). For larger volumes graduated centrifugation tubes are used and the results read directly. Merthiolate or sodium azide should be added as preservative. It is also possible to store the antigen-coupled beads at –20°C or to freeze-dry* them.

2.2.5. *Handling of bead suspensions*

All glassware should be siliconized to prevent adherence of protein-coupled agarose beads. Pipetting of bead suspensions in our laboratory is performed with Eppendorf (Fa. Eppendorf, Hamburg, F.R.G.) micropipettes immediately after thorough mixing with a Vortex shaker.

2.2.6. *Staining and washing procedures*

Staining and washing of beads can easily be performed with a home-made device. Plastic tubes with an inner diameter of 10 mm, at the bottom of which filters are mounted retaining particles with a diameter of more than 40 μm (Pharmacia, Uppsala) are pressed firmly onto silicone rubber discs to achieve complete caulking. 100 μl of a thoroughly mixed bead suspension and 100 μl of the appropriate antiserum or conjugate are incubated in these tubes by continuous shaking. After incubation, the tubes are lifted from the silicone rubber discs, so that the stained beads can be easily washed with a repipetting device. Washing is performed with 3 × 3 ml PBS within 15 min followed by incubation overnight at 4°C with 3 ml PBS of high ionic strength (0.65 M NaCl) after the last incubation. After the last washing the beads are transferred with a micropipette to a slide, mixed with mounting fluid**, covered with a cover glass and sealed with paraffin.

---

* For freeze drying, beads should be suspended in a 2.5% (w/v) lactose and 2.5% (w/v) dextran T 10 (Pharmacia, Uppsala) solution in PBS.

** $NaHCO_3$ 0.0715 g, Na_2CO_3 0.016 g, distilled water to 10 ml, glycerol to 100 ml = mounting fluid, pH 9.0.

An alternative procedure which facilitates staining and washing of large numbers of test samples has been proposed by Haaijman and Brinkhof [16]. They use the wells of flat-bottomed microtest plates (System Cooke; Greiner, Würtingen, F.R.G.; cat. No. M 220–29 ART) as reaction vessels which allow the performance of 96 assays with one plate. To each well 50–100 μl of a thoroughly mixed bead suspension and 50–100 μl of the appropriate antiserum or conjugate dilution are added. Attention should be paid to the homogeneity of the bead suspension. When large experiments are performed it is advisable to slowly stir the suspension with a magnetic stirrer during pipetting.

Washing of beads after incubation can best be performed as described by Schauenstein et al. [40] and chapter 4 of this volume for membrane fluorescence studies with eight- or twelve-channel dispenser and eight- or twelve-channel aspiration manifolds. For adding the washing fluid (PBS with 0.65 M NaCl, 100–200 μl/well) the "multi-channel reagent dispenser" (Microtiter Dynatech, cat. No. AM 58) can be used. For aspirating the washing fluid either a "dispenser manifold 8 tip" (Microtiter Dynatech cat. No. MA 3004) or a "dispenser manifold 12 tip" (Microtiter Dynatech cat. No. MA 3005) is attached to a water suction vacuum pump and in this way used as an aspiration manifold. The depth of immersion of the aspiration manifold is adjusted by means of layers of tape wound around both poles of the comb and is best calibrated to give a residual volume of 50 μl in each well after suction. There is no need to spin the plates after the addition of washing fluid. The plate simply may be left standing for 5–10 min after adding the washing fluid. The supernatant may then be aspirated without disturbing the beads lying on the bottom of the wells. Successive incubations can be carried out in the same plate. During incubation plates are sealed with adhesive tape (plate sealers, Microtiter Dynatech cat. No. M 30).

Staining and washing of beads in microtest plates has two main advantages when large series of experiments are performed: a) a comprehensive range of semi- and fully automatic equipment for pipetting, diluting, transferring, etc. is commercially available (Titertek, Flow Lab. Irvine, U.K., and Microtiter, Dynatech Zug, Switzerland); and b) readings of the results can be performed directly in the plate through the plate bottom when an inverted fluorescence microscope is available (for details see below). For this purpose 50 μl of mounting fluid are added to each well after the last washing and the plate is then covered with a dark cover.

For the demonstration of antibodies in antisera etc., the smallest quantity of beads should be used which still leaves sufficient amounts of beads (for measurements) after the incubation-, washing- and transfer procedures. This produces the highest degree of sensitivity. For each protein the optimal antigen or antibody concentration for coupling has to be found. Reference values for the proteins used so far can be seen from literature listed in Table 2.I. In all our experiments an incubation time of 2 h was found to be sufficient. Under certain circumstances longer incubation periods may, however, be necessary.

For the DASS system all available and suitable fluorescent dyes can be used. We have so far used fluorescein isothiocyanate (FITC), tetramethylrhodamine isothiocyanate (TRITC), and in some experiments 4-acetamido-4′-isothiocyano-stilbene-2,2′-disulfonic acid (SITS) and all three fluorochromes worked. Direct as well as indirect staining techniques can be used. Poor quality conjugates which give high background values with tissue sections usually also give non-specific binding values with the DASS system. Conjugated $F(ab)_2$ fragments of antibodies also in the DASS system seem to give better results. When quantitative evaluation of results is performed the indirect techniques seem to be 4–10 times more sensitive than the direct technique. The higher non-specific binding values of the indirect technique make visual evaluation more difficult, however. For visual reading therefore at least part of the gain in specific staining is lost due to an increase of non-specific staining above the visual threshold.

The complement fluorescence technique using fluorochrome-labelled anti-C3 antibodies for the demonstration of C3 bound from fresh serum as complement source to antibodies previously attached to the antigenic substrate cannot be used, when either Sepharose or Sephadex are used as carriers. Both carriers directly bind C3 from fresh serum via the alternate pathway of complement activation [24].

2.2.7. Alternatives

An alternative method to the direct measurement of fluorescent antibodies or antigens bound to an inert carrier has been described by Aalberse [1]. He quantified the binding of IgG to anti-IgG-coated paper discs with a second layer of fluorochrome-labelled anti-IgG antibody (junction technique) by eluting the fluorescein with 0.1 NaOH after excessive washing of the complex. The fluorescence intensity was then measured in the fluid phase. Aalberse was able, with this technique, to quantify IgG at a concentration range of approximately 20–200 ng/ml. To my knowledge no further applications of this method have been reported so far.

A more direct approach was recently undertaken by Sedlacek et al. [41]. These authors used films of polymethylmathacrylate (Plexiglas) with a plane surface to which various proteins can be coupled as artificial substrates for immunofluorescence and called this technique: fluorescence immunoassay with plane surface (FIAPS). The autofluorescence of this material was found to be negligible and the non-specific binding of protein only minimal. The quality criteria for the carrier material (binding homogeneity, optical quality, batch to batch variation) used in this type of assay are critical, but when appropriately controlled such materials certainly will be of interest in the future. That the focusing problem of such measurement can be solved in practice has been shown by International Diagnostic Tests (IDT, Boehringer, Ingelheim, F.R.G.) with the commercially available FIAX test system which also uses antigens and antibodies coupled to not further defined plane surfaces as artificial substrates.

TABLE 2.I

REPORTED APPLICATIONS OF THE DASS SYSTEM

Reference	System	Determination of
Van Dalen et al. [47]	DASS, SBM and visual reading	Anti-IgG, -IgM, -Ova conjugates, direct technique
Knapp and Ploem [27]	DASS, SBM	Anti-IgG, -Ova conjugates and antisera, IgG, direct and indirect technique
Capel [7]	DASS, SBM and visual reading	Anti-IgG conjugates, IgG direct technique
Knapp et al. [28]	DASS, SBM	Anti-human collagen antibodies, indirect technique
Deelder and Ploem [10]	DASS, SBM and visual reading	Anti-*Schistosoma mansoni* antibodies, indirect technique
Deelder and Ploem [11]	DASS, SBM	Anti-*Fasciola hepatica* antibodies, indirect technique
Knapp et al. [29]	DASS, SBM	Specificity testing of anti-human IgG, IgM and IgA conjugates
Capel [8]	DASS, SBM and visual reading	Anti-IgG antisera, IgE concentration in serum, IgE anti-cat dander antibodies in serum
Capel and Aalberse [9]	DASS, SBM	IgE concentration in serum, IgE anti-allergen antibodies in serum
Knapp and Ludwig [26]	DASS, SBM	Anti-human thyroglobulin antibodies in serum
Haaijman et al. [20]	DASS, SBM	Human IgG, mouse IgM and Ova quantification
Streefkerk et al. [44]	DASS, SBM and visual reading (beads attached to slides)	Anti-*Schistosoma mansoni* and anti-bovine Ig antibodies
Bloemmen et al. [4]	DASS, SBM	Specificity testing of anti-mouse Ig class and subclass conjugates
Haaijman and Brinkhof [16]	DASS, SBM	Ig class and subclass levels in murine serum

Reference	System	Determination of
Haaijman [15]	DASS, SBM	Antibodies against LPS, HSA, Rauscher leukemia virus, and simian sarcoma viral antigens in murine serum. MTV antigens in milk C-type viral antigens in cell cultures
Koch et al. [30]	DASS, SBM	Putative human C-type oncornavirus
Haaijman and Slingerland-Teunissen [8]	DASS, SBM	Anti-DNP, -Ova, -C1q conjugates, FITC-protein A
Deelder et al. [14]	DASS, ADM method	Anti-*S. mansoni* antibodies
Pehamberger et al. [32]	DASS, ADM method	Anti-gliadin antibodies
Raybould and Chantler [36]	DASS, SBM and visual reading	Anti-IgG, -IgM, -IgA-fibrinogen, -C3, -*Salmonella* (polyv.) conjugates

DASS, defined antigenic substrate spheres system; SBM, single bead measurements; ADM, aperture defined microvolume; LPS, lipopolysaccharide; HSA, human serum albumin.

2.3. EVALUATION OF RESULTS

2.3.1. Visual reading

Residual levels of non-specific fluorescence make visual discrimination of positive and negative results sometimes difficult. It can be facilitated, however, by admixing earmarked negative (coated with an unrelated antigen or antibody) beads to the preparation, before starting the staining and washing procedure. Negative beads for instance can be earmarked with TRITC when FITC-labelled conjugates and selective filtering are used [47]. Another possibility to facilitate visual reading was recently described by Raybould and Chantler [36] and will be discussed in section 2.5.

Whenever visual readings are performed the possibility of attaching the beads to slides before staining and washing should be considered. In this way a very low number of beads is sufficient for testing and the time-consuming transfer of stained and washed beads from tubes or microtest plate-wells to slides can be avoided. Streefkerk et al. [44] used gelatin-coated slides to achieve firm adherence of antigen-coupled beads to glass slides.

2.3.2. Measurement of fluorescence intensity

Most investigators so far used microfluorometers to measure the fluorescence intensity of stained beads. The fluorescence intensity distribution of individual beads within one preparation follows a normal distribution. The fluorescence intensity of a number of different beads should therefore be determined and averaged. An alternative described below is the measurement of the fluorescence intensity of packed beads using the aperture-defined microvolume (ADM) method recently described by Deelder et al. [14].

2.3.2.1. Instrumentation

Beads which have been transferred to slides after staining and washing can be read and measured with an ordinary fluorescence microscope. For those beads left in the flat-bottomed microplates after staining and washing and for the ADM method an inverted fluorescence microscope is needed.

Suitable microscopes with appropriate microfluorometers are commercially available from a number of different firms. Fully equipped automatic microfluorometers are available from Leitz (MPV II and MPV compact), Reichert (Univar equipped for fluorometry) and Zeiss (MPM 03 and SF fluorometer). But there are also many other possibilities to adapt microscopes for this purpose. In our experiments we are using a Reichert Immunopan microscope and a Leitz Diavert microscope, both equipped for epi-illumination, a Reichert microphotometer provided with a Philips photomultiplier XP 1010 and a digital voltmeter (Weston, 1240). To achieve a fixed and as short as possible an interval between the onset of the excitation and the triggering of the voltmeter in order to avoid variable fading of the fluorescence, we have automated our microscopes using relatively inexpensive pneumatic components as described in detail by Haaijman and Wijnants [19]. The sequence of operations which has to be performed for every individual measurement can be summarized as follows: 1) location of the desired object (e.g. one bead) with bright field- or phase-contrast illumination; 2) closing the substage illumination path; 3) opening the photomultiplier; 4) opening the epi-illumination path; 5) starting the voltmeter; 6) reset to starting situation. It is evident from this enumeration that apart from the fading problem also the number of handlings which have to be performed for every measurement demand automation.

2.3.2.2. Measurement of individual beads

Under the CNBr activation conditions described above the antigens are usually coupled in the direct vicinity of the surface. Therefore the fluorescence intensity is (relatively) independent of the bead size when only a plug of individual beads is measured. For this purpose a measuring diaphragm with a field size smaller than the field size of the bead should be used for quantitation. The fluorescence measurement obtained from an object is always the sum of the actual fluorescence of the object and the background fluorescence. The background fluorescence is greatly dependent on the diameter of the measuring diaphragm. Objects with low fluorescence intensity, therefore, theoretically should be measured with a measuring diaphragm as small as possible in order to minimize the background interference. With very small measuring diaphragms, however, even minimal inhomogeneities of the bead material can substantially influence the result. We therefore usually used a field size of the measuring diaphragm which was about 50% smaller than the smallest beads included in the fluorescence intensity measurements.

From each preparation, depending on the variation of the individual values, the fluorescence intensity of 5–10 beads should be measured. The background is measured from an empty part of the preparation. Three background measurements are usually taken per preparation. The fluorescence intensity can be expressed in relative units and/or referred to an external or internal standard.

2.3.2.3. Standards for the measurement of fluorescence intensity

In absorption spectrophotometry, the concentration of a given substance in solution is found by comparing the light transmittance of the test solution with that of the diluent. For fluorometry a blank value as used in absorption measurement does not exist, because the background ideally gives a zero reading. Therefore, the fluorescence intensity of a sample should be compared with that of a fluorescent standard sample. The fluorescent standard sample can be an internal standard, e.g. the fluorescence intensity obtained with a standard conjugate which is included in all experimental series and to which all values are referred. In addition, external standards are frequently used.

The most convenient, external standard is the uranyl glass (GG 17 of Schott and Gen., Mainz, F.R.G.) standard [38] and, although it has many limitations (discussed in detail by Haaijman and Van Dalen [17], it is still widely used by many investigators. In addition to the uranyl glass a wide variety of other standards for fluorescence intensity measurements have been described [22, 34, 39, 42, 45, 48, 49]. The use of FITC- and TRITC-labelled Sephadex beads as external standards recently described by Haaijman [17] seems to be very promising. An internal immunological standard has to be conducted in every experiment, so that all values obtained can be referred to this standard preparation. Whenever possible this internal laboratory standard should be tested against and related to one of the internal biological reference preparations (see the corresponding chapter in this book).

2.3.2.4. The aperture-defined microvolume (ADM) method

The relatively time-consuming fluorometric evaluation of individual beads is a limiting factor for the applicability of the DASS system for a large series of experiments. Deelder et al. [14] recently proposed a method which circumvents this problem. This method is based on the principle that the incident light beam projected by a microscope objective illuminates a microvolume in the form of a cone: an aperture-defined microvolume. With this technique one measurement in a layer of sedimented beads suffices to obtain a mean value of the fluorescence intensity of stained beads in one preparation. With this technique measurements are performed in the following way: after the washing procedure following the antiserum and/or conjugate incubation step, the supernatant buffer is aspirated until a final volume of about 20 μl is reached and the beads are transferred with a micropipette to a Terasaki type tray (Cooke Microtiter tray, cat. No. M 220-55 ART). After sedimenting the beads either by centrifugation or by letting them stand in the bench for some time, the fluorescence intensity of sedimented beads can be measured with a photometer attached to an inverted microscope equipped for transmitted and incident illumination. For measurements an objective with a sufficiently long working distance should be used. The measuring diaphragm is first focused on the border between the bottom and the wall of the first well and then centered in the middle of the first well. The Terasaki tray can then either be automatically read-out with a mechanical scanning stage (Leitz and Zeiss scanning stages for microtest plates), connected to a small bench table computer (e.g. HP 97S), or it can also be read by manually moving the tray and centering the measuring diaphragm in the middle of each well. The automatic version allows the measurement of a total Terasaki tray (60 wells) in about 1–2 min. By hand it can be done in about 10–30 min. Deelder et al. [14] showed that this technique has a high reproducibility and the same sensitivity as individual bead measurements for the detection of *Schistosoma mansoni*-specific antibodies and antigen. We had the same experience when using the ADM method for the detection of anti-gliadin antibodies in patients' sera [32].

Comment. Measurements performed in this way are highly reproducible when an optimal focusing position is chosen. Minor focusing differences from well to well do not seem to significantly influence the result. It is necessary to have a sufficiently thick layer of beads present in each well of the Terasaki tray in order to obtain bead volume independent measurements. The minimal volume required is 5–10 μl packed beads, but it may vary from objective to objective. The use of two conjugates with different fluorochromes is possible and can be used, for instance, for the simultaneous screening for IgM and IgG antibodies. Transferring the beads after staining and washing in either tubes or the larger 96-well microtest trays to the Terasaki trays is still a time-consuming factor. This might possibly be solved in the future by performing the whole test in larger 96-well microtest trays with wells of the V type, but with a small flat bottom (about 2 mm). It would then be possible to perform all staining and washing procedures, and also the reading of the results in one tray and the whole procedure could be fully automated.

2.4. APPLICATIONS

In principle, the DASS system and other artificial substrates can be used for any fluorescent binding assay, provided one of the constituents can be covalently coupled to an inert carrier and antisera against the binding constituent are available. So far, however, the DASS system has been used mainly for the demonstration and quantification of antibodies and antigens. Sepharose-coupled antigens are used for the quantitation of antibodies and coupled antibodies for the quantitation of antigens. The sensitivity of the technique has been found to be comparable to radioimmunoassay (RIA) and enzyme immunoassay (EIA) techniques. Considerable efforts were also made to use this system for the characterization and standardization of fluorochrome-labelled conjugates.

Most of the applications of the DASS system which have been reported in the literature up to now are listed in Table 2.I. The DASS system has contributed significantly to a better understanding and especially a better (quantitative) characterization of the various parameters which influence the outcome of immunofluorescence experiments. In our opinion it is also an invaluable tool for the characterization and standardization of fluorochrome-labelled reagents and for the performance of immunoassays on a research scale. For routine applications of the DASS system the main disadvantage, so far, has been the time-consuming fluorometric evaluation of the test results.

2.5. FURTHER DEVELOPMENTS

In our opinion the two most urgent steps for further developments to be taken in this field are a) to find still better carrier materials and coupling procedures, and b) to further facilitate and automate the performance of the incubation, washing and reading procedures. Better carrier materials and coupling procedures would be of major importance for the visual evaluation of results, since the human eye is very sensitive in discriminating between absolutely negative and weak fluorescence but rather poor in discriminating between a weak non-specific staining and a not very strong specific fluorescence, which can easily be differentiated by microfluorometry. We never had problems with non-specific staining when direct staining techniques were used, e.g. for the characterization of conjugates. We do have problems, however, when we use an indirect staining technique, e.g. for the demonstration of antibodies in human sera. In this case the non-specific staining is much stronger and the patients' sera have to be diluted considerably.

Raybould and Chantler [36] have recently proposed the use of sodium metaperiodate-activated cross-linked Sepharose 4B beads blocked with rhodamine-bovine serum albumin prior to reduction instead of CNBr activated Sepharose 4B beads. They found that this procedure gives negligible variation in staining of individual beads and a reddish-orange non-specific fluorescence as compared to a bright yellow-green specific fluorescence when non-selective filter systems and FITC-labelled reagents are used. Under these conditions the authors find it easy to visually assess the results of their experiments. In addition to this procedure there are many other possibilities open which have to be evaluated. One possibly interesting alternative might be, for instance, the use of aminoethyl-polyacrylamide beads to which proteins can be coupled with a soluble carbodumine. With growing interest in affinity chromatography and related techniques a variety of suitable substrate carriers will probably be available in the near future. For immunofluorescence studies the ideal carrier material should primarily fulfill two criteria: a) the non-specific binding of Ig to the carrier material should be as low as possible; and b) the density of reactive antigens or antibodies per square unit should be as high as possible.

Visual reading is certainly important for small-scale experiments and for small laboratories where only qualitative or semi-quantitative results are needed. For large-scale experiments not only measurements of individual beads but also visual reading of all the results are too laborious. For this type of assay automation is needed. When fully automated the fluoroimmunoassay can, however, compete with the radioimmunoassay and the enzyme immunoassay both of wich also have disadvantages. Several steps in this direction have already been taken. One very promising development in this direction is the previously described ADM method for automatically reading the results in the DASS system. With the commercial availability of suitable trays allowing the performance of the whole test in the same plate this method seems to be ready for use in large-scale experiments. Another modification to which the ADM method could be applied is the combination of fluorometry and enzyme technology by using enzymes with a fluorogenic substrate in enzyme immunoassays. With the enzyme β-D-galactosidase and the substrate methylumbelliferyl galactoside, for instance IgG at a level of 0.1 ng can be detected [24]. Other methods which might be of value in the future are the fluorescence immunoassays using plane surface solid phases like the FIAPS as described by Sedlacek et al. [41] and discussed in section 2.2.7 and the commercially available FIAX test kits (IDT Europe, Division of Boehringer, Ingelheim, F.R.G.).

In addition to substrate and automation improvements tremendous progress has already been made in recent years and further advance can be expected in the near future by increasing the sensitivity of fluoroimmunoassays with better instrumentation and new fluorophores. It actually seems to be possible to develop fluoroimmunological methods which are even more sensitive than the radioimmunoassay [43, 50].

REFERENCES

1 Aalberse, R.C. (1973) Quantitative fluoroimmunoassay. Clin. Chim. Acta *48,* 109–111.

2 Allen, J.C. (1963) Immunofluorescence applied to protein solutions. J. Lab. Clin. Med. *62,* 517–524.

3 Bergquist, N.R., Holubar, K., Diaz, G.A. and Beutner, E.H. (1972) The manufacture of protein microphoreses by suspension polymerization. Int. Arch. Allergy Appl. Immunol. *43,* 791–799.

4 Bloemmen, F.J., Radl, J., Haaijman, J.J., Van den Berg, P., Schutt, H.R.E. and Hijmans, W. (1976) Microfluorometric evaluation of the specificity of fluorescent antisera against mouse immunoglobulins with the defined antigen substrate spheres (DASS) system. J. Immunol. Methods *10,* 337–355.

5 Brandtzaeg, P. (1972) Evaluation of immunofluorescence with artificial sections of selected antigenicity. Immunology *22,* 177–183.

6 Camargo, M.W. and Ferreira, A.W. (1970) A microscopic immunofluorescence technique with soluble protein fixed to cellulose particles. Int. Arch. Allergy Appl. Immunol. *39,* 292–300.

7 Capel, P.J.A. (1974) A quantitative immunofluorescent method based on the covalent coupling of protein to Sepharose beads. J. Immunol. Methods *5,* 165–178.

8 Capel, P.J.A. (1975) The defined antigen substrate spheres (DASS) system and some of its applications. Ann. N.Y. Acad. Sci. *254,* 108–118.

9 Capel, P.J.A. and Aalberse, R.C. (1975) A quantitative immunofluorescence method for the determination of IgE antibodies in comparison with the radioallergosorbent test (RAST). J. Immunol. Methods *7,* 77–84.

10 Deelder, A.M. and Ploem, J.S. (1975) An immunofluorescence reaction for *Schistosoma mansoni* using the defined antigen substrate spheres (DASS) system. J. Immunol. Methods *4,* 239–251.

11 Deelder, A.M. and Ploem, J.S. (1975) An immunofluorescence reaction for *Fasciola hepatica* using the defined antigen substrate spheres (DASS) system. Exp. Parasitol. *37,* 173–178.

12 Deelder, A.M., Snoijink, J.J. and Ploem, J.S. (1975) Experimental optimization of the DASS system for immunodiagnosis of some helminth infections. Ann. N.Y. Acad. Sci. *254,* 119–136.

13 Deelder, A.M., Snoijink, J.J. and Ploem, J.S. (1975) Immunoprecipitation and class-specific immunofluorescence titration of human serum antibodies to *Schistosoma mansoni* antigens. Z. Parasitenkd. *46,* 195–201.

14 Deelder, A.M., Tanke, H.J. and Ploem J.S. (1978) Automated quantitative immunofluorescence using the aperture defined microvolume (ADM) method. *In* Knapp, W., Holubar, K. and Wick, G. (eds.), Immunofluorescence and Related Staining Techniques (Elsevier/North-Holland Biomed. Press, Amsterdam) pp. 31–44.

15 Haaijman, J.J. (1977) Quantitative immunofluorescence microscopy-methods and applications. Thesis, University of Leiden.

16 Haaijman, J.J. and Brinkhof, J. (1977) A microfluorometric assay for immunoglobulin class and subclass levels in murine serum. J. Immunol. Methods *14,* 213–224.

17 Haaijman, J.J. and Van Dalen, J.P.R. (1974) Quantitation in immunofluorescence microscopy. A new standard for fluorescein and rhodamine emission measurements. J. Immunol. Methods *5,* 359–374.

18 Haaijman, J.J. and Slingerland-Teunissen, J. (1978) Equipment and preparative procedures in immunofluorescence microscopy: quantitative studies. In Knapp, W., Holubar, K. and Wick, G. (eds.), Immunofluorescence and Related Staining Techniques (Elsevier/North-Holland Biomed. Press, Amsterdam) pp. 11–29.

19 Haaijman, J.J. and Wijnants, F.A.C. (1975) Inexpensive automation of the Leitz Orthoplan microfluorometer using pneumatic microcomponents. J. Immunol. Methods *7,* 255–270.

20 Haaijman, J.J., Bloemmen, F.J. and Ham, C.M. (1975) Microfluorometric immunoassays with antigens bound to Sepharose beads. Ann. N.Y. Acad. Sci. *254,* 137–150.

21 Haaijman, J.J., Van den Berg, P. and Brinkhof, J. (1977) Immunoglobulin class and subclass levels in the serum of CBA mice throughout life. Immunology *32,* 923–927.

22 Jongsma, A.P.M., Hijmans, W. and Ploem J.S. (1971) Quantitative immunofluorescence. Standardization and calibration in microfluorometry. Histochemie *25,* 329–343.

23 Kato, H., Fukui, H., Hamaguchi, Y. and Ishikawa, E. (1976) Enzyme-linked immunoassay: conjugation of the F(ab)′ fragment of rabbit IgG with β-D-galactosidase from *E. coli* and its use for immunoassay. J. Immunol. *116,* 1554-1560.

24 Kato, K., Hamaguchi, Y., Fukui, H. and Ishikawa, E. (1976) Enzyme-linked immunoassay. Conjugation of rabbit anti-(human immunoglobulin G)antibody with β-D-galactosidase from *Escherichia coli* and its use for human immunoglobulin G assay. Eur. J. Biochem. *62,* 285–292.

25 Knapp, W. (1974) Interaction of the third component of complement (C3) with cross-linked dextran. I. Binding of C3 from normal human serum to cross-linked dextran as defined by quantitative immunofluorescence. Z. Immunitaetsforsch. *148,* 213–224.

26 Knapp, W. and Ludwig, H. (1976) Microfluorometric demonstration of thyroglobulin antibodies with the defined antigen substrate spheres (DASS) system. Z. Immunitaetsforsch. *151,* 61–68.

27 Knapp, W. and Ploem, J.S. (1974) Microfluorometry of antigen–antibody interactions using the defined antigen substrate spheres (DASS) system. Sensitivity, specificity and variables of the method. J. Immunol. Methods *5,* 259–273.

28 Knapp, W., Menzel, J. and Steffen, C. (1974) Microfluorometric evaluation of anti-collagen antibodies with the defined antigen substrate spheres (DASS) system. Z. Immunitaetsforsch. *148,* 132–141.

29 Knapp, W., Haaijman, J.J., Schuit, H.R.E., Van den Berg, P., Ploem, J.S. and Hijmans, W. (1975) Microfluorometric evaluation of conjugate specificity with the defined antigen substrate spheres (DASS) system. Ann. N.Y. Acad. Sci. *254,* 94–107.

30 Koch, G., Nooter, K., Bentvelzen, P. and Haaijman, J.J. (1977) Serological characterization of a putative human C-type oncornavirus by means of the Sepharose bead immunofluorescence assay. Eur. J. Cancer *13,* 1397–1403.

31 Paronetto, F. (1963) The fluorescent antibody technique applied to titration and identification of antigens in solutions or antisera. Proc. Soc. Exp. Biol. Med. *113,* 394–397.

32 Pehamberger, H., Menzel, J., Holubar, K. and Knapp, W. (1978) Demonstration of gliadin antibodies with quantitative immunofluorescence (Workshop Report Immunodermatology). In Knapp, W., Holubar, K. and Wick, G. (eds.), Immunofluorescence and Related Staining Techniques (Elsevier/North-Holland Biomed. Press, Amsterdam) p. 271.

33 Ploem, J.S. (1967) The use of a vertical illuminator with interchangeable dichroic mirrors for fluorescence microscopy with incident light. Z. Wiss. Mikrosk. *68,* 129–142.

34 Ploem, J.S. (1971) Standards for fluorescence microscopy. In Holborow, E.J. (ed.), Standardization in Immunofluorescence (Blackwell Scientific Publ., Oxford) pp. 137–154.

35 Porath, J., Axen, R. and Ernback, S. (1967) Chemical coupling of proteins to Sepharose. Nature (London) *215,* 1491–1492.

36 Raybould T.J.G. and Chantler, S. (1979) Comparison of activation and blocking procedures in the use of defined antigen substrate spheres (DASS) system for quantitative and visual assessment of conjugate activity. J. Immunol. Methods *27,* 309–318.

37 Richards, F.F. and Koningsberg, W.H. (1973) Speculations. How specific are antibodies? Immunochemistry *10,* 545–553.

38 Rigler, R. (1966) Microfluorometric characterization of intracellular nucleic acids and nucleoproteins by acridine orange. Acta Physiol. Scand. *67,* Suppl. 267.

39 Ruch, F. (1970) Principles and some applications of cytofluorometry. In Wied, G.L. and Bahr, G.F. (eds.), Introduction to Quantitative Cytochemistry, Vol. 11 (Academic Press, New York) pp. 431–450.

40 Schauenstein, K., Wick, G. and Kink, H. (1976) The micromembrane-fluorescence test: a new semi-automated technique based on the microtiter system. J. Immunol. Methods *10,* 143–150.

41 Sedlacek, H.H., Mück, K.F., Rehkopf, R., Baudner, S. and Seiler, F.R. (1979) A new method for fluorescence immunoassay using plane surface solid phases (FIAPS). J. Immunol. Methods *26,* 11–24.

42 Sernetz, M. and Thaler, A.A. (1970) A capillary fluorescence standard for microfluorometry. J. Microsc. *91,* 43–52.

43 Soini, E. and Hemmilä, I. (1979) Fluoroimmunoassay: present status and key problems. Clin. Chem. *25,* 353–361.

44 Streefkerk, J.G., Deelder, A.M., Kors, N. and Kornelis, D. (1975) Antigen coupled beads adherent to slides: a simplified method for immunological studies. J. Immunol. Methods *8,* 251–256.

45 Thomson, L.A. and Hageage, G.J. (1975) Evaluation of exication light sources for incident immunofluorescent microscopy. Appl. Microbiol. *30,* 616–624.

46 Toussaint, A.J. and Anderson, R.I. (1965) Soluble antigen fluorescent antibody technique. Appl. Microbiol. *13,* 552–558.
47 Van Dalen, J.P.R., Knapp, W. and Ploem, J.S. (1973) Microfluorometry on antigen–antibody interactions in immunofluorescence using antigens covalently bound to agarose beads. J. Immunol. Methods *2,* 383–392.
48 Velapoldi, R.A., Travis, J.C., Cassat, W.A. and Yap, W.T. (1975) Inorganic ion-doped glass fibres as microspectrofluorometric standards. J. Microsc. *103,* 293–303.
49 Walker, P.J. and Watts, J.M.A. (1970) Permanent fluorescent test slides. J. Microsc. *92,* 63–65.
50 Wieder, I. (1978) Background rejection in fluorescence immunoassay. In Knapp, W., Holubar, K. and Wick, G. (eds.), Immunofluorescence and Related Staining Techniques (Elsevier/North-Holland Biomed. Press, Amsterdam) pp. 67–80.

Wick et al. (eds) Immunofluorescence Technology. Selected Theoretical and Clinical Aspects © Elsevier Biomedical Press, 1982

CHAPTER 3

The use of lasers to determine the fluorescence characteristics of fluorescein derivatives in immunofluorescence assays

K. SCHAUENSTEIN, G. BÖCK and G. WICK

Institute for General and Experimental Pathology, University of Innsbruck, 6010 Innsbruck, Austria

3.1. INTRODUCTION

This chapter deals with the practical and theoretical aspects of the application of laser light for excitation in the immunofluorescence (IF) technique. Lasers are known to emit extremely homogeneous and monochromatic light up to very high energies. The possible great advantages of this kind of illumination for the IF method were first discussed in 1966 by Mansberg and Kusnetz [12], at a time when lasers emitting the proper wavelengths (i.e. visible blue and green) still had to be developed. With the introduction of argon lasers tunable to emit lines at 488 nm and 514 nm, this idea became realizable, and the first report on IF with lasers appeared in 1971 by Kaufman et al. [9] followed by others [1, 17, 21]. Since that time lasers have been nearly exclusively used in the fluorescence-activated cell sorter (FACS) [2], where the usually weak fluorescence signals obtained from cell membrane stainings must be strong enough to enable the physical separation of cell populations on the basis of fluorescence. Another rather sophisticated IF technique involving focussed laser light is the fluorescence-photobleaching-recovery technique (FPR) [4, 18] as pointed out in chapter 4 on membrane fluorescence and later on in this article.

The general use of this light source for routine equipment is still hampered by its relatively high expense. These problems, however, might be solved in the near future, as large numbers of various laser types emitting light of any wavelength and energy are already on the market, and it seems therefore justifiable to point out the great practical advantages of lasers as compared with the usual mercury vapour bulbs.

Section 3.3 of this chapter discusses data obtained with a laser microfluorometer concerning the fluorescence kinetics (i.e. fading and recovery) of fluorescein isothiocyanate (FITC) during short-time excitation. Since bleaching of fluorescence is known to be positively correlated to the excitation energy applied, the illumination with the energy-rich laser light was found to be of great value for this kind of work. Analysis of FITC fluorescence bleaching was recently found to provide information about the nature of binding of conjugates to antigenic substrates.

3.2. PRACTICAL ASPECTS

The modern types of fluorescence microscope which are generally used for IF work have reached a high level of perfection concerning the filter systems and the optical performance. In particular the introduction of epi-illumination systems [13] brought about a large step towards better efficiency. The fluorescence excitation using the conventional mercury arcs is, however, still a problem in several respects: a) they are relatively short-lived and expensive; b)

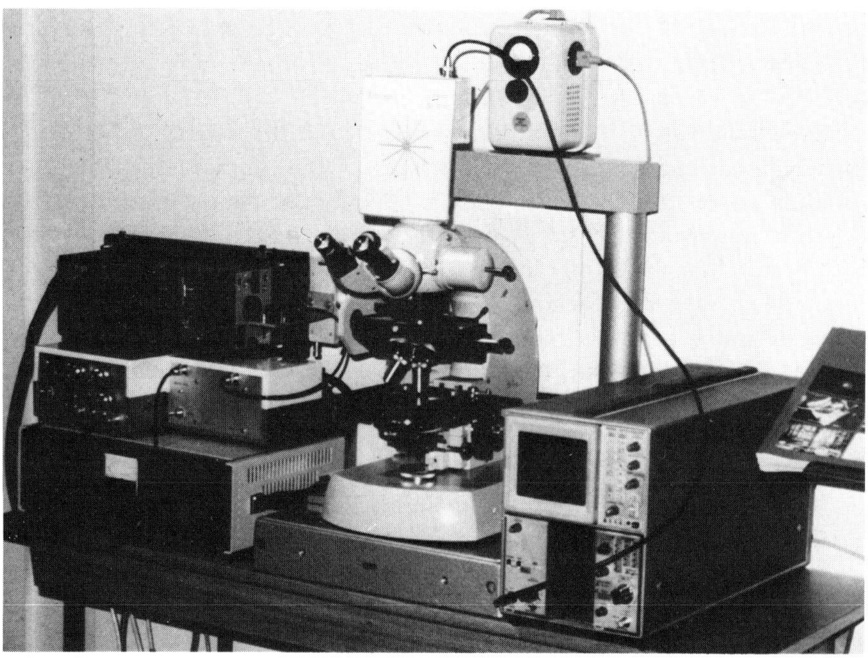

Fig. 3.1. Laser fluorescence microscope. A continuously working argon ion laser of 10 mW energy (left) is attached to a fluorescence microscope (middle) to serve as incident light source. The intensity of fluorescence signals is measured by a photodiode on top of the microscope and is displayed on a storage oscilloscope (right).

Hg emits very low energies at the excitation maximum of FITC, i.e. 491 nm, which has to be filtered out entailing further loss of light energy; and c) the radiation intensity is not optimally constant, which is important for quantitative IF work.

Concerning the economic point of view, it should be mentioned that small argon laser tubes have lifetimes about 10-fold longer than those of mercury lamps (200 h) without any loss of irradiation energy. The cost of 10 Hg arcs, on the other hand, amounts to more than 50% of the price of a complete 10 mW argon laser model, which is perfectly apt for IF work. Taken together with the other advantages of this light source, as outlined below, it is certainly justified to recommend it for laboratories with a high turnover of Hg lamps and for any IF work dealing with low fluorescence intensities.

Fig. 3.1 shows a laser fluorescence microscope as it is used in this laboratory [14]. An argon ion laser (162; Spectra Physics, Mountain View, CA) is fitted on an optical bench to a fluorescence microscope (Zeiss Forschungsmikroskop) to serve as an incident light source. Excitation times are regulated by electronically gated acousto-optical shutters (Fig. 3.2). In the microscope the laser beam is deflected by a dichroic mirror and focussed by the objective into the plane of the object. The emitted green fluorescence passing the mirror and a barrier filter is quantified by a fast photodiode, the signal of which can be recorded by means of a storage oscilloscope. For work with rhodamine (tetramethylrhodamine isothiocyanate, TRITC) conjugates the laser can be tuned to the second wavelength, i.e. 514 nm, and a dichroic mirror with the respective optical properties (reflection of light with a wavelength shorter than 514 nm, transmission of light with a wavelength greater than 600 nm) can be used. In the present adjustment the laser illuminated area of the whole visual field is about 250 μm^2 to which a total energy of 2.5×10^3 W·cm^{-2} of 488 nm light is delivered.

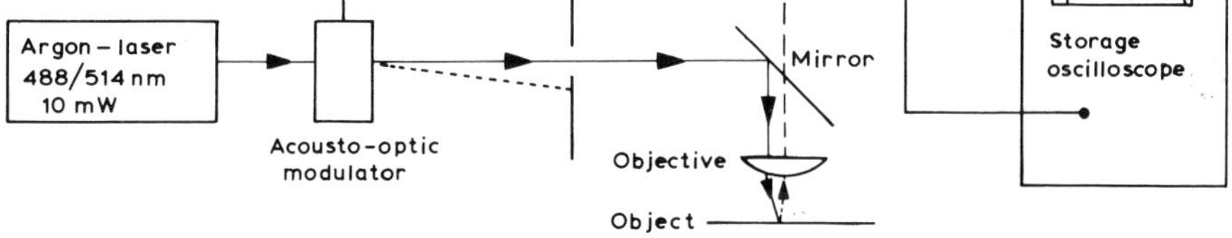

Fig. 3.2. Schematic representation of the laser microscope set-up. For the generation of short light pulses (range of μs) an acousto-optical modulator was introduced. An electronically operated pulse generator activates a high frequency source, the impulse of which alters the optical properties of the crystal in the modulator leading to a slight deflection of the laser beam (------) onto a diaphragm. (------, fluorescence).

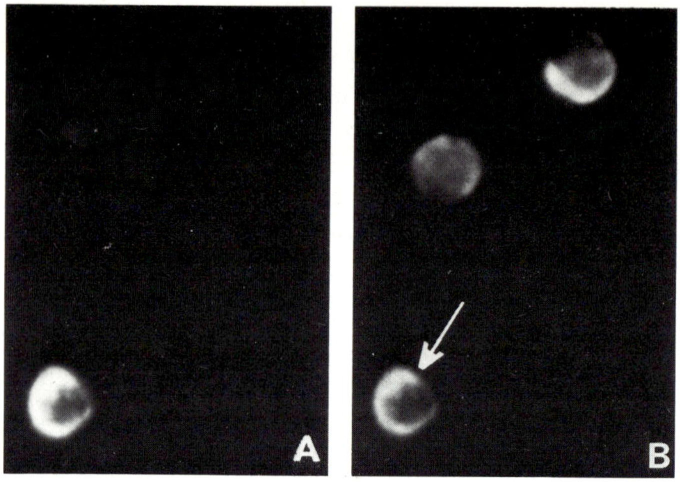

Fig. 3.3. Comparison of fluorescence intensities obtained with laser and mercury lamps in microphotography. A) Chicken plasma cell in the spleen stained with FITC anti-chicken IgG and exposed to 10 pulses of a laser light beam of 0.01 s duration (not illuminating the whole field). B) The same cell (arrow) and surrounding cells illuminated with mercury light for 120 s. Note the strong intensity of the plasma cell, which was pre-exposed to laser light.

To illustrate the intensity differences compared with Hg bulbs, Fig. 3.3 shows plasma cells treated with specific, fluorescent anti- immunoglobulin (Ig) conjugate, and illuminated with normal Hg vapour bulbs, and with the Argon ion laser, respectively. The cell in Fig. 3.3A was exposed to 10 laser pulses each of 0.01 s duration. In order to obtain comparable fluorescence intensity with the Hg lamp, the cells in Fig. 3.3B had to be exposed for 120 s. After this time a great deal of the fluorescence is irreversibly faded [5, 7]. Thus, in the present system, fluorescence intensity is increased by a factor of the order of 10^3. As will be described in the following section, bleaching of this strong fluorescence is almost 100% reversible after a dark interval. Thus, using short-excitation pulses of laser light, it is not only possible to overcome fluorescence intensity problems in microfluorometry, but also, thanks to the recovery phenomenon, to take repeated photographs from one and the same positively stained object.

The high constancy of laser irradiation (see Instruction Manual, Model 162, CW Argon Laser, Spectra Physics, Mountain View, CA) should be pointed out once more. The practical importance of this feature obviously concerns not only quantitative microfluorometric work, where the system can be calibrated by means of fluorescent glass standards, but especially the more commonly used evaluation of IF results by the eye of the observer.

3.3. STUDIES ON BLEACHING AND RECOVERY OF ANTIBODY-BOUND FITC

3.3.1. The bleaching effect

The rapid bleaching of fluorescence of fluorescein dyes, like FITC, during continuous excitation is one of the most prominent problems of the IF

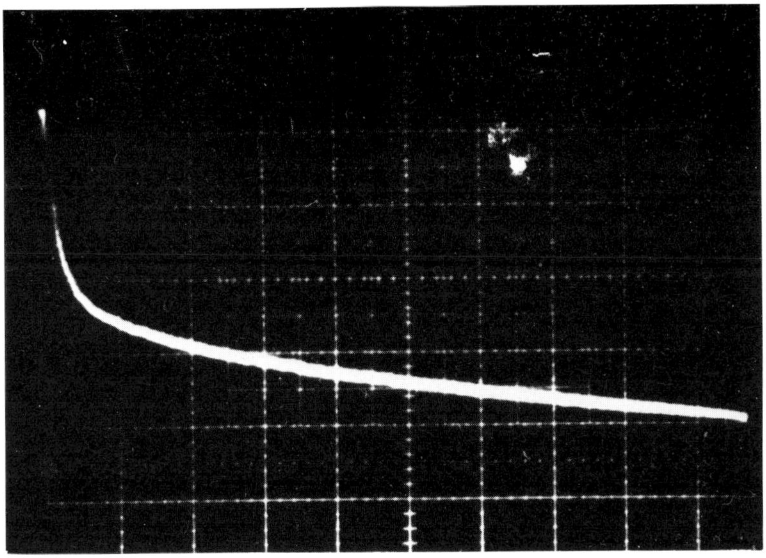

Fig. 3.4. Fluorescence bleaching of free FITC in aqueous solution. Time base 200 μs. Note the rapid initial fading during the first 100 μs of excitation.

technique. This process was first studied with conventional light sources in 1960 by Goldman [5], and he showed that it is linearly correlated to the energy of excitation. Therefore, the enhanced fluorescence emission intensity achieved by the higher excitation energy of lasers must be expected to bleach to a high degree in a very short time. As was shown earlier [14], the correlation of the excitation energy to the bleaching rate is still linear at the energies applied by the 10 mW argon laser. Fig. 3.4 shows the fluorescence intensity of free FITC in aqueous solution monitored over an excitation period of 2 ms. A rapid initial loss of about 40% of the original intensity is observed during the first 100 μs of excitation. Thus, for the study of these fluorescence kinetics it turned out to be essential to use very fast shutters, photometers, and recording devices.

3.3.2. The recovery effect

Kaufman et al. [9] were the first to describe the partial recovery of fluorescence upon repeated short-laser illuminations interspaced by longer dark intervals. This finding was confirmed by Bergquist [1] and by ourselves [17, 21]. Using equipment similar to that described above, the recovery phenomenon was demonstrated on biological substrates, namely indirect IF to detect antinuclear antibodies (ANA) on rat liver nuclei, and autoantibodies against thyroglobulin on sections of human colloid goiter. Furthermore, it was shown that this effect was negatively correlated to the length of excitation and positively to the dark interval. Fig. 3.5A shows the fluorescence kinetics of FITC bound to Sephadex G-25 beads during two short illuminations of 3 ms with a dark interval of 3 ms. A marked recovery of initial fluorescence is

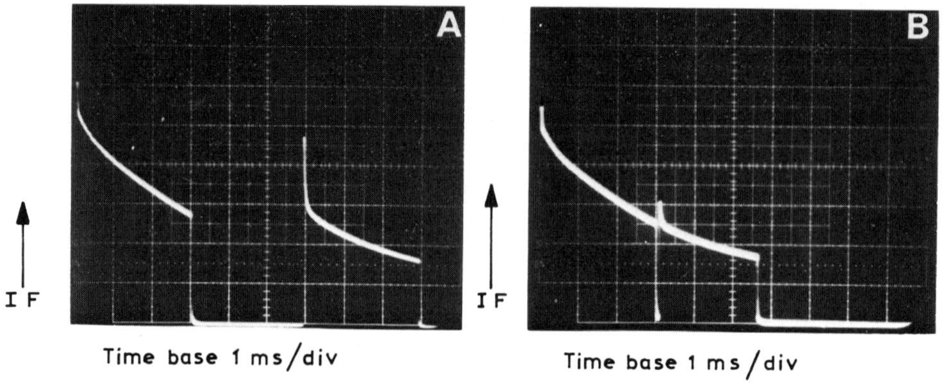

Fig. 3.5. Recovery of faded fluorescence. The substrate is FITC-coated Sephadex beads. A) Two pulses of 3 ms with a 3 ms dark interval. Recovery of about 60% of initial fluorescence. B) Two pulses of 3 ms with a 100 μs dark interval. No significant fluorescence recovery.

obtained, whereas only little recovery is seen when the dark interval is reduced (Fig. 3.5B). The practical implications of this effect for the IF method are twofold: 1) as pointed out in section 3.2, the recovery effect allows repeated photography of fluorescent staining, and 2) the application of a rotating diaphragm to interrupt the laser beam in a stroboscope-like manner can drastically slow down the rapid photobleaching process, provided the speed and the slit of this diaphragm can be adjusted to give the optimal excitation/dark interval conditions for maximal recovery of the respective fluorescence intensity under investigation.

It should be stressed that this type of fluorescence recovery has nothing to do with the one described in the FPR technique, where small areas of fluorescently labelled living cells are irreversibly bleached by means of a focussed laser beam, and the reappearance of fluorescence gives information about the lateral mobility of the respective surface structure in the cell membrane. This attractive technique has been applied for lymphocyte surface markers and surface receptors for hormones such as insulin and epidermal growth factor [4, 18].

3.3.3. The influence of the microenvironment of the FITC molecule on its bleaching properties

The general sensitivity of fluorescence phenomena towards changes in the environment of the fluorochrome molecule is well documented [20]. With respect to the IF method, this matter was investigated for FITC by several authors [6, 10, 14, 16, 19], because of its practical significance for quantitation and standardization of the technique. More recently, it became evident that the bleaching characteristics of FITC, as expressed by the shape of fluorescence intensity curves, are particularly sensitive towards alterations of the milieu of the dye. In a recent paper, Hirschfeld [8] has shown the bleaching characteristics of several fluorescent dyes to differ significantly according to

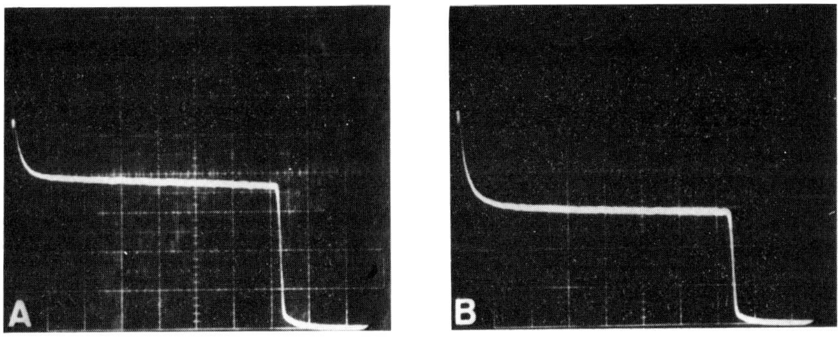

Fig. 3.6. Effect of binding of FITC to protein macromolecules (immunoglobulin) on bleaching characteristics. A) Free FITC. B) FITC bound to immunoglobulin. Note the enhanced bleaching (time base 0.2 ms/div.).

whether they are excited in the free form or chemically bound to macromolecules. Regarding FITC, it was found that binding to antibody molecules considerably enhanced the fluorescence bleaching as compared with the free dye molecules in aqueous solution. This is in agreement with previous observations of our own [14] and is illustrated in Fig. 3.6A, B.

In further attempts to make use of this effect for the IF technique, the bleaching properties of antibody-bound FITC were assayed in direct IF tests after either non-specific adsorption or specific immunological binding of these conjugates to antigenic substrates. Fig. 3.7 shows the immunological system; G-25 dextran beads (superfine) were coated with one of two different antigens: bovine serum albumin (BSA) or rabbit immunoglobulin (RIg). Direct IF tests were performed with suspensions of these antigen-coated carriers with various dilutions of FITC-labelled rabbit anti-BSA and FITC-swine anti-RIg conju-

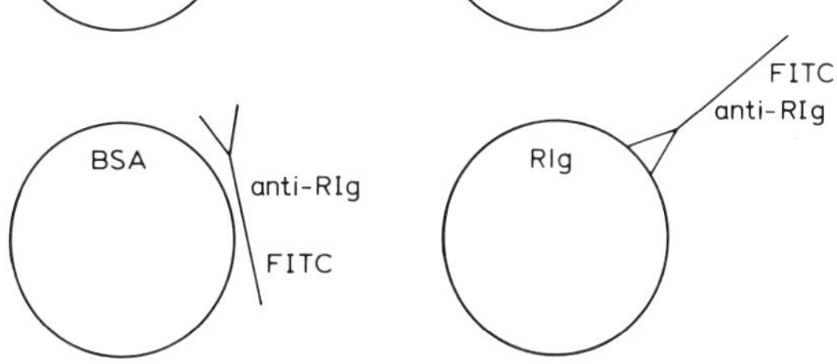

Fig. 3.7. Immunological system for the evaluation of the effect of specific and non-specific binding of antibody conjugates on FITC bleaching properties. G-25 superfine beads were coated with two different antigens (BSA, bovine serum albumin, RIg, rabbit immunoglobulin) and treated with various dilutions of FITC-labelled anti-BSA and anti-RIg antibodies.

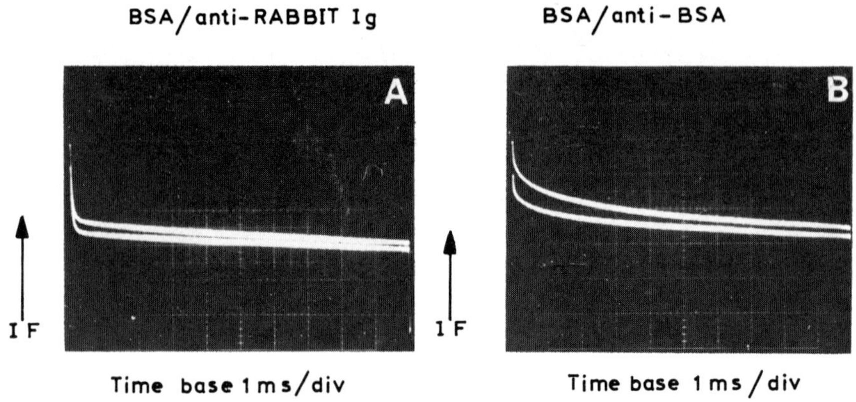

Fig. 3.8. FITC bleaching characteristics as a possible monitor for the specificity of FITC antibody binding. A) Bleaching curves for FITC anti-RIg non-specifically bound to a BSA-coated Sephadex bead. B) Suppressed fluorescence bleaching of FITC anti-BSA antibody bound to its homologous antigen. Illumination time = 10 ms. Dark interval between pulses (curves) was 1s. (Reproduced from Schauenstein et al. [15] with permission of the publisher.)

gates. Fig. 3.8A depicts the bleaching curves for FITC anti-RIg non-specifically bound to BSA-coated dextran beads. The shape of these curves is quite similar to that found for the free FITC antibody conjugate (see Fig. 3.6). In contrast, the specific immune reaction of a conjugate with its homologous antigen (e.g. anti-BSA with BSA-coated beads) was found to significantly suppress the bleaching process in the first millisecond of excitation as shown in Fig. 3.8B. Analogous results were obtained in the second system. Preliminary mathematical analysis of these data revealed that the shape of both types of bleaching curves fitted hyperbolic functions. The factor expressing the function per unit time was found to differ for non-specifically and specifically bound conjugates with a ratio of about 1 : 10 [15]. More detailed analyses are presently in progress.

3.4. DISCUSSION AND CONCLUSIONS

The use of laser light in the IF technique has attractive features for both practical and theoretical aspects. One problem still to be solved is the small visual field that is illuminated by the focussed laser beam in the present equipment, which restricts its application to a certain degree. Expansion of the beam by optical means is possible but accompanied by profound loss of energy/area delivered, which in principle could be compensated for by the use of more expensive lasers with higher energies. Another, more elegant way to overcome this problem would be to scan the visual field with the focussed laser beam by means of tunable electronic devices. This could combine the use of cheap lasers with the advantages of the recovery phenomenon. This problem is currently being studied in our laboratory.

The studies of the bleaching characteristics of FITC seem to be promising for the development of methods to discern between specific and non-specific staining in IF assays. It has to be mentioned, however, that this work is still preliminary and several theoretical questions remain to be answered. Bleaching of FITC, as it is observed under the present conditions, seems to involve at least two different processes occurring in parallel: a) the rapid initial loss of fluorescence intensity during the first microseconds of excitation, which appears to be reversible; and b) a more gradual bleaching process most probably caused by irreversible photodecomposition of the dye and increasing with higher energies or longer times of continuous excitation. The first rapid and reversible process turned out to be highly sensitive to changes in the chemical and physical microenvironment of the dye molecule. Changing the concentration of e.g. glycerol in the embedding medium has been shown to lead not only to quenching of the initial intensity [14], but also to similar effects to those described in section 3.3.3 (to be published). It is therefore of crucial importance to work under strictly standardized conditions for this kind of experiment.

Studies are currently in progress to investigate the photochemical mechanisms underlying the short-time fluorescence kinetics of antibody-bound FITC. In an extensive study using the flash photolysis technique in combination with kinetic spectrophotometry, Lindquist [11] showed that free fluorescein in aqueous solution was quantitatively converted into a transient triplet state followed by the formation of short-lived radicals as a result of single high-power light flashes. The decay of these intermediates was found to be accompanied by the recovery of the ground state of the fluorescein molecule, which may sufficiently explain the recovery of FITC fluorescence observed in the present system. With regard to the observed alterations of short-time bleaching of antibody-bound FITC, it would be important to know which of the various rapid intermediate reactions is most affected by the specific immune reaction of the conjugate with its antigen.

Recent direct IF systems with biological antigenic substrates, i.e. smears of bone marrow and spleen to detect single Ig-producing plasma cells, gave bleaching data which were in perfect agreement with those described for the bead system. Thus, the analysis of short-time fluorescence kinetics appears to be a useful tool for improving the specific information obtainable from IF assays in general.

ACKNOWLEDGEMENTS

Part of the work referred to in this paper was supported by the Austrian Research Council (project No. 4114) and the Legerlotz-Foundation, Innsbruck. We acknowledge the permission by the publishers to reproduce Fig. 3.8.

REFERENCES

1 Bergquist, N.R. (1973) The pulsed dye laser as a light source for the fluorescent antibody technique. Scand. J. Immunol. *2,* 37–44.

2 Bonner, W.A., Hulet, H.R., Sweet, R.G. and Herzenberg, L.A. (1972) Fluorescence activated cell sorting. Rev. Sci. Instrum. *43,* 404–409.

3 Cuatrecasas, P. (1970) Protein purification by affinity chromatography. J. Biol. Chem. *245,* 3059–3065.

4 Dragsten, P., Henkart, P., Blumenthal, R., Weinstein, J. and Schlessinger, J. (1979) Lateral diffusion of surface immunoglobulin, Thy-1 antigen and a lipid probe in lymphocyte plasma membrane. Proc. Natl. Acad. Sci. U.S.A. *76,* 5163–5167.

5 Goldman, M. (1960) Antigenic analysis of Entamoeba hystolytica by means of fluorescent antibody. 1. Instrumentation for microfluorometry of stained amoebae. Exp. Parasitol. *9,* 25–36.

6 Haaijman, J.J. (1977) Quantitative Immunofluorescence Microscopy – Methods and Applications. Institute for Experimental Gerontology of the Organization for Health Research TNO, Rijswijk (Z.H.), The Netherlands.

7 Herzog, F., Albini, B. and Wick, G. (1973) Comparison of filters used in immunofluorescent staining procedures with fluorescein-isothiocyanate (FITC) conjugates. J. Immunol. Methods *3,* 211–220.

8 Hirschfeld, T. (1979) Fluorescence background discrimination by prebleaching. J. Histochem. Cytochem. *27,* 96–101.

9 Kaufman, G.I., Nester, J.F. and Wasserman, D.E. (1971) An experimental study of lasers as excitation sources for automated fluorescent antibody instrumentation. J. Histochem. Cytochem. *19,* 476–496.

10 Klugerman, M.R. (1966) Chemical and physical variables affecting the properties of fluorescein isothiocyanate and its protein conjugates. J. Immunol. *95,* 1165–1173.

11 Lindquist, L. (1960) A flash photolysis of fluorescein. Ark. Kemi *16,* 79–138.

12 Mansberg, H.P. and Kusnetz, J. (1966) Quantitative fluorescence microscopy: fluorescent antibody automatic scanning techniques. J. Histochem. Cytochem. *14,* 260–273.

13 Ploem, J.S. (1967) The use of vertical illuminators with interchangeable dichroic mirrors for fluorescence microscopy with incident light. Z. Wiss. Mikrosk. *68,* 129–142.

14 Schauenstein, K., Böck, G. and Wick, G. (1978) Factors influencing fluorescence properties of free and protein bound fluorochromes. Macro- and microfluorometric observations. *In* Knapp, W., Holubar, K. and Wick, G. (eds.), Immunofluorescence and Related Staining Techniques (Elsevier/North-Holland, Amsterdam) pp. 81–95.

15 Schauenstein, K., Böck, G. and Wick, G. (1980) Short time bleaching of fluorescein isothiocyanate. A possible parameter for the specific binding of conjugates in immunofluorescence. J. Histochem. Cytochem. *28,* 1029–1031.

16 Schauenstein, K., Schauenstein, E. and Wick, G. (1978) Fluorescence properties of free and protein bound fluorescein dyes. I. Macrospectrofluorometric measurements. J. Histochem. Cytochem. *26,* 277–283.

17 Schauenstein, K., Wick, G., Herzog, F. and Steinbatz, A. (1975) Investigation of the recovery phenomenon in immunofluorescence after laser excitation. J. Immunol. Methods *8,* 9–15.

18 Schlessinger, J., Schecter, Y., Willingham, M.C. and Pastan, I. (1978) Direct visualization of binding, aggregation, and internalization of insulin and epidermal growth factor on living fibroblastic cells. Proc. Natl. Acad. Sci. U.S.A. *75,* 2659–2663.

19 Steinbach, G. and Von Mayersbach, H. (1976) Characterization of fluorescein isothiocyanate. II. Absorption and fluorescence after conjugation to human and rabbit γ-globulin and bovine serum albumin. Acta histochem. *55,* 110–124.

20 Van Duuren, B.L. (1963) Effects of the environment on the fluorescence of aromatic compounds in solution. Chem. Rev. *63,* 325–354.

21 Wick, G., Schauenstein, K., Herzog, F. and Steinbatz, A. (1975) Investigation of the recovery phenomenon after laser excitation in immunofluorescence. Ann. N.Y. Acad. Sci. *254,* 172–174.

Wick et al. (eds) Immunofluorescence Technology. Selected Theoretical and Clinical Aspects © *Elsevier Biomedical Press, 1982*

CHAPTER 4

Membrane immunofluorescence

K. SCHAUENSTEIN and G. WICK

Institute for General and Experimental Pathology, University of Innsbruck, 6010 Innsbruck, Austria

4.1. INTRODUCTION

The detection of antigenic structures on the outer plasma membrane of isolated cells is one of the essential experimental approaches in basic and applied immunological research. The numerous techniques developed for the various kinds of cell surface structures can be grouped as follows.

1. Cellular techniques which are based either on cytoadherence, such as rosette assays with untreated or sensitized red blood cells, the mixed hemagglutination technique for the detection of cell surface determinants on tissue sections [27], and cell affinity chromatography [11, 21], or on functional cellular assays in vitro, such as the mixed lymphocyte reaction and the cell-mediated cytotoxicity assay for the detection of "lymphocyte-defined" antigenic determinants of the major histocompatibility complex.

2. Serological techniques which make use of the complement-dependent cytotoxic activity of antibodies against cell surface determinants as assessed, e.g., by trypan blue exclusion or the ^{51}Cr release assay [15]. More refined techniques consist in the immunoprecipitation of radiolabelled surface proteins and analysis by polyacrylamide gel electrophoresis after solubilization of the membranes by non-ionic detergents [10].

3. Serological staining methods which use antibodies coupled to various

marker molecules or radioactive isotopes to visualize the specific immune reaction on the surface of cells in the light, fluorescence, or electron microscope.

Among these techniques, membrane immunofluorescence (MeIF), i.e. the detection of cell surface determinants by means of fluorochrome-labelled (most frequently fluorescein isothiocyanate (FITC)) antibodies, has gained substantial importance due to several positive, practical and theoretical aspects, the most prominent of which are: a) easy and uncomplicated performance, b) high sensitivity, c) the possibility of quantification by microfluorometers, d) evaluation of living cells enabling the direct follow-up of kinetics of determinants in the membrane, e) simultaneous detection of two surface antigens by means of double staining methods, and f) the possibility of cell sorting according to antigenic properties by means of the fluorescence-activated cell sorter (FACS).

The present chapter describes the usual procedure for MeIF tests and also a time- and reagents-saving semi-automated micromethod developed in this laboratory. The evaluation of MeIF in the fluorescence microscope and by means of microfluorometers is discussed, including theoretical and practical aspects of the different staining patterns which are a reflection of the distribution of membrane antigens detected.

4.2. METHODS

4.2.1. Usual procedure

As with any other IF assay, MeIF can be performed in a direct or indirect manner (sandwich or antiglobulin technique); the latter is supposed to be more sensitive than the direct systems, as a larger number of labelled antibody molecules is bound per antigenic site [6]. Furthermore, for the detection of specific antigen receptors on the surface of lymphocytes, MeIF can be carried out in a reversed way using the respective antigen labelled with fluorescein or tetramethylrhodamine isothiocyanate (FITC or TRITC) as reagent. The usual MeIF procedure as originally described by Möller [12] is performed in test tubes. For direct assays small volumes (0.05–0.1 ml) of the cell suspension (optimal concentration for lymphocytes: 1–2 $\times$ 10^7/ml) are mixed with the same volume of FITC antibody and incubated at the required temperature (see below) for 30 min. Thereafter the cells are washed (3–5 times) to remove excess free conjugate from the medium. For indirect assays, the first incubation is carried out with an unlabelled antibody, which, after washing, is followed by a second incubation step with the FITC-labelled anti-immunoglobulin conjugate. Optimal conjugate dilutions should be determined for each system by means of chessboard titrations [29] to minimize non-specific staining effects. After removal of free conjugate by further washing the cells are ready for evaluation. They are either observed immediately in a viable state (e.g. by direct mounting of a small drop of the stained cell suspension with a cover slip) or spread onto slides, air-dried, fixed (e.g. ethanol/ether, 1 : 1), and mounted in buffered glycerol (glycerol/PBS, 9 : 1). Fixation of cells in suspension can be accomplished by incubation in 2% formaldehyde for 4–6 h followed by two washes with phosphate-buffered saline (PBS) containing 0.02 M NaN_3 (I. Zan-Bar, personal communication). Cells fixed by this method retain their morphological features and keep for several weeks in suspension (at 4°C), which is of particular practical importance for work with the FACS.

4.2.2. The micro-membrane fluorescence test

Using the conventional procedure with its time-consuming washing processes, a maximum of about 80–100 indirect MeIF preparations (= tubes) per day can be performed by one experienced person. It was mainly for this reason that a semi-automated microassay (MMF) was developed in this laboratory, using units of the Microtiter System® [20]. This technique makes it possible to perform MeIF on several hundred preparations within a few hours and also contributes to standardization, as a large number of samples is processed under exactly the same conditions. Furthermore, it economizes on cells and reagents as only a quarter of the usual volume (i.e. 25 μl) is used. Fig. 4.1 shows the various parts of the equipment. The test procedure has been described in earlier publications [16, 20]. Briefly, the antiserum or conjugate is diluted in a serial manner in V-bottomed Microtiter plates using calibrated

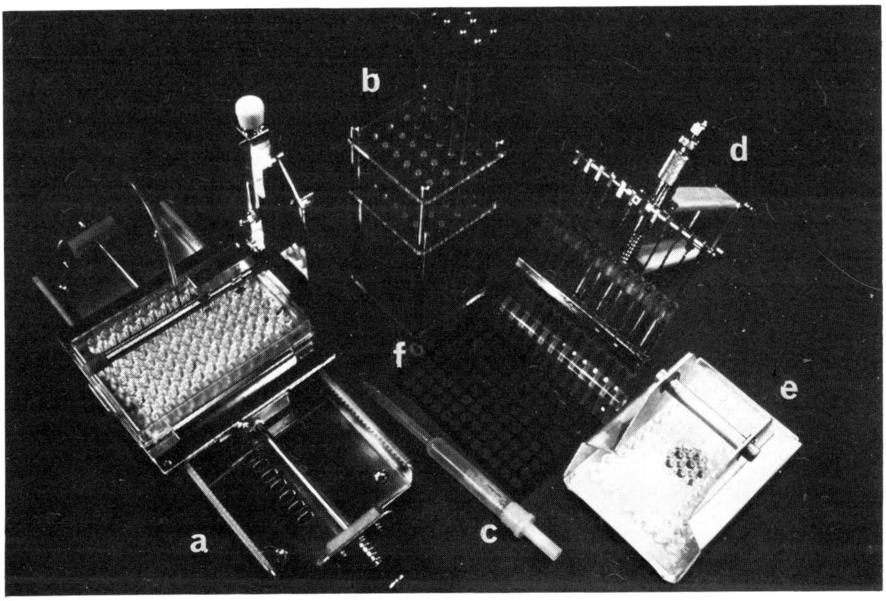

Fig. 4.1. Equipment for the micro-membrane fluorescence assay. a) Coombs rinser; b) microdiluter, 25 μl volume; c) dropper pipette, 25 μl; d) multiple dispenser; e) centrifuge carrier for Microtiter plates; f) Cooke® "anti-glare shield", which can be used as a slide for large numbers of samples.

dropper pipettes and microdiluters of 25 μl volume. 25 μl of the cell suspension (optimal concentration for lymphocytes 5–10 × 10^6/ml) are added to the antibody dilutions and incubated at the required temperature for 30 min. For the washings, the plates are placed in centrifuge carriers for Microtiter plates which are available for various centrifuge types, and centrifuged for 3 min at 700 × *g*. Between the centrifugations the supernatants are removed by a single, sharp flick of the wrist and the medium is refilled (0.1 ml/well) by means of a Coombs rinser (Cooke AM 57). Exact withdrawal of the washing fluid to a residual volume of 25 μl is of obvious importance at two steps of the indirect procedure: 1) before the addition of the conjugate, and 2) before the distribution of the stained cells on the slides. It is accomplished by connecting the dispenser comb of the Coombs apparatus to a water suction pump and immersing it into the wells to a defined depth, which is determined by layers of tape wound around both poles of the comb, as depicted in Figs. 4.2 and 4.3.

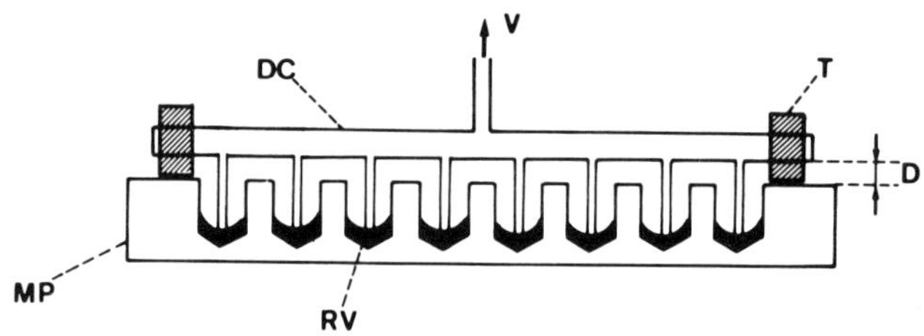

Fig. 4.2. Defined withdrawal of supernatants. The depth of immersion is adjusted by layers of tape wound around both poles of the dispenser comb. DC, dispenser comb; T, tape; D, distance defined by layers of tape; MP, microtiter plate (V-profile); RV, residual volume (0.025 ml); V, vacuum pump.

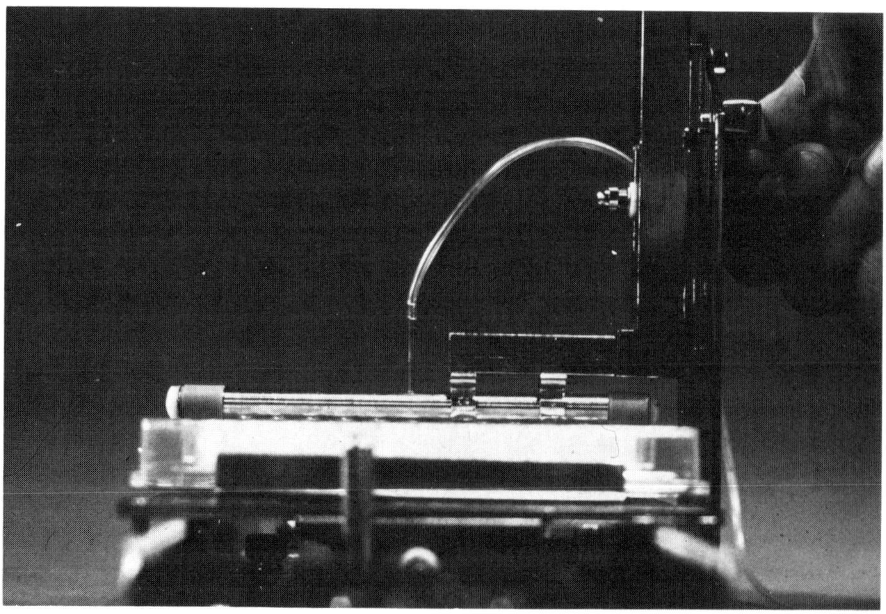

Fig. 4.3. Withdrawal of supernatants using the adapted Coombs rinser attached to a vacuum pump.

After the last wash, the stained cell suspensions are either fixed by 2% formaldehyde, as described above, or transferred onto slides (Cooke microprint 10 spots, CL 100) by means of a multiple dispenser pipette, air-dried, fixed, mounted in buffered glycerol and stored at 4°C. A modification of this microtechnique has been developed for the detection of circulating immune complexes using Raji cells [2].

4.2.3. Evaluation of MeIF tests

Readings of MeIF tests are performed with normal IF microscopes, using incident light excitation facilities. Optimal magnifications are 400–1000 ×. For the unbiased enumeration of positive and negative subpopulations in a given total of cells, it is advisable to first count cells of a visual field at a normal, transmitted light illumination using dark-field or phase-contrast condensors. Thereafter, the number of fluorescent cells is determined by incident light fluorescence excitation. Relative quantitative information can be obtained either by determining the titer of an antiserum on various cells at identical conditions or by measuring relative fluorescence intensities using a microfluorometer. By these means it is possible to compare the expression of a certain antigen on the surface of cells of different origin or stages of differentiation [18]. It should be remembered that comparison of quantitative IF data is not possible unless experiments are performed with the same serological reagents and under strictly identical conditions. Various physico-chemical factors such as temperature, pH, composition of the mounting medium, etc. have been described to profoundly alter the fluorescence properties of free and bound fluorescein dyes [19, 28]. Another factor, which considerably influences the quantitative outcome of MeIF with living cells is the expression of the different staining patterns on the membrane, as is outlined below. For quantitative studies the formation of caps, which may be followed by rapid disappearance of the respective surface determinants, should therefore be prevented by the addition of 0.02 M sodium azide to the medium and washing fluid.

A unique methodological advantage of MeIF is the possibility to evaluate stained cell suspensions by means of the FACS [5]. This instrument, which is described in detail in a separate chapter of this volume, enables both rapid distribution analysis and physical separation of cell subpopulations according to cell size and relative fluorescence intensity.

4.3. MEMBRANE DETERMINANTS DETECTABLE BY MeIF

It is beyond the scope of this chapter to deal with all the different membrane antigens that have been detected and studied by the MeIF method. In genetical terms three kinds of antigenic determinants can be serologically detected on the surface of living cells of humans or animals. 1. Heteroantigens, i.e. determinants recognized by antibody raised in a different species. These antigens comprise mainly strong species- and organ-specific determinants. Conventional heteroantisera usually are very strong reagents with high titres. To render them specific for one certain antigen, however, requires tedious and time-consuming absorption procedures. 2. Alloantigens, i.e. determinants defined by inter-strain immunization within one and the same species. Membrane structures studied by this approach are blood group antigens, different alleles of various lymphocyte markers, and the determinants of the major histocompatibility complex (MHC). Alloantibodies, although strictly specific for a given gene product without the necessity of absorption are usually of rather weak staining capacity in comparison with heteroantibodies. With the advent of the monoclonal antibody technique [8] these problems, however, seem to be solved. 3. Surface determinants that are recognized in syngeneic conditions, i.e. they appear in one given individual. Their occurrence is usually accompanied by certain pathological conditions, such as autoimmune processes (autoantigens) or malignant transformation (tumor-associated antigens).

4.4. STAINING PATTERNS

The following three types of staining patterns on the single cell can be observed in MeIF tests [4]: A) ringshaped, homogeneous; B) aggregates, spots

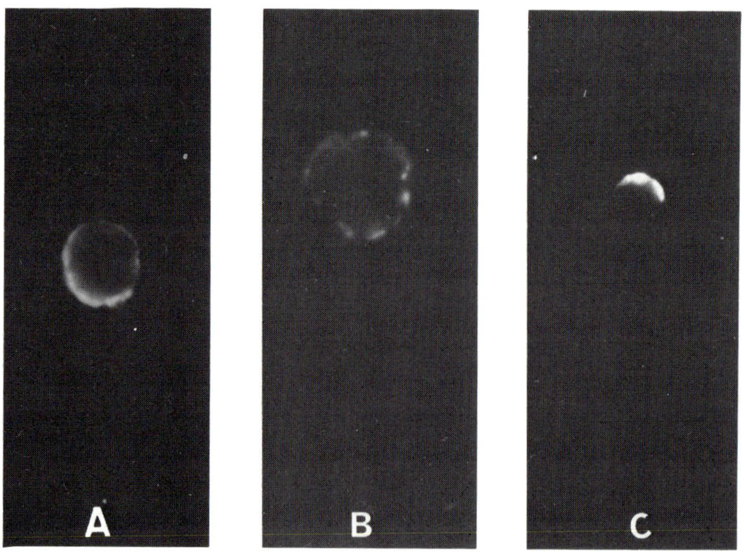

Fig. 4.4. Staining patterns obtained in membrane immunofluorescence. A) Homogeneous, ringlike (indirect assay with turkey anti-bursa cell antiserum on chicken bursa cells). B) Patches and spots (human chronic lymphatic leukemia cell stained with TRITC-labelled anti-κ-light-chain antibody). C) Cap (human thymus cell indirectly stained with horse anti-human thymocyte antibody).

and patches; and C) caps (Fig. 4.4). The expression of these three different forms is dependent on many variables, e.g. cell type investigated, the reagents applied, certain experimental conditions, etc. In the following section, some basic theoretical aspects of the kinetics of cell surface antigens underlying the different distribution types will be discussed. Most of these investigations were performed using the MeIF method. Furthermore, it will be shown how to make use of the different staining patterns for the study of steric correlations of two different membrane antigens.

4.4.1. Theoretical aspects of the kinetics of cell surface determinants

Membrane antigens are generally protein or glycoprotein molecules embedded to various degrees in the lipid bilayer of the plasma membrane as shown in Fig. 4.5. Under normal conditions the distribution of these molecules can be expected to have a fairly random character [25], although natural clustering to various degrees has been described for certain membrane determinants [1].

The MeIF staining pattern reflecting the random distribution of a surface determinant is the ringshaped, homogeneous one. This picture is obtained under any experimental conditions with erythrocytes of various species. It has been attributed to the fact that membrane determinants of these cells are a priori anchored by spectrin fibres, a protein which is lacking in the plasma membrane of other cells [24]. Homogeneous staining of nucleated cells (e.g. lymphocytes) can be seen in MeIF tests using monovalent Fab fragments of antibody and/or conjugates [13, 26]. Furthermore, it is also observed with very high concentrations of divalent or polyvalent antibody, provided the density of the detected antigen on the membrane is high enough.

Fluorescent "patches" or "spots" are normally obtained with nucleated cells using lower concentrations of di- or polyvalent antibodies. This pattern

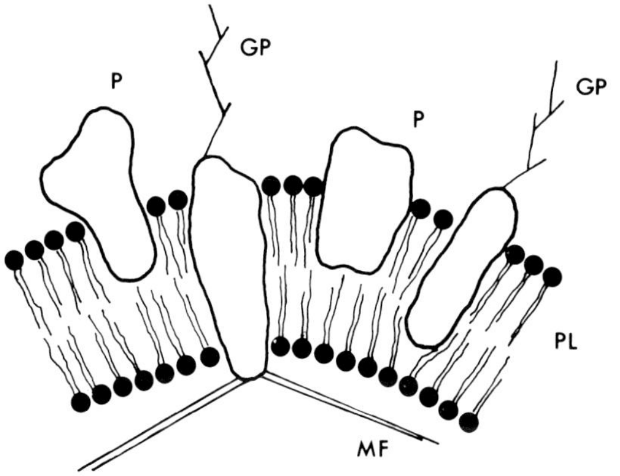

Fig. 4.5. Current model of the cell membrane. Protein (P) and glycoprotein (GP) macromolecules are embedded in the phospholipid bilayer (PL). Molecules reaching the inner membrane surface may come in contact with elements of the cytoskeleton such as microfilaments (MF).

corresponds to passive aggregation of surface antigens, a process also called redistribution, which is metabolically independent as it occurs also in the cold (4°C) and in the presence of sodium azide (0.02 M) or other inhibitors of cellular metabolism [13]. There is strong evidence that the redistribution of antigen receptors of B lymphocytes (i.e. surface immunoglobulin) also occurs in vivo upon encounter with antigen and may be the triggering signal for B-cell activation and proliferation [26]. The formation of patches, or spots, has been used for the estimation of the mean density of a surface determinant according to whether it is obtained in an indirect or direct MeIF assay [7]. Since an antibody molecule is known to span a distance of 140 Å, it can be expected that redistribution will occur in a direct assay in cases where the mean minimal distance of the respective surface structures does not exceed this value. Accordingly, for the indirect system a mean minimal distance of 420 Å could be sufficient to allow aggregate formation.

Capping – in contrast to aggregation – is a phenomenon which can be inhibited by conditions or substances that block the cellular metabolism (e.g. cold or NaN_3). Furthermore, this process was shown to also be influenced by Ca^{2+} and substances affecting the contractile microfilaments of the cytoskeleton like cytochalasin B and D. Cytochalasin B, an agent blocking the microfilaments, strongly inhibits capping, whereas cytochalasin D, which activates them, is able to disrupt preformed caps [22]. Due to the possibility of evaluating living cells, capping can be directly studied and followed up by MeIF. It is supposed to consist in the confluence of redistributed (= aggregated) surface molecules in a semi-lunar manner. Thus, "patches" and "spots" would be a prerequisite for cap formation. Electron microscopic studies revealed caps to occur preferentially on a characteristic cell pole near the Golgi apparatus [22]. Incubation of stained cells at capping conditions for longer time periods was shown to result in the formation of so-called "hand mirror forms", the fluorescent cap being the "handle", and later on in the disappearance of the detected antigen from the surface by either ingestion or shedding of the immune complexes [9]. When these cells, "stripped" of the respective antigen, are further incubated at optimal metabolic conditions, a resynthesis of this determinant can be observed on the cell surface. Stripping and resynthesis of membrane determinants may be used as a proof of their cellular origin, ruling out the possibility of passive adsorption from the environment.

4.4.2. Double staining and co-capping

As pointed out in the introduction this chapter, another great advantage of MeIF compared with other related techniques is the possibility of simultaneously studying two surface determinants on one and the same living cell by means of double-staining methods. This is possible owing to the availability of fluorochromes with different excitation and fluorescence emission characteristics, the most widely used of which are FITC (green fluorescence excited by visible blue) and TRITC (red fluorescence excited by visible green). A third suitable compound, the blue fluoresceing 4-acetamido-4′-isothiocyano-stilbene-2,2′-disulfonic acid (SITS), was described in 1975 by Rothbart et al. [14]. Information about steric relationships between two surface antigens can be obtained by differential capping in combination with the double-staining technique as outlined below.

4.4.2.1. Methods

A crucial prerequisite for any successful IF double-staining experiment is to exclude unwanted cross-reactions between the different antisera and conjugates applied. This problem arises mainly in situations where two indirect MeIF tests have to be combined. Accordingly, care has to be taken to select a combination of reagents prepared from different species as schematically depicted in Fig. 4.6 for a double-staining assay for two different surface determinants (denoted Lp and B) on chicken B lymphocytes [18]. The two different MeIF tests are usually performed in a sequential manner, particularly where double staining should be combined with a co-capping experiment. In these cases the first step is done under conditions optimal for the formation of caps, i.e. incubation with conjugate in a 37°C water bath for about 20 min. At this stage it is important to keep to a certain incubation time, as in certain systems the disappearance of capped immune complexes from the surface may occur to a considerable degree even within such short times. In order to physically separate the two antigens in the membrane, the second assay is carried out under conditions preventing capping, i.e. at 4°C or by addition of 0.01–0.02 M NaN_3 to the medium. After the last wash, the preparations are ready for evaluation either in the living state or fixed and mounted in buffered glycerol.

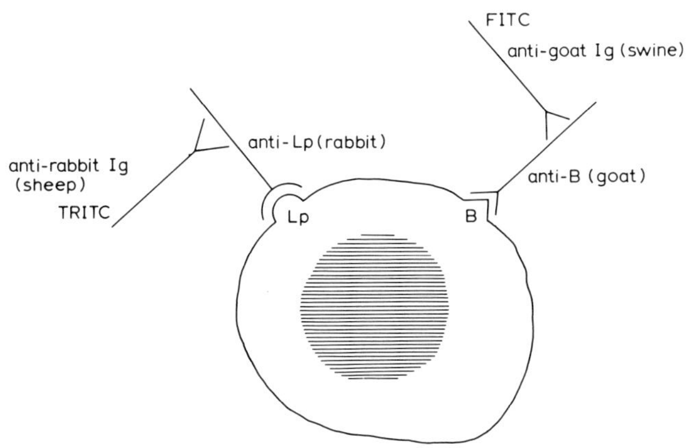

Fig. 4.6. Schematic representation of two independent, indirect membrane immunofluorescence systems for the simultaneous detection of two different surface determinants (B and Lp) on chicken B lymphocytes.

4.4.2.2. *Evaluation*

The distribution of two types of surface determinants in a certain cell population is examined by the same kind of evaluation as for MeIF reading, i.e. counting cells in normal light illumination followed by sequential fluorescence examination with both wavelengths. A crucial factor for optimal distinction of green and red MeIF staining lies in the optical system, i.e. the filter combinations. Furthermore, the general fluorescence properties of the two fluorochromes used have to be considered. The green fluorescence of FITC usually appears much stronger than the red one of TRITC. It is necessary therefore in many cases to use TRITC conjugates in higher concentrations than those with FITC in order to be in comparable sensitivity ranges for both test systems. The fluorescence of FITC, on the other hand, is, in contrast to TRITC, subject to strong fading within a short time period (see chapter 3), which has to be taken into account for prolonged observations and microphotography.

Fig. 4.7 shows an example of a double-staining co-capping experiment designed to demonstrate the sterical independence of two different surface structures on the plasma membrane of peripheral chicken lymphocytes: chicken spleen cells were first treated with a specific goat anti-chicken thymus

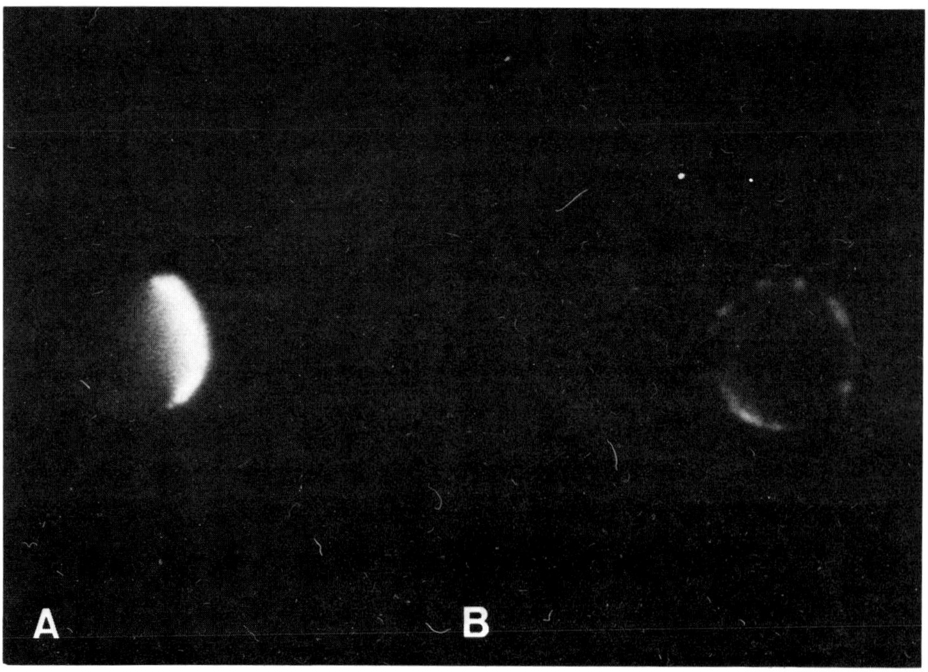

Fig. 4.7. Co-capping experiment with chicken splenic lymphocytes to demonstrate the independent expression of two surface determinants (T, Lp). A) Cap obtained with anti-T (goat) and FITC-labelled anti-goat Ig (swine). B) Patchy staining of the same cell at non-capping conditions (0.02 M NaN_3) with rabbit anti-Lp and sheep anti-rabbit Ig TRITC.

cell serum, the reaction of which was visualized by means of a swine anti-goat Ig FITC conjugate under conditions allowing cap formation (37°C, 20 min). In the second step, the same cell suspension was subjected to an indirect assay with a rabbit antiserum specific for a surface determinant (Lp), which is present on a subpopulation of peripheral chicken lymphoid cells, and a sheep anti-rabbit Ig TRITC conjugate in the presence of 0.02 M NaN_3. The sterical independence of both detected antigens is obvious.

4.5. CONCLUSIONS

Since its introduction in 1961 by Möller [12], MeIF has become a standard technique both in immunological routine diagnostics (e.g. determination of B and T cells in the peripheral blood, detection of autoantibodies against cell surface antigens, etc.) and for basic cell membrane research.

Recent developments dealing with the quantitative determination of the lateral mobilities of various membrane structures on various cell types make use of the bleaching properties of FITC and measure the recovery of fluorescence after total bleaching by laser irradiation as a parameter for the lateral diffusion of the respective membrane determinant [3]. This fluorescence photobleaching recovery technique (FPR) may provide more detailed insight into kinetic events on the cell surface during activation and differentiation.

Another subject of more recent investigations is the absolute quantitation of MeIF results by means of cytofluorometers or the FACS. Besides the solution of certain problems inherent to fluorescence [17], one of the most important steps towards this goal is certainly the application of monoclonal antibodies derived from immune hybridomas [8]. These reagents, being optimally homogeneous and specific, are expected to react with their homologous antigens at constant molecular ratios, thus enabling the calibration of quantitative systems and the determination of absolute antigen concentrations on the surface of living cells.

ACKNOWLEDGEMENT

Part of the work mentioned in this paper was supported by the Austrian Cancer Research Fund.

REFERENCES

1 Abbas, A.K., Ault, K.A., Karnowsky, M.J. and Unanue, E.R. (1975) Non-random distribution of surface immunoglobulin on murine B lymphocytes. J. Immunol. *114*, 1197–1204.

2 Albini, B., Ossi, E., Penner, E. and Andres, G.A. (1979) A micromethod for the detection of circulating immune complexes using Raji cells. Immunobiology *156*, 191.

3 Dragsten, P., Henkart, P., Blumenthal, R., Weinstein, J. and Schlessinger, J. (1979) Lateral diffusion of surface immunoglobulin, Thy-1 antigen, and a lipid probe in lymphocyte plasma membranes. Proc. Natl. Acad. Sci. U.S.A. *76,* 5163–5167.

4 Greaves, M.F., Owen, J.J.T. and Raff, M.C. (1973) T and B Lymphocytes. Origin, Properties, and Roles in Immune Responses (Excerpta Medica, Amsterdam/American Elsevier Publ., New York) pp. 48–52.

5 Herzenberg, L.A. (1978) The fluorescence activated cell sorter (FACS): a retrospective and prospective view. *In* Knapp, W., Holubar, K. and Wick, G. (eds.), Immunofluorescence and Related Staining Techniques (Elsevier North-Holland, Amsterdam) pp. 99–110.

6 Holborow, E.J. (1970) Standardization in Immunofluorescence (Blackwell Scientific Publ., Oxford).

7 Karnovsky, M.J. and Unanue, E.R. (1973) Mapping and migration of lymphocyte surface macromolecules. Fed. Proc. *32,* 43–54.

8 Köhler, G. and Milstein, C. (1975) Continuous cultures of fused cells secreting antibody of predefined specificity. Nature (London) *256,* 495–497.

9 Loor, F., Forni, L. and Pernis, B. (1972) The dynamic state of the lymphocyte membrane. Factors affecting the distribution and turnover of surface immunoglobulins. Eur. J. Immunol. *2,* 203–212.

10 Marchalonis, J.J. and Cone, R.E. (1973) Biochemical and biological characteristics of lymphocyte surface immunoglobulin. Transplant. Rev. *14,* 3–49.

11 Matthews, N., Rolland, J.M. and Nairn, R.C. (1976) Lymphoid cell fractionation by aggregated immunoglobulin-agarose columns. J. Immunol. Methods *9,* 323–335.

12 Möller, G. (1961) Demonstration of mouse isoantigens at cellular level by the fluorescent antibody method. J. Exp. Med. *114,* 415–434.

13 Raff, M.C. and De Petris, S. (1973) Movement of lymphocyte surface antigens and receptors: The fluid nature of the lymphocyte plasma membrane and its significance. Fed. Proc. *32,* 43–54.

14 Rothbart, P.H., Olthoff, J.G. and Mul, N.A.V. (1975) Experience with a new fluorochrome. Ann. N.Y. Acad. Sci. *254,* 65.

15 Sanderson, A.R. (1964) Application of iso-immune cytolysis using radiolabelled target cells. Nature *204,* 250.

16 Schauenstein, K. (1977) A new rapid modification for membrane fluorescence tests based on the microtiter system. Microsc. Acta *80,* 31–36.

17 Schauenstein, K. (1978) Workshop report on application of immunofluorescence flow cytophotometry and quantitative immunofluorescence. *In* Knapp, W., Holubar, K. and Wick, G. (eds.), Immunofluorescence and Related Staining Techniques (Elsevier North-Holland, Amsterdam) pp. 257–270.

18 Schauenstein, K. (1979) Surface characteristics of chicken peripheral B and T lymphocytes defined by specific heteroantisera. Dev. Comp. Immunol. *3,* 321–340.

19 Schauenstein, K., Bock, G. and Wick, G. (1978) Factors influencing fluorescence properties of free and protein bound fluorochromes. Macro- and microfluorometric observations. *In* Knapp, W., Holubar, K. and Wick, G. (eds.), Immunofluorescence and Related Staining Techniques (Elsevier North-Holland, Amsterdam) pp. 81–95.

20 Schauenstein, K., Wick, G. and Kink, H. (1976) The micro membrane fluorescence test (MMF): a new rapid semiautomated technique based on the Microtiter system. J. Immunol. Methods *10,* 143–150.

21 Schlossman, S.F. and Hudson, L. (1973) Specific purification of lymphocyte populations on a digestible immunoadsorbent. J. Immunol. *110,* 313–315.

22 Schreiner, G.F. and Unanue, E.R. (1976) Calcium sensitive modulation of Ig capping: evidence supporting a cytoplasmic control of ligand–receptor complexes. J. Exp. Med. *143,* 15–31.

23 Schreiner, G.F. and Unanue, E.R. (1977) Membrane and cytoplasmic changes in B lymphocytes induced by ligand–surface immunoglobulin interaction. Adv. Immunol. *24,* 37–165.

24 Singer, S.J. (1974) The molecular organisation of membranes. Ann. Rev. Biochem. *43,* 805–833.

25 Singer, S.J. and Nicolson, G.L. (1972) The fluid model of the structure of cell membranes. Science *175,* 720–731.

26 Taylor, R.B., Duffus, W.P.H., Raff, M.C. and De Petris, S. (1971) Redistribution and pinocytosis of lymphocyte surface immunoglobulin molecules induced by anti-immunoglobulin antibodies. Nature New Biol. *233,* 225–229.

27 Thunold, S., Tonder, O. and Wiig, J.N. (1973) Localisation in mouse lymphoid tissue of receptors for immunoglobulin. Scand. J. Immunol. *2,* 135–142.

28 Van Duuren, B.L. (1963) Effects of the environment on the fluorescence of aromatic compounds in solution. Chem. Rev. *63,* 325–354.

29 Wick, G., Baudner, S. and Herzog, F. (1978) Immunofluorescence (Medizinische Verlagsgesellschaft, Marburg).

Wick et al. (eds) Immunofluorescence Technology. Selected Theoretical and Clinical Aspects © *Elsevier Biomedical Press, 1982*

CHAPTER 5

Fluoro-immuno-cytoadherence (FICA): a simple and versatile method for the demonstration and characterization of antigen-binding cells

H. WOLF and G. WICK

Institute for General and Experimental Pathology, University of Innsbruck Medical School, A-6020 Innsbruck, Austria

5.1. INTRODUCTION

The demonstration of antigen-binding cells (ABC) for experimental and clinical purposes is now commonly performed using immuno-cytoadherence techniques which employ antigen-coated erythrocytes as indicator particles for rosette formation [20, 24]. Additional methods are immunofluorescence with fluorochrome-labelled antigen preparations [32] and isotope-labelling procedures [4, 21]. Rosette formation enjoys the broadest application because it does not involve any special requirements, such as the use of fluorescence microscopes or the handling of isotopes and the development of autoradiographs. Antigen-coated indicator red blood cells (RBC) adhere to surface receptors of the ABC in question and thus result in the formation of characteristic rosettes which can be evaluated under conventional microscopes. Using RBC of different species, which can be distinguished by size or shape and are coated with different antigens, multiple populations of ABC can be demonstrated simultaneously by this method [30]. Nevertheless, for this purpose RBC of various species must always be available, antigen-coating procedures are rather tedious and time-consuming and the antigens carrying RBC have only a limited shelf-life. Furthermore, exact quantification of the degree of coating is often difficult.

In this chapter we describe a simple and versatile method based on the preparation of stable antigen-coated particles which allows for the demonstration of ABC and affords the simultaneous possibility for specificity control. The method was named fluoro-immuno-cytoadherence (FICA) [30]. It is based on the combination of two principles. 1. The so-called defined antigenic substrate spheres (DASS) system [18, 38], where antigens are covalently coupled to carrier particles (e.g. agarose or cross-linked dextran). Such particles have successfully been used for quantitative evaluation of direct and indirect immunofluorescence tests and this method is described in detail in chapter 2 of this volume. 2. The principle of affinity chromatography [47], where cell suspensions can be depleted of, or enriched for, various subpopulations by virtue of the adherence of certain cells to the surface of ligand-coated carrier particles after passage over appropriate columns and subsequent elution.

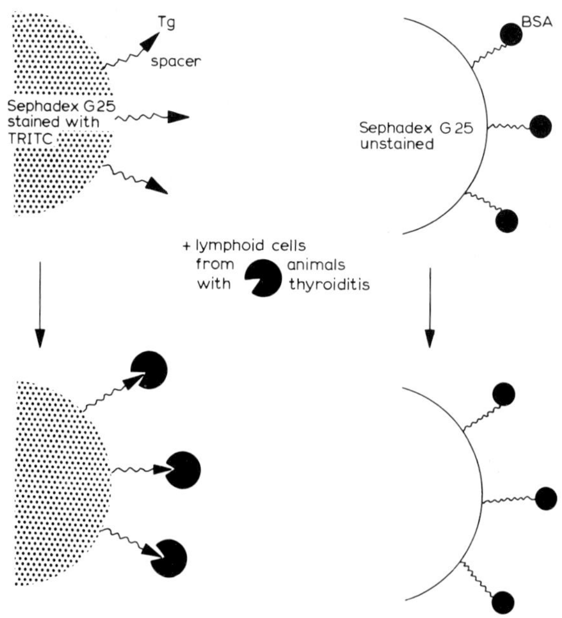

Fig. 5.1. Principle of FICA method. The Tg- and BSA-coated beads are mixed with lymphocyte suspension to be analysed for the presence of antigen-binding cells. Cells with the appropriate surface receptor will adhere to the respective bead population leaving beads coated with a control antigen unaffected. The two (or three) different kinds of beads can be identified by their color.

For FICA, antigens are coupled to the surface of fluorescent beads via a molecular spacer chain. The specificity and degree of antigen coating can be assessed by immunofluorescence as detailed later in this chapter. The antigen-coated beads are then mixed with the cell suspension to be analysed. Lymphoid cells possessing receptors for any of the antigens presented on a given kind of beads will adhere to these and form "inverted" rosettes around them (Fig. 5.1). Beads stained with a certain fluorochrome (e.g. fluorescein isothiocyanate, FITC) and coated with a given antigen can be mixed with differently stained (e.g. tetramethylrhodamine, TRITC) beads carrying another antigen and, if desired, with unstained particles coated with a third antigen. After addition of the lymphoid cell suspension to be analyzed, the evaluation can be done under a fluorescence microscope equipped for the two–wavelength method, permitting simultaneous specificity control (Fig. 5.2). If no fluorescence microscope is available, the different types of antigen-laden indicator beads can also be mixed with aliquots of the cell suspension in separate tubes and the rosetting cells in each tube can then be counted by conventional microscopy (Fig. 5.3).

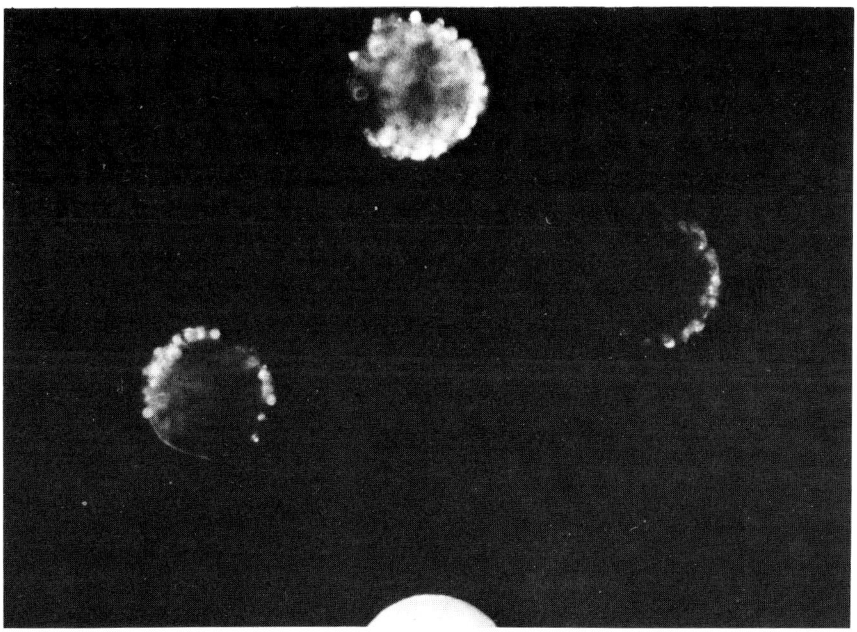

Fig. 5.2. Appearance of FICA tests, monitored by fluorescence microscopy. Antigens, e.g. Tg and BSA, are coupled onto the surface of different charges of spacer-armed Sephadex G-25 beads. The type of coating is visualized by different fluorescent dyes. Addition of lymphocytes to a mixture of both kinds of beads resulted in adherence to those beads coated with the respective antigen, identified by its color of fluorescence. In this case sensitized lymphoid cells (counterstained with acridine orange for better visualization) adhere to Tg-coated, non-fluorescent beads. At the bottom a cross-section of a BSA-coated, red fluorescent control bead without adherent cells in seen. (Reproduced from Richter and Wick [30] with permission from the publisher.)

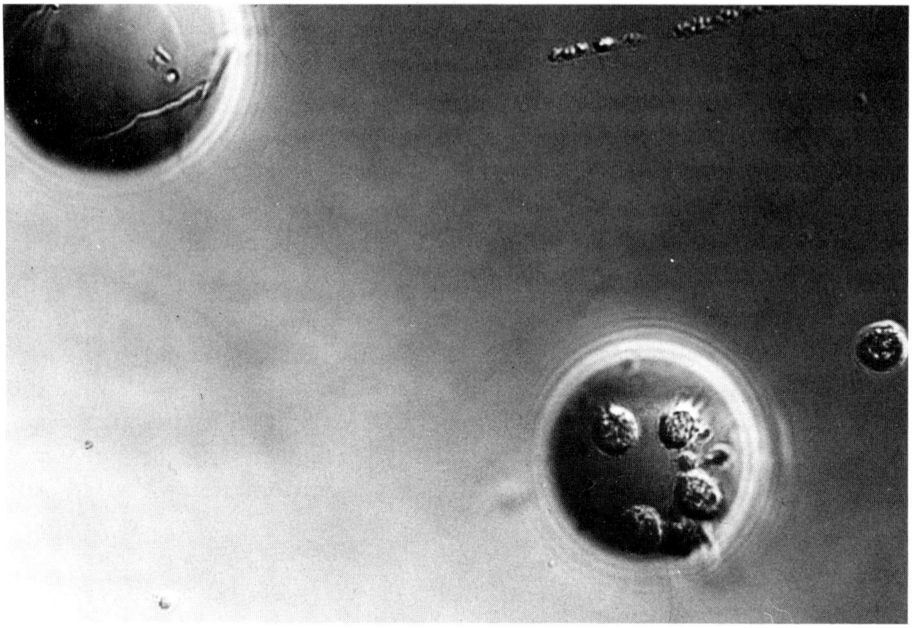

Fig. 5.3. Appearance of FICA tests, monitored under phase contrast. Tg-coated bead forming rosette with lymphocytes specific for Tg. In the left upper corner a BSA-coated control bead is present.

Several requirements had to be fulfilled before acceptance of this method for routine use in experimental and clinical diagnostic work: appropriate beads had to be selected which preferably could be lyophilized; the beads had to be of rather uniform size; the ligands had to be coupled to the surface of the beads in a manner which allowed for an optimal presentation of antigen determinants of lymphoid cell receptors. This latter goal was achieved by selection of an appropriate "spacer" chain, because conventionally coated beads, e.g. via cyanogen bromide (CNBr) activation alone, did not lend themselves to the formation of specific and stable rosettes. It was furthermore desirable to devise a method where activated, spacer-armed, uncoated particles remain stable for long periods of time and always ready for ligand coupling. Finally, antigen-coated beads also should have a long shelf-life.

First we will describe the preparation of spacer-armed antigen-coated beads, including some modifications which have been introduced since the original description of the FICA technique. Also two examples of the application of FICA, viz. the demonstration of thyroglobulin-binding cells (Tg-BC) in an experimental animal model and in human Hashimoto thyroiditis, will be presented and, finally, it will be shown that beads prepared for FICA can also be used for affinity chromatographic enrichment of ABC.

5.2. FICA METHODOLOGY

5.2.1. *Method of bead preparation*

In recent years many different methods have been developed for the isolation and fractionation of cell populations according to their surface properties or receptors using affinity chromatography. This technique is based on the immobilization of the relevant substance, e.g. antigen, to a chromatographic bed material.

A variety of matrices, including polyacrylamide [9], porous glass [2, 34], polyvinyl-alcohol, polysaccharides [25, 28, 44], and other polymers [39], as well as a variety of coupling methods for ligands, such as CNBr [10], carbodiimide [11], oxirane [36], benzoquione [6], divinylsulfone [37], have been reported.

The most widely employed chromatographic support is based on the use of polysaccharide matrices, e.g. Sephadex G-type (Pharmacia, Uppsala, Sweden), a modified dextran obtained by biopolymerization of the glucose residues of sucrose. Due to the degree of cross-linking and thus of swelling properties, it is possible to prepare the gels with different molecular permeability thresholds, which allow for the selection of the best conditions for molecular chromatography [25]. Furthermore, because of its high content of OH groups, this material is also well suited for the preparation of immunoadsorbents [44].

For the affinity chromatographic separation of ABC [30], it is helpful to attach the relevant ligand not directly to the supporting matrix but rather via a spacer chain. The length of the spacer is critical. If it is too long, this may be responsible for unspecific – mostly hydrophilic – interactions and decreases the selectivity of the separation [23]. Too short a spacer is ineffective due to the possible steric interference between the matrix and material binding to the ligand and because of the experience that small ligands, e.g. substrates for enzymes or haptens, should be at a distance of at least 15–25 Å from the matrix backbone to be fully accessible.

The decision as to which immobilization method is best suited for a particular ligand may be based on the operational conditions, such as temperature, pH, contact time, and the performance of chromatography by columns or the batch method. FICA was originally developed for studies on the effector mechanisms of spontaneous, hereditary autoimmune thyroiditis in an animal model for human Hashimoto thyroiditis, the Obese strain (OS) of chickens. For the demonstration of active and passive Tg-BC in OS chickens, it is possible to use red blood cells from Normal White Leghorn (NWL) chickens as indicator [32]. The coating of these cells with the appropriate antigen, in this case Tg, can best be done with the chromium chloride method [19], and the so prepared cells can be stored for maximally one week at 4°C. Proper specificity and efficiency of antigen coating must be verified using reference sera in passive hemagglutination.

For the investigation of ABC in patients with Hashimoto thyroiditis and other autoimmune diseases, normal human red blood cells (blood group O), which are usually selected for low background values, were not optimally suited because of their tendency to aggregate and to lyse during the coating procedure with chromium chloride ($CrCl_3$). In order to replace these indicator cells by a stable and reproducible antigen-presenting system, Sephadex G-25 superfine, with a dry bead diameter of 10–40 μm and a relative density of 1.12 g/ml, was originally selected for its size characteristics and the convenience of chemical activation and ligand coupling. To get uniformly sized particles the beads were first swollen either in distilled water for 3 h at room temperature or by boiling for 1 h, and could then be fractionated by consecutive passage through 50 and 28 μm mesh steel sieves. Other methods, such as density centrifugation or viscosity-dependent procedures, were found to be less successful. The resulting preparation of beads, with a mean diameter of 26 ± 7 μm, was quite useful for the FICA method, but had the disadvantage of rather small yields. Now beads with a uniform diameter are commonly available, such as latex particles with different calibrated sizes (e.g. polymeres from Rhône-Poulenc, Paris, France).

5.2.2. Activation of beads

The introduction of CNBr for activation of beads of a polysaccharide nature [3, 27], as well as the modification of polyacrylamide gels via azide formation [15], initiated the rapid development of biospecific chromatography. CNBr reacts with the hydrophilic support in the following way [26]:

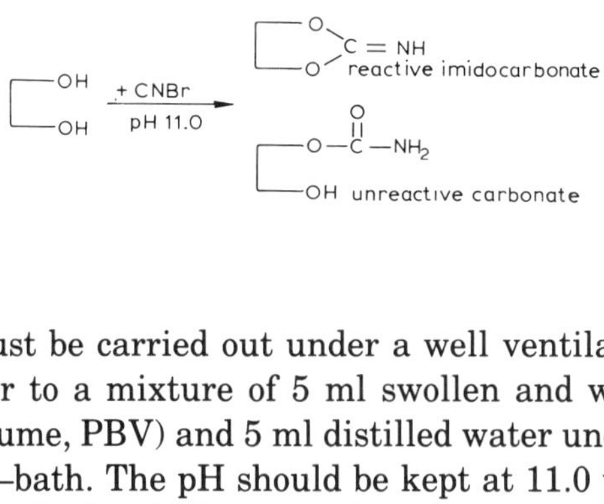

This reaction must be carried out under a well ventilated fume cupboard by adding 1 g CNBr to a mixture of 5 ml swollen and washed Sephadex G-25 (packed bead volume, PBV) and 5 ml distilled water under gentle stirring and cooling in an ice–bath. The pH should be kept at 11.0 with 3 N NaOH. After 8–12 min the beads should be washed under suction on a Büchner funnel (coarse disc No. 3) five times with ice-cold distilled water in order to remove excess CNBr. The spacer is then attached onto the CNBr-activated beads.

5.2.3. Spacer

Step 1. Preparation of 3,3′-diaminodipropylamine-Sephadex. The first part of the spacer 3,3′-diaminodipropylamine is coupled to the CNBr-activated beads by the following reaction:

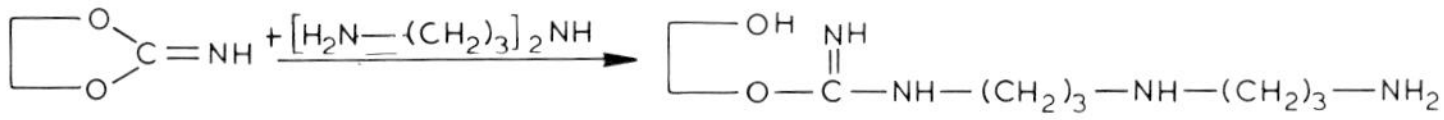

isourea derivative

isourea derivative
An aqueous 2 mM solution of the diamine is brought to pH 10 to obtain the amino groups in the reactive unprotonated state and for each ml of PBV 1 ml of this material is added. After vertical rotation for 16 h at 4°C and extensive washing with ice-cold distilled water this material, i.e. the ω-aminoalkyl-Sephadex, is then ready for further elongation of the spacer chain.

Step 2. Preparation of the carboxylic terminal derivative. One ml of succinic anhydride is then added per ml of PBV in an equal volume of distilled water at 4°C.

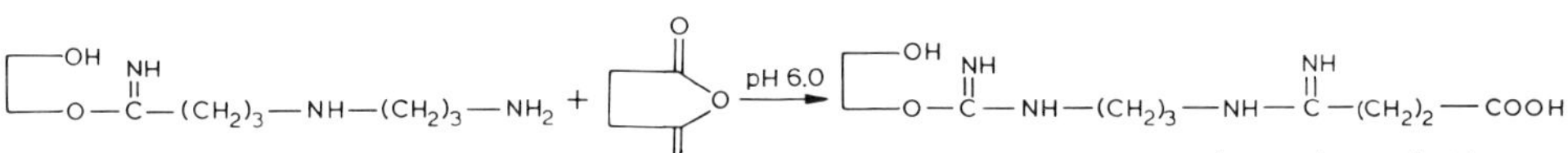

carboxylic terminal derivative

The pH must be adjusted to, and maintained at, 6.0 with 5 N NaOH. When no further change in pH occurs the incubation is continued without rotation for 5 h at 4°C. As can be shown by means of color reaction with sodium trinitrobenzenesulfate (Merck, Darmstadt, F.R.G.), the amino groups react quantitatively with the anhydride. In the presence of a water-soluble carbodiimide, e.g. 1-ethyl-3-(3-diamino-propyl)-carbodiimide (Fluka, Buchs, Switzerland), these Sephadex beads carrying carboxyl groups could be coupled to primary amino group-bearing compounds at pH 5.0.

Step 3. Preparation of the *N*-hydroxylsuccinimide ester:

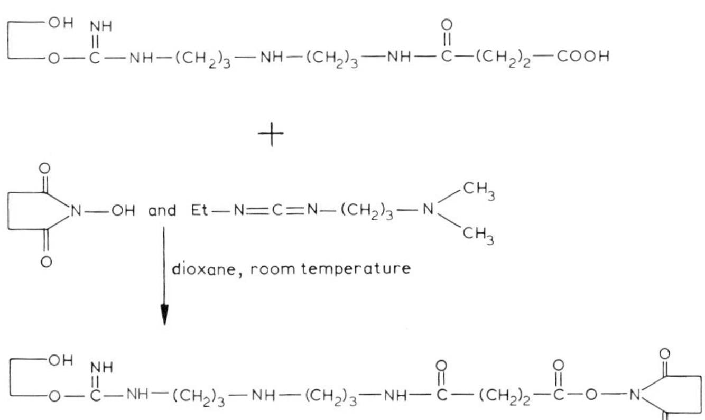

activated ester

The carboxylic terminal-Sephadex is next washed five times with 0.1 N NaOH, distilled water and finally dehydrated by washing with water-free dioxane (Merck, Darmstadt, F.R.G.). Solid *N*-hydroxysuccinimide (0.1 M) (Merck, Darmstadt) is added to the bead/dioxane suspension (1/2, v/v) followed by addition of 0.1 M *N*-ethyl-*N*-(3-dimethylaminopropyl)carbodiimide (Fluka, Buchs, Switzerland). The mixture is gently stirred for at least 1 h after consecutive washings with 5 PBV of dioxane, 5 PBV of 95% methanol and again with 5 PBV of dioxane; the beads can be stored in highly purified and sodium-dried dioxane for longer than one year in an air-tight protected bottle. To keep the beads water-free, it is of advantage to add a molecular sieve, 4 Å (Merck, Darmstadt, 5708 Perlform). The so prepared spacer-armed, activated beads can be used immediately without additional manipulation for the coupling of proteins or any other ligand-containing primary amino groups. As soon as the activated beads come into contact with aqueous solutions of such ligands, avid attachment will take place.

5.2.4. Coating with ligands

In the case of Tg and bovine serum albumin (BSA) optimal coupling was found to occur upon addition of 4 mg protein in physiological saline to each ml of activated packed beads at 4°C overnight with vertical rotation. The activated beads could be transferred directly with a wide bore pipette into the aqueous protein solution. We used antigen preparations such as BSA (Behring Werke AG, Marburg, F.R.G.), chicken Tg (Ch-Tg) purified from a saline-thyroid extract by chromatography on concanavalin A-Sepharose and human Tg (h-Tg) prepared by ammonium sulfate precipitation combined with molecular sieve chromatography on Sephadex G-200.

5.2.5. Deactivation of the ligand-coupled product

Proper deactivation and thus blocking of remaining free sites of antigen-coated beads is an important step for the final outcome of FICA tests. Despite the relative ease of ligand binding to activated sites, not all available binding sites for spacer arms are occupied. In the case of large molecular substances being fixed to the matrix the density of excess reactive groups is particularly important. For the present purpose the routinely used compounds, glycine and ethanolamine, were found to be insufficient, when used alone. However, a preincubation with an appropriate (non-cross-reacting "nonsense") normal serum or purified protein before the deactivation procedure eliminates this problem. If this co-coupling is performed with a fluorochrome-labelled protein, simultaneous staining of the beads can be obtained by this procedure. For this purpose rabbit γ-globulin for work in the above-mentioned avian system, and chicken γ-globulin for study in the mammalian system can be labelled with FITC or TRITC. To 0.5% solutions of these conjugates in 5 ml PBS unlabelled rabbit or chicken γ-globulin is added to a final concentration of 4%. In experiments with only two different antigen-coated bead preparations, one is labelled with the FITC conjugate and the other left unstained. In the case of three antigens, the additional type of beads is labelled with the TRITC-conjugate. Possible active sites remaining after the coupling procedure are deactivated with the 4% rabbit or chicken γ-globulin solution (5 ml/ml PBV) under vertical rotation at 4°C for 8 h. The final deactivation is done conventionally by means of 1 M glycine, ethanolamine (1 ml/ml PBV), or mercaptans when introduction of additional nitrogen is to be avoided. More recently it has been found to be of advantage to store antigen-coated beads in a buffer (phosphate-buffered saline; PBS) containing 0.5% of the antigens to maintain a sufficient degree of coupling over long periods (months) of time.

5.2.6. Performance of tests

5.2.6.1. Test for specificity of coating

The specificity tests are done by direct immunofluorescence (DIF) or indirect immunofluorescence (IIF) at room temperature using the semi-automated membrane fluorescence micro-method [35] and following the recommendations of Capel and Aalberse [7] (Fig. 5.4). This procedure is based on the commercially available Microtiter^{TM} equipment and further details of this method may be found in chapter 4 of this volume. For the IIF specificity

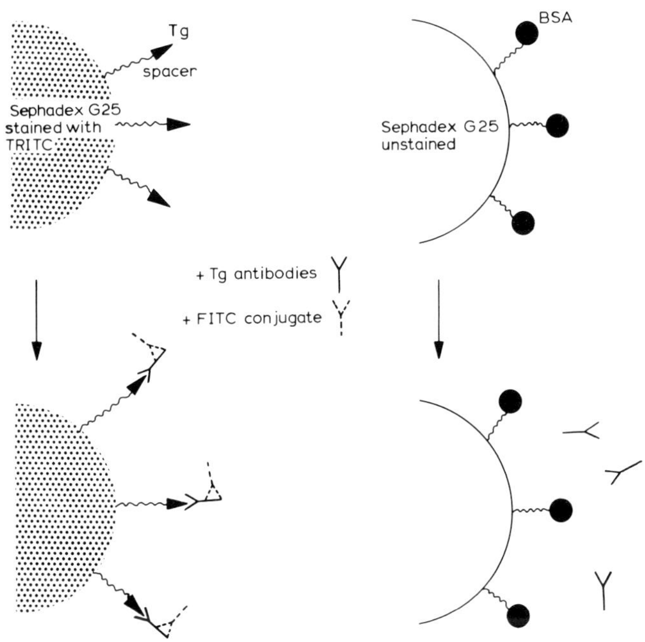

Fig. 5.4. Specificity control for antigen-coated beads. Specificity of antigen coating is checked on beads either labelled with TRITC and coated with Tg or unlabelled and coated with BSA. In the example shown the FITC conjugate binds only to the Tg-coated beads (visualized by means of the two-wavelength method).

tests the following two antisera were used: 1) a rabbit anti-BSA serum showing a titer of 1 : 4096 in passive hemagglutination; 2) an OS serum (OS-139) containing Tg-autoantibodies with a hemagglutination titer of 1 : 2048. In the present example, two FITC-labelled anti-Ig conjugates were used and characterized according to the guidelines of Beutner et al. [5]: a) a goat anti-rabbit IgG (Behringwerke AG, Marburg, F.R.G., Lot. No. 458 F) with a F/P ratio of 3.0, 15 standard precipitation units by chessboard titration; b) a rabbit anti-chicken IgG produced in this laboratory with a F/P ratio of 2.3, eight standard precipitation units, and an optimal working dilution of 1 : 32.

5.2.6.2. Experimental protocol

The experimental protocol for the FICA is as follows. 25 μl of the bead suspension (5% v/v) are delivered to each well of a "V-bottom" microtiter plate (Cooke Engineering Comp., Alexandria, VA); this volume corresponds to 1.2–1.3 × 10^5 beads/well. The plates are then centrifuged at 400 × g (5 min), washed six times with PBS, the final supernatant discarded and 150 μl of the conjugate dilution added to each well. After a further incubation of 2 h at 4°C, followed by six additional washings, the beads are resuspended in 150 μl saline and one drop from each well transferred onto glass slides, e.g. Teflon-coated multiwell Cooke slides (Cooke Engineering Comp.). The preparations are finally mounted in buffered glycerol (glycerol/PBS, 9 : 1; pH 7.2). Observations are made using a fluorescence microscope appropriately equipped for vertical illumination [14].

5.3. DIAGNOSTIC APPLICATION OF FICA

5.3.1. Demonstration of Tg-BC in peripheral blood of OS chickens with hereditary spontaneous autoimmune thyroiditis (SAT)

OS chickens spontaneously develop autoimmune thyroiditis within the first few weeks of life [42, 43]. Based on the data from extensive studies during the last 15 years this strain can be considered as the best model for human Hashimoto thyroiditis which it resembles in all morphologic, serologic and functional aspects [42, 43]. The thyroid glands of OS chickens become severely infiltrated by lymphoid cells, mainly plasma cells, and many germinal centers arise within these infiltrated organs. Circulation of in vivo bound autoantibodies to Tg (Tg-AAb) occur in a high percentage of OS birds [42], while AAb to thyroid microsomal antigens and to non-thyroid antigens are observed in lower frequency [17, 31]. Due to the fact that SAT develops in an avian species, with its clearcut anatomical and functional separation of the B- and T-dependent portions of the immune system, the OS is optimally suited for the study of the role of B and T cells in the natural history of this disease. B cells, or the antibodies produced by these, seem to play a major role among the effector mechanisms leading to infiltration and finally to complete destruction of the thyroid glands. Thus, neonatal or in ovo bursectomy leads to a significant decrease of the frequency and severity of SAT and of the occurrence of circulating Tg-AAb [40]. On the other hand, neonatal thymectomy entails the development of more severe SAT [41]. The number of B cells is significantly higher in the periphery of OS as compared to normal control chickens [1]. Conventional rosette tests using chicken RBC coated with normal chicken Tg by the tannic acid procedure revealed an increase of Tg-BC in the peripheral blood and spleen of OS chickens with peak values well before maximum degree of SAT and circulation of Tg-AAb titers were usually obtained [29]. Carefully controlled inhibition experiments showed that Tg-BC consisted of two major populations: B cells actively synthesizing their own Tg receptors ("active" rosette-forming cells, RFC) and T cells with passively acquired receptors ("passive" RFC) [29, 31]. In both cases the presence of active Tg-BC may be a prerequisite for the later development of SAT and perhaps even constitute precursors of a population of effector cells [32].

It was against this background that FICA with chicken Tg-coated Sephadex G-25 beads was used as a simple tool for the enumeration and possible later enrichment of Tg-BC from the peripheral blood of OS chickens. Table 5.I gives a comparison of data obtained with conventional rosette tests and the FICA method analysing suspensions of peripheral blood lymphocytes from untreated NWL, BSA-immunized NWL and OS birds with SAT [30]. While chicken RBC or beads with control antigens give only background values both in the conventional rosette assay and in FICA, significant numbers of ABC could be detected in the homologous systems. The FICA affords considerably more ABC (note that the number of RFC are given per 10^4 peripheral blood lymphocytes, while FICA-positive cells relate to 10^3 lymphoid cells), but also shows higher background levels as compared to the rosette test.

TABLE 5.I

COMPARISON OF ROSETTE TESTS WITH FICA TEST

Groups of chickens (n = 4)	Mean number of RFC/10^4 PBL		Mean number of FICA-positive cells/ 10^3 PBL		Serum titers in passive hemagglutination ($\log_2$)	
	Tg	BSA	Tg	BSA	Tg	BSA
NWL non-immune	2.5	2.5	7.0	8.8	<1	<1
NWL–BSA	3.5	39.0	8.3	27.2	<1	11
OS	16.0	3.0	16.0	6.0	6.0	<1

RFC/10^4 PBL, No. of lymphocytes forming rosettes with antigen-coated RBC/10^4 peripheral blood lymphocytes.
FICA/10^3 PBL, No. of lymphocytes adhering to antigen-coated beads/10^3 peripheral blood lymphocytes. NWL, Normal White Leghorn chickens; OS; Obese strain chickens. (Data from Richter and Wick [30].)

TABLE 5.II

THYROID SEROLOGY AND ANTIGEN-BINDING CELLS IN HASHIMOTO PATIENTS
(Data from Richter et al. [33].)

Patients	n	Sex (F/M)	Mean age (range)	Serology					Antigen-binding cells (FICA)/10^3 PBL[e]	
				Tg-AAb		IIF	Microsome-AAb			
				Passive HA[a]	IIF(CA_1)[b]	CA_2[c]	Passive HA[a]	IIF[d]	Tg	BSA
Hashimoto thyroiditis	24	22/2	57 (35–78)	17/24	17/24	2/24	18/24	13/24	25.2 ± 7.8	5.0 ± 1.4
Non-Hashimoto, non-Graves disease goiter	12	9/3	45 (19–64)	1/12	ND[f]	ND	0/12	ND	6.6 ± 4.9[g]	4.2 ± 1.3
Normal + other controls	10	8/2	32 (21–45)	0/10	ND	ND	0/10	ND	3.9 ± 1.7[h]	3.8 ± 1.5

[a] Titer 20 in tanned cell hemagglutination test.
[b] Titer 10 in IIF on methanol-fixed, frozen sections of a human colloid goiter.
[c] Same as in b; sera absorbed with human thyroglobulin.
[d] Titer 10 in IIF on unfixed, frozen sections of human thyrotoxic goiter.
[e] Mean No. of lymphocytes/10^3 PBL adhering to antigen-coated beads; only two or more cells adhering to a single bead counted as positive.
[f] Not done.
[g] Statistically significant difference to Hashimoto group ($P<0.005$).
[h] Statistically significant difference to Hashimoto group ($P<0.001$).

No correlation exists between the titer of circulating antibodies and the total number of ABC. This fact will be also demonstrated in the human example cited below.

5.3.2. Demonstration and characterization of Tg-BC in the peripheral blood of Hashimoto thyroiditis patients

This section will serve to demonstrate a) the applicability of the FICA method to a human system in general, b) the enumeration of Tg-BC in the peripheral blood of patients with Hashimoto thyroiditis, c) the possible significance of Tg-BC for the diagnosis of Hashimoto thyroiditis, and d) the possibility to further characterize Tg-BC by means of a combination of FICA with other serological techniques [48]. To this goal the number of Tg-BC in individual Hashimoto patients was compared to the serological findings and, where possible, the cytology of needle biopsy material; groups of non-Hashimoto, non-Graves disease goiter patients and age- and sex-matched healthy individuals served as controls. For these experiments FITC-labelled Tg-coated and unlabelled BSA-coated beads were employed. The overall picture in the three groups with respect to conventional thyroid AAb serology and Tg-BC is given in Table 5.II. Seven of the Hashimoto patients were serologically negative and only one patient of the non-Hashimoto, non-Graves disease goiter group showed Tg-AAb in a titer of 1 : 40. It is evident that elevated numbers of Tg-BC were only found in the Hashimoto group. Interestingly, all 24 patients in this group displayed this phenomenon irrespective of their serological data. As a matter of fact two patients who were originally classified in the second group had elevated numbers of Tg-BC and negative serology. A fine needle biopsy finally confirmed the diagnosis "Hashimoto thyroiditis". It seems, therefore, that the demonstration of Tg-BC is a better diagnostic parameter for Hashimoto disease than Tg-AAb determination alone. Specificity controls were done by preincubation of Hashimoto patients' peripheral blood lymphocytes with Tg or rabbit IgG and subsequent performance of FICA. Table 5.III exemplifies some of these data. Table 5.IV gives the results of six selected patients which emphasize the lack of correlation between the occurrence and titer of AAb to Tg, the second colloid antigen (CA_2) or thyroid microsomal antigens and the number of Tg-BC found in FICA assays. In a more detailed discussion of these data, we also demonstrated that lymphoid cells which passively absorbed their receptors are included in the total number of Tg-BC, but make up only a minor portion of these.

5.4. ATTEMPTS TO ENRICH ABC BY AFFINITY CHROMATOGRAPHY

Some methods for enrichment or depletion of mammalian B and T cells are well established [22]. In contrast to the work with relatively abundant cell

TABLE 5.III

INHIBITION OF ANTIGEN-BINDING CELLS IN FICA
(Data from Richter et al. [33].)

Preincubation [a] of lymphocytes	PBS		2% Tg		2% Rabbit γ-globulin		2% Tg + 2% rabbit γ-globulin	
Antigen coating	Tg	BSA	Tg	BSA	Tg	BSA	Tg	BSA
No. antigen-binding cells/10^3 PBL								
Expt.1	26	8	8	9	20	4	ND[b]	ND
Expt.2	30	7	8	7	23	3	4	2

[a] 45 min at room temperature followed by addition of antigen-coated beads.
[b] Not done.

populations (e.g. total B or T cells) less data are available for separation of such small subpopulations as ABC. We compared the usefulness of several enrichment techniques of ABC in the chicken system using BSA as a model antigen. It is shown that affinity chromatography with BSA-coated polyacrylamide beads proved to be the method of choice for this purpose, while FICA beads are less useful due to the firm adhesion of ABC to this material.

5.4.1. Animals, immunization procedure, and cell harvesting

Normal White Leghorn chickens from a local breeder were used throughout. The birds were immunized intravenously by an injection of 4 mg BSA in 2 ml PBS, pH 7.2, and boosted weekly in the same manner until sacrifice. Citrated blood (3.8% sodium citrate, 1 : 10 v/v) was obtained by heart bleeding and the buffy coat lymphocytes were isolated by centrifugation (7 min, 400 × *g*). After two washings of the cells with PBS, adherent cells were removed by passing the suspension through a nylon wool column (Leukopak Leukocyte Filter, Fenwal Labs., Deerfield, IL) for 60 s, a procedure previously shown to avoid the concomitant retention of B cells. The so treated peripheral blood lymphocytes (PBL) were pooled with spleen cells from the same animal for further analysis. Splenic lymphocytes were prepared by mincing spleen fragments on ice and consecutively passing them through 80 – 200 mesh stainless steel sieves followed by a 60 s passage through a nylon wool column. The combined lymphocyte suspension was adjusted to a concentration of 1–4 × 10^8 cells/ml. For use in affinity chromatography the medium was supplemented with 5% heat-inactivated (30 min, 56°C), ultracentrifuged (56,000 × *g*, 90 min) normal chicken serum (NCS) absorbed with pooled chicken RBC (1/5, v/v).

TABLE 5.IV

TYHROID SEROLOGY AND Tg-BINDING IN HASHIMOTO PATIENTS/SELECTED REACTION PATTERNS
(Data from Richter et al. [33].)

Patients	Age	Sex	Serology					Antigen-binding PBL/10^3 [e]	
			Tg-AAb			Microsome-AAb			
			Passive HA[a]	IIF (CA_1)[b]	IIF-CA_2[c]	Passive HA[a]	IIF[d]	Tg	BSA
W.M.	65	F	250,000	80	10	20,480	20	18	6
F.A.	69	F	40,960	40	10	40,960	10	31	3
C.R.[f]	50	F	40	40	10	320	10	20	5
P.A.	60	F	250,000	80	10	80,000	40	22	5
S.M.[f]	63	F	20	20	10	10	10	39	4
K.J.	65	F	20	10	10	20,480	40	28	7

[a] Titer in tanned cell hemagglutination tests.
[b] Titer in IIF on methanol-fixed, frozen sections of a human colloid goiter.
[c] Same as b; sera absorbed with thyroglobulin.
[d] Titer in IIF on unfixed, frozen sections of human thyrotoxic goiter.
[e] No. of lymphocytes adhering to beads/10^3 PBL.
[f] Needle biopsy.

5.4.2. Enrichment techniques

Three essential methods were used, based on the following principles.

1. Separation of rosetting and non-rosetting cells by density centrifugation [16].

2. Adherence to chemically modified ligands. ABC adhere to antigen covalently bound to gelatine [12] or non-covalently attached to plastic surfaces like polystyrene, polyphenyl or cellulose nitrate [8, 13].

3. Column affinity chromatography where antigen is chemically bound, e.g. to a cross-linked polysaccharide bead matrix [45].

Affinity chromatography was studied most extensively in the course of these experiments and seems to be the method of choice for obtaining a high yield of ABC [48]. Pilot studies showed satisfactory flow properties of all the columns tested when 2×10^8 lymphocytes were applied in 1 ml aliquots. All experiments were performed at 22°C because no temperature dependence for the degree of enrichment was found in preliminary investigations. The effluent, however, was collected on ice. To keep cells viable it proved to be necessary to add 5% NCS (inactivated at 56°C for 30 min, ultracentrifuged at $56{,}000 \times g$ for 90 min, absorbed 1/5, v/v, with pooled chicken RBC) to the medium.

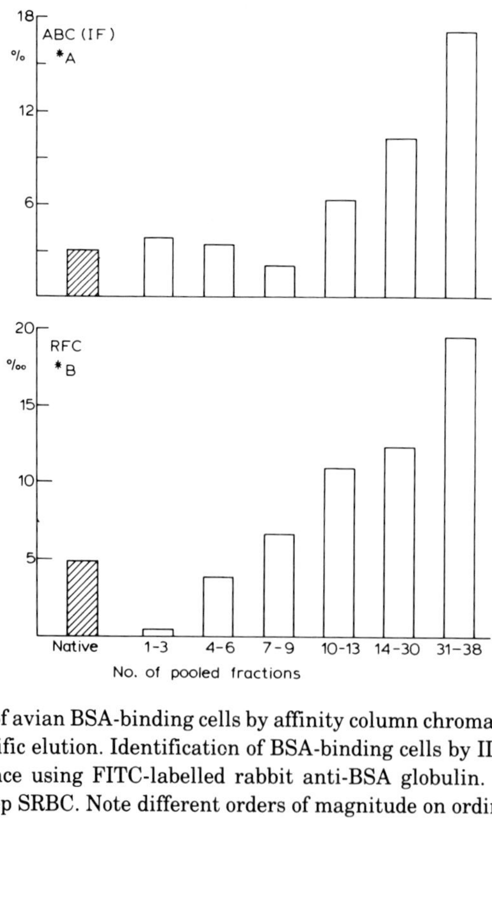

Fig. 5.5. Enrichment of avian BSA-binding cells by affinity column chromatography on Sepharose 6B beads without specific elution. Identification of BSA-binding cells by IIF or rosette formation. *A) Immunofluorescence using FITC-labelled rabbit anti-BSA globulin. *B) Rosette formation using BSA-coated sheep SRBC. Note different orders of magnitude on ordinate scales. (Data from Wolf et al. [48].)

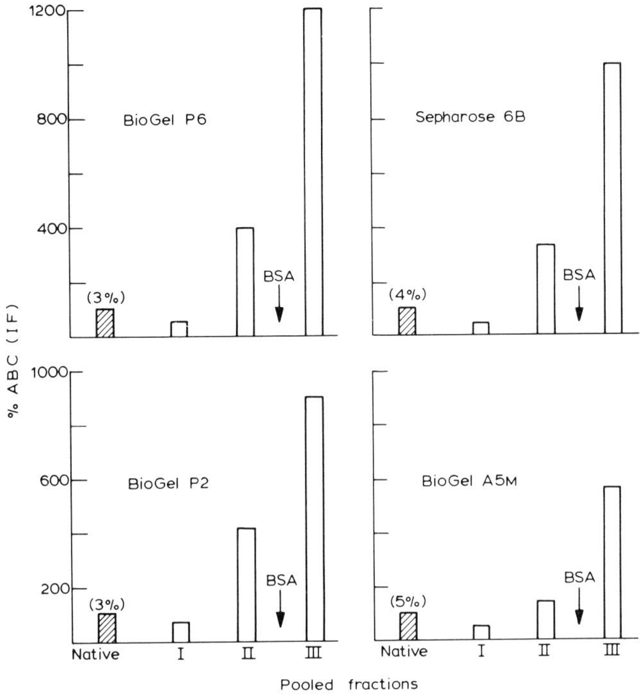

Fig. 5.6 Comparison of different affinity chromatography matrices for the enrichment of avian antigen-binding cells, detected using IIF. Antigen: BSA. Conjugate. rabbit anti-BSA globulin, FITC-labelled. Fraction I: early effluent. Fraction II: late effluent. Fraction III: BSA-eleuted cells. (Data from Wolf et al. [48].)

Chromatography with Sepharose 6B resulted in a delay rather than a stable binding of ABC, as there was about a fivefold enrichment in the last fraction without specific elution (Fig. 5.5). As shown in this diagram indirect immunofluorescence proved to be about 10 times more sensitive than rosette formation. The specificity of this delay was demonstrated by the failure to enrich BSA–ABC using a control column coated with an unrelated antigen (human Ig). Furthermore, lymphocytes sensitized against chicken Tg were not enriched by passage over BSA columns. The degree of enrichment, as detected by indirect immunofluorescence, could be further improved by specific elution with 0.5% BSA followed by mechanical agitation.

Comparing the different column matrices (see Fig. 5.6) Bio-Gel P6 constantly gave the best result. The reason for these differences seems to be the uniformly covalent binding of antigen to polyacrylamide beads but not to agarose. Hemagglutinating inhibition assays of the column effluent fluid before specific elution showed that the passage of lymphoid cells results in a release of antigen from agarose but not from polyacrylamide beads (Table 5.V). This was true even though relatively low (4 mg/ml) BSA concentrations, just sufficient for complete saturation of activated beads, were used. In the last series of experiments BSA was bound to Sephadex G-25 via the spacer

TABLE 5.V

HAEMAGGLUTINATION INHIBITION (HAI) TESTS
(Data from Wolf et al. [48].)

BSA column [a]	Log$_2$ titer of standard rabbit anti-BSA serum diluted in [b]				
	PBS	PBS + 5% NCS	Fraction 2	Fraction 8	BSA 0.5%
Polyacrylamide (Bio-Gel P6)	9	9	9	9	1
Agarose (Sepharose 6B)	9	9	5	7	1

[a] Column volume: 2.5 cm^3 in 9 mm diameter column.
[b] Column washed in PBS, equilibrated in PBS + 5% NCS. 2–3 $\times$ 10^8 cells in 1 ml applied. Collection in 8 ml fractions effluent buffer harvested at each step of procedure and tested in HAI.

described for the FICA method. This procedure makes the antigen better attainable for lymphocyte receptors and, therefore, a more stable binding is achieved. However, elution of adherent cells by the conventional method (antigen + mechanical agitation) was unsuccessful. Attempts using different ionic strength salt solution (0.2–2.0 M NaCl), low pH buffers (pH 6.0–3.0), Tween 20 (0.1%), distilled water, or 5 mM EDTA amounted to a threefold maximum degree of enrichment only.

In summary, it is shown that in a direct comparison between the methods using spacer-armed Sephadex G-25 and EDTA elution or polyacrylamide beads (Bio-Gel P6) with specific elution, the latter enrichment procedure is still superior. Variation of the spacer length in the FICA technique, however, may even render the FICA technique equally suitable for the enrichment of ABC. Furthermore, these findings, although unrewarding for the purification or enrichment of ABC by affinity chromatography with spacer-armed beads, emphasize the usefulness of this method for the preparation of very stable rosettes which are not even disrupted by rather harsh chemical or mechanical treatment.

5.5. CONCLUSIONS

FICA has proven to be a simple and specific method for the determination of ABC. This has been exemplified both in experimental systems and for the clinical diagnosis of human autoimmune thyroiditis by the enumeration of Tg-BC. Tg-BC seem to be specific diagnostic markers for ongoing autoimmune thyroiditis and – at least in our hands – a more reliable criterium for the diagnosis of Hashimoto thyroiditis than conventional thyroid serology. FICA is a versatile method applicable to any protein ligand. Activated, spacer-armed, uncoated beads can be stored for many months without loss of activity and are immediately ready for coupling. Antigen-coated beads are likewise stable for at least one year. Taking advantage of the two-wavelength immunofluorescence techniques three ligands can be tested simultaneously (FITC-stained, TRITC-stained and unstained beads). However, unlimited numbers of ligands can be included in the test, if each assay is performed in a separate tube and read on separate slides using a conventional microscope. Finally the spacer-armed, ligand-coupled beads which are prepared for FICA are also useful for the electron microscope analysis of ABC and the enrichment or depletion of such cells in column affinity chromatography.

ACKNOWLEDGEMENTS

This work was supported by the Austrian Research Council (project Nos. 1997 and 3120).

REFERENCES

1 Albini, B. and Wick, G. (1974) Proportional increase of bursa cells in chickens of the Obese strain. Nature (London) *249,* 653–654.

2 Arkles, B.T. and Briningar, W.S. (1975) Respiratory properties of rat liver mitochondria immobilized on an alkylsilylated glass surface. J. Biol. Chem. *22,* 8856–8862.

3 Axén, R., Porath, J. and Ernbach, S. (1967) Chemical coupling of peptides and proteins to polysaccharide by means of cyanogen halides. Nature (London) *214,* 1302–1304.

4 Bankhurst, A.D. and Wilson, J.D. (1971) Detection of antigen-binding cells by combined rosette formation and autoradiography. Nature New Biol. *234,* 154–155.

5 Beutner, E.H., Sepulveda, M.R. and Barnett, E.V. (1968) Quantitation studies of immunofluorescent staining. Relationships of characteristics of unadsorbed anti-human IgG conjugates to their specific and nonspecific staining proteins. Bull. W.H.O. *39,* 587–606.

6 Brandt, J., Andersson, L.O. and Porath, J. (1975) Covalent attachment of proteins to polysaccharide carriers by means of benzoquinone. Biochim. Biophys. Acta *386,* 196–202.

7 Capel, P.J.A. and Aalberse, R.C. (1975) A quantitative immunofluorescence method for the determination of IgE antibodies in comparison with the radioallergosorbent test (RAST). J. Immunol. Methods *7,* 77–84.

8 Catt, K.J. and Traeger, G.W. (1967) Solid-phase radioimmunoassay in antibody-coated tubes. Science *158,* 1570–1571.

9 Cuatrecasas, P. (1970) Protein purification by affinity chromatography. J. Biol. Chem. *245,* 3059–3065.

10 Cuatrecasas, P., Wilchek, M. and Anfinsen, C.B. (1968) Selective enzyme purification by affinity chromatography. Proc. Natl. Acad. Sci. U.S.A. *61,* 636–643.

11 Golub, E.S., Mishell, R.J., Weigle, W.O. and Dutton, R.W. (1968) A modification of the hemolytic plaque assay for use with protein antigens. J. Immunol. *100,* 133–137.

12 Haas, W. and Layton, J. (1975) Separation of antigen-specific lymphocytes. J. Exp. Med. *141,* 1004–1014.

13 Herrmann, J.E. and Collins, M.F. (1979) Quantitation of immunoglobulin adsorption to plastics. J. Immunol. Methods *10,* 363–366.

14 Herzog, F., Albini, B. and Wick, G. (1973) Comparison of filters used in immunofluorescent staining procedures with fluorescein isothiocyanate (FITC) conjugates. J. Immunol. Methods *3,* 211–220.

15 Inman, J.K. (1974) Covalent linkage of functional groups, ligands and proteins to polyacrylamide beads. *In* Colowick, S.P. and Kaplan, N.O. (eds.), Methods in Enzymology, *Vol. 34* (Academic Press, New York) pp. 30–58.

16 Jondal, M. (1976) SRBC rosette formation as a human T lymphocyte marker. Scand. J. Immunol. *5,* Suppl. 5, 69.

17 Khoury, E.L., Bottazzo, G.F., Wick, G. and Roitt, I.M. (1979) Humoral autoimmune response in the Obese strain of chickens: organ specific reactivity to thyroid and gastric cellular antigens. *In* Proceedings of the Serono Symposium on Autoimmune Aspects of Endocrine Disorders, Pisa, Italy 1979 (in press).

18 Knapp, W. and Ploem, J.S. (1974) Microfluorometry of antigen–antibody interactions in immunofluorescence using the defined antigen substrate spheres (DASS) system. Sensitivity, specificity and variables of the method. J. Immunol. Methods, 259–273.

19 Kofler, R. and Wick, G. (1977) Some methodological aspects of the chromium chloride method for coupling antigens to erythrocytes. J. Immunol. Methods *16,* 201–209.

20 Modabber, F., Morikawa, S. and Coons, A.H. (1970) Antigen binding cell in normal mouse thymus. Science *170,* 1102–1104.

21 Naor, D. and Sulitzeanu, D. (1969) Binding of ^{125}I-BSA to lymphoid cells of tolerant mice. Int. Arch. Allergy Appl. Immunol. *36,* 112–119.

22 Natvig, J.B., Perlmann, P. and Wigzell, H. (eds.) (1976) Lymphocytes: Isolation, Fractionation and Characterization (Universitetsforlaget, Oslo).

23 O'Carra, P., Barry, S. and Griffin, T. (1974) Interfering and complicating adsorption effects in bioaffinity chromatography. *In* Jakoby, W.B. and Wilchek, M. (eds.), Methods in Enzymology, *Vol. 34* (Academic Press, New York) pp. 108–126.

24 Perrudet-Badoux, A. and Frei, P.C. (1969) On the mechanism of "rosette" formation in human and experimental thyroiditis. Clin. Exp. Immunol. *5,* 117–125.

25 Porath, J. and Flodin, P. (1959) Gel filtration: a method for desalting and group separation. Nature (London) *183,* 1657–1659.

26 Porath, J. and Axén, R. (1976) Immobilization of enzymes to agar, agarose and sephadex supports. *In* Colowick, S.P. and Kaplan, N.O. (eds.), Methods in Enzymology, *Vol. 44* (Academic Press, New York) pp. 19–45.

27 Porath, J., Axén, R. and Ernback, S. (1967) Chemical coupling of proteins to agarose. Nature *215,* 1491–1492.

28 Porath, J., Jonson, J.C. and Lååas, T. (1971) Agar derivatives for chromatography electrophoresis and gel-bound enzymes. Desulphated and reduced cross-linked agar and agarose in spherical bead form.

29 Richter, E. and Wick, G. (1975) Thyroglobulin binding lymphoid cells in Obese strain (OS) chickens. J. Immunol. *114,* 757–761.

30 Richter, E. and Wick, G. (1977) Fluoro-immuno-cytoadherence (FICA): a new method for the identification and enumeration of antigen-binding cells. Z. Immunitaetsforsch. *152,* 351–362.

31 Richter, E., Sundick, R. and Wick, G. (1975) Heteroagglutinins and spontaneous rosette-forming cells in Obese strain (OS) chickens. Z. Immunitaetsforsch. *149,* 61–68.

32 Richter, E., Wick, G. and Schauenstein, K. (1975) The nature of active and passive thyroglobulin binding lymphoid cells in Obese strain (OS) chickens. Eur. J. Immunol. *5,* 554–559.

33 Richter, E., Wick, G., Zambelis, N., Ludwig, H. and Schernthaner, G. (1978) Demonstration of thyroglobulin-binding peripheral blood cells in Hashimoto patients by fluoroimmunocytoadherence. Clin. Immunol. Immunopathol. *11,* 178–189.

34 Robinson, P.J., Dunnhill, P. and Lilly, M.D. (1971) Porous glass as a solid support for immobilization or affinity chromatography of enzymes. Biochim. Biophys. Acta *242,* 659–661.

35 Schauenstein, K., Wick, G. and Kink, H. (1976) The micro-membrane-fluorescence test: a new semiautomated technique based on the microtiter system. J. Immunol. Methods *10,* 143–150.

36 Sundberg, L. and Porath, J. (1974) Preparation of adsorbents for biospecific affinity chromatography. J. Chromatog. *90,* 87–98.

37 Uy, R. and Wolf, F. (1977) 1,4-Butanediol diglycidyl ether coupling of carbohydrates to sepharose. Affinity adsorbents for lectins and glycosidases. Anal. Biochem. *81,* 98–107.
38 Van Dalen, J.P.R., Knapp, W. and Ploem, J.S. (1973) Microfluorometry on antigen–antibody interaction in immunofluorescence using antigen covalently bound to agarose beads. J. Immunol. Methods *2,* 383–392.
39 Vieth, W.R. and Venkatasubramanian, K. (1976) Collagen immobilized enzyme system. Choice of collagen as support matrix. *In* Colowick, S.P. and Kaplan, N.O. (eds.), Methods in Enzymology, *Vol. 47* (Academic Press, New York) pp. 243–263.
40 Wick, G., Kite, J.H., Cole, R.K. and Witebsky, E. (1970) Spontaneous thyroiditis in the Obese strain of chickens. III. The effect of bursectomy on the development of the disease. J. Immunol. *104,* 45–53.
41 Wick, G., Kite, J.H. and Witebsky, E. (1970) Spontaneous thyroiditis in the Obese strain of chickens. IV. The effect of thymectomy and thymo-bursectomy on the development of the disease. J. Immunol. *104,* 54–62.
42 Wick, G., Sundick, R.S. and Albini, B. (1974) Review: the Obese strain (OS) of chickens. An animal model with spontaneous autoimmune thyroiditis. Clin. Immunol. Immunopathol. *3,* 272–300.
43 Wick, G., Boyd, R., Hála, K., De Carvalho, L., Kofler, R., Müller, P.U. and Cole, R.K. (1981) The Obese strain (OS) of chickens with spontaneous autoimmune thyroiditis: review of recent data. Curr. Top. Microbiol. Immunol. *91,* 109–128.
44 Wide, L. and Porath, J. (1966) Radioimmunoassay of proteins with the use of Sephadex-coupled antibodies. Biochim. Biophys. Acta *130,* 257–259.
45 Wigzell, H. and Andersson, B. (1969) Cell separation on antigen-coated columns. Elimination of high rate antibody-forming cells and immunological memory cells. J. Exp. Med. *129,* 23–27.
46 Witebsky, E., Kite, J.H., Wick, G. and Cole, R.K. (1969) Spontaneous thyroiditis in the Obese strain of chickens. I. Demonstration of circulating autoantibodies. J. Immunol. *103,* 708–715.
47 Wolf, H., Gattringer, C. and Wick, G. (1977) Enrichment of avian antigen binding cells (ABC) by affinity chromatography. *In* Hoffman-Ostenhoff, O., Breitenbach, M., Koller, F., Kraft, D. and Scheiner, O. (eds.), Affinity Chromatography (Pergamon Press, New York) pp. 313–316.
48 Wolf, H., Gattringer, C. and Wick, G. (1979) Avian antigen binding cells: enrichment methods. J. Immunol. Methods *25,* 77–88.

Wick et al. (eds) Immunofluorescence Technology. Selected Theoretical and Clinical Aspects © *Elsevier Biomedical Press, 1982*

CHAPTER 6

Automated methods in immunofluorescence studies

J.S. PLOEM

Department of Histochemistry and Cytochemistry, University of Leiden, 2333 AL Leiden, The Netherlands

6.1. INTRODUCTION

Automated methods in immunofluorescence microscopy (IFM) are based on fluorescence intensity measurements of cells or cellular components. For fluorescence intensity measurements a variety of instruments have been developed permitting more or less automated measuring procedures of fluorescent objects [14, 20, 21, 26, 27, 31, 32, 35, 51, 57–59]. More recently, microfluorometers have been adapted to inverted fluorescence microscopes [12, 18, 23, 41]. Inverted microscopes (Fig. 6.1) are used if fluorescence has to be measured from stained cells in tissue culture tubes or in immunological test trays.

Scanning microfluorometry has been introduced for the measurement of fluorescence intensities in multiple small spots (e.g. 0.25–0.5 μm) in the microscopic preparation [34, 41]. This method can provide information about the distribution of fluorescence intensities within a cell from which morphological information can be extracted; this information may serve for the recognition of certain cellular structures or organelles. In such scanning microfluorometers stepping stages [52, 63] or vibrating mirrors [30] are used to

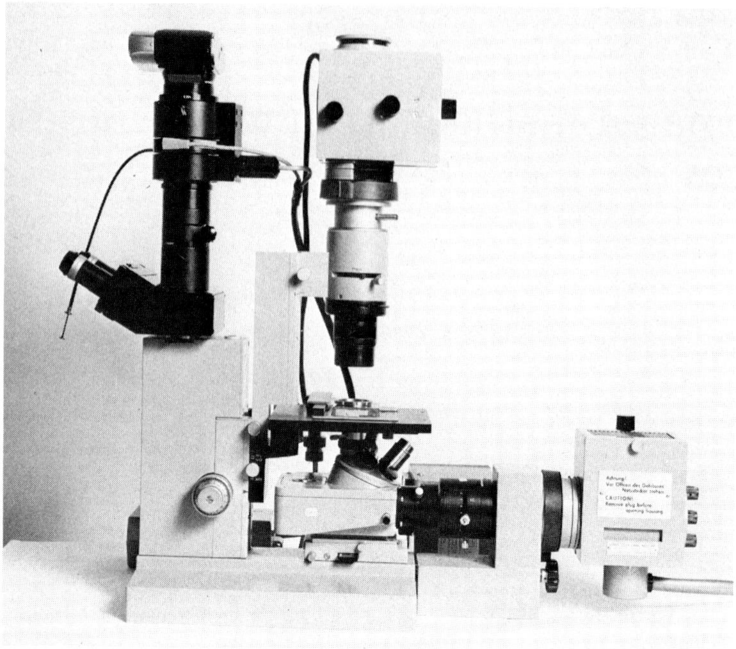

Fig. 6.1. Inverted fluorescence microscope. The vertical illuminator, including exchangeable dichroic mirror sets, is mounted below the stage. A high-pressure mercury light source directs its light into the inverted fluorescence vertical illuminator. Excitation light is then projected onto stained cells grown on the lower cover glass in a tissue culture chamber which can be seen on the microscope stage. Above the microscope stage a mounting for a long-focus phase condenser system and an additional Tungsten light source are positioned. Fluorescent images can be seen through the eyepieces or photographed using a trinocular head.

obtain rapid measurements from a large number of small spots in the specimen. A more recent development is high-speed scanning using TV systems [1, 37, 42]. A conventional plumbicon or vidicon tube can be used for strongly fluorescent stains. Relatively weak fluorescent stains have to be scanned with a TV tube equipped with an image intensifier [55]. Mini- and microcomputers are used to control the operation of high-speed stepping stages or vibrating mirrors and the signal processing. As technical developments have been impressive in the last decade, the performance/price ratio and the speed of mini- and microcomputers have improved considerably. This makes the pattern recognition approach in automated immunofluorescence a much more realistic proposal than a few years ago.

IFM is widely used in many biomedical routine applications, and the intensity of the fluorescence is typically indicated with –, ±, +, ++ and +++. The use of microfluorometry has facilitated the comparison of the results of the immunofluorescence reaction [15, 27, 50, 51]. Quantitative methods are increasingly being used in experimental work, since modern microfluorometers equipped with minicomputers are well suited to perform large numbers of readings [12, 33]. Automated immunofluorescence tests, however, are still in an experimental phase. The main reason for this is that quantitative measurements by automated machines are more dependent on the specificity and the potency of reagents than semi-quantitative observations by laboratory workers. In several applications unwanted fluorescence cannot be avoided and this appears to be an especially difficult problem for automated systems. The human observer seems better able to deal with unwanted fluorescence by using his powerful capacity for pattern recognition. The recently developed possibility to produce monoclonal antibodies through fusion of antibody-producing cells with a plasma cell tumor line is therefore very promising for quantitative IF studies [19]. Schauenstein and Wick [51] conclude that efforts to improve quantitative IFM have to concentrate on a) the quality of immunological reagents, b) the enhancement of sensitivity by the introduction of high energetic illumination devices combined with fast recording equipment on the one hand and the rejection of non-specific background on the other, and c) further automation of the performance and evaluation of the IF test.

In flow cytometry – using strong excitation with a laser light source of IF-stained cells in a fluid stream, with or without fluorescence-activated cell sorting – automation has reached a high degree of perfection. Flow cytometers are described in another chapter of this volume.

This chapter deals with the main microscopic set-ups for automation or semi-automation in quantitative immunofluorescence. To illustrate the possibilities of this instrumentation for routine or research applications, a few examples of quantitative automated fluorescence studies are described.

6.2. SEMI-AUTOMATED MICROFLUOROMETRY

Microfluorometry is essentially a method for measuring low concentrations of fluorescent reaction products, as linearity between the intensity of emitted fluorescence light and the concentration of the fluorescent reaction product only exists at low local absorbances [44]. Provided that the optical configuration is optimal, a favourable signal to noise ratio can be obtained even at very low concentrations.

To compare fluorescence values from one preparation to another, standards must be used for calibration of the microfluorometer and for evaluation of the specimen staining. Background readings are unsuited as reference values since they are composed of the dark current of the photomultiplier, unwanted excitation light and autofluorescence. Moreover, measurement values from a stained IF reaction product will change in a non-linear way with changes in the voltage supply and electronic amplification. Two types of standards should therefore be used: those intended for calibration of optical and electronic parts of the microscope and those intended to serve as a reference standard for a certain IF-stained specimen.

Fluorescent phosphor crystals and uranyl glass belong to the first type of

						2	2						
			3	9	15	18	18	14	7	2			
		5	18	32	36	38	37	35	28	14	3		
	5	21	35	41	44	46	45	44	40	32	16	2	
2	15	35	42	47	49	49	50	48	46	41	30	10	
5	27	41	48	52	52	52	53	52	48	45	38	21	3
9	32	43	49	52	55	55	55	54	50	46	41	27	5
11	33	45	50	53	55	55	57	54	51	48	43	29	5
8	32	43	49	53	54	54	57	54	50	47	41	26	4
5	25	41	46	50	53	54	52	52	48	46	38	19	2
2	14	36	42	46	48	48	51	50	47	45	41	29	9
	4	20	35	41	44	45	45	53	39	31	14	2	
		4	16	28	34	37	35	33	23	11	3		
			2	5	10	13	13	9	4	2			
						2	2						

Fig. 6.2. Printout by the computer terminal of the measured values obtained with a scanning microfluorometer from a bead homogeneously stained with FITC according to Haaijman and Van Dalen [17]. A step size of 0.5 μm was used.

standard. Standards of microscopical dimensions containing, or stained with, the same fluorochrome as the specimen to be measured can be used as reference values if the amount of fluorochrome in such standards is exactly known. The first examples of such standards were defined as microdroplets of a known diameter [36]. Microcapillaries filled with a defined amount of fluorochrome solution [22, 56] and Sepharose beads (Fig. 6.2) of known dimensions [17] serve the same purpose and are more practical to use. For additional calibration in IF procedures the DASS (defined antigen substrate spheres) system can be used [10, 16].

There are, in addition, other sources of error in microfluorometry which should, if possible, be avoided. These errors are: fading, quenching, re-absorbance of fluorescence light if emission and excitation spectra overlap, and the inner filter effect, e.g. occurring in heavily stained sections when deep layers cannot be reached by the exciting rays because the exciting light has already been absorbed in the superficial layers [5, 44].

For a review of quantitative fluorescence microscopy, the reader is referred to Ploem [38].

6.2.1. Instrumentation

Microscope stands for microfluorometry are best equipped with two types of illumination: substage transmitted and incident illumination. Incident illumination is most suited for fluorescence intensity measurements [46, 47], as the functions of illumination and observation of the specimen are combined in one objective. When exact focussing of the objective is maintained, excitation conditions will be reproducible during movement of the microscopic slide on the microscope stage. As soon as a new part of the specimen is focussed, it is automatically placed in the optimal position for measurement. The more

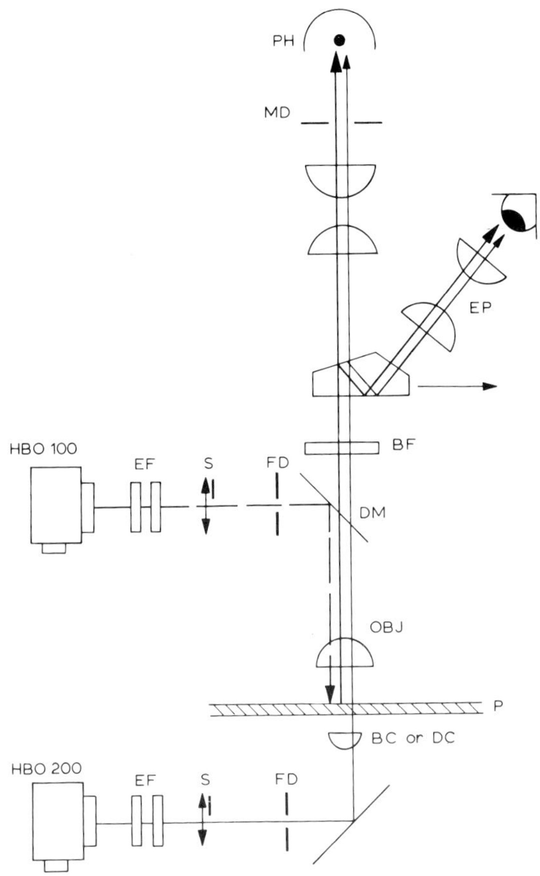

Fig. 6.3. Schematic diagram of a microfluorometer enabling incident illumination, using a vertical illuminator and substage illumination with a bright or dark field condenser. This microscope should be used if objects to be measured cannot be identified without their fluorescence. In that case very weak fluorescence should be excited by means of substage excitation, using very dense filtering with a condenser of low numerical aperture. When the object is localised by using low power eyepieces (e.g. 4×) which enable visualisation of very dimly fluorescing objects, strong incident illumination can be used for measuring the objects. The excitation with a substage condenser should be kept short by employing a shutter(s) in the substage lightpath. Symbols: HBO 100 is a direct-current highly stabilized light source. HBO 200 is a classical mercury high-pressure lamp operated on alternating current. Excitation filters in both incident and transmittent lightpaths are indicated with EF. S, shutter; FD, field diaphragm; BC, bright field condenser; DC, dark field condenser; OBJ, objective; DM, dichroic mirror in vertical illuminator; BF, barrier filter; EP, eyepieces; MD, measuring diaphragm of microfluorometer part; PH, photomultiplier.

laborious alignment of the substage condenser with the alignment of the objective and the requirement for reproducible focussing of the condenser are thus avoided and the condenser can then be used as a second illuminating system to search for fluorescent objects to be measured (Fig. 6.3). Two illumination light paths may also be employed in those applications where a fluorescent and absorbent stain are combined in one specimen or when fluorescent double staining is used [9, 43].

A mercury high pressure lamp can provide substage illumination of very low light intensity, using thick excitation filters and a condenser of low numerical aperture. If low power objectives with high numerical aperture (NA) and eyepieces with low magnification (e.g. 4×) are used in combination with this illumination [40], fluorescent objects can be searched for and centered in a measuring diaphragm. In other words, when very effective fluorescence light collection is used the intensity of the excitation light can be kept relatively low. This low light intensity limits the fading of the objects to be measured. During the search for these objects, the substage field diaphragm is kept fully opened to illuminate the whole field. A HBO 100 mercury high-pressure arc operated on a highly stabilised DC power supply provides the epi-illumination which is concentrated on the specimen by means of a vertical illuminator. The HBO 100 lamp is used for measurement. The field diaphragm of the vertical illuminator is kept only slightly larger than the measuring

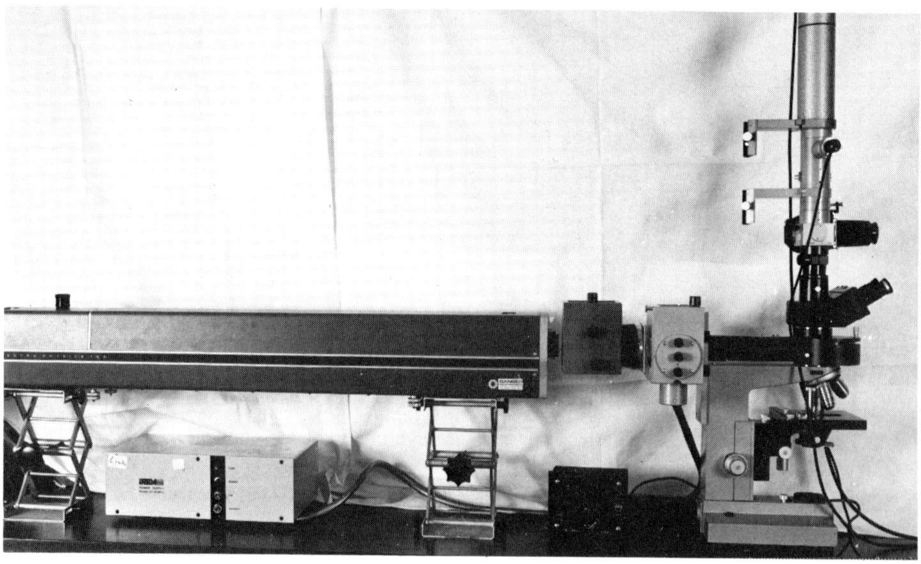

Fig. 6.4. A fluorescence microscope with a vertical illuminator is depicted. The microscope uses two light sources: one is an argon ion laser which can be recognised as the elongated structure behind the microscope. A mercury lamp is attached for auxiliary fluorescence illumination. The microscope is equipped with a measurement device for fluorescence and a photomultiplier (MPV-2, Leitz). For both the laser excitation and the excitation by the mercury lamp incident illumination is used. Care should be taken that the lens coatings are not damaged by the strong laser excitation. A beam extender is often necessary for this purpose.

diaphragm to prevent unnecessary fading of the remaining microscope field by the strong epi-illumination.

Besides high-pressure lamps, lasers are increasingly used to excite fluorescence (Fig. 6.4). The strong blue and green lines of laser light sources have enabled microfluorometry of very weakly fluorescing, small objects [2, 25, 49, 64]. Another advantage of using very short exposure times is that fading is reported to be much less [3, 51].

In modern automated microscopes, the light paths can be alternately switched on and off by means of electronically operated shutters [48]. During the period of searching the substage electronical shutter is open. The measuring operation is started by pressing a button that initiates the electronic circuit. The shutter in the transmitted light path is now closed and the shutter in the incident light path opened for a very short period which can be varied between 0.001 and 1 s. Connection of the microfluorometer microscope to simple signal analysing and recording units such as a digital voltmeter and a papertape device provides automated data output of the measured values. These data can then be fed to a computer for e.g. histogram prints of the recorded fluorescence intensity measurements [43]. In more sophisticated, modern but relatively simple instruments, signal acquisition and data handling are performed with microcomputers [13, 45].

				23		24	45	62	66	53	24						
			39	40				48	81	86	69	72	55	49	35		
		42	26						39	54	69	49	64	58	69	45	
	39	33		26						39	44	50	47	57	69	74	
28	66	29			23					37	39	52	48	55	59	00	26
58	63									25	38	41	48	52	67	71	41
73	42	25								29	41	48	44	55	57	79	39
55	52	41	27							35	48	45	46	45	46	73	55
62	76	51	34	23		24		24	30	39	47	39	54	54	60	80	41
	59	53	53	38	36	38	34	34	32	40	51	48	54	50	62	71	
	52	58	55	35	42	45	37	44	43	52	52	51	50	65	78	62	
	32	58	42	50	42	45	50	51	42	48	67	51	53	65	75	35	
		59	42	49	49	35	41	47	51	63	45	57	61	70	62		
		27	45	42	44	41	42	62	52	55	72	72	69	82	46		
			41	48	51	60	62	70	66	66	60	66	80	60			
					26	49	59	68	83	76	80	64	51				
									27	25							

Fig. 6.5. Computer printout of a human plasma cell stained with FITC-marked immunoglobulin against heavy chains. Each figure presents a measured fluorescence intensity in an area of about 0.5 μm in the cell. It should be noted that the fluorescence in the area of the nucleus is much lower than in the rest of the cell. To obtain an isolation of the cell from its background the lowest threshold for the printout has been set at 23 relative fluorescence units as measured by the microfluorometer scanning microscope. Each spot is measured after movement of the stage in X or Y direction of 0.5 μm, using a stage provided with stepping motors under the control of a computer. These measurements were performed during a visit of Albert Coons to our Leiden laboratory.

6.3. SCANNING MICROFLUOROMETRY

Scanning microfluorometry can contribute to a better interpretation of IF specimens if the objects of interest cannot be sufficiently isolated from the background and centered in the field of a measuring diaphragm for measurement with a conventional microfluorometer. This may occur quite often, as patterns in IF specimens may be complex (Fig. 6.5). By scanning each individual point in a human plasma cell, which has been stained with a FITC-marked antibody against heavy chains, a computer printout can be obtained showing the fluorescence distribution in the cell. The only way to isolate the interesting structures from the background consists of subtraction of uninteresting background regions of the whole microscope field by selecting a threshold in the digitalized image of the entire field that has been stored in the computer. The parts of the image above this threshold then represent the objects to be studied and the areas below the chosen threshold represent the background (Fig. 6.6). The signal to noise ratio in the IF specimen, however, is sometimes not sufficient for a separation of the interesting objects from the background of the specimen. Mathematical treatment of the individual measured points in the specimen with computer programs can be used for enhancement of the image contrast [53].

Scanning techniques are also necessary if a statistical evaluation of the IF reaction product in a large number of microscope fields is required in order to obtain a representative sampling of the entire IF specimen. Furthermore,

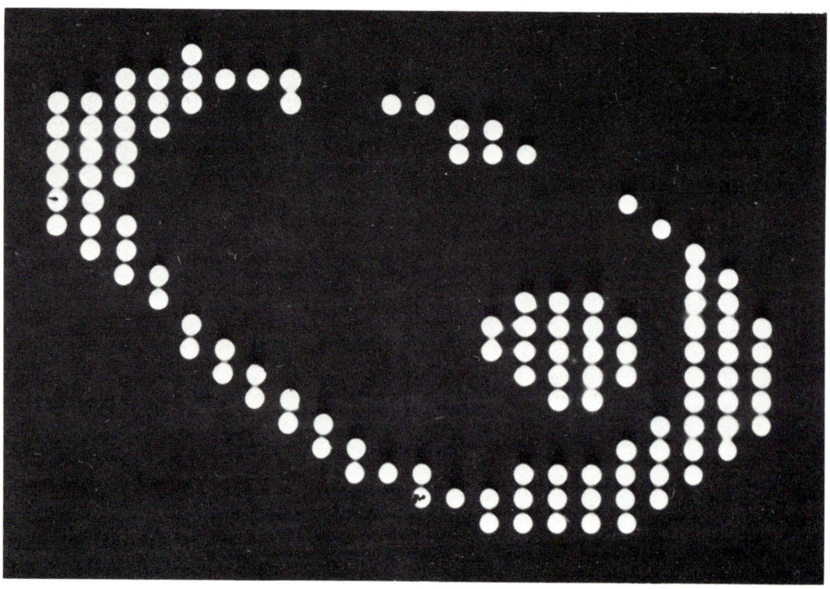

Fig. 6.6. The screen display of a human lymphocyte showing fluorescence of methyl green, used as a staining method for RNA in the cytoplasm and the nucleolus. The shape of the lymphocyte has been distorted by the geographical arrangement of the computer display. All points above a certain threshold are indicated as white points.

scanning fluorometry may contribute to the possibility of measuring moderate differences in the intensity of the IF staining for a better interpretation of the IF test. Scanning microfluorometers can be divided into object-plane scanners, such as stage scanners [34, 54, 63, 65], image-plane scanners, such as vibrating mirror scanners [30], and TV scanners.

Kaufman and his collaborators [24, 25], used an image-plane scanner with an argon-ion laser as an excitation light source. The vibrating mirror performed a two-dimensional raster scan. Subsequently the fluorescence map of the microscope field was stored in the computer memory. By using a series of simple algorithms on these images, it was possible to distinguish IF-stained treponemas from debris. These studies, although not tested in large-scale routine screening programmes, showed that an automated pattern recognition instrument is capable of replacing the human observer in some IF applications. In the meantime, laser and computer technology have improved considerably [39]. Hence it can be expected that much more efficient machines of similar design may presently be constructed.

Schipper et al. [53] used microfluorometric scanning in the quantification of neuronal and extraneuronal fluorescence (Fig. 6.7). The microfluorometric

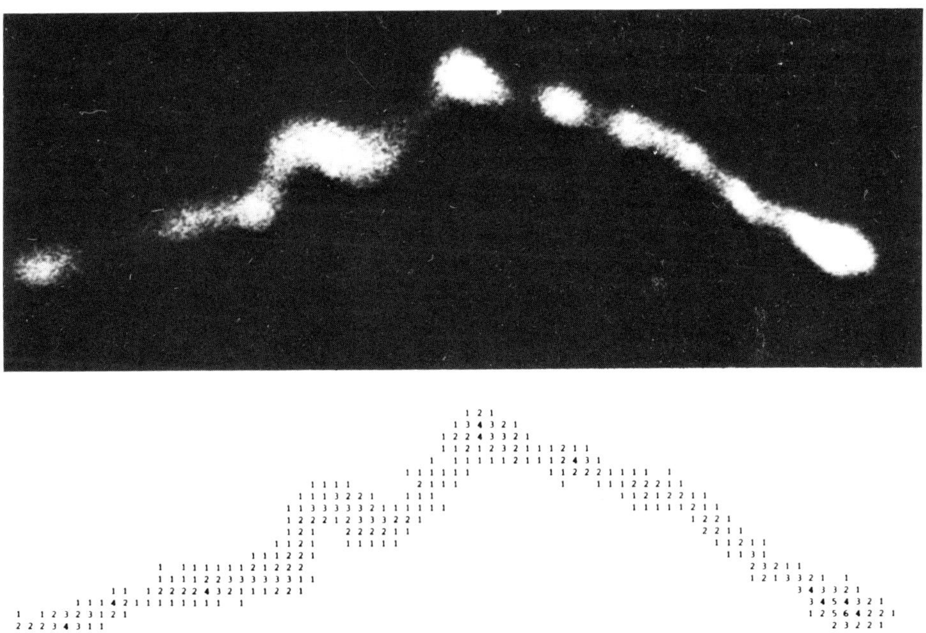

Fig. 6.7. Upper part: the formaldehyde-induced fluorescence (FIF) of an individual axon is photographed in the fluorescence microscope. It can be noted that most of the FIF is distributed in various concentrations (varicosities) along the axon axis. Lower part: the result is shown from the same axon measured with a scanning microfluorometer. Each point represents a 0.5 μm spot in the specimen. Each value represents the relative fluorescence value measured by the computer-operated instrument. In this example it is clearly not feasible to put measuring diaphragms around this type of structures; they are irregular in shape and distribution and must be isolated from the background by computer calculations.

scanning was performed with a microfluorometer (Leitz, MPV II) equipped with a 0.5 μm measuring spot and a 0.5 μm scanning stage, which was controlled by a PDP 12 computer. Mathematical analysis of the histograms of the scan areas (50 × 50 μm) resulted in detailed information on neuronal and extraneuronal fluorescence intensities. Especially in preparations with a poor contrast, scanning methods in combination with mathematical histogram analysis provide better results than microfluorometry alone (Fig. 6.8). Programmes that may be used for controlling the scanning process and the data handling are, e.g., APAMOS (Zeiss) or HIDACSYS [61].

Recently, FITC-marked antibodies have also been made against some neurotransmitter substances. These can be measured by scanning microfluorometry in a similar way.

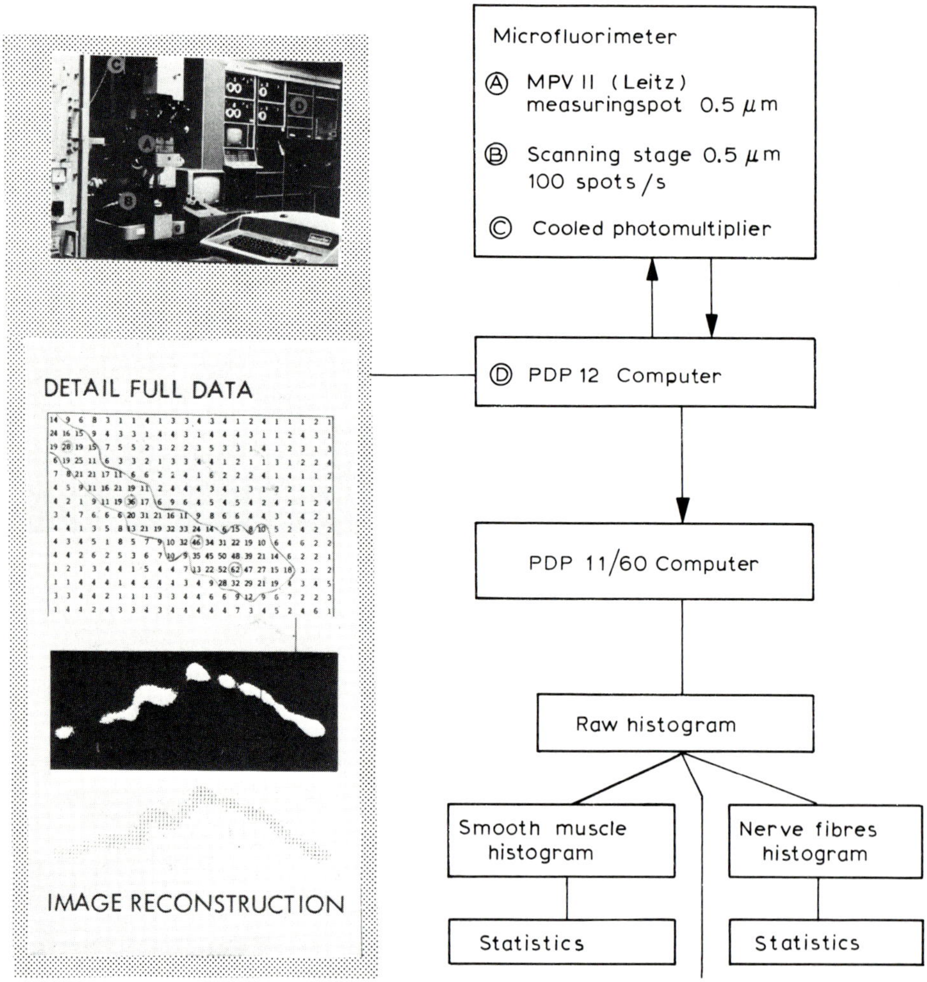

Fig. 6.8. A schematic diagram is made of the method used to obtain image reconstruction of structures which present formaldehyde-induced fluorescence. The diagram is self-explanatory.

6.4. AUTOMATED FLUORESCENCE MEASUREMENTS IN MULTIPLE WELLS OF IMMUNOLOGICAL TEST TRAYS USING SCANNING STAGES

The visual assessment of fluorescence intensities in a large number of wells of immunological test trays proved to be unsatisfactory due to its subjectivity. Therefore, automated measurements using microcomputers have been introduced. The measurement of fluorescence of cells, particles or fluid in wells of immunological microtitration trays is illustrated by the defined antigen substrate spheres system (DASS) and the aperture-defined microvolume method (ADM).

6.4.1. The use of inverted fluorescence microscopes for measuring micro beads as IF models

Capel [7], Knapp and Ploem [28] and Van Dalen et al. [60] introduced a quantitative immunofluorescence model system based on the covalent binding of antigen or antibody to cyanogen bromide (CNBr)-activated agarose beads (DASS system). Capel [8] and Haaijman [16] have done an extensive study on the performance of these beads as standards and their possible applications. The system was originally described for the specificity testing of conjugates [4, 29] but was soon applied to other immunological studies, such as the determination of immunoglobulin levels [8], the demonstration of specific antibodies against e.g. parasite antigens [10, 11], and the determination of circulating antigens [16].

Although the DASS system offers a number of advantages, it has, in contrast to a technique like the enzyme-linked immunosorbent assay (ELISA), the disadvantage that it requires time-consuming fluorometric evaluation of the results if only a standard incident light microfluorometer is used. Haaijman and Wijnants [18] described the use of a semi-automated, inverted fluorescence microscope for the measurement of individual beads sedimented at the bottom of a flat-bottom microtitration tray. In this way the time-consuming transfer of the beads to microscope slides could be avoided. The fluorescence values of 96 samples (five beads per sample were measured) could be determined in 1 h. In a further development it was found possible to perform a large number of measurements of beads sedimented at the bottom of a microtitration tray, using a computer-operated scanning stage mounted on an inverted fluorescence microscope [45].

6.4.2. The aperture-defined microvolume (ADM) method for measuring fluorescence

By applying the principle of the ADM method [12, 41], in which an incident beam of light, focussed by a microscope objective, illuminates a microvolume of fluid in the form of a cone, the measurement of individual beads was no longer necessary. The shape of the cone in the fluid is determined by the aperture and the focal length of the microscope objective used.

The ADM principle was applied originally to the instrumental calibration of microfluorometers, using a uranyl glass to measure the fluorescence excited by an incident light beam through an objective oiled to the uranyl glass in an epi-illumination system [22, 36]. The fluorescence emitted from the illuminated cone of the uranyl glass inside the uranyl glass is measured. The maximum reading is obtained with the objective just touching the glass.

It was found that the fluorescence readings in solid or fluid volumes are relatively independent of the position of the focal plane of the objective, provided that the focal plane falls within the measured sample. Deelder et al. [12] proved that measurements in bead volumes of 8 μl or more in Terasaki-type microtitration plates were independent of the volume of fluid in the wells and of small variations in the position of the objective. At present the read-out of bead volumes in microtitration or Terasaki-type microtitration trays can be performed automatically, since several manufacturers have introduced microscope scanning stages that can hold Terasaki and microtitration trays of normal size (Leitz, Märzhäuser, Zeiss) (Fig. 6.9).

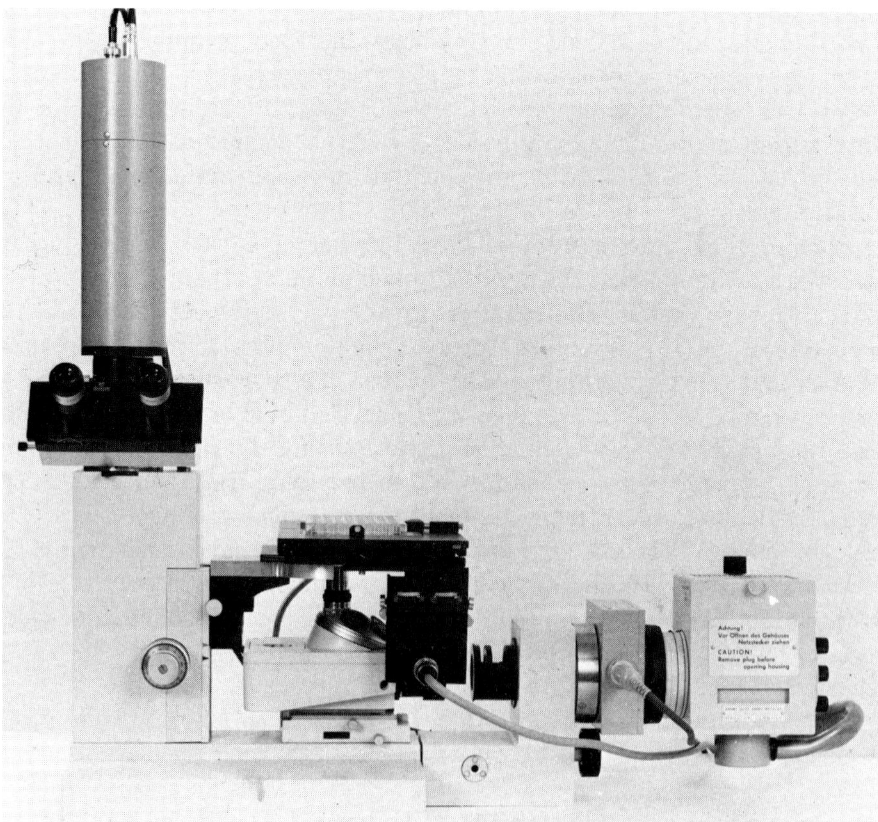

Fig. 6.9. A microfluorometer used for the microtiter scanning system consisting of an inverted microscope (Diavert, Leitz), a photomultiplier and a computer-controlled scanning stage (Märzhäuser, West-Germany).

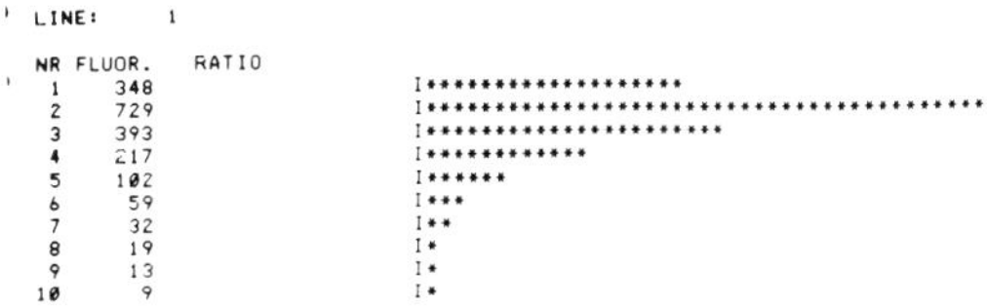

Fig.6.10. Printout of fluorescence intensities measured in one row (10 wells) of a microtitration tray filled with a 2-fold dilution series of 4-methylumbelliferone (MUF). Concentration in well (No. 2) = 1000 ng MUF/ml.

To enhance the applicability of automated ADM measurements in immunofluorescence procedures, the microfluorometer and a scanning stage have been interfaced to a LSI-11 microcomputer to measure the wells of a microtitration plate sequentially and to produce the results either in a histogram format or as a printout of the scan through the plate. The scan will yield a matrix of measurement values that can be printed row by row, column by column, or with a histogram for each row or column respectively (Fig. 6.10). The computer programmes to run the system can be stored in cheap ultraviolet light erasable read-only memories (PROMS) and do not require the relatively expensive paper tape, floppy disks or larger disks. This makes the resulting microfluorometer/microcomputer combination much more suited for a routine-oriented environment.

The ADM method can be carried out rapidly and is highly reproducible, as was demonstrated by Deelder et al. [12]. They found that, when all wells of a Terasaki type tray are filled with 10 μl of a suspension of monodisperse polystyrene FITC-labelled beads and the tray is scanned automatically, the standard deviation of the measurements was less than 2.5% of the mean value. The time needed for the automated scanning was about 1 min.

6.4.3. Application of the ADM method to Schistosoma mansoni diagnosis

Initially, Deelder and Ploem [10] assessed circulating antibody to *S. mansoni* by measuring the fluorescence of individual FITC-labelled beads which were coupled to antigen and incubated either with serum of patients infected with *S. mansoni* or with control sera. The fluorescence was measured in microtitration or Terasaki-type trays with the aid of an inverted microscope microfluorometer.

The ADM method proved to be much simpler. Comparative studies of the ADM-measuring method with individual measurements on *S. mansoni* antigen-coupled beads incubated with infected and control sera showed a good correlation between individual bead measurements and the ADM method.

6.4.4. Application of the ADM method to a fluorescent ELISA technique

Recently it has been shown [13] that an automated microfluorometer can be applied to the measurement of fluorescence levels of immunogalactosidase assays with a fluorogenic substrate. By performing 100 measurements in each well of a Terasaki-type tray and by calculating the mean value of these measurements very accurate results were obtained. With regard to the minimum detectable fluorescence level, it appeared that a concentration of 4 ng 4-methylumbelliferone (MUF)/ml could still be measured. This is about the same sensitivity as is reached in a cuvette-type spectrofluorometer. These findings correspond to the results of Josselin-De Jong et al. [23], who also observed a minimum detectable level of 4 ng MUF/ml when using an inverted microscope microfluorometer.

By constructing the microfluorometer system as flexibly as possible, it can also be applied to individual bead measurements and for the measurements of fluorescence in layers of sedimented agarose beads in the DASS system. Furthermore, the apparatus can be used for the quantitative determination of absorbance values for ELISA-type reactions with a chromogenic substrate, if a transmitted light path is included. Comparison of immunogalactosidase assays with an immunofluorescence test (FITC conjugate) and an immunoperoxidase test – in the DASS and ELISA respectively – showed, apart from an about 4-fold increase in sensitivity due to the use of a fluorogenic instead of a chromogenic substrate, a total increase in sensitivity of about 10–100-fold. This is possibly caused by the quality of the galactosidase conjugates and the apparently high turnover of the substrate by the enzyme.

Since the sensitivity is about the same as a radioimmunoassay (RIA)-type reaction, the application of immunogalactosidase assays seems promising for, e.g., the screening of determinants on cell surfaces and for the assessment of cell products such as specific antibodies produced by monoclonal hybridomas.

6.4.5. Automated scanning of cytotoxicity tests

The same instrumental set-up as described for the scanning of immunological test trays can be applied to cytotoxicity tests [6]. Wells of Terasaki-type trays are filled with carboxyfluorescein diacetate-labelled target cells and effector cells. After incubation, the residual fluorescence in the carboxyfluorescein diacetate-labelled cells is measured. For more detailed information about this method, the reader is referred to the papers by Bruning et al. [6] and Van de Poel et al. [62].

With a similar methodology, measurement of the antibody-dependent cellular cytotoxicity on the basis of carboxyfluorescein fluorochromasia should be possible.

6.5. TV SCANNING AND IMAGE ANALYSIS

Fast image analysing systems are now being manufactured by many industries (e.g. Quantimet from Imanco, TAS from Leitz). The TV scanning system in our own laboratory (LEYTAS) consists of a microscope, a Plumbicon

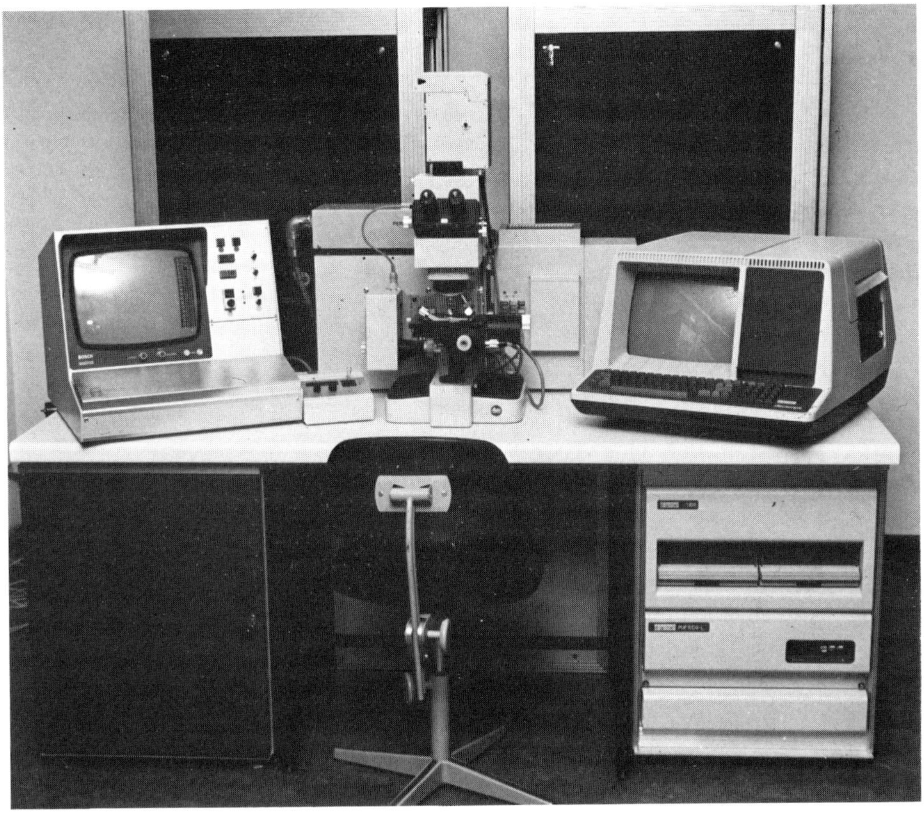

Fig. 6.11. Photograph of the Leyden Television Analysis System (LEYTAS). In the middle is the fully automated microscope with the automatic magnification changer. Positioning of the stage and autofocus system are under computer control. At the right bottom of the table you can see the LSI microcomputer provided with two floppy disks for memory support and introduction of the programming. On the table at right is the computer terminal allowing instructions to the hardwired logic of the Leitz TAS system. Algorithms for the system have been developed by Serra and Meyer in Fontainebleau. Basic hardwired system, TAS, is supplied by E. Leitz in Germany.

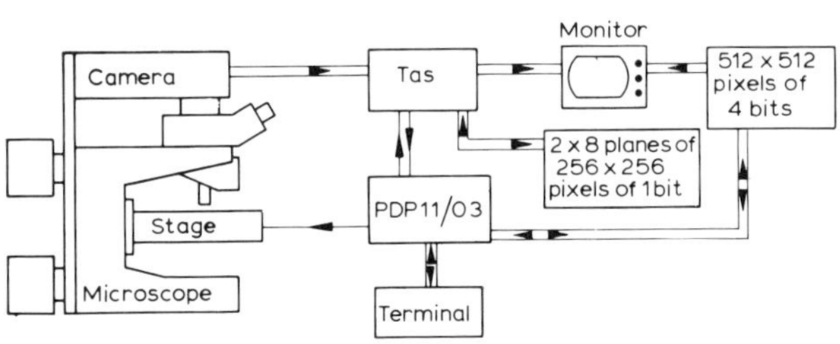

Fig. 6.12. Schematic diagram of the LEYTAS configuration.

TV camera, the texture analysing system (TAS), a buffer memory, and a minicomputer (Figs. 6.11 and 6.12). Microscope functions and focussing are fully automated. Many pattern recognition operations can be performed on an entire microscopic field of about 200 × 200 μm with a spatial resolution of 0.5

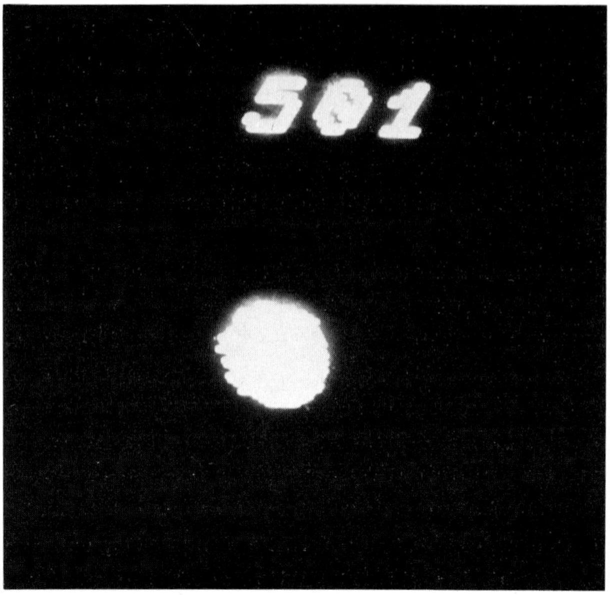

Fig. 6.13. On the TV screen of the LEYTAS system, all the points of a FITC-stained nucleus in an ANF test are shown beyond a certain threshold. The measured nucleus is given in relative surface units by the TAS logic. This type of measurement can be carried out quickly over the whole field. Basic frame analysing rate of such a system is 20 ms for an entire microscopic field.

μm in less than a second. Preliminary experiments in the analysis of fluorescence images with a Plumbicon TV camera have shown that the signal to noise ratio of the TV-scanned fluorescence images is favourable if the fluorescence image is sufficiently bright. For instance, we were able to obtain TV images of sufficient brightness and good contrast in antinuclear factor (ANF) tests. For excitation of the FITC-stained nucleus (Fig. 6.13), a HBO 100 mercury lamp was used in combination with a KP 490 filter and a 40×, NA 1.30 objective in an epi-illumination system. The intermediate image of the objective is then directly projected into the vidicon tube without using an eyepiece. With special TAS procedures it is possible to automatically select nuclei above certain preselected thresholds, while fluorescent debris is eliminated. These results indicate that stronger light sources such as lasers or very sensitive TV tubes will enable selection of small or weaker fluorescing objects and distinguish those from fluorescent debris.

Recent research in our laboratory involves the selection of red blood cells detected with a FITC-labelled antibody to hemoglobulin S in a blood smear. This research was instigated by the following biological problem. It has been shown that point mutations may cause the occurrence of rare sickle cells in the peripheral blood of normal individuals. They occur, however, in an extremely low frequency (1 in 10^7 red blood cells). Thus in order to judge whether a person or an animal has been exposed to an increased mutation risk, a very large quantity of blood cells would have to be counted. For visual counting a period of weeks has to be reckoned with, since at least 10^8 red blood cells have to be screened manually for the occurrence of a few sickle cells. These sickle cells can now be searched for with LEYTAS, that is equipped with a sensitive TV tube. The weak FITC fluorescence of the labelled sickle cells proved to be sufficiently strong for a TV image, if an especially sensitive camera, the Silicon Intensified Target Camera (SIT Camera; 4804/H Series; RCA electronic components, U.S.A.), was used.

The procedure for counting the blood cells and selecting the positive cells, which is under study at present, is as follows. The red blood cells are counted by LEYTAS, using their absorption image at 405 nm. This absorption image is also used for a focussing algorithm. During the automated focussing, the vertical position of the scanning stage is recorded. After scanning one line of fields (e.g. 150 fields of 250 × 250 μm) and calculating the position of the stage in these fields, the illumination will be changed to epi-illumination by electronic shutters and a computer-operated vertical fluorescence illuminator. The same fields in one scan line of the stage will be screened again, but now for the occurrence of cells positive for sickle cell hemoglobulin. The excitation light is generated from a HBO mercury lamp. Excitation filters are KP 490 and BG 38. A 510 nm dichroic mirror is used and a 530 AL filter is implemented as a fluorescence selection filter. Fig. 6.14 shows the analogue TV image of the absorption of erythrocytes. Although the contrast between erythrocytes and the background is not optimal, a counting can be performed automatically by setting thresholds. This counting of erythrocytes in Fig. 6.14 is depicted in Fig. 6.15. Fig. 6.16 shows two cells with FITC fluorescence after

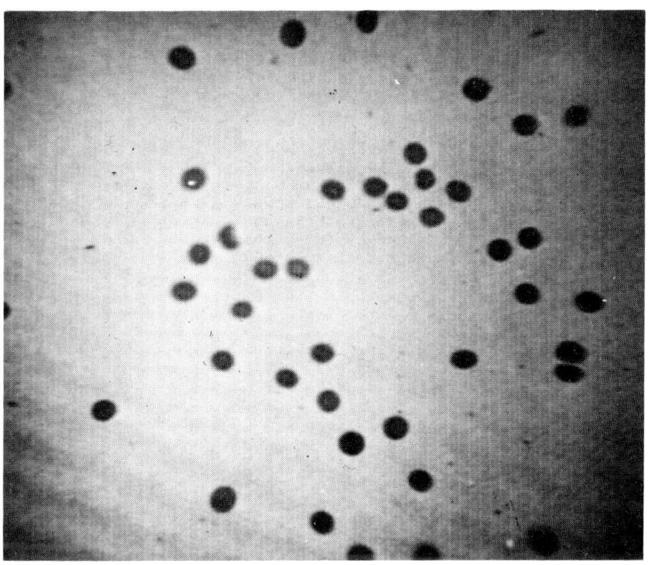

Fig. 6.14. Analogue image of a TV screen of the LEYTAS system with the absorbance of hemoglobulin of red blood cells at 405 nm.

incubation with FITC-labelled antibody against hemoglobulins. The cells are detected by TAS algorithms.

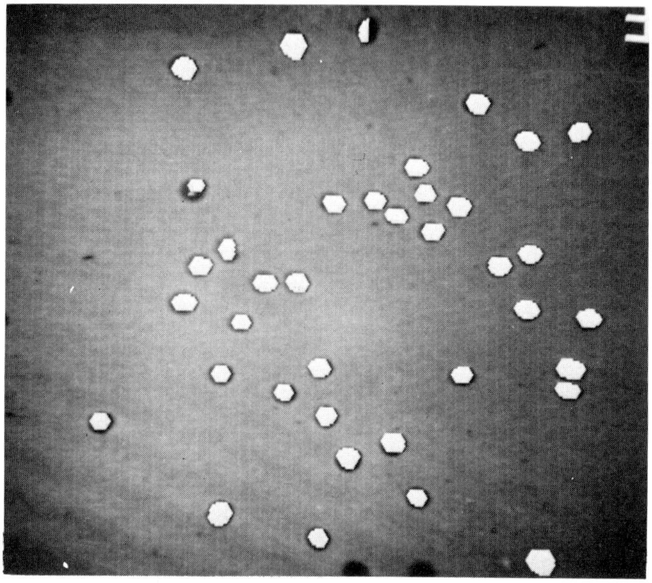

Fig. 6.15. Presents the same field of view as in Fig. 6.14 and shows the detection of the red blood cells which can now be counted rapidly by TAS logic.

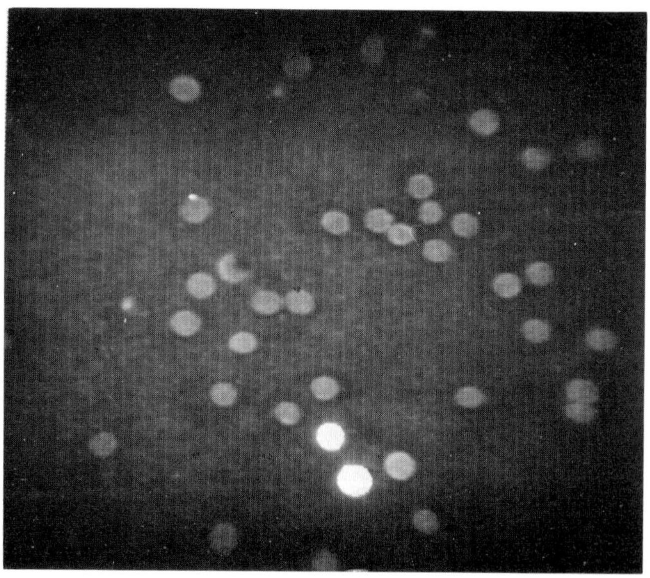

Fig. 6.16. The same microscopic field is shown but now illuminated with an epi-illuminator to detect two red cells which demonstrate FITC antibody directed against hemoglobulins. These rare events can be counted and compared with the total number of erythrocytes.

REFERENCES

1 Al, I., Cornelisse, C.J., Pearson, P.L. and Ploem, J.S. (1978) Automated chromatin analysis using the Leyden television analysis system (Leytas). Acta Histochem. Suppl.-Band *XX,* 211–215.

2 Bergquist, N.R. (1973) The pulsed dye laser as a light source for the fluorescent antibody technique. Scand. J. Immunol. *2,* 37–44.

3 Bergquist, N.R. and Nilsson, P. (1975) Laser excitation of fluorescent copolymerized immunoglobulin beads. Ann. N.Y. Acad. Sci. *254,* 157–162.

4 Bloemmen, F.J., Radl, J., Haaijman, J.J., Van den Berg, P., Schuit, H.R.E. and Hijmans, W. (1976) Microfluorometric evaluation of the specificity of fluorescent antisera against mouse immunoglobulins with the defined antigen substrate spheres (DASS) system. J. Immunol. Methods *10,* 337–355.

5 Boehm, N. and Sprenger, E. (1968) Fluorescence cytophotometry: a valuable method for the quantitative determination of nuclear Feulgen-DNA. Histochemie *16,* 100–118.

6 Bruning, J.W., Kardol, M.J. and Arentzen, R. (1980) Carboxyfluorescein fluorochromasia assays. I. Non-radioactively labeled cell-mediated lympholysis. J. Immunol. Methods *33,* 33–44.

7 Capel, P.J.A. (1974) A quantitative immunofluorescence method based on the covalent coupling of protein to sepharose beads. J. Immunol. *5,* 165–178.

8 Capel, P.J.A. (1979) Complement fixation studies with the DASS system. Thesis, Amsterdam.

9 Cornelisse, C.J. and Ploem, J.S. (1976) A new type of two-color fluorescence staining for cytology specimens. J. Histochem. Cytochem. *24,* 72–81.

10 Deelder, A.M. and Ploem, J.S. (1974) An immunofluorescence reaction for *Schistosoma mansoni* using the defined antigen substrate spheres system (DASS). J. Immunol. Methods *4,* 239–252.

11 Deelder, A.M. and Ploem, J.S. (1975) An immunofluorescence reaction for *Fasciola hepatica* using the defined antigen substrate spheres (DASS) system. Exp. Parasitol. *37,* 173–178.

12 Deelder, A.M., Tanke, H.J. and Ploem, J.S. (1978) Automated quantitative immunofluorescence using the aperture defined microvolume (ADM) method. *In* Knapp, W., Holubar, K. and Wick, G. (eds.), Immunofluorescence and Related Staining Techniques (Elsevier/North-Holland, Amsterdam) pp. 31–44.

13 Deelder, A.M., Koper, G., De Water, R., Tanke, H.J., Rotmans, J.P. and Ploem, J.S. (1980) Automated quantitative measurement of immunogalactosidase procedures with a fluorogenic substrate (using the aperture defined microvolume measurement method). Application to *Schistosoma mansoni* immunodiagnosis. J. Immunol. Methods *36,* 269–285.

14 Goldman, M. (1967) An improved microfluorometer for measuring brightness of fluorescent antibody reactions. J. Histochem. Cytochem. *15,* 38–45.

15 Goldman, M. (1971) Microfluorimetry in the antigenic analysis of closely related microorganisms. Ann. N.Y. Acad. Sci *177,* 439–445.

16 Haaijman, J.J. (1977) Quantitative immunofluorescence microscopy. Methods and applications. Thesis, Leiden.

17 Haaijman, J.J. and Van Dalen, J.P.R. (1974) Quantification in immunofluorescence microscopy. A new standard for fluorescein and rhodamine emission measurement. J. Immunol. Methods *5,* 359–374.

18 Haaijman, J.J. and Wijnants, F.A.C. (1975) Inexpensive automation of the Leitz orthoplan microfluorometer using pneumatic components. J. Immunol. Methods *7,* 255–270.

19 Herzenberg, L.A. (1978) The fluorescence activated cell sorter (FACS): a retrospective and prospective view. *In* Knapp, W., Holubar, K. and Wick, G. (eds.), Immunofluorescence and Related Staining Techniques (Elsevier/North-Holland, Amsterdam) pp. 99–109.

20 Hijmans, W., Jongsma, A.P.M. and Ploem, J.S. (1971) Kwantitatieve immunofluorescentie bij de ANF-test met humane granulocyten. Ned. T. Geneesk. *115,* 1925.

21 Irvine, W.J., Chan, M.M.W. and Williamson, W.G. (1969) The application of microphotometry to the indirect immunofluorescent antibody technique using the human gastric parietal cell

antigen-antibody system. Clin. Exp. Immunol. *4,* 607–617.
22 Jongsma, A.P.M., Hijmans, W. and Ploem, J.S. (1971) Quantitative immunofluorescence. Standardization and calibration in microfluorometry. Histochemie *25,* 329–343.
23 Josselin-De Jong, J.E., Jongkind, J.F. and Ywema, H.R. (1980) A scanning inverted microfluorometer with electronic shutter control for automatic measurements in micro-test plates. Anal. Biochem. *102,* 120–125.
24 Kaufman, G.I. and Nester, J.F. (1972) Automation of the fluorescent treponemal antibody-absorption test. J. Histochem. Cytochem. *20,* 255–260.
25 Kaufman, G.I., Nester, J.F. and Wasserman, D.E. (1971) An experimental study of lasers as excitation sources for automated fluorescent antibody instrumentation. J. Histochem. Cytochem. *19,* 469–476.
26 Killander, D., Levin, A., Inoue, M. and Klein, E. (1970) Quantification of immunofluorescence on individual erythrocytes coated with varying amounts of antigen. Immunology *19,* 151–156.
27 Killander, D., Hellstrom, U., Johansson, N., Klein, E., Levin, A. and Perlmann, P. (1973) Immunofluorometric determinations of surface immunoglobulins of individual normal and malignant human lymphoid cells. *In* Thaer, A.A. and Sernetz, M. (eds.), Fluorescence Techniques in Cell Biology (Springer Verlag, Berlin–Heidelberg–New York) pp. 163–181.
28 Knapp, W. and Ploem, J.S. (1974) Microfluorometry of antigen–antibody interactions in immunofluorescence using the defined antigen substrate spheres (DASS). J. Immunol. Methods *5,* 259–273.
29 Knapp, W., Haaijman, J.J., Schuit, H.R.E., Radl, J., Van den Berg, P., Ploem, J.S. and Hijmans, W. (1975) Microfluorometric evaluation of conjugate specificity with the defined antigen substrate spheres (DASS) system. Ann. N.Y. Acad. Sci. *254,* 94–107.
30 Mansberg, H.P. and Kusnetz, J. (1966) Quantitative fluorescence microscopy. Fluorescent antibody automatic scanning techniques. J. Histochem. Cytochem. *14,* 260–273.
31 Nairn, R.C., Herzog, F., Ward, H.A. and De Boer, G.R.B. (1969) Techniques: microphotometry in immunofluorescence. Clin. Exp. Immunol. *4,* 697–705.
32 Neurath, A.R. (1965) Fluorometric estimation of antigens (antibodies). Z. Naturforsch. *20,* 974–976.
33 Pachmann, K. and Killander, D. (1976) Simultaneous quantification of two antigens in mixture in individual cells by microimmunofluorometry. J. Immunol. Methods *12,* 67–79.
34 Piller, H. (1977) Microscopic Photometry (Springer Verlag, Berlin–Heidelberg–New York).
35 Ploem, J.S. (1970) Quantitative immunofluorescence. *In* Holborow, E.J. (ed.), Standardization in Immunofluorescence (Blackwell Scientific Publ., Oxford) pp. 63–73.
36 Ploem, J.S. (1970) Standards for fluorescence microscopy. *In* Holborow, E.J. (ed.), Standardization in Immunofluorescence (Blackwell Scientific publ., Oxford) pp. 137–153.
37 Ploem, J.S. (1976) Automation of immunofluorescence. *In* Rapid Methods and Automation in Microbiology, 2nd International Symposium, Cambridge, pp. 193–196.
38 Ploem, J.S. (1977) Quantitative fluorescence microscopy. *In* Meek, G.A. and Elder, H.Y. (eds.), Analytical and Quantitative Methods in Microscopy (Cambridge University Press) pp. 55–89.
39 Ploem, J.S. (1980) Appropriate technology for the quantitative assessment of the final reaction product of histochemical techniques. *In* Trends in Enzyme Histochemistry and Cytochemistry, Ciba Foundation Symp. *73* (New Series) pp. 275–303.
40 Ploem, J.S., De Sterke, J.A., Bonnet, J. and Wasmund, H. (1974) A microspectrofluorometer with epi-illumination operated under computer control. J. Histochem. Cytochem. *22,* 668–677.
41 Ploem, J.S., Tanke, H.J., Al, I. and Deelder, A.M. (1978) Recent developments in immunofluorescence microscopy and microfluorometry. *In* Knapp, W., Holubar, K. and Wick, G. (eds.), Immunofluorescence and Related Staining Techniques (Elsevier/North-Holland, Amsterdam) pp. 1–10.
42 Ploem, J.S., Vrolijk, J., Al, I. and Pearson, P.L. (1979) Mechanical and electronical means for image acquisition. *In* Pressmann, N.J. and Wied, G.L. (eds.), The Automation of Cancer Cytology and Cell Image Analysis (Tutorials of Cytology, Chicago) pp. 287–288.
43 Ploem-Zaaijer, J.J., Beyer-Boon, M.E., Leyte-Veldstra, L. and Ploem, J.S. (1979) Cytofluorometric and cytophotometric DNA measurements of cervical smears stained using a new bi-

color method. *In* Pressman, N.J. and Wied, G.L. (eds.), The Automation of Cancer Cytology and Cell Image Analysis (Tutorials of Cytology, Chicago) pp. 225–235.

44 Prenna, G., Mazzini, G. and Cova, S. (1974) Methodological and instrumental aspects of cytofluorometry. Histochem J. *6*, 259–278.

45 Reuter, W.G. (1980) Mikroskopphotometrie für den Routinebetrieb. Labor Praxis in der Medizin, Vogel Verlag Wuerzburg, Heft 1.

46 Rost, F.W.G. (1972) Fluorescence microscopy. *In* Pearse, A.G.E. (ed.), Histochemistry, Theoretical and Applied (Churchill Livingstone, Edinburgh–London) pp. 1171–1206.

47 Ruch, F. (1970) Principles and some applications of cytofluorometry. *In* Wied, G.L. and Bahr, G.F. (eds.), Introduction to Quantitative Cytochemistry, *Vol. 2* (Academic Press, New York–London) pp. 431–450.

48 Ruch, F. and Leeman, U. (1973) Cytofluorometry. *In* Neuhoff, V. (ed.), Molecular Biology, Biochemistry and Biophysics, *Vol. 14,* Micromethods in Molecular Biology (Springer Verlag, Berlin–Heidelberg–New York) pp. 329–346.

49 Sacchi, C.A., Svelto, O. and Prenna, G. (1974) Pulsed tunable lasers in cytofluorometry. Histochem. J. *6*, 251–258.

50 Schauenstein, K. (1978) Application of immunofluorescence flow cytometry and quantitative immunofluorescence. *In* Knapp, W., Holubar, K. and Wick, G. (eds.), Immunofluorescence and Related Staining Techniques (Elsevier/North-Holland, Amsterdam) pp. 257–270.

51 Schauenstein, K. and Wick, G. (1980) Quantitative immunohistochemistry. Acta. Histochem. Suppl. Band *XXII,* 101–110.

52 Schipper, J., Tilders, F.J.H. and Ploem, J.S. (1978) Microfluorometric scanning of sympathetic nerve fibres, an improved method to quantitate formaldehyde induced fluorescence of biogenic amines. J. Histochem. Cytochem. *26,* 1057–1066.

53 Schipper, J., Tilders, F.J.H., Groot Wassink, R., Boleij, H.F. and Ploem, J.S. (1980) Microfluorometric scanning of sympathetic nerve fibres: quantification of neuronal and extraneuronal fluorescence with aid of histogram analysis. J. Histochem. Cytochem. *28,* 124–132.

54 Schothorst, A.A., Suurmond, D. and Ploem, J.S. (1977) In vitro studies on the protoporphyrin uptake and photosensitivity of normal skin fibroblasts and fibroblasts from patients with erythropoietic protoporphyria. J. Invest. Dermatol. *69,* 551–557.

55 Sedlacek, H.H. and Gundlach, H. (1976) The use of television cameras equipped with an image intensifier in the immunofluorescence microscopy. Behring Inst. Mitt. *59,* 64–70.

56 Sernetz, M. and Thaer, A.A. (1970) A capillary fluorescence standard for microfluorometry. J. Microsc. *91,* 43–52.

57 Taylor, C.E.D. (1975) Quantitative immunofluorescence studies. A contribution towards standardization. Laboratorium *2,* 333–337.

58 Taylor, C.E.D. and Heimer, G.V. (1975) Quantitative immunofluorescence studies. Ann. N.Y. Acad. Sci. *242,* 151–156.

59 Taylor, C.E.D., Heimer, G.V. and Lidwell, D.M. (1971) Use of a fibre optic probe for quantitative immunofluorescence studies. Lancet *1,* 785–786.

60 Van Dalen, J.P.R., Knapp, W. and Ploem, J.S. (1973) Microfluorometry on antigen–antibody interaction in immunofluorescence using antigens covalently bound to agarose beads. J. Immunol. Methods *2,* 383–392.

61 Van de Ploeg, M., Van den Broek, K., Smeulders, A.W.M., Vossepoel, A.M. and Van Duijn, P. (1977) Hidacsys: computer program for interactive scanning cytophotometry. Histochemistry *54,* 273–288.

62 Van der Poel, J.J., Kardol, M., Goulmy, E., Blokland, E. and Bruning, J.W. (1981) Carboxy fluorescein fluorochromasia CML. Comparative study. Immunol. Lett. *2,* 187–193.

63 Wasmund, H. (1976) Computergesteuertes Scanning-Mikroskop für die Analyse von Einzelzellen. Leitz-Mitt. Wiss. Tech. *VI, 6,* 217–223.

64 Wick, G., Schauenstein, K., Herzog, F. and Steinbatz, A. (1975) Investigations of the recovery phenomenon after laser excitation in immunofluorescence. Ann. N.Y. Acad. Sci. *254,* 172–174.

65 Zimmer, H.G. (1973) Microphotometry. *In* Neuhoff, V. (ed.), Micromethods in Molecular Biology (Springer Verlag, Berlin–Heidelberg–New York) pp. 297–328.

Wick et al. (eds) Immunofluorescence Technology. Selected Theoretical and Clinical Aspects

CHAPTER 7

Immunofluorescence measurements by flow cytometry

JAN W.M. VISSER and GER J. VAN DEN ENGH

Radiobiological Institute TNO, and Department of Radiobiology of the Erasmus University, Rijswijk, The Netherlands

---

7.1. INTRODUCTION

The development of flow cytometry* and flow sorting has contributed significantly to the progress in immunofluorescence microscopy. Immunologists who first started to employ this technique rapidly learned that the instruments offer important advantages such as rapidity, flexibility and quantitation, but also that they had to encounter unexpected artifacts [23]. New methods for antiserum and cell handling which overcame the initial problems and which also opened doors to new immunofluorescence techniques had to be developed. Flow cytometers can presently be employed in a variety of studies. In the area of immunofluorescence, they are used to measure antibody binding to cells and to sort subpopulations of cells which differ in amount of binding. They are employed for studies of lymphocyte differentiation [21, 25], hybrid isolation [7], haemopoietic stem cell characterization [3, 16], isolation of fetal cells [12], isolation of ghost-containing cells [26], expression of virus-specific antigens (e.g. ref. 15), and optimization of maintenance of monoclonal antibody-producing cell lines [2, 10, 30, 46]. In addition, flow cytometers can be used to quantitate or detect antibodies in sera [6], to elucidate membrane structures by the study of energy transfer after immunofluorescent labelling [5] and to determine cell cycle parameters of subpopulations of cells which react with a specific antiserum [22]. Calibrated flow cytometers can be used to calibrate other immunological tests like the complement-dependent cytotoxicity assay and immunoelectron microscopy.

The flow cytometers reach limits in their applicability in immunofluorescence if large numbers of cells have to be sorted and also if absolutely no cell loss is a requirement of the experiment. Flow cytometers cannot be used to study immunofluorescence in tissues. Up to now, no reports have been published of immunoabsorbance measurements by flow cytometers. However, since work on light scatter disturbances by immunoenzymatic staining is in progress [20], it may be expected that immunoabsorbance measurements will also be possible in the near future.

In the present chapter we will describe instrumental and preparative methods for immunofluorescence with flow cytometers. Analysis and sorting will be treated separately as much as possible. Some applications in experimental and clinical studies will be considered and methods for quantitating all results will be described. Other reviews with a similar purpose of introduction

---

* Flow cytometry = pulse cytophotometry = flow cytofluorography = flow cytofluorometry.

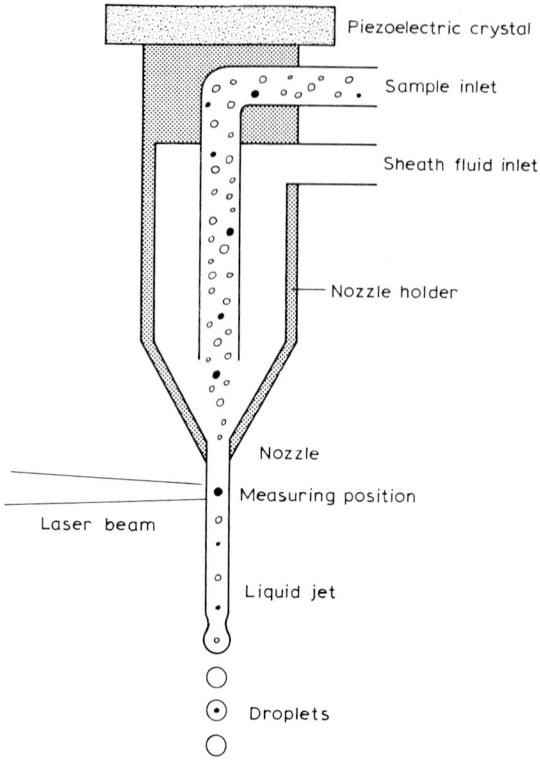

Fig. 7.2. Schematic diagram of one type of flow cell in use in flow cytometers. In this type, the measuring point is in the liquid jet below the nozzle; in other types, the measuring point can be inside an optically well-defined cuvette. If the flow cytometer is not of the sorting type, the piezoelectric crystal is not necessary and the liquid jet may be replaced by tubing.

In all types of flow cytometers, an intersection point is constructed where the excitation light beam and the light-collecting lenses are in focus. The cells contained in a stream of fluid traverse this intersection point one by one. If a fluorescent cell crosses the intersection, it produces a flash of scattered and fluorescence light of the duration of the time period of illumination. Light-collecting lenses and mirrors transport this flash of light from the cell to

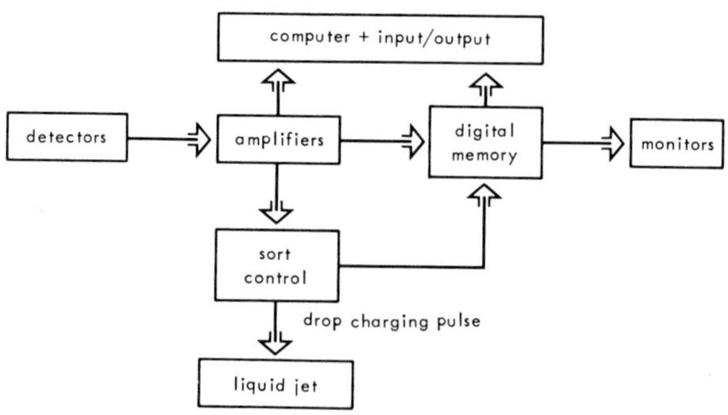

Fig. 7.3. Schematic outline of the electronic signal processing in flow cytometers.

optical transducers, which may be shielded by optical filters to distinguish scatter from fluorescence.

The alternating current (AC) part of the electronics output of the transducers is amplified and processed through electronic analyzers (Fig. 7.3). By this means, only the light flashes from cells and not the continuous background light from unbound dyes in the jet or from room light are amplified and processed. Depending on the dimensions of the spot of excitation light, two types of electronic processors are in use. If the spot of excitation light is larger than the cells, then the peak height of the detected pulse is generally determined; this is then linearly proportional to the total amount of light scattered or emitted as fluorescence into the light-collecting lens by the cell which crosses the intersection. If the light spot is smaller than the cells, then the pulse is generally integrated to obtain a linear proportionality between machine output and cell fluorescence. The proportionality constants can be calculated from calibration of the device and so the machine output can be directly related to the number of fluorescent molecules and to the size of the cells. Table 7.I summarizes the typical features of flow cytometers.

TABLE 7.I

TYPICAL VALUES FOR FLOW CYTOMETERS

Analysis	
Nozzle diameter (= maximum cell diameter)	50–80 μm
Smallest particles detected by scatter	0.5 μm diameter
Variation coefficient for scatter measurements	0.5–2%
Lower threshold for fluorescence measurements[a]	10^3 FITC molecules
Variation coefficients for fluorescence measurements	1–3%
Cell speed at measuring point	10 $m \cdot s^{-1}$
Time duration of measurement	2–5 μs/cell
Time duration of signal processing	2–30 μs/cell
Maximal cell rate for analysis[b]	$10^4 \cdot s^{-1}$
Optimal cell rate for analysis	$10^3 \cdot s^{-1}$
Sorting	
Droplet frequency	20–40 kHz
Maximal cell rate for "pure" sorting[b]	$10^3 \cdot s^{-1}$
Maximal cell rate for "raw" sorting[b]	$10^4 \cdot s^{-1}$

[a] See Appendix A (p.00).
[b] See Section 7.8.1 (p.00).

The possibility to sort with flow cytometers originates from an invention in which a stream of ink droplets could be electrically charged and deflected in a strong electrostatic field to produce letters or curves on paper [38]. As explained above, the cells in flow cytometers are contained in a stream of liquid by which they are guided through a measuring point. The liquid stream breaks into droplets when led into the air (Fig. 7.2). The drop size and the distance between the drops can be controlled by choice of the diameter of the nozzle through which the stream comes into the air, by the pressure on the liquid stream and, most importantly, by a piezoelectric transducer which is connected to the nozzle. The piezoelectric tranducer oscillates with a steady frequency and this causes a constant frequency of droplet formation. The presence of this control makes it possible to know exactly the time duration between the measurements of a cell during its traversal of the laser beam and the arrival of that cell at the droplet break-off point. And, consequently, it can be known which droplets contain cells that are to be separated from other cells. The separation procedure is as follows. If a cell to be sorted arrives at the droplet break-off point, the liquid jet is electrically charged during the formation of a set number of droplets. Therefore, the cell will be contained in a droplet which is charged. This charged droplet is deflected from the main stream in a strong electrostatic field. By control of the droplet charge and the electrostatic field, the deflected droplets can be positioned accurately. They can be collected in a separate tube, on a slide, in a culture dish away from the main stream, etc.

The investigator determines which cells are to be sorted. Therefore, he sets the machine to measure optical properties of the cells by which differences between cells are distinguished. For each property, he defines the signal heights above and below which the machine triggers droplet charging. Thus, if cells are run through the machine, those which cause signals within the set limits will be deflected. Generally, the droplets can be charged positively or negatively so that they can be deflected into two opposite directions. Therefore, in each run, two subpopulations of cells can be separated from the undeflected stream simultaneously.

TABLE 7.II

LASER LINES SUITABLE FOR IMMUNOFLUORESCENCE EXCITATION

Fluorochrome	Laser line (nm)	Laser type
SITS	351–364[a]	High power argon ion
	334–356[a]	High power krypton ion
FITC	488	Argon ion
	483	High power krypton ion
TRITC	488	High power argon ion
	515	Argon ion
	458–515[a]	Argon ion
	531	Krypton ion
	521	High power krypton ion
XRITC	515	High power argon ion
	568	Krypton ion
	521–568[a]	Krypton ion

[a]Multiline mode.

7.2.2. Instrumental requirements for immunofluorescence measurements with flow cytometers

7.2.2.1. Lasers

Flow cytometers designed to measure immunofluorescence use lasers as light sources. The laser is generally of the argon ion type, with powerful lines at 488 and 515 nm, which are suitable wavelengths for the excitation of fluorescein isothiocyanate (FITC) and also – though less efficiently – of tetrametylrhodamine isothiocyanate (TRITC) (Table 7.II). Krypton ion lasers are also in use. Their 531 and 568 nm lines are more suitable for excitation of TRITC; the 568 nm line is especially useful for the excitation of the rhodamine derivative XRITC (tetra-*N*-cyclopropylrhodamine isothiocyanate). Flow cytometers may also be equipped with two lasers tuned at different wavelengths for independent and more efficient excitation of FITC and TRITC or XRITC. In addition, in two laser systems autofluorescence by cells may be decreased by preillumination [13].

7.2.2.2. Filters

Since cells scatter light in all directions when they pass the laser beam, the photomultiplier (PM) by which fluorescence is measured has to be shielded by optical filters. Most absorbing glass filters are found to be fluorescent themselves; if they are excited by light scatter from the cell, they emit a pulse of fluorescence. The PM cannot distinguish such a fluorescence pulse from one which originates from the cell. Of the absorbing glass filters tested, only Schott KV ones were found to have a low fluorescence yield; however, at present, there is no KV filter with the required wavelength specificity. Therefore, the filters to be used for immunofluorescence are of the interference type. Such filters are generally mounted on a layer of absorbing glass. If so, the filter has to be placed with its interference layers directed to the cell and as far away from the PM as possible, in order to minimize contributions from filter fluorescence to the signal.

In general, the fluorescence of filters can be detected by comparing the signals from unstained cells measured with the filters at varying distances from the PM. Table 7.III gives a list of filters in use for immunofluorescence measurements in flow cytometers. For simultaneous measurements of red and green fluorescence or perpendicular light scatter and fluorescence, it is of advantage to use dichroic beam splitters. It is sometimes useful to make use of the polarization direction of the laser light in order to improve the specificity of the measurements. The perpendicular light scatter, which causes most artifacts in immunofluorescence measurements by flow cytometers, is polarized into the same direction as the laser light. Fluorescence is generally depolarized. Thus, by placing a polarizing filter in between the liquid jet and the light-collecting objective, most of the perpendicular scatter light can be blocked by proper rotation of the filter, whereas almost half of the fluorescence is transmitted.

TABLE 7.III

IMMUNOFLUORESCENCE FILTERS USED IN FLOW CYTOMETRY

Fluorochrome and excitation	PM type	Filter (combination)
FITC (488 nm)	S20	520 or 530 nm long pass filters[a] far away from PM
FITC + PI (488 nm)	S20 S11	PI: 590 nm long pass filter[b] FITC: (510–550) nm band pass filter[c] + dichroic 580 nm beam splitter[d]
TRITC (515 nm or multiline)	S20	550 nm long pass filter[e] far away from PM
TRITC + FITC (488 nm)	S20 S11	TRITC: 590 nm long pass filter[b] FITC: (510–550) nm band pass filter[c] + dichroic 580 nm beam splitter[d]
TRITC + FITC (515 nm or multiline)	S20 S11	TRITC: 590 nm long pass filter[b] FITC: 550 nm long pass filter[e] far away from PM + dichroic 580 nm beam splitter[d]

[a] 5200 cut-on Ditric.
[b] Schott OG-590.
[c] Pomfrett 488 nm rejecting interference filter.
[d] Melles Griot edge filters, Zeiss FT 580.
[e] Schott kV-550.

7.2.2.3. Lenses

The laser is focused onto the liquid jet by a lens or lens system. The size of the focal spot determines the intensity of light at that spot. If cells are weakly fluorescent, it may be useful to replace the laser light-focussing lens by one which has a shorter focal distance. This decreases the size of the illuminated area and increases the intensity at the measuring position. Care must be taken not to diminish the size of the illuminated area in the liquid jet below the cell size if one employs a flow cytometer which does not integrate the PM signals. Furthermore, with diminished focal spots most flow cytometers become more sensitive to displacements of cells from the central axis of the liquid jet. Therefore, the ratio of the sheath to sample fluids in the jet should be maximal with minimal focal spot dimensions.

7.2.2.4. Photomultipliers

Mainly S-20 type photomultipliers are used in flow cytometers. If red and green fluorescence are to be measured simultaneously (e.g. FITC- and TRITC-labelled cells), green fluorescence may be detected by an S-11 type PM. This type is not as sensitive in the red spectral region as the S-20, which may help to distinguish between red and green fluorescence. Perpendicular light scatter is also generally measured by photomultipliers. If fluorescence is measured simultaneously, perpendicular light scatter is best measured by an S-11 type PM, and fluorescence by an S-20 type.

7.2.3. Calibration

Fluorescence and light scatter measurements by flow cytometers can be quantitated by comparison with measurements obtained with beads of known dimensions and known content of fluorescent molecules (e.g. ref. 43). Appendix A (section 7.10) describes a method for preparing such beads to calibrate forward light scatter and FITC and TRITC fluorescence measurements. Photomultipliers can be calibrated by use of the same beads. It must be kept in mind that the response of photomultipliers may depend upon the spectrum of the light measured; a change of filters may alter the sensitivity. The calibration beads may be used also to optimize the machine and to detect artifacts. By using such beads, it could be determined that freshly isolated unstained thymocytes produce artificial signals which are equivalent to 1–2 $\times$ 10^3 FITC molecules (FACS II; excitation 488 nm; 1 W). Above this threshold differences of 200–300 FITC molecules per cell could be distinguished. For TRITC, these figures were a factor of 3 higher (excitation at 514.5 nm; 1 W).

7.2.4. Signal processing and display

Data may be presented in a variety of ways (e.g. ref. 28). For quantitative work, the "histogram" or frequency distribution of the fluorescence intensities per cell is most adequate (Fig. 7.4). For immunofluorescence measurements, transformation to a logarithmic intensity scale may be of great advantage (Fig. 7.4). This transformation can be performed by processing the signals through logarithmic amplifiers [10] or by computation. The former method is generally used in flow sorters.

7.3. PREPARATION OF ANTISERA AND FLUOROCHROME

Antisera for flow cytometry can generally be prepared as for fluorescence microscopy [10]. The quantities of antisera required for extensive analysis are larger, because more cells are measured and, after measurements, the cells are generally not saved for a second measurement. Immunofluorescence measurements by flow cytometers may also require more control measurements than those made by fluorescence microscopes. Therefore, more types of antisera may be needed.

to flow cytometry have been written by Herzenberg et al. [11], Horan and Wheeless [14], Mullaney et al. [29], Steinkamp [35], and the first book dedicated to this topic has been recently published [27].

7.2. INSTRUMENTS

Several types of flow cytometers are currently available [27]; however, not all of them are suitable for use in immunofluorescence studies. In this section, we will first present the principles of flow cytometry and sorting. We will then outline the instrumental requirements for measurements of immunofluorescence.

7.2.1. The principle of flow cytometry and sorting

In simple terms, flow cytometers can be regarded as fluorescence microscopes where the movable stage has been replaced by a stream of fluid in which the cells are passed through the illuminated focal spot of the objective and where the oculars, eyes and brains are replaced by photomultipliers and electronic signal processors. Figs. 7.1 and 7.2 show schematic diagrams of the optical and flow parts of a flow cytometer fitted for immunofluorescence measurements. Fig. 7.3 gives a schematic outline of the electronics of such a device.

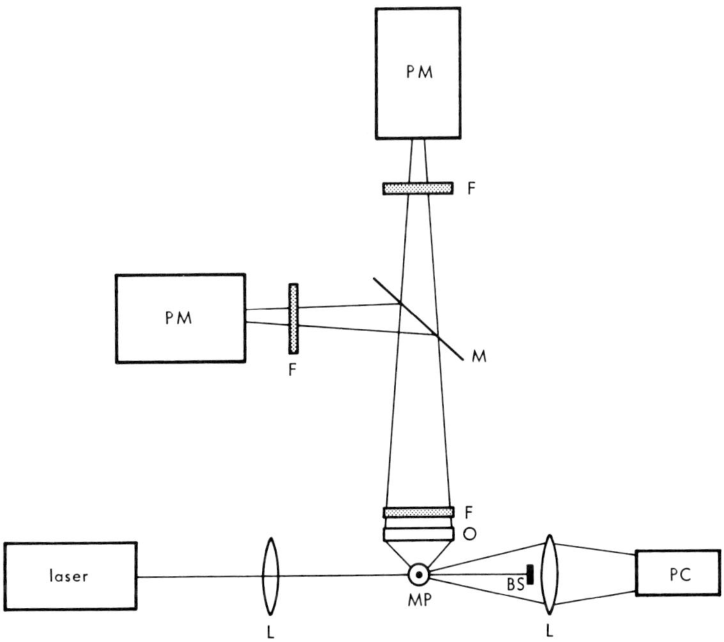

Fig. 7.1. Schematic diagram of a flow cytometer as viewed from the top. L, lens; MP, measuring position; BS, beam stop; O, objective; F, filter; M, beam splitting mirror; PC, photocell; PM, photomultiplier.

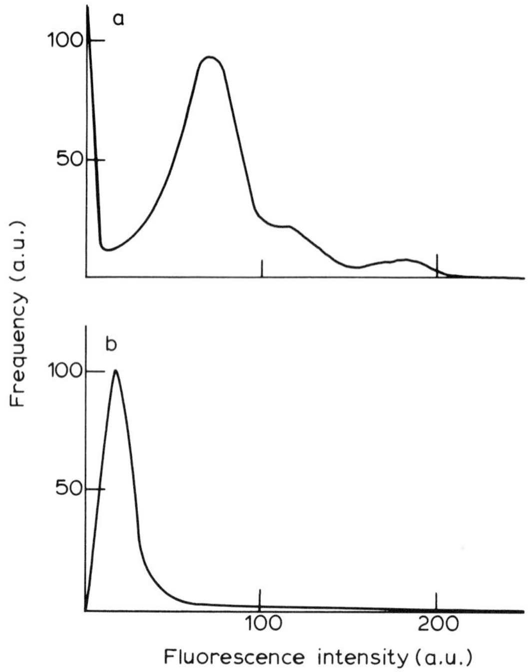

Fig. 7.4. Frequency distribution of the fluorescence intensity of mouse spleen cells labelled with biotin-conjugated monoclonal anti-Thy-1,2 and subsequently with FITC-avidin. a) Logarithmic intensity scale. b) Linear intensity scale.

7.4. PREPARATION AND LABELLING OF CELL SUSPENSIONS

7.4.1. Single cell suspensions

Flow cytometers are readily blocked by aggregates of cells, debris or very large cells. There are several methods for disrupting tissues into single cell suspensions. For membrane immunofluorescence, the employment of enzymatic methods must be avoided. Generally, the following procedure yields satisfactory single cell suspensions:

a) cut tissue into small pieces with lancet or scissors (e.g. in a watch glass) and add cold (0–4°C) medium (volume ratio 1 : 1);

b) transfer this suspension onto a nylon filter (mesh width: 100–200 μm) on top of a glass filter;

c) rinse repeatedly with cold medium and gently press the suspension through the filter;

d) pass the suspension through needles of decreasing diameter, starting with gauges 17–19 and ending with gauges 25–27. For many tissues (e.g. mouse bone marrow, spleen, thymus, lymph node), the use of needles can be replaced by gentle pipetting and vortexing. Sonication is sometimes useful; however, this may result in considerable cell kill.

7.4.2. *Fixation*

For membrane immunofluorescence, the cells can be fixed by adding diluted formaldehyde to the suspension (final concentration: 0.04% v/v); the suspension is kept in the cold (0–4°C) for 10 min, washed, and the cells are suspended in medium. Cells which are fixed according to this mild treatment have to be measured within 24 h. Fixation for storage for longer periods can be done by using higher concentrations of formaldehyde (final concentration: 4% v/v). The cells must be washed prior to use.

7.4.3. *Labelling*

There is a variety of procedures for the labelling of cells. In our laboratory, good results have consistently been obtained by employing the procedure outlined in Table 7.IV. This procedure does not require large amounts of antisera and, if cells are carefully resuspended after each step, the number of aggregates is generally negligible.

TABLE 7.IV

LABELLING OF CELLS WITH FLUORESCEINATED ANTIBODY FOR FLOW CYTOMETRY

1. Suspend cells at $2 \times 10^7 \cdot ml^{-1}$ in HBSS[a]
2. Add 5–10 μl of properly diluted antiserum to 25 μl cell suspension
3. Leave at 4°C for 30 min
4. Wash twice with 3 ml HBSS
5. If direct labelling, proceed with step 9
6. For indirect labelling, centrifuge and add 5–10 μl properly diluted fluoresceinated anti-immunoglobulin to the cell pellet
7. Leave at 4°C for 45 min
8. Wash twice with 3 ml HBSS
9. Resuspend in 1 ml HBSS
10. Store at 0–4°C until measurement
11. Add 10 μl propidium iodide ($5\ mg \cdot ml^{-1}$) shortly before measurement

[a] Hanks' balanced salt solution of correct osmolarity and containing 0.1% sodium azide and 1% bovine serum albumin.

Antigens bound to fluorescent beads may serve as markers for antibody-secreting cells. Especially for control of the cultures of monoclonal antibody (MAb)-producing cells such antigen–bead complexes are very powerful [10]. Beads may also be used to determine the concentration of certain antibodies in sera by flow cytometers. Activated beads are incubated with serum and subsequently with the fluorescent antibody against the antibody under study. The amount of fluorescence per bead then is a measure of antibody concentration in the serum [6, 14]. This procedure can also be performed with test cells [1].

7.4.4. *Capping*

To avoid energy transfer mechanisms, capping should be prevented before and during the measurements. The sodium azide in the medium, the low temperatures and, if necessary, the fixation all serve this purpose.

7.4.5. *Aggregation*

Labelling often induces aggregation of cells. The amount of aggregation generally depends on the antiserum concentration. Therefore, to diminish aggregation, the antiserum used for labelling cells can be diluted. If the fluorescence intensity becomes too low as a result of the dilution, and if there are still aggregates, the following can be of help. Shortly before measurements, the aggregates can be disrupted by forcing the cell suspension gently through 25–27 gauge hypodermic needles. During the measurement of a cell suspension in a flow cytometer, cells may aggregate again in the sample compartment. If this occurs, change the sample regularly and pipette or "needle" the suspensions shortly before measurements.

7.4.6. *Washing*

Debris may be removed prior to the measurements as described by Shortman et al. [34] by layering the cell suspension (1–2 ml) on top of 1 ml

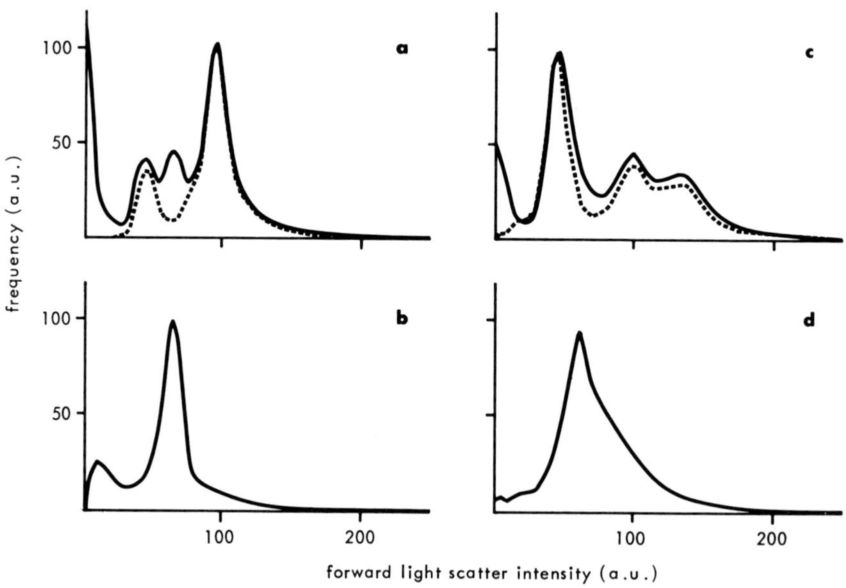

Fig. 7.5. Frequency distributions of forward light scatter intensities of mouse thymocytes (a, b) and mouse bone marrow cells (c, d). a, c) Solid lines represent all cells, dashed lines represent viable cells which did not take up propidium iodide. b, d) The scatter histogram of the dead cells which fluoresce red due to propidium iodide uptake. Each curve is normalized to its own peak value.

serum in a test tube. After 15 min, large debris will have sedimented into the serum. The cell suspension is removed and again layered on top of 1 ml serum and centrifuged. Now, the cells will be in the serum, while the small debris is in the top layer. The top layer is removed and medium added to the serum containing the cells; the cells are washed and suspended in medium containing sodium azide (0.1% v/v) at 0–4°C until use.

7.5. DEAD CELLS

In immunofluorescence measurements, flow cytometers have great difficulty in recognizing dead cells if no precautions are taken. If cells of a uniform size are studied, dead cells can be distinguished from living cells because of their lower intensity of forward light scatter (Fig. 7.5a, b). The non-specific immunofluorescence of the dead cells can then be excluded by electronical selection [23]. Generally, however, cell suspensions contain cells of different sizes. The dead cells in such a suspension cannot all be distinguished from the living cells by forward light scatter (Fig. 7.5 c,d). Several methods can be used to make the distinction. If a few drops of propidium iodide (final concentration: 50 $\mu g \cdot ml^{-1}$) are added to the suspension shortly before measurements, all nucleated dead cells with membrane damage will fluoresce brightly red. Living cells, dead cells with intact membranes and cells without nuclei do not

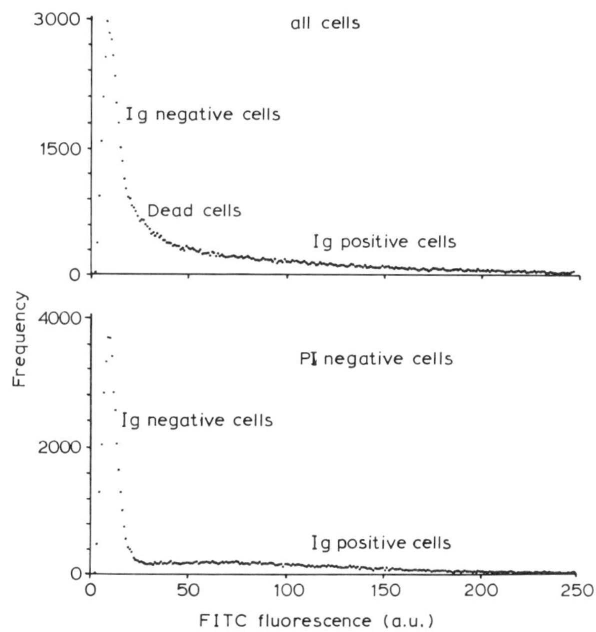

Fig. 7.6. Frequency distributions of green immunofluorescence intensities of mouse spleen cells labelled with an anti-immunoglobulin serum conjugated with FITC. Upper curve: all cells. Lower curve: only cells without propidium iodide fluorescence.

fluoresce after this treatment. By simultaneous measurements of red fluorescence from propidium iodide and of green fluorescence from FITC, the green immunofluorescence from living cells can be distinguished from that of dead cells which fluoresce green and red (Fig. 7.6).

7.6. CYTOTOXICITY ASSAY

The propidium iodide exclusion method can be used to determine the live/dead cell ratio after complement-mediated cytotoxicity tests. As a counterstain for living cells, fluorescein or bisbenzimide H33342 or H33662 can be used. Fluorescein can be brought into cells by incubation with fluorescein diacetate (FDA). Esterases split off fluorescein, which leaks out of dead cells much more rapidly than out of living cells. H33342 and H33662 stain intracellular DNA of both viable and dead cells and fluoresce blue if excited by ultraviolet light.

7.6.1. Procedure with FDA and propidium iodide

a) Dissolve FDA in acetone (5 mg·ml^{-1});
b) add 25 μl to 10 ml medium at 40°C and stir vigorously for 15 min;
c) filter the suspension (0.45 μm Millipore);
d) add 1 ml of this FDA solution to 1 ml cell suspension;
e) add 20 μl of a propidium iodide solution of 0.05 mg·ml^{-1};
f) keep at room temperature for 15 min (thymocytes) to 45 min (bone marrow and lymph nodes);
g) determine the ratio of red fluorescent cells (dead cells) to green fluorescent cells (living cells). This measurement can be performed by using a fluorescence microscope or a flow cytometer (Fig. 7.7).

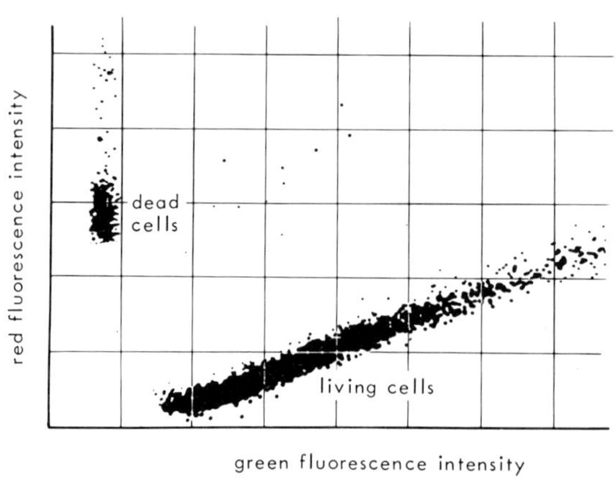

Fig. 7.7. Dot display of red versus green fluorescence intensity of thymocytes stained with propidium iodide and FDA as described in the text.

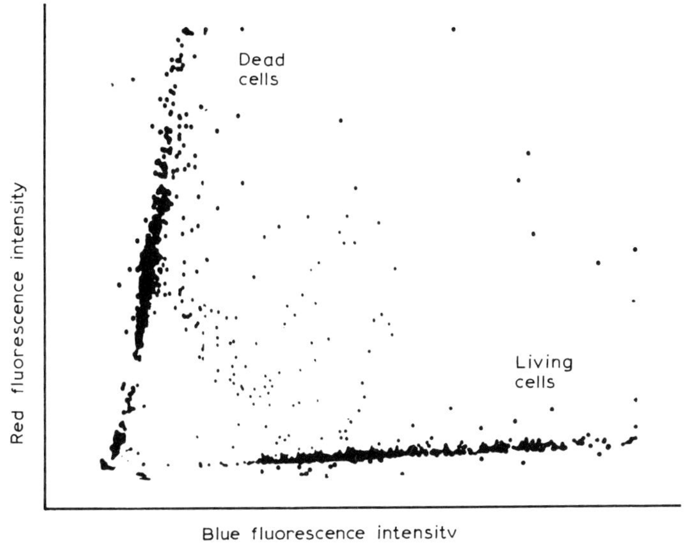

Fig. 7.8. Dot display of red versus blue fluorescence intensity of mouse bone marrow cells stained with propidium iodide and H33342 as described in the text.

7.6.2. Procedure with bisbenzimide derivatives

H33342 and H33662 may be used if cell cycle parameters are studied in combination with a cytotoxicity test or other immunological experiments [22, 36].

For this purpose: a) take 1 ml cell suspension (3×10^6 cells·ml^{-1} suspended in a medium of pH 7.0–7.5 and add 0.1 ml H33342 or H33662 of 200 μg·ml^{-1}; b) leave at 37°C for 1 h; c) add 10 μl propidium iodide of 5 mg·ml^{-1} and measure. UV excitation (350–360 nm) excites both the bisbenzimide and propidium iodide. The living cells fluoresce blue (maximum at 470 nm), while dead cells fluoresce blue and red (Fig. 7.8). The blue fluorescence of the dead cells is weaker than that of the living cells due to the energy transfer from the bisbenzimide to propidium iodide [36].

7.7. IMMUNOFLUORESCENCE MEASUREMENTS WITH FLOW CYTOMETERS

7.7.1. General considerations

The optimal cell concentration and the minimal volume of cell suspension are different for all types of flow cytometers. The optimal concentration depends on the following. The resolution of the device is partly dependent on the position of the cells in the liquid stream when they pass the laser beam. This position is best controlled if the contribution from sample fluid to that stream is minimal, i.e. the ratio of sheath fluid to sample fluid is maximal.

This minimal amount of sample fluid has to contain enough cells to measure at a reasonable rate without much coincidence. In the FACS, we therefore generally run cell samples containing about 3 × 10^6 cells/ml. The smallest volume usually is 0.5 ml. However, a device has been recently constructed by which very small aliquots (10 μl) can be processed by the flow cytometer [39]. The device is commercially available (Becton Dickinson FACS Systems, Sunnyvale, CA).

During analysis, cells sediment in the sample tube. Large cells sediment more rapidly than small cells. Therefore, the sample has to be stirred repeatedly to measure a random selection of cells. Alternatively, the sample tube has to be emptied completely in each measurement.

7.7.2. Sterilization of the instrument

If cells are to be cultured after separation, the sorter has to be sterilized prior to the experiment in order to avoid bacterial or other contamination of the sorted fractions. Sterilization may be accomplished as follows:
a) run water through tubing to remove saline;
b) flush all tubing with ethanol (with or without Hibitane 0.5% v/v);
c) flush with cold boiled water to remove Hibitane, ethanol and air bubbles;
d) fill tubing with sterile sheath fluid. Sterility during sorting is made more certain by gently blowing sterile air above the collection tubes.

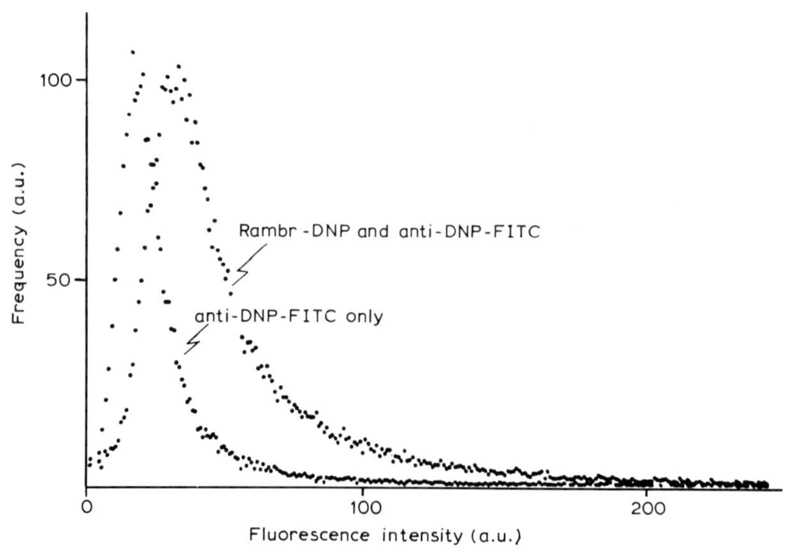

Fig. 7.9. Frequency distribution of the fluorescence intensity of BC3 mouse bone marrow cells labelled with a fluoresceinated anti-dinitrophenol (DNP) serum after labelling with a DNP-conjugated rabbit anti-mouse brain antiserum (Rambr-DNP). Control cells were not labelled with Rambr-DNP.

7.7.3. *Control measurements*

Several controls must be run in the same experiment to take full advantage of flow cytometers. This is mainly due to the fact that "negative" cells may also give rise to a detectable signal. This signal may be caused by autofluorescence, by light scatter and by noise (see next section). Therefore, the most important control is a measurement of the fluorescence signals of cells not binding antiserum. Ideally, these cells should be prepared in a similar manner to that of the cells under study. This is possible only for some studies, e.g. for measurement of the binding of specific antisera against specific mouse strains, cells from other mouse strains can serve as controls. Ideally, the control cells should have the same light scatter properties as the cells under study. With cells that are labelled directly it is appropriate to measure the immunofluorescence for various dilutions of the antiserum. With indirect labelling, the appropriate control for "negative" cells is a sample containing the cells under study which were treated in a similar way to the indirectly labelled ones except for the first antiserum incubation: cells should be kept at 37°C without the first antiserum present for the same time period as that of the cells with antiserum (Fig. 7.9).

If two or more fluorochromes are used, controls should include cells that are incubated with only one of each fluorochrome. FITC has a long tail of fluorescence emission into the red spectral region, which can interfere with measurements of TRITC immunofluorescence [24]. Controls of cells stained with FITC only may serve to quantitate the amount of FITC fluorescence detected by the photomultiplier which is set to measure red fluorescence from TRITC. The opposite situation, TRITC fluorescence detected by the green sensitive photomultiplier, should also be checked by the use of a control consisting of cells which are labelled with TRITC antiserum only.

7.7.4. *Background analysis*

A good control for most samples is the measurement of noise. The noise may originate from laser light fluctuations, photomultipliers, room light or debris in sheath or sample fluid. If the flow cytometer is triggered by the forward light scatter signal to measure the fluorescence signal (as is usually the case), the device will also attribute a certain value to the noise from the fluorescence detection system if the cell does not fluoresce at all. The noise can be quantitated by triggering the flow cytometer randomly or, better still, by triggering the device to measure "fluorescence" when no cells are illuminated (Fig. 7.10).

7.7.5. *Simultaneous light scatter measurements*

Simultaneous measurements of light scatter are very helpful. As mentioned above (Section 7.5), dead cells can sometimes be distinguished from

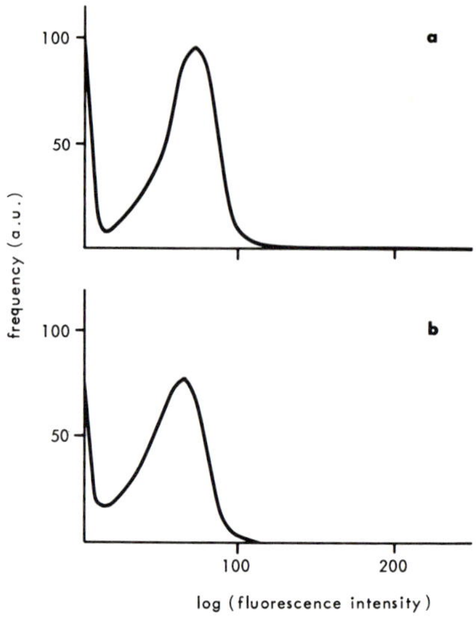

Fig. 7.10. Frequency distributions of fluorescence intensity signals of unstained BC3 mouse spleen cells (a) and of the fluid jet (b). The latter distribution was obtained by triggering the flow cytometer to measure fluorescence 10 μs after the detection of a cell. The distribution of control AKR mouse spleen cells which are negative in Thy-1,2, labelled as described for Fig. 7.4, was similar to that shown in a.

living cells on the basis of forward light scatter measurements. Debris may also be detected by light scatter, and by electronic windows the contribution of debris to the fluorescence measurement may be eliminated.

Furthermore, since forward light scatter intensity is a measure of size, simultaneous scatter measurements may reveal subpopulations of cells with equal immunofluorescence intensity but different sizes and, if the scatter detector is calibrated, simultaneous measurements may be used to determine the number of bound antibodies per unit volume or membrane area. This sometimes decreases the number of subpopulations found, since cells increase in size during the cell cycle, exposing more binding sites in G_2/M than in G_0/G_1 (Fig. 7.11).

7.8. SORTING AND FURTHER TREATMENTS

Several factors may be of influence when cells are to be sorted in a flow cytometer: the desired purity and recovery, the time duration, the number of cells to be sorted, the viability, etc. This section may be of help in deciding how to set up a sorting experiment.

7.8.1. Purity and recovery

In sorting flow cytometers, cells pass the measuring point ideally one by one and can be deflected shortly afterwards in droplets (Fig. 7.12). During the

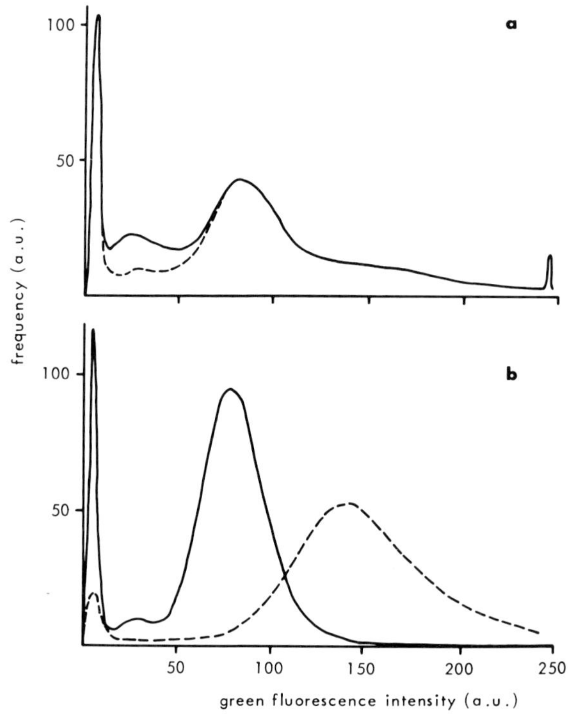

Fig. 7.11. Frequency distributions of fluorescence intensities of mouse thymocytes labelled with an anti-Thy-1 antiserum, and subsequently with anti-rabbit immunoglobulin FITC. Upper curves: all cells (——); cells which did not show red propidium iodide fluorescence (– – –). Lower curves: thymocytes with forward light scatter intensities of 65–75 arbitrary units (a.u.) (the majority of the cells) (——); cells with forward light scatter intensities of 110–120 a.u. (– – –), which have twice the volume of the majority of the cells [44].

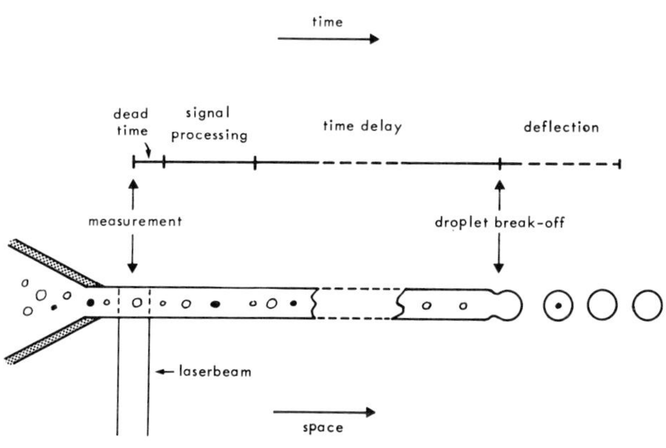

Fig. 7.12. Schematic outline of coupling between time and space for signal processing in a sorting flow cytometer.

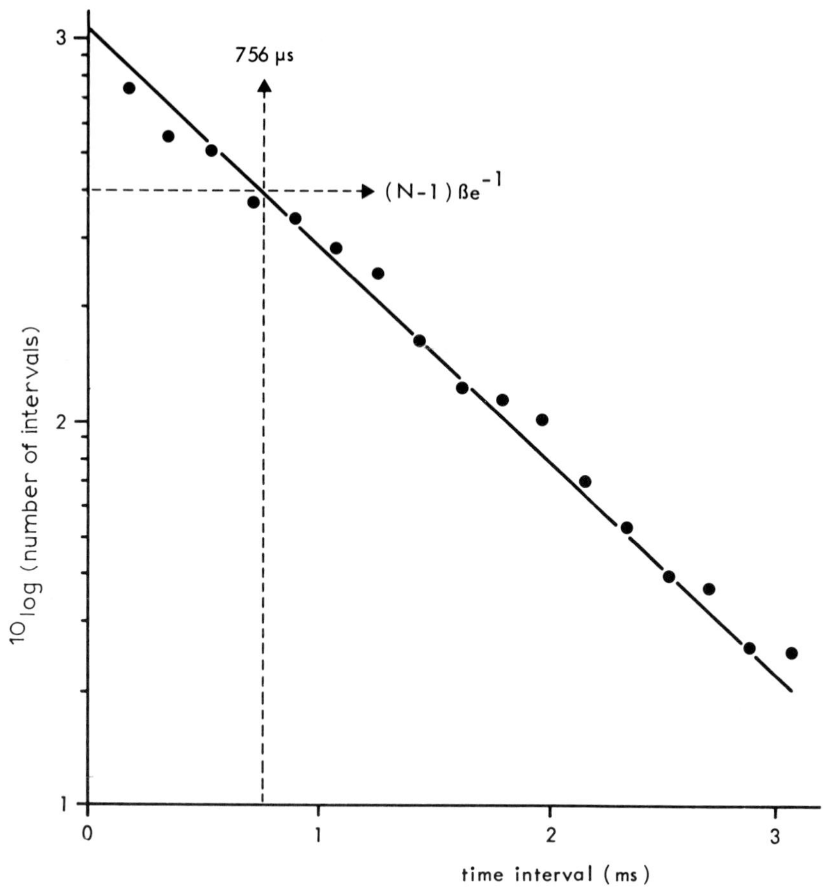

Fig. 7.13. Example of a frequency distribution of time intervals between cells in a FACS II flow cytometer.

measurement of a cell and for some microseconds afterwards, most flow cytometers are "blind" for other cells. Subsequently, the device requires 2–30 µs to analyse the detected light pulse. During this period, other cells can be detected but not analysed. Thereafter, the cell flows to the drop break-off point, where it arrives 0.1–1.0 ms after the measurement. Other cells can be detected and analysed during this period. Consequently, depending on the rate at which cells are fed into the measuring position, a number of cells is neither detected nor analysed by the device.

Most sorting flow cytometers are provided with electronics which can be set to prevent sorting of a certain cell if it is closely followed or preceded by another one which is not to be sorted into the same direction. Therefore, a choice can be made between purity and recovery to some extent. The arrival of cells at the measuring point is at random. As can be seen from Fig. 7.13, the distribution can be described by the function:

$$F(t) = (N-1)\,\beta\, e^{-\beta t}$$

where F is the frequency, N is the total number of cells measured for the distribution curve, β the mean number of arrivals per unit of time (β^{-1} is the mean time interval), and t is the length of the time interval between the cells*. Therefore, as expected, the arrival of cells at the measuring position and the time intervals between cells are distributed according to the Poisson statistics.

This knowledge allows accurate prediction of cell loss and sorting purity for the various settings of the flow cytometer. We have to distinguish the following three possibilities in our device (a FACS II, Becton Dickinson FACS Systems, Sunnyvale, CA).

1. Cells follow each other within the dead time of the machine (3 μs). This time duration is similar to that of the cell's traversal through the laser light beam. Therefore, the device does not distinguish the cells separately. The measured pulse will be a combination of the pulses of the cells. This phenomenon may thus contribute to the impurity of the sort. The incidence of such events is generally low: the probability equals $[1-\exp(-\beta\, t_d)]$, where t_d equals 3 μs (Appendix B, Section 7.11). So, with $\beta = 10^4 \cdot s^{-1}$ (a high rate), the probability is only 3%, with $\beta = 10^3 \cdot s^{-1}$, it is 0.3%**.

2. Cells follow each other during the analysing time which, in our device, equals 12 μs with the pulse height analyser off and 22 μs with the analyser on. In this situation, the sorter detects another cell but does not analyse it. For this event, our sorter has the option "abort" which, if set at "on", prevents deflection of cells spaced shorter than the analysing time. Here, the investigator has to decide between impurity and recovery. The probability of the event equals $[1-\exp(-\beta\, t_a)]$, where t_a is the analysing time (Appendix B). With t_a = 12 μs and $\beta = 10^4 \cdot s^{-1}$ the probability equals 11%; with $\beta = 10^3 \cdot s^{-1}$ it equals 1.2%. Therefore, with abort at "on" and 10^4 cells/s, about 20% of the desired cells are not deflected. With abort "off" and 10^4 cells/s the sorted fraction contains unwanted cells. The percentage of unwanted cells also depends on the fraction of all cells to be sorted**.

3. Cells follow each other with a time duration longer than the analysing time but short enough for the cells to be deflected in the same droplets.

---

* Due to discretization in the pulse height analyser for our sorter the value of $(N-1)$, β cannot be read directly from the intersection with the y-axis in Fig. 7.13. The intersection in this figure gives the sum of all time intervals shorter than one channel of the analyser. In this experiment, one channel was equivalent to 18 μs, N equaled 46,500, β equaled 1323 s^{-1}; therefore

$$\int_0^{18\,\mu s} (N-1)\,\beta\, e^{-\beta t} dt = 0.0235 \times 46500 = 1094$$

which is indeed the intersection with the y-axis.

** The contribution of the event to the impurity depends on the fraction of all cells which is desired, e.g. if 90% of the cells are to be sorted into a certain direction, the probability that an unwanted cell follows a wanted cell is only 10%. Consequently, the contribution to impurity is much smaller than if, e.g. only 10% of the cells are sorted, where 90% of the closely following cells are unwanted. Therefore, to accurately determine the impurity and cell loss, the probabilities found by the Poisson statistics must be multiplied by the fraction of desired cells.

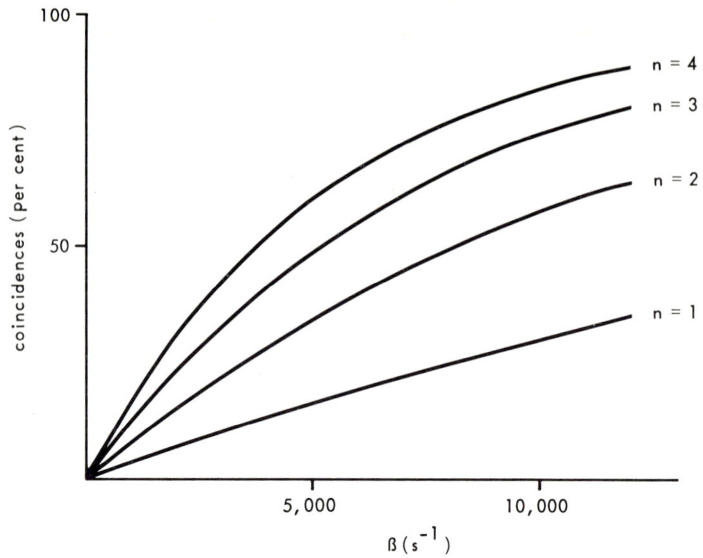

Fig. 7.14. Dependence of coincidence on cell rate (β) in a flow cytometer for different numbers of droplets deflected per wanted cell (n). Curves are calculated by use of Eqn. (2), Appendix B.

Clearly, this time duration is dependent on the number of droplets deflected per cell and on the drop frequency. The probability of this event equals $1-\exp[-(2n-1)\,\beta f^{-1}-\beta\, t_a]$, where n is the number of droplets deflected per cell and f is the droplet frequency (Appendix B). With $f = 4 \times 10^4 \cdot s^{-1}$, $n = 2$, $t_a = 12$ μs and $\beta = 10^4 \cdot s^{-1}$, this probability equals 58%; for $\beta = 10^3 \cdot s^{-1}$, it equals 8% (Fig. 7.14). Here too, the investigator has to make a choice between purity and recovery. Many wanted cells may be lost if pure sorting is required at high cell rates ("coincidence in" mode in the FACS II) and the contamination of the deflected cells by unwanted cells may be high at high cell rates. Also here, the degree of contamination depends on the fraction of wanted cells in the unseparated cell suspension.

7.8.2. Processing of high cell numbers

If many cells are to be sorted pure and without significant loss, the following procedure is recommended. First, sort at a high rate ($10^4 \cdot s^{-1}$) all wanted cells plus their coincident neighbours. Then centrifuge the sorted, collected fraction, suspend the cells at the appropriate sample concentration and re-run the cells through the sorter at a rate which is low enough for the required recovery for a pure sort. Using the relations given in Section 7.8.1, it can be calculated that, by a two-run procedure, a subpopulation of 10% can be sorted in an almost pure state and with less than 10% loss out of 10^7 cell within 1 h. In a single run, this would take almost 3 h. It is clear that this time difference becomes greater at higher cell numbers. It will also become greater if the fractions to be sorted are smaller and if less cell loss is required.

7.8.3. *Other causes of impurity and cell loss*

A number of causes of cell loss other than those mentioned in Section 7.8.1 have been described in the literature. Stovel [37] discovered that large cells in the nozzle may disturb the droplet formation. This disturbance results in random droplet formation and consequently, in possible cell loss. Stöhr and Vogt-Schaden [36] have observed cell kill by laser excitation employing the H33662 stain as described in Section 7.6.2. We have detected cell kill by laser light in the FACS with cells that were stained with H33342 after incorporation of bromodeoxyuridine (BrdU) [45]. No kill was observed without BrdU incorporation.

Another cause of impurity and cell loss is the uncertainty of the cell position after measurement. During the time between measurement and droplet formation, the cell may drift away with respect to its original position in the liquid jet. The longer the time, the further away this diffusion occurs. If the time between measuring and drop break-off points is long, impurities can be prevented by charging more droplets per cell. However, this may increase cell loss: as discussed above (Section 7.8.1), the recovery decreases if more droplets are deflected per cell. As is shown in Fig. 7.15, more than 90% of the cells can be caught by charging only one droplet per cell if the deflection pulse is given at the right time point. We generally charge two or three drops per cell to anticipate minor changes in the time duration between measurement and arrival at the break-off point during a run.

A most important cause of cell loss is drying out of the collection tube wall. This loss can be prevented by rinsing the collection tube wall where the deflected droplets arrive with some drops of medium containing 5–20% serum prior to and after the sorting. Alternatively, siliconized collection tubes can be

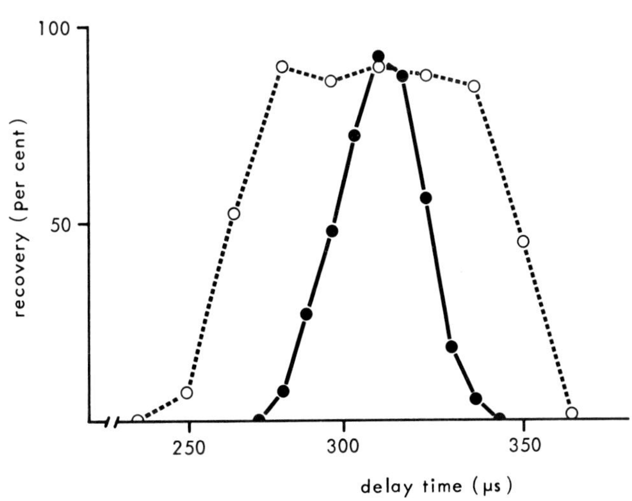

Fig. 7.15. Dependence of the recovery of sorting on the time duration between measurement and droplet charging. ●—●, One droplet deflected per cell; ○—○, three droplets deflected per cell.

used. The use of plastic tubes is not recommended. The plastic may become charged locally at the spot where the charged droplets fall and then repulse the charged droplets, resulting in cell loss.

Finally, we would like to mention here two causes of cell loss which are specific for larger cells. Firstly, sedimentation in the sample tube may affect the recovery. Repeated stirring is the only solution presently known to overcome or prevent this loss. Secondly, several flow cytometers are equipped with a filter in the sample feed line. These filters may catch the large cells. Therefore, such filters should be used only with reservations.

7.8.4. Collecting

The deflected droplets are usually collected in glass tubes. For various purposes, other collection vials, plates or slides can be used. A device for collecting known numbers of deflected cells in separate wells of microtest plates is commercially available (Becton Dickinson FACS Systems, Sunnyvale, CA). Collection on microscope slides has been done since the earliest days of flow sorting. Due to the necessary saline in the sheath fluid, the morphology of air-dried samples on microscope slides is poor, unless some serum is added to the drop on the slide prior to drying. If enough cells are available, it is recommended to sort cells for morphological studies in glass tubes and process them from there as usual. It may be worth mentioning here that, with three droplets deflected per cell and with a nozzle of 50 μm diameter, the cell concentration in a collection tube should be about $5 \times 10^5 \cdot ml^{-1}$

Another collector for deflected droplets may be filtration paper. This is being used for sorted cells which have been radioactively labelled prior to the sorting. The filtration paper can be processed as usual in liquid scintillation counters.

Special collectors have also been described for further analysis of small sorted fractions by Pipkin et al. [31]. The wider the field of application of cell sorters, the more heterogeneous will the collection of collector devices probably be. It may save time to construct your own optimal collector. For most purposes of further cell handling, collecting in glass tubes gives adequate results. Only if the cell positioning capability of the sorter is is used, e.g. for sorting single cells in separate wells of microtest plates, is it really necessary to employ other collectors.

7.9. SOME ILLUSTRATIVE EXAMPLES

7.9.1. Experimental hematology

The stem cells of blood are of low incidence, even in haemopoietic organs like bone marrow. Still, their membrane characteristics can be determined by the following procedure. Bone marrow cells are labelled with fluoresceinated

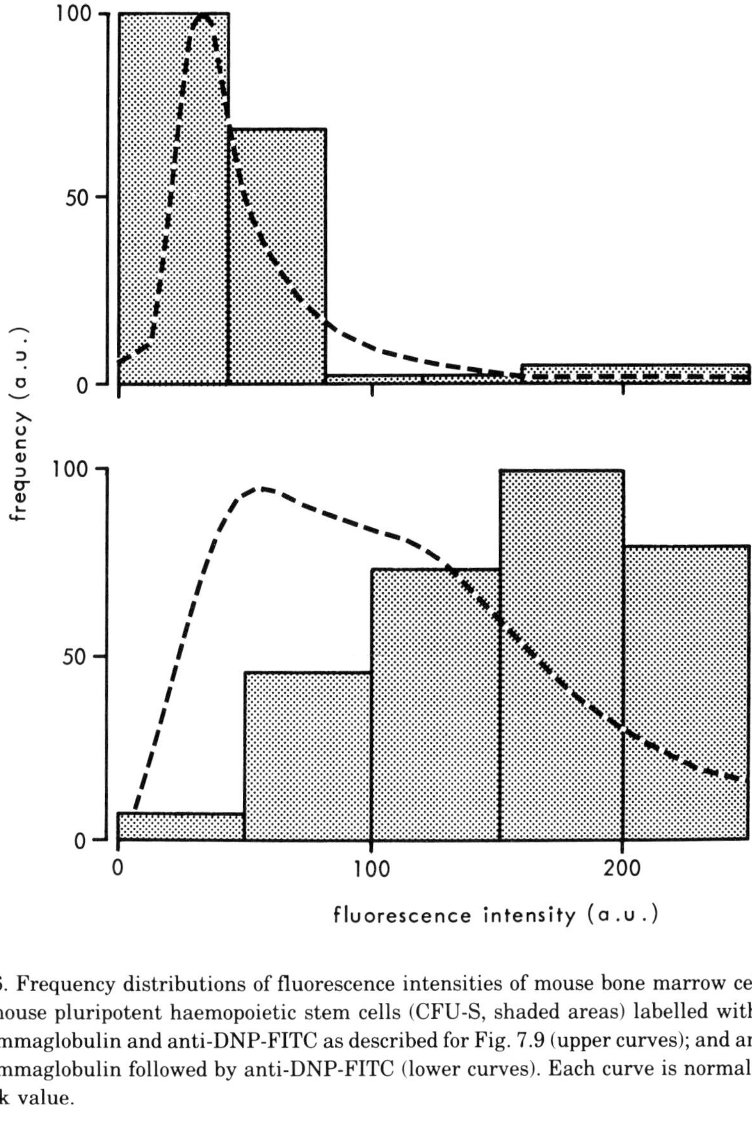

Fig. 7.16. Frequency distributions of fluorescence intensities of mouse bone marrow cells (– – –) and of mouse pluripotent haemopoietic stem cells (CFU-S, shaded areas) labelled with: Rambr-DNP-gammaglobulin and anti-DNP-FITC as described for Fig. 7.9 (upper curves); and an anti-H2-DNP-gammaglobulin followed by anti-DNP-FITC (lower curves). Each curve is normalized to its own peak value.

antibody. The cells are then separated into subpopulations differing in fluorescence intensity by the use of a cell sorter. The number of stem cells in each subpopulation is then determined by in vivo and in vitro culture assays which make use of the colony-forming capacity of stem cells. Fig. 7.16 shows the result of such a procedure for mouse bone marrow labelled with anti-Ia and with anti-Thy-1. It can be concluded from these results that the pluripotent haemopoietic stem cell of the mouse contains more Ia-antigens than the average bone marrow cells and that this stem cell bears no θ-antigens.

A problem with in vivo assays is the presence of the antibody on the cells after the sorting. The immune system of the host mouse is likely to kill the labelled cells; or, alternatively, the homing of the cells may be affected by the label. In the above experiments, the label was removed by papain treatment after sorting and prior to injection into the host mice [41]. Since only a mild treatment with papain did not affect the in vivo assay with unlabelled control bone marrow cells, the labelling with antibody had to also be at low concentrations. Therefore, the distributions of the fluorescence intensities (i.e. the amount of antibody per cell) shown in Fig. 7.16 do not show as much difference between "positive" and "negative" cells as can be obtained with higher concentrations of antibody. As pointed out by Böhn [4], however, affinities can be assessed accurately only at low concentrations. Therefore, we have devoted several sections of this chapter to stressing that controls and background noise should be included in the experiments.

7.9.2. Morphological studies

Human tonsil cells were labelled with anti-IgA FITC. About 18% of the cells were found to be positive (Fig. 7.17). The negative cells were separated from the positive cells by a cell sorter in a two-run procedure. After this, no anti-IgA-positive cells could be detected in the negative fraction. This fraction was subsequently labelled with combinations of anti-IgD, anti-IgM and anti-IgG, bound to FITC and/or TRITC. These preparations were examined by fluorescence microscopy for relative numbers of fluorescent cells. Using this procedure, it was possible to assay the simultaneous occurrence of three different Ig subclasses on a single cell; this is not easily possible without a cell sorter, because of the availability of only two useful fluorescent dyes for antibody staining. The problem in this experiment was the low incidence of some of the Ig subclass combinations (less than 2%), whereas the loss of wanted cells in the cell sorter was about 20%. It could be shown that this loss was not likely to be selective for a specific subpopulation of tonsil cells. However, due to

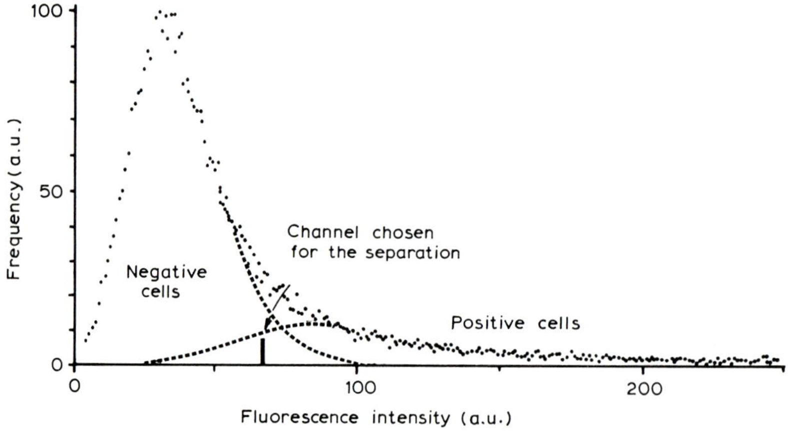

Fig. 7.17. Frequency distribution of the fluorescence intensity of human tonsillar cells labelled with FITC-labelled Fab fragments of a sheep immunoglobulin fraction directed against human IgA. Theoretical curves (---) for the distribution of "positive" and "negative" cells are indicated.

this loss, no conclusive evidence could be obtained from the experiment. The results, however, were in accordance with data obtained later by other methods [42].

7.9.3. Clinical applications

At present, clinical applications of flow cytometers almost always employ only the analysing capability of the device. Sorting of subpopulations of enough cells, e.g. to transplant into patients, by a flow cytometer sorter takes too long to be of practical use. The analysing power of flow cytometers for immunofluorescence studies in patients has been employed extensively by Greaves and Janossy and coworkers. They have reported adequately on this work (e.g. refs. 17, 18, 32); hence we refer to the literature with respect to this subject. So far, the sorting power of the technique has been employed in immunofluorescence studies with patients only to separate fetal cells from the peripheral blood of pregnant women [12]. It is likely that other applications will be found in the future. The sorter is capable in principle of separating one special cell out of many others and of positioning that cell accurately. Further progress in cell culturing and genetic engineering will enable clinicians to grow as many replicates of that one cell as needed.

7.10. APPENDIX A: CALIBRATION BY FLUORESCENT BEADS

To prevent blockage of the flow system, beads smaller than about 50 μm must be selected. Sephadex G-25 superfine beads (Pharmacia Fine Chemicals, Uppsala) are swollen (24 h, in 2 M NaOH) and subsequently sieved to remove the largest beads. Sieving may be performed wet, using two layers of nylon gauze of 50 μm mesh width. Sieving twice gives best results. The beads are then provided with amino groups by heating them to 80°C with 100 $mg{\cdot}ml^{-1}$ aminoethylsulphuric acid in 2 M NaOH for 24 h. Subsequently, staining is performed for 45 min with FITC or TRITC, the concentrations in the staining solution ranging from 10^{-6} to 10^{-2} $mg{\cdot}ml^{-1}$.

The extinction of single FITC- or TRITC-stained beads can be derived from measurements of the extinctions of suspensions containing 1×10^5–5×10^6 beads/ml. The extinction of the beads incubated with higher concentrations than 10^{-4} $mg{\cdot}ml^{-1}$ dye can be determined by the following procedure. Suspend the beads at a known concentration in buffered glycerol (1 part phosphate-buffered saline to 9 parts of glycerol) at pH 7.8 in 1 cm cuvettes. Determine the extinction at 498 and 600 nm for FITC and at 555 and 650 nm for TRITC in a spectrophotometer provided with strongly scattering material in between cuvette and photodetector [33]. Determine also the extinction of a cuvette with a similar concentration of unstained beads at the same wavelengths. Subtract from the extinction value with stained beads the values with unstained beads and subsequently, for FITC, from that at 498 nm that at 600 nm and, for

TRITC, from the value at 555 nm that at 650 nm. The resultant values are the extinctions of the suspensions corrected for light scatter, for FITC at 498 nm and for TRITC at 555 nm.

Next, determine the size distribution of the beads by a calibrated microscope or a Coulter counter. From these data, the extinction of a single absorbing spherical particle can be derived by calculations as described by Duysens [8]:

$$T_p = 1 - \frac{E_{sus}}{p \log e} \qquad (1)$$

where T_p is the average transmission of a single particle, E_{sus} is the extinction of the suspension, and p is equal to the total cross-sectional area of all particles in the cuvette divided by the area of the side of the cuvette which is perpendicular to the light beam and as far as the cuvette is filled. Furthermore:

$$T_p = 2[1-(1+\alpha_p)\, e^{-\alpha_p}]/\alpha_p^2 \qquad (2)$$

where $\alpha_p = (\log e)\, E_p$ and E_p is the extinction of a particle for a beam passing through the center of that sphere. From E_p the concentration of FITC or TRITC in the beads can be calculated by application of Beer's law, if the specific molar absorbances (ϵ) are known. According to Van Dalen and Haaijman [40], the molar absorbance of bound FITC at 498 nm and pH 7.8 is $6.9 \times 10^4\ M^{-1} \cdot cm^{-1}$ and that of TRITC at 555 nm and pH 7.8 is $4.8 \times 10^4\ M^{-1} \cdot cm^{-1}$. The size of the beads is known from measurements. Since E_p is the extinction through the center of the sphere, the diameter of the sphere must be taken as optical path length applying Beer's formula. Therefore, $c = E_p/d$, with c as the concentration and d as the diameter.

The absolute number of dye molecules per bead is dependent on the volume of the bead. The distribution of the sizes of the beads is known; therefore, the average number of fluorescent molecules can be calculated. If the distribution of sizes of beads is rather heterogeneous, the calculations described by Latimer and Eubanks [19] should be employed. With the sieved Sephadex beads, however, the difference between the results of the calculations described above and those of the more precise calculations of Latimer and Eubanks is less than 3%.

After determination of the number of dye molecules per bead for several concentrations of dye in the incubation medium, run aliquots of beads through the flow cytometer and measure fluorescence and light scatter intensities under controlled conditions (temperature, pH, PM power, gain, filters, laser power). The fluorescence intensity per bead should be dependent on the number of dye molecules per bead only. This can be tested in the range of dye concentrations where the extinction can be measured. If this condition is fulfilled, the number of dye molecules per bead for the lower concentration can be obtained by extrapolation or from the fluorescence measurements (Fig. 7.18).

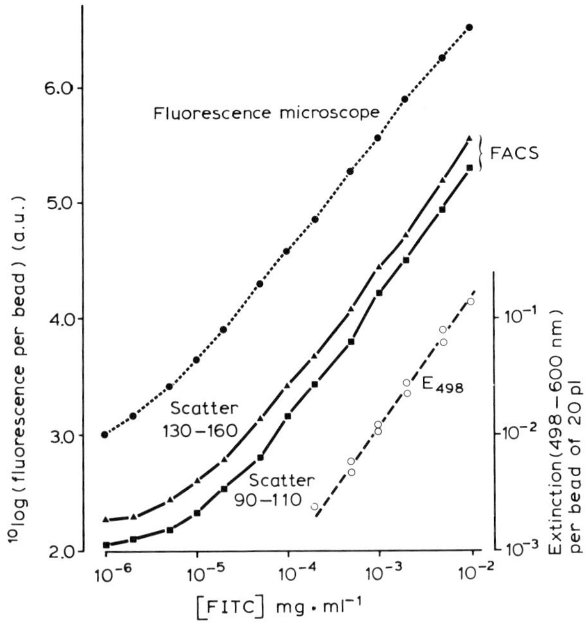

Fig. 7.18. Relative fluorescence intensities and extinctions of small aminoethyl Sephadex beads stained for 45 min in various concentrations of FITC. Measurements by an automated fluorescence microscope [9] (●); measurements by a FACS II of beads with scatter intensities of 130–160 a.u. (▲) and of 90–110 a.u. (■); extinction of individual beads calculated as described in Appendix A from absorbance measurements with bead suspension (○).

By measuring a sample of beads with a known fluorochrome content in each series of immunofluorescent measurements, the results can be expressed in absolute values (Fig. 7.19, right-hand scale) and so different series of measurements can be compared quantitatively. From Fig. 7.19, it can also be derived that "negative" cells produce signals in our FACS which are equivalent to 2×10^3 FITC molecules.

7.11. APPENDIX B: CALCULATIONS TO DETERMINE RECOVERY AND PURITY OF SORTING

7.11.1. Poisson statistics

The distribution function of Poisson statistics is:

$$f(t) = \beta e^{-\beta t}. \tag{3}$$

The expected average value of t equals therefore:

$$t = \int_0^{\infty} t f(t)\, dt = \beta^{-1} \tag{4}$$

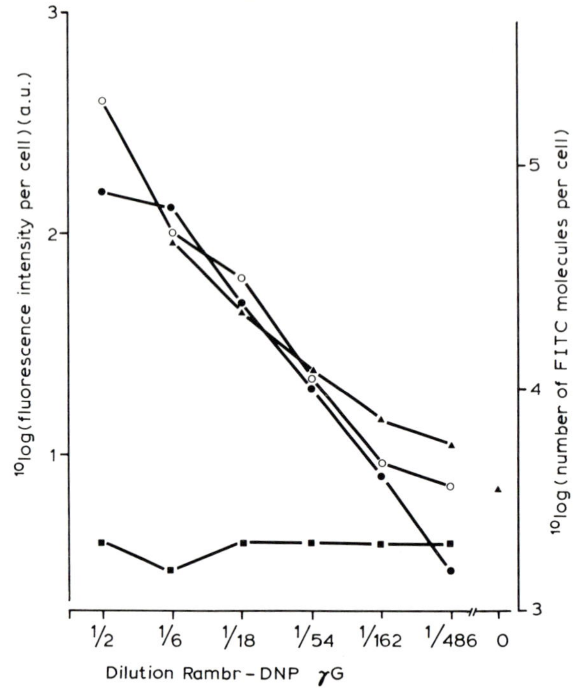

Fig. 7.19. Median fluorescence intensities of mouse thymocytes incubated with various concentrations of Rambr-DNP-gammaglobulin and FITC-labelled rabbit anti-chimpanzee albumin DNP. Anti-DNP-FITC dilutions: 1/6 (▲); 1/18 (○); 1/54 (○); no anti-DNP-FITC (■). The fluorescence intensity scale was calibrated by the use of FITC beads.

and the probability that n events happen within a time period, T equals:

$$P_n(\beta,t) = \int_0^T f(t)\mathrm{d}t\, P_{n-1}[\beta(T-t)] = \frac{(\beta T)^n}{n!}e^{-\beta T} \tag{5}$$

The chance that $n = 0$ or P_0 is therefore:

$$P_0(\beta,T) = e^{-\beta T}$$

7.11.2. Coincident arrival of cells

In a flow cytometer in which the arrival of the cells at the measuring position is described by the Poisson statistics, the probability that a cell is not followed by another cell with a time interval shorter than T is equal to the probability of no cells during T, P^-, is given by:

$$P^- = e^{-\beta T} \tag{7}$$

Consequently, the probability for coincidence, P^+, equals:

$$P^+ = 1-e^{-\beta T} \tag{8}$$

If coincidence of both preceding and following cells is recognized by the flow cytometer, the square of P_f can be taken as the total probability of no coincidence. The probabilities for coincidences of more than two cells can be calculated from Eqn. 5. This event is of importance in sorting with flow cytometers if both β (the cell rates) and the number of deflected droplets per cell are high.

7.11.3. Sorting of coincident cells

For pure sorting in flow cytometers, it is necessary that only droplets are deflected which contain wanted cells. Therefore, the sorting device has to recognize unwanted cells preceding and following a wanted cell within the time duration of the deflection pulse. For various reasons, a longer time duration is taken in most devices. In our FACS II, it is checked whether another cell follows or precedes the wanted cell within a time duration of $(2n-1)/2f$, where n is the number of droplets deflected per cell and f is the droplet frequency. During this time, the sorter also determines whether coincident cells are wanted or not. If they are, they can also be deflected.

There is also a probability that the cells are too close to both be analysed. This probability equals $[1-\exp(-\beta\ t_a)]$, where t_a is the time duration for analysis.

The total probability then that cells are possible impurities in the deflected droplets equals:

$$1 - \exp\left[\frac{-(2n-1)\beta}{f} - \beta\ t_a\right] \qquad (9)$$

For $f = 4 \times 10^4 \cdot s^{-1}$ and $t_a = 12.5\ \mu s$, which are realistic figures this can be written more simply as:

$$1-\exp\left[-(2n-\tfrac{1}{2})\beta/f\right].$$

ACKNOWLEDGEMENTS

Most of the work discussed here is part of a study on the regulation of haemopoiesis which is supported by a programme grant of The Netherlands Foundation for Medical Research (FUNGO) which is subsidized by The Netherlands Organization for the Advancement of Pure Research (ZWO).

We are indebted to all who are or have been involved in this study through several years.

REFERENCES

1 Aaij C., Von dem Borne A.E.G.Kr., Verheugt F.W.A. and Engelfriet C.P. (1978) The use of continuous flow fluorometry in immunohaematology. *In* Knapp, W., Holubar, K. and Wick, G. (eds.), Immunofluorescence and Related Staining Techniques (Elsevier/North-Holland Biomedical Press, Amsterdam) pp. 137–146.

2 Arnold B., Battye F.L. and Miller J.E.A.P. (1979) An improved method for selecting T-cell hybridomas by the fluorescence-activated cell sorter. J. Immunol. Methods *29,* 353–360.

3 Basch R.S., Janossy G. and Greaves M.F. (1977) Murine pluripotential stem cells lack Ia-antigen. Nature *270,* 520–522.

4 Böhn B. (1976) High-sensitivity cytofluorometric quantitation of lectin and hormone binding to surfaces of living cells. Exp. Cell Res. *103,* 39–46.

5 Chan S.S., Arndt-Jovin D.J. and Jovin T.M. (1979) Proximity of lectin receptors on the cell surface measured by fluorescence energy transfer in a flow system. J. Histochem. Cytochem. *27,* 56–64.

6 Cram L.S. and Forslund J.C. (1974) A quantitative method for evaluating fluorescent antibodies and the conjugation process. Immunochemistry *11,* 667–672.

7 Dorman B.P., Shimizu N. and Ruddle F.H. (1978) Genetic analysis of the human cell surface: antigenic marker for the human X chromosome in human–mouse hybrids. Proc. Natl. Acad. Sci. U.S.A. *75,* 2363–2367.

8 Duysens L.N.M. (1956) The flattening of the absorption spectrum of suspensions, as compared to that of solutions. Biochim. Biophys. Acta *19,* 1–12.

9 Haaijman J.J. (1977) Quantitative immunofluorescence microscopy: methods and applications. Ph.D. Thesis, University of Leiden, Leiden, The Netherlands.

10 Herzenberg L.A. and Ledbetter J.A. (1979) Monoclonal antibodies and the fluorescence-activated cell sorter: complementary tools in lymphoid cell biology. *In* Kaplan, J.G. (ed.), The Molecular Basis of Immune Cell Function (Elsevier/North-Holland Biomedical Press, Amsterdam) pp. 315–330.

11 Herzenberg L.A., Sweet R.G. and Herzenberg L.A. (1976) Fluorescence-activated cell sorting. Sci. Am. *234,* 109–117.

12 Herzenberg L.A., Bianchi D.W., Schröder J., Cann H.M. and Iverson G.M. (1979) Fetal cells in the blood of pregnant women: detection and enrichment by fluorescence-activated cell sorting. Proc. Natl. Acad. Sci. U.S.A. *76,* 1453–1455.

13 Hirschfield T. (1979) Fluorescence background discrimination by prebleaching. J. Histochem. Cytochem. *27,* 96–101.

14 Horan P.K. and Wheeless Jr. L.L. (1977) Quantitative single cell analysis and sorting. Science *198*, 149–157.

15 Horan M., Horan P.K. and Williams C.A. (1975) Quantitative measurement of SV40 T-antigen production. Exp. Cell Res. *91,* 247–252.

16 Hunt S.V. (1979) The presence of Thy-1 on the surface of rat lymphoid stem cells and colony-forming units. Eur. J. Immunol. *9,* 853–859.

17 Janossy G., Francis G.E., Capellaro D., Goldstone A.H. and Greaves M.F. (1978) Cell sorter analysis of leukemia-associated antigens on human myeloid precursors. Nature *276,* 176–178.

18 Janossy G., Hoffbrand A.V., Greaves M.F., Ganeshaguru K., Pain C., Bradstock K.F., Prentice H.G., Kay H.E.M. and Lister T.A. (1980) Terminal transferase enzyme assay and immunological membrane markers in the diagnosis of leukemia: a multiparameter analysis of 300 cases. Br. J. Haematol. *44,* 221–234.

19 Latimer P. and Eubanks C.A.H. (1962) Absorption spectrophotometry of turbid suspensions. A method of correcting for large systematic distortions. Arch. Biochem. Biophys. *98,* 274–285.

20 Leary J.F. and Todd P. (1977) Laser cytophotometric detection of variations in spatial distribution of concanavalin A cell surface receptors following viral infection. J. Histochem. Cytochem. *25,* 908–912.

21 Ledbetter J.A., Rouse R.V., Micklem H.S. and Herzenberg L.A. (1980) T cell subsets defined by expression of Lyt-1, 2, 3 and Thy-1 antigens. J. Exp. Med. *152,* 280–295.

22 Loken M. (1980) Simultaneous quantitation of Hoechst 33342 and immunofluorescence on viable cells using a fluorescence activated cell sorter. Cytometry *1,* 136–142.
23 Loken M.R. and Herzenberg L.A. (1975) Analysis of cell populations with a fluorescence-activated cell sorter. Ann. N.Y. Acad. Sci. *254,* 163–171.
24 Loken M.R., Parks D.R. and Herzenberg L.A. (1977) Two-color immunofluorescence using a fluorescence-activated cell sorter. J. Histochem. Cytochem. *25,* 899–907.
25 Mathieson B.J., Sharrow S.O., Campbell P.S. and Asofsky R. (1979) An Lyt differentiated thymocyte subpopulation detected by flow microfluorometry. Nature *277,* 478–480.
26 Mekada E., Yamaizumi M. and Okada Y. (1978) An attempt to separate mononuclear cells fused with human red blood cell-ghosts from a cell mixture treated with HVJ (Sendai virus) using a fluorescence activated cell sorter (FACS II). J. Histochem. Cytochem. *26,* 62–67.
27 Melamed M.R., Mullaney P.F. and Mendelsohn M.L. (eds.) (1979) Flow Cytometry and Sorting (J. Wiley, New York).
28 Miller M.H., Powell J.I., Sharrow S.O. and Schultz A.R. (1978) Rapid data collection, analysis and graphics for flow microfluorometry instrumentation. Rev. Sci. Instrum. *49,* 1137–1142.
29 Mullaney P.F., Steinkamp J.A., Crissman H.A., Cram L.S., Crowell J.M., Salzman G.C. and Martin J.C. (1976) Laser flow microphotometry for rapid analysis and sorting of mammalian cells. Ann. N.Y. Acad. Sci. *267,* 176–190.
30 Parks D.R., Bryan V.M., Oi V.T. and Herzenberg L.A. (1979) Antigen-specific identification and cloning of hybridomas with a fluorescence-activated cell sorter. Proc. Natl. Acad. Sci. U.S.A. *76,* 1962–1966.
31 Pipkin J.L. Jr., Hinson W.G. and Hunziker J. (1980) A collection device for small electronically sorted samples from flow cytometers. Anal. Biochem. *101,* 230–237.
32 Révész T. and Greaves M. (1975) Ligand-induced redistribution of lymphocyte membrane ganglioside GM1. Nature *257,* 103–106.
33 Shibata K. (1958) Spectrophotometry of intact biological materials. Absolute and relative measurements of their transmission, reflection and absorption spectra. J. Biochem. *45,* 599–623.
34 Shortman K., Williams N. and Adams P. (1972) The separation of different cell classes from lymphoid organs. V. Simple procedures for the removal of cell debris, damaged cells and erythroid cells from lymphoid cell suspensions. J. Immunol. Methods *1,* 273–287.
35 Steinkamp J.A. (1977) Multiparameter analysis and sorting of mammalian cells. *In* Catsimpoolas, B. (ed.), Methods of Cell Separation, *Vol. 1,* Chap. 7 (Plenum Press, New York–London).
36 Stöhr M. and Vogt-Schaden M. (1980) A new dual staining technique for simultaneous flow cytometric DNA analysis of living and dead cells. *In* Laerum, O.D. et al. (eds.), Flow Cytometry IV (Universitetsforlaget, Bergen) pp. 96–99.
37 Stovel R.T. (1977) The influence of particles on jet breakoff. J. Histochem. Cytochem. *25,* 813–820.
38 Sweet R.G. (1965) High frequency recording with electrostatically deflected ink jets. Rev. Sci. Instrum. *36,* 131–136.
39 Sweet R.G., Stovel R.T., Nozaki T. and Moore W.A. (1979) Small sample delivery system. *In:* Automated Cytology VII. Abstract II-18 (Engineering Foundation, New York).
40 Van Dalen J.P.R. and Haaijman J.J. (1974) The determination of the molar absorbance coefficient of tetramethyl rhodamine isothiocyanate relative to fluorescein isothiocyanate. J. Immunol. Methods *5,* 103–106.
41 Van den Engh G.J. and Platenburg M.G.C. (1978) Suppression of CFU-S activity by rabbit-anti-mouse brain serum can be overcome by treatment with papain. Exp. Hematol. *6,* 627–630.
42 Vessière-Louveaux F.M.Y.R., Hijmans W. and Schuit H.R.E. (1980) Presence of multiple isotopes on the surface of human tonsillar lymphocytes. Eur. J. Immunol. *10,* 186–191.
43 Visser J.W.M., Haaijman J.J. and Trask B.J. (1978) Quantitative immunofluorescence in flow cytometry. *In:* Knapp, W., Holubar, K. and Wick, G. (eds.), Immunofluorescence and Related Staining Techniques (Elsevier/North Holland Biomedical Press, Amsterdam) pp. 147–160.
44 Visser J.W.M., Van den Engh G.J. and Van Bekkum D.W. (1980) Light scattering properties of murine hemopoietic cells. Blood Cells *6,* 391–407.

45 Visser J.W.M., Bol S.J.L. and Van den Engh G.J. (1981) Characterization and enrichment of murine hemopoietic stem cells by fluorescence activated cell sorting. Exp. Hematol. *9*, 644–655.

46 Williams A.F., Galfré G. and Milstein C. (1977) Analysis of cell surfaces by xenogeneic myelomo-hybrid antibodies: differentiation antigens of rat lymphocytes. Cell *12*, 663–673.

Wick et al. (eds) Immunofluorescence Technology. Selected Theoretical and Clinical Aspects © *Elsevier Biomedical Press, 1982*

CHAPTER 8

Production of monoclonal antibodies for the analysis of the ontogeny of the murine lymphoid system by flow cytometry

J.J. HAAIJMAN

Institute for Experimental Gerontology TNO, Rijswijk, The Netherlands

8.1. INTRODUCTION

Monoclonal antibodies are secreted by plasmacytoma cells in which the genetic information for the specified antibody has been introduced by fusion with spleen cells of immunized donors. The technique was first described by Köhler and Milstein [10] who were able to immortalize mouse spleen cells producing antibodies directed against sheep red blood cells. They used polyethylene glycol to fuse spleen cells of an immunized mouse with an aminopterin-sensitive plasmacytoma line growing in tissue culture. Hybrid cells were selected on the basis of their aminopterin resistance. Fusion is possible between plasmacytoma and spleen cells of the same species and of closely related species. Mouse–mouse hybridizations have been used most frequently up to now for monoclonal antibodies against non-murine antigens. For anti-mouse antibodies immune rat spleen cells were fused with mouse plasmacytomas [12] and with rat plasmacytoma cells [5].

Monoclonal antibodies produced by hybridomas recognize only one antigenic determinant (epitope) and are monospecific by definition. The method of their preparation offers the possibility of dissecting the antibody repertoire of a given donor against a given epitope. It thus becomes possible to use the full recognition capability of the vertebrate immune system. Hybridoma antibodies differ from conventional antisera in that they consist of one molecular-defined immunoglobulin species with one constant and one variable part for heavy and light chains. Monoclonal antibodies have already been proven to be invaluable in the detection of antigenic determinants within complex antigen systems such as cell surface markers. Before the introduction of monoclonal antibodies cell surface determinants could only be demonstrated with alloantisera provided that the antigens showed allelic differences, or by conventional xenogeneic antisera. Alloantisera are generally weak and difficult to obtain in sufficient quantities, especially in the mouse system. Xenogeneic antisera are often stronger but show varying degrees of unwanted specificities. Hybridoma antibodies, however, can be produced in large quantities and their apparent specificity is only determined by the presence or absence of the antigenic determinant they recognize. Before going into details with regard to the application of monoclonal antibodies in the detection of cell surface antigens, the techniques of producing these antibodies will be illustrated with one example: the generation of a monoclonal rat antibody directed against mouse IgM.

8.2. THE GENERATION OF MONOCLONAL RAT ANTI-MOUSE IgM

Lewis rats were immunized intraperitoneally with a mixture of 50 μg of CBPC 112 (IgM of the "b" allotype) and 50 μg HPC 76 (IgM of the "a" allotype) precipitated on alum and given together with 2×10^9 killed *Bordetella pertussis* organisms. The purified proteins were kindly provided by Dr. V.T. Oi (Department of Genetics, Stanford University, CA). A booster injection with the same amount of antigen was given 3 days prior to fusion. The Lou/Ws1/M derived hypoxanthine–aminopterin–thymidine (HAT)-sensitive 210 RC Y3. Ag1.2.3. (abbreviated Y3) [5] myeloma line was used as the parent line. The plasmacytoma line was obtained from the Medical Research Council by the courtesy of Dr. C. Milstein (Department of Biochemistry, University of Cambridge, U.K.). Hybridization was carried out essentially according to the protocol of Oi and Herzenberg [15]. In brief, for fusion 10^8 Y3 cells were co-centrifuged with 10^8 spleen cells from an immunized rat. Polyethylene glycol 1500 (PEG; Merck, A.G., Darmstadt, F.R.G.); 50% in RPMI 1640 tissue culture medium (Flow Laboratories, Irvine, Scotland) was added slowly and allowed to react with the cells for 1 min. The PEG was then slowly diluted in 240 ml of HAT-containing RPMI medium with 15% fetal calf serum (FCS). The suspension was plated into ten 24-well Costar plates (Costar Division, Cambridge, MA) and these were incubated at 37°C in 7% CO_2. The culture medium was changed every 7 days. Clones of growing cells were apparent only after 21 days of culture. Supernatants were tested with solid-phase radioim-

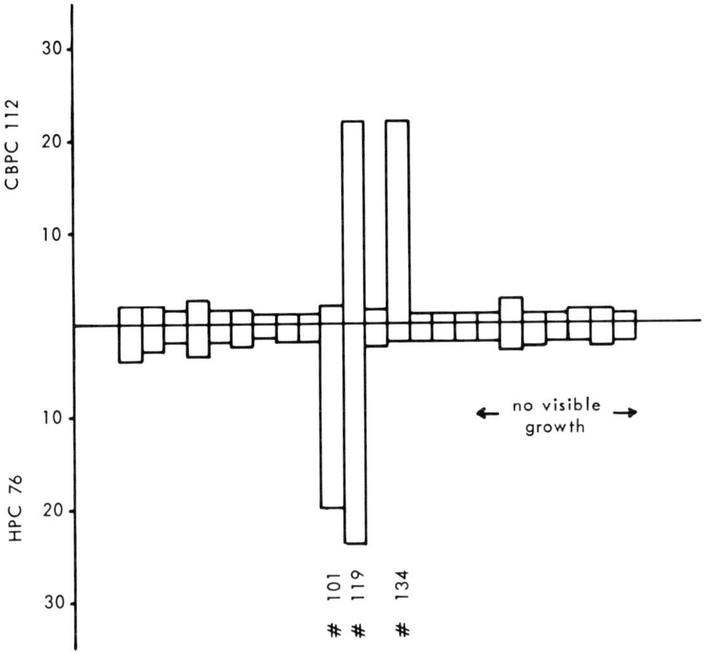

Fig. 8.1. Initial screening of supernatants of the 151 hybridization. 96-well polyvinyl plates were coated with 30 μl CBPC112 or HPC76 (each 100 μg/ml in 0.01 M Tris-HCl, pH 8.5) per well for 1 h. Plates were rinsed three times with 1% BSA in PBS (RIA buffer, containing also 0.02% NaN_3). 20 μl of supernatants diluted 1 : 2 in RIA buffer were added to individual wells and incubated for 1 h. After washing with RIA buffer 20,000 c.p.m. of ^{125}I -labeled rabbit anti-rat IgG (RARA IgG) was added. 1 h later the plates were again washed and the amount of radioactivity bound to individual wells was determined by γ-counting. Shown is the ratio between wells incubated with supernatant and those incubated with RIA and ^{125}I-labelled RARA IgG alone. Supernatants from wells showing no visible growth served as a second control.

munoassay (RIA) for the presence of anti-IgM, using an oligospecific rabbit anti-rat immunoglobulin (kindly provided by Dr. R.L. Coffman, Department of Pathology, Stanford University, CA) labeled with I^{125} as the second step. The rabbit antiserum had been affinity-purified and extensively absorbed to remove any antibody cross-reacting with mouse immunoglobulins. Test results are shown in Fig. 8.1. CBPC 112 and HPC 76 were used as the target antigens in the assay.

Only three out of 23 tested supernatants showed reactivity in the RIA with one or both antigen preparations. Supernatant 101 reacted only with the HPC 76 myeloma, supernatant 134 only with the CBPC 112, and supernatant 119 with both proteins. Supernatants 101 and 134 were tentatively classified as anti-idiotypic and 119 as a possible anti-IgM. For further characterization the supernatants were tested on an array of purified myeloma proteins of various classes and subclasses. They failed to react (Table 8.I) to any significant degree with MOPC 21 (IgG_1, "a" allotype), MOPC 245T (IgG_1, "b" allotype), GPC 8 (IgG_{2a}, "a" allotype), and CBPC 101 (IgG_{2a}, "b" allotype). The cultures 101, 119 and 134 were transferred via hypoxanthine–thymidine (HT) medium to

TABLE 8.I

CHARACTERIZATION OF SUPERNATANTS FROM HYBRIDIZATION 151

Antigen	Heavy chain	Allotype	Supernatant No.			
			101	119	125	134
CBPC 112	IgM	b	2.9[a]	26.7	3.4	28.3
HPC 76	IgM	a	23.6	28.6	3.9	2.8
MOPC 104E	IgM	a	2.9	53.0	4.1	1.9
351E4A12	IgM	b	5.2	18.0	1.8	1.7
NMS (SJL/J)	–	b	1.0	1.6	0.9	1.0
NMS (BALB/c)	–	a	1.4	6.5	1.1	1.4
MOPC 21	IgG_1	a	1.1	1.4	1.0	0.9
MOPC 245T	IgG_1	b	1.3	1.2	2.1	1.1
CBPC 101	IgG_{2a}	b	1.5	2.9	0.9	2.0
GPC 8	IgG_{2a}	a	1.5	2.0	1.2	2.3

[a] Ratio c.p.m. supernatant/c.p.m. background.

normal medium and expanded into flasks before subcloning. Subcloning was done with the fluorescence-activated cell sorter (FACS) modified according to Parks et al. [18] to deposit single live cells into individual wells of 96-well microtitration plates. Subclones were derived from all three initial cultures. They were expanded in 24-well Costar plates and eventually grown in flasks. To purify antibody, batches of antibody-rich supernatant were passed over a goat anti-rat immunoglobulin–Sepharose column. Elution was first with 0.02 M glycine-HCl, pH 3.2, followed by 0.02 M glycine-HCl, pH 2.3. Because the binding activity on a mg of protein basis was much higher in the pH 3.2 eluted fraction, reported experiments were performed with this fraction only. Purified antibody preparations were analysed in double diffusion with anti-class and -subclass-specific antisera. The 101 antibody proved to be an IgG_{2c}, 119 an IgG_{2a} and 134 an IgG_1 antibody, respectively. The 119 antibody was characterized for its chain composition by first growing the hybrid cells in the presence of ^{35}S-labeled methionine. The radioactive antibody was subjected to two-dimensional gel electrophoresis according to Jones [9]. In the first dimension the reduced antibodies were separated on the basis of isoelectric point, and in the second dimension according to size.

The Y3 light chain was still synthesized clearly by the 119 cells and the antibody was classified as HLK according to the nomenclature of Köhler and Milstein [10]. Large-scale production of the 119 antibody was obtained by growing the cells as a tumor in Lou rats. No measures were taken to elicit the formation of ascites; instead, the fully grown (subcutaneous) tumor was suspended in RPMI 1640 medium. The cells were stored in liquid nitrogen and the supernatant was treated with ammonium sulphate in order to precipitate the immunoglobulins. Fig. 8.2 shows a comparison between the supernatant derived from the tumor and that from tissue culture. The first one contained

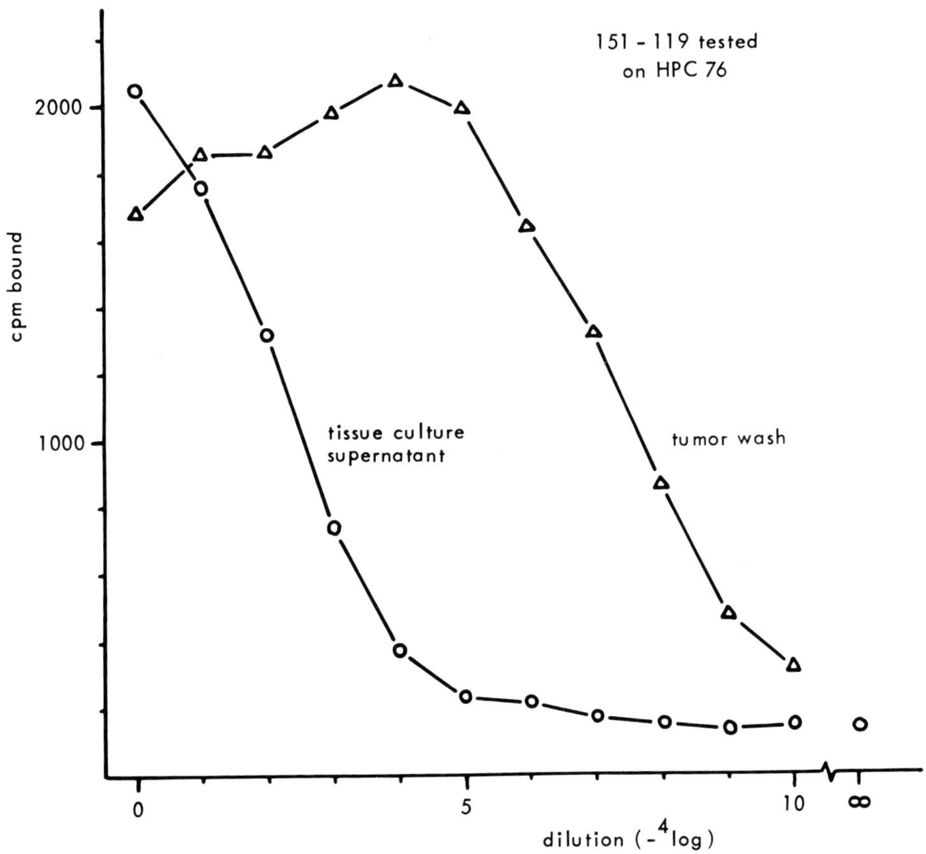

Fig. 8.2. Large-scale production of rat anti-mouse IgM. The 151-119 cells were grown in Lou rats (see text) as a tumor. Polyvinyl plates were coated with HPC 76 protein to measure the relative amount of anti-IgM in antibody-rich supernatant and the tumor wash. (For assay see legend Fig. 8.1.)

about 1000-fold more antibody (as judged from the titration curves) than the second one. One trial to grow the 119 cells in Lewis hosts failed to yield a measurable tumor.

Remarks

1. The choice of the Lewis rat as the immunized donor was only determined by logistics. The Lou/Ws1/M strain appeared rather difficult to breed and too few animals were available at the time this experiment was initiated. Ideally, the Lou × Lewis hybridoma cells should be grown in the appropriate F_1. Mild irradiation of hosts belonging to other strains, however, may prove equally satisfactory.

2. The fusion protocol presented here differs in two important aspects from that given by Oi and Herzenberg [15]: a) the cells were plated into full-strength HAT medium immediately after fusion; and b) the concentration of plated cells was much lower, e.g. 10^6/ml instead of 2×10^7/ml. The purpose of

these modifications was to reduce both the need for repeated feeding of the cultures and the likelihood of more than one fusion event per individual well. Fazekas de St. Groth and Scheidegger [4] reported in extenso on this type of variables in the hybridization technique.

3. No feeder cells were used during either the initial period after fusion or subcloning. Fazekas de St. Groth and Scheidegger [4] found a significant increase in the number of positive cultures if macrophages were added on days −1, 0 or 1 of fusion.

4. Although a small number of wells with growing cells after HAT selection makes it highly improbable that these wells contain more than one clone, subcloning in our view is obligatory if the antibody is to be prepared in bulk. It seems advisable to reclone a given cell line (especially with the HLK chain composition) at least once every 6 months in order to exclude the selective propagation of fast growing, non-producing, variants.

5. Testing supernatants from fusion experiments is the most time-consuming part of the monoclonal antibody technique. Testing should be performed only on supernatants from wells with clear cell growth, which are supernatants that turn yellow about 2–3 days after adding new medium. In the initial testing the immunizing antigen should be used as the target and a polyvalent anti-immunoglobulin as the second step. In later stages of the characterization, more discriminative targets and second steps should be used. In our hands, the solid-phase RIA proved sufficiently sensitive and reproducible to find the relevant cultures; however, promising developments have recently been reported, using enzyme-linked immunosorbent assay (ELISA) techniques [11]. These techniques allow visual inspection of the end product and appear to be very suitable, especially for initial screening in which a quantitative assay is not mandatory.

6. Purification of antibodies from hybridoma supernatants is best achieved by affinity chromatography, using conventional heteroantisera preferably of not too high an affinity. This allows the elution of bound antibodies under relatively mild conditions, resulting in antibody preparations of high quality. Because the passage of large volumes of supernatant through Sepharose columns is time-consuming, one might employ a concentration step first. Promising in this respect is the method in which the cells are grown in 5%, instead of 15%, serum-containing medium. The spent medium in which cells have been growing is concentrated either by vacuum or by pressure. Volume reductions of 20–40-fold are easily achieved. Ammonium sulphate or sodium sulphate precipitation may help to reduce the volume another 20-fold. Normally, the last step is not necessary, and the vacuum or pressure concentrated supernatants are passed over the columns directly.

7. If production of large quantities of antibody-containing supernatant is aimed at, it is advisable to try to adapt the cells to newborn calf serum (NCS) instead of FCS. This will reduce the cost of production by a factor of approximately 4. Most cells will grow equally well in NCS and FCS. However, some lines proved to be resistant to the change. Fazekas de St. Groth and

Scheidegger [4] selected a variant from the well-known Sp2/0 line, which will grow in either FCS, NCS or horse serum. According to their report hybridomas derived with this variant (F/O) are equally amenable.

8.3. TECHNIQUES FOR THE USE OF MONOCLONAL ANTIBODIES WITH IMMUNOFLUORESCENCE

Several methods will be introduced and discussed in this section pertinent to the use of rat and mouse monoclonal antibodies in immunofluorescence. Most of the data shown were obtained with the FACS (FACS II, Becton, Dickinson and Company, Mountain View, CA) equipped with a logarithmic amplifier. The logarithmic transformation of the photomultiplier output has two advantages.

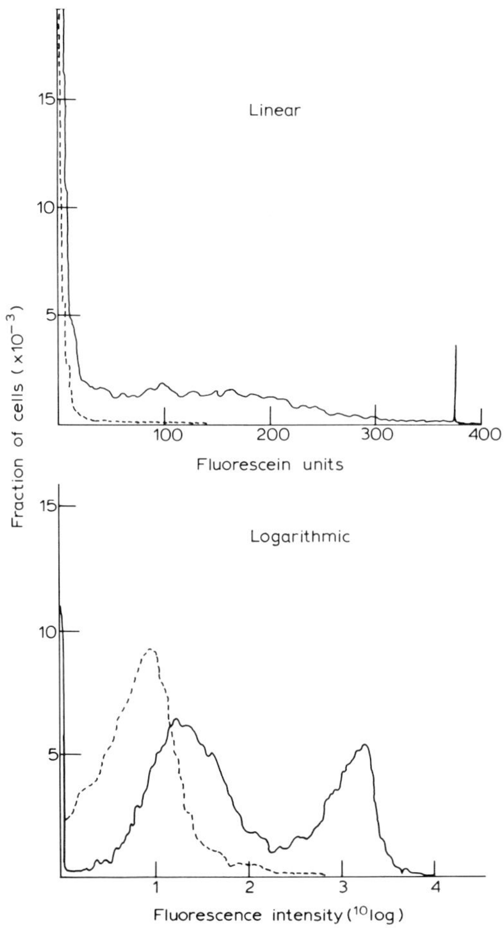

Fig. 8.3. Comparison between linear and logarithmic FACS analysis. 10^6 BALB/c spleen cells (8 weeks of age) were incubated with 1 μg FITC-conjugated rat anti-mouse Thy-1 (59-AD2.2). The FACS histograms of 10^4 cells each were obtained after linear and logarithmic processing of the photomultiplier output. Dashed lines: unstained cells.

1. The density of most cell surface antigens appears to be logarithmically distributed resulting in Gaussian-like histograms. Moreover, the width of the distribution is considerably reduced, which allows a better discrimination between various populations. In Fig. 8.3 a comparison is shown for the staining of mouse spleen cells with directly conjugated rat anti-Thy-1. One set of curves (unstained cells were used as the control) was obtained with the regular linear amplifier and in the other set logarithmic transformation was used. Clearly, the logarithmic amplifier is superior in revealing two separate populations. The smaller the population of positive cells, the more important this feature becomes.

2. Another advantage of logarithmic amplification is the accommodation of a large range of fluorescence intensities within a single histogram. In other words, the most dull and the most bright cells are generally on scale. This fact proved to be very important in the study of the representation of IgM on the cell surface (see below).

8.3.1. Preparation of cells for FACS analysis

Cell suspensions were made by the regular methods into medium consisting of RPMI 1640, 5% heat-inactivated and filtered FCS, 0.1% NaN_3 and 10 mM Hepes. After washing, the cells were counted using the acridine orange–ethidium bromide method [18]: appropriately diluted cell suspensions were mixed 1 : 1 (v/v) with a solution containing 5 μg/ml acridine orange and 100 μg/ml ethidium bromide (alternatively, propidium iodide may be used). Under the fluorescence microscope the living and dead cells show up green and red, respectively. The fluorescence is strong enough to allow admixing of low levels of transmitted light for the visualization of the hemocytometer grid. The fluorescence microscope is best equipped with a 150 W halogen lamp, KP 490 excitation filters and a LP 520 barrier filter. The cell suspensions were adjusted to 2–4 $\times$ 10^7 cells/ml. Twenty-five to 50 μl of cell suspension (10^6 cells) were incubated with 50 μl of reagent in individual wells of 96-well microtitre plates (Dynatech Laboratories Inc., Alexandria, VA, cat. No.: 1-220-24). Washing of cells between successive reagents was done by adding medium followed by centrifugation at relatively low speed (3 min at 800 r.p.m.). Two wash cycles were performed routinely. The cells were taken up in 1 ml of medium after the last wash and were ready for FACS analysis.

Remarks

1. It is essential for FACS analysis to have cell preparations with as few dead cells as possible, since these cells will accumulate dye indiscriminately. Specific guidelines are difficult to give because these will change with every organ studied. It appears of importance to always handle the cells on ice and allow as little time as possible between collection of the cells and eventual analysis. The medium seems to have little influence on viability. Good results were obtained both with the RPMI and with buffered saline.

2. Removal of red blood cells is normally unnecessary if one is working with spleen, thymus, lymph node or bone marrow suspensions. The FACS allows the discrimination of red blood cells, lymphocytes and larger cells on the basis of scatter signals. Under certain circumstances (for instance if samples have to be sorted) it is obligatory to remove red cells. All normal methods such as NH_4Cl, glycerol or distilled water treatment are applicable in FACS work. No significant difference in yield or quality of the preparations was observed. A note of caution may apply to distilled water; in some experiments a selective loss of a certain subpopulation was found.

Lymphocytes from peripheral blood can only be studied adequately with the FACS if the red blood cells are removed. Centrifugation over a layer of Lympholyte-M (Flow Laboratories, Irvine, Scotland) appears to be the most suitable method.

3. The number of cells per incubation should be held constant relative to the amount of antibody added to allow comparisons on fluorescence quantities. It is therefore advisable to express the amount of added antibodies in $\mu g/10^6$ cells instead of a dilution of a given antibody preparation.

4. Regular RPMI 1640 contains phenol red which is fluorescent under green excitation. This fluorescence is seen as a small dircct current (DC) shift of the fluorescence signals and is negligible under almost all circumstances.

8.3.2. Incubation schemes

8.3.2.1. Direct techniques

Quite a few monoclonal antibodies can be used directly fluoresceinated. An example was already shown in the case of rat anti-mouse Thy-1 (Fig. 8.3). The following conjugation method (see also Goding [6]) may be employed: 1–2 mg of antibody in 2 ml of buffer is dialysed against 0.1 M $NaHCO_3$, for at least 4 h. 50 µg of fluorescein isothiocyanate (FITC) or tetramethylrhodamine isothiocyanate (TRITC) is added dissolved in dimethyl sulphoxide (1 mg of fluorochrome/ml DMSO). The solution is added in small aliquots and mixed thoroughly with the protein solution. The mixture is allowed to stand for 4 h at room temperature or 8 h at 4°C. It is then desalted on a prewashed PD10 disposable column (Pharmacia Fine Chemicals, Uppsala) using 3 ml of eluting buffer. Washing of the column is done with 1% bovine serum albumin (BSA) in phosphate-buffered saline (PBS). As a precaution 0.02% NaN_3 is added. The column is normally eluted with this buffer also. The disposable, calibrated columns preclude the use of extensive equipment for locating the labeled materials.

8.3.2.2. Indirect techniques

1. Anti-immunoglobulin sandwich. The most widely used form of the indirect technique is still the anti-immunoglobulin method where a labeled antiserum is employed directed against the immunoglobulins (Ig's) of the species in which the specific antibody was prepared. In the murine system this sandwich can be used if the monoclonal antibodies directed against cell surface determinants were derived either from rat × rat or rat × mouse fusions. An example of the former is the already described rat anti-mouse IgM. Binding of this antibody to murine B cells was successfully demonstrated by using a fluorescent mouse anti-rat Ig. Using a mouse second step has the advantage that no additional binding to Fc receptors (except that of the rat monoclonal) is to be expected [12]. In practice, SJL/J mice were immunized intraperitoneally with purified rat IgG emulsified in complete Freund's adjuvant. Immunization was repeated three times. The bleeds of several donors were pooled and subjected to ammonium sulphate precipitation, followed by fractionation over Sepharose-bound protein A. The drop-through fraction (primarily IgG_1 antibodies) was used for conjugation. Choice of either the IgG_1 or IgG_2 fraction seems not to be crucial. Good staining was also obtained with the latter. However, a possible advantage is that the IgG_1 antibodies will not bind complement, which makes it less likely that stained and sorted cells will be lysed in vivo upon transfer. Non-murine (for instance rabbit or goat) anti-rat Ig preparations are often able to give satisfactory results also. Care should be taken to remove all possible cross-reactivity with murine Ig which can generally be accomplished by repeated passage over Sepharose-bound normal mouse serum (NMS) (use pooled sera of several allotypes). Affinity purification on Sepharose bound rat Ig is advisable prior to absorption of unwanted specificities. Originally, binding of the rat × mouse hybridoma proteins directed against mouse cell surface determinants was demonstrated with the mouse anti-rat Ig sandwich [12]. The technique has been superceded lately by the direct technique (see e.g. ref. 13).

2. *Hapten sandwiches.* The normal anti-Ig technique is unapplicable if allogeneic hybridoma antibodies are used. Conjugated anti-(sub)class specific antisera can be used in a few cases, e.g. anti-IgG, anti-IgG_1 or anti-IgG_{2a}, if the substrate is thymus. With spleen or bone marrow this solution is unattractive because the direct binding to B-cell populations may confuse the interpretation of the results. This is even more the case if the antigens studied are confined to the B cells such as IgD or Ia antigens. In these cases the hapten sandwiches which were introduced by Wofsy et al. [23] provide the only workable solution. Haptens are conjugated to antibodies and binding of these antibodies to cells is followed with a fluorescently labelled anti-hapten antibody. A few of these systems have been worked out: nitroiodophenol (NIP), dinitrophenol (DNP), arsanilic acid (ARS), and lactose (Lac). The performance of all four systems seems to be quite similar. DNP may not be advisable since some anti-DNP antibodies have been shown to react with nuclear factors (Dr. J. Radl, personal communication). Conjugation of NIP with antibodies using NIP succinimide requires the same procedure as that described for fluorescein and rhodamine. Conjugation of ARS and Lac involves a more complex chemistry although, recently, active intermediates have become available commercially. The most promising member of the hapten sandwich group is the biotin–avidin method [2, 8]. The binding between biotin and avidin is exceedingly strong and

specific. Biotin may be conjugated to protein in a similar way as for the regular fluorochromes, using the biotin succinimide available from Pierce (Rockford, IL). Avidin is available through Sigma (St. Louis, MO) and can be labelled normally (it may be advisable to test the biotin binding of various avidin batches before conjugation, since some avidin batches may perform better than others; Dr. D.R. Parks, personal communication). Labelled avidin can also be purchased directly (Vector Labs., Burlingame, CA; Becton, Dickinson and Co., Mountain View, CA).

Remarks

1. The direct technique is to be preferred wherever applicable because of its simplicity and unambiguity in the interpretation of the results. The direct technique, however, is generally slightly less sensitive than the indirect techniques. Another problem with the direct technique is the choice of the appropriate controls. The regularly used unstained cell preparation is, of course, unsatisfactory. Some investigators use immunoglobulin preparations of hybridomas with unknown antigen-binding activity but which are of the same class as the test hybridoma. It is evident that individual peculiarities of particular preparations may go unnoticed in this way. The only proper controls in direct techniques are substrate controls.

2. The direct technique generally gives less bright staining than the indirect techniques. On the other hand, the signal to noise ratio is often better.

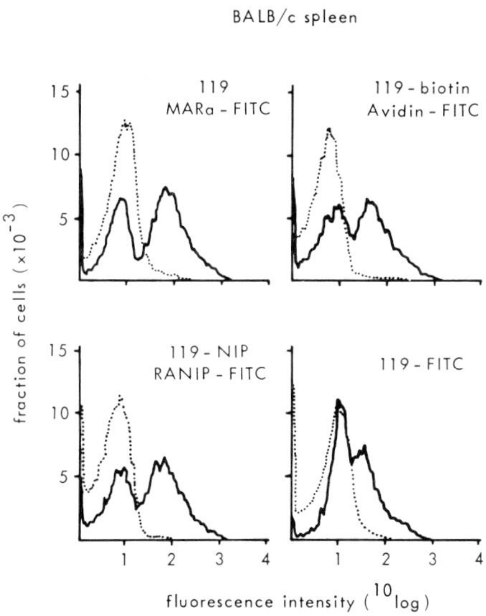

Fig. 8.4. Demonstration of surface IgM by several immunofluorescence techniques. The monoclonal rat anti-mouse IgM (151-119) was conjugated with biotin succinimide, NIP succinimide or FITC; for the anti-Ig technique unlabelled antibody-rich supernatant was used. Dashed lines represent cells incubated with the second step only: FITC-conjugated mouse anti-rat IgG (MARa/FITC), FITC-conjugated avidin, and FITC-conjugated rabbit anti-NIP (RANIP/FITC), respectively. In the case of the direct technique, unstained cells were used as the controls.

In some cases the amplification provided by the second step cannot be omitted. Fig. 8.4 illustrates this for the already described anti-IgM. IgM is represented on mature murine B cells only in very small quantities. With an anti-Ig second step it was possible to obtain a good distinction between positive and negative cells. Directly conjugated anti-IgM, on the other hand, only revealed the cells with the largest density of IgM, even though this preparation proved to be very suitable for visualizing IgM-containing plasma cells in cytocentrifuge preparations of spleen and bone marrow, indicating that the antigen-binding activity of the antibody was not destroyed during labeling. NIP- and biotin-conjugated anti-IgM are also shown with their appropriate controls in Fig. 8.4. In our hands, the anti-Ig technique was best suited for revealing IgM-positive cells. Of course these results relate only to this particular antigen–antibody system and the conclusions cannot be generalized.

3. The biotin–avidin system is advisable over other hapten sandwich techniques because of the ease of conjugation and the very low background fluorescence caused by avidin alone. Regular RPMI contains small amounts of biotin which do not seem to interfere to any significant degree.

4. Double staining experiments provide special problems in working with monoclonal antibodies because these are frequently derived from the same animal species. Antibodies directly conjugated with fluorescein and rhodamine are optimal if the signal to noise ratio allows such a choice. In a single laser FACS system (argon laser), using a combination of the 488 and 515 nm lines, the excitation of rhodamine (excitation maximum: 550 nm) is evidently suboptimal; in addition, the fluorescein emission is sacrificed by about 50% because strong filtering of the emission is needed to exclude the 515 excitation light from entering the photomultiplier. Dual laser systems have been installed now in a few laboratories in which 488 excitation for FITC is provided with an argon laser and the 550 excitation for TRITC either by a krypton laser or by a pulsed dye laser. It is too early to decide which excitation for rhodamine will prove the most durable.

The emission spectrum of fluorescein overlaps that of rhodamine, albeit only to a small extent. If a cell stained only with fluorescein-labeled antibody is hit by the 488 nm laser it will generate a small signal in the "red" photomultiplier channel. This contamination is proportional to the signal received by the "green" photomultiplier and may be suppressed electronically [14]. Recently, systems are under development in which the cells are excited sequentially by fluorescein and rhodamine excitation. An alternative solution is the introduction of dyes of the rhodamine class, the emission spectrum of which lies more in the 700 nm range instead of the 600 nm range as for TRITC.

8.4. THE USE OF MONOCLONAL ANTIBODIES TO STUDY THE ONTOGENY OF VARIOUS CELL SUBPOPULATIONS IN THE MOUSE

Relevant data will be summarized in this section on the development of various cells in spleen, thymus, lymph nodes and bone marrow, characterized by cell surface determinants recognized by monoclonal antibodies. Evidently, a comprehensive review of the available literature is out of place here. Rather, a highly personal selection is given.

8.4.1. The ontogeny of T cells

T cells in the mouse are characterized by the Thy-1 marker. Monoclonal antibodies directed against Thy-1 may be divided into those recognizing allelic determinants on the Thy-1 molecules (alleles of Thy-1 are called Thy-1.1 of which the type strain is AKR/J, and Thy-1.2 which is carried by almost all other strains) and those reacting with framework determinants which are common to Thy-1.1 and Thy-1.2. Several monoclonals of each variety have been described and are commercially available. Using conventional antisera, Cantor and Boyse [3] were able to divide the Thy-1-positive cells on the basis of the representation on the cell surface of the Lyt antigens. These authors used a cytotoxic method followed by a functional assay of the remaining cells. They came to the conclusion that helper T cells carry the Lyt-1 antigen and that Lyt-2 is present on suppressor and cytotoxic T cells. For the sake of clarity we omit the Lyt-3 designation, since under normal circumstances Lyt-3 appears to be present on all Lyt-2-positive cells [13]. The largest subpopulation of Thy-1-positive cells, however, carried both markers (viz. Lyt-1,2$^+$) and were hypothesized to be the precursors of both Lyt-1$^+$ and Lyt-2$^+$ cells. In line with this hypothesis was the observation that neonatal spleen contains Lyt-1,2$^+$ cells only, the frequency of which was high (up to 30% of all nucleated cells) and decreased during the first few weeks. The more mature Lyt-1$^+$ and Lyt-2$^+$ populations started to appear only in the third week of life. After the preparation of monoclonal anti-Lyt reagents and the application of FACS analysis it became clear that the division according to Lyt-1 phenotype was quantitative rather than qualitative [13]. Helper T cells and suppressor/cytotoxic T cells appeared to carry a high density and a low density of Lyt-1, respectively. Lyt-2 was shown to be present on a much smaller population of peripheral T cells than originally assumed on the basis of the results obtained

TABLE 8.II

DEVELOPMENT OF SPLENIC T CELLS IN BALB/c MICE

Age (days)	Thy-1	Lyt-1	Lyt-2	Lyt-2/Thy-1
10	3[a]	5	1	0.33
20	6	10	2	0.33
35	22	26	8	0.36
56	26	29	10	0.38
140	28	34	12	0.43

[a] Positive cells as percent of total nucleated cells.

with the cytotoxicity experiments; only about 30–40% Thy-1$^+$ cells are also positive for Lyt-2.

In view of these discrepancies it was of interest also to re-examine the ontogeny of Lyt subclasses in the spleen of mice. In Table 8.II the ratio is given between the frequency of Lyt-2- and Thy-1-positive cells as a function of age. It is evident that no large decrease in this ratio was observed. This would be expected if all neonatal T cells were of the Lyt-1,2$^+$ variety and would differentiate within the spleen in the course of time into Lyt-2$^-$ and Lyt-2$^+$ cells. Ledbetter et al. [13] studied the density of Thy-1 and Lyt antigens in various organs. They found that in the course of differentiation from cortical thymocyte via medullary thymocyte to peripheral T lymphocyte, Thy-1 decreases in density, Lyt-1 increases and Lyt-2 remains relatively constant. Using this technique, we have compared the antigen density profiles of nursling T cells in spleen with those of adult splenic T cells (Fig. 8.5). No clear

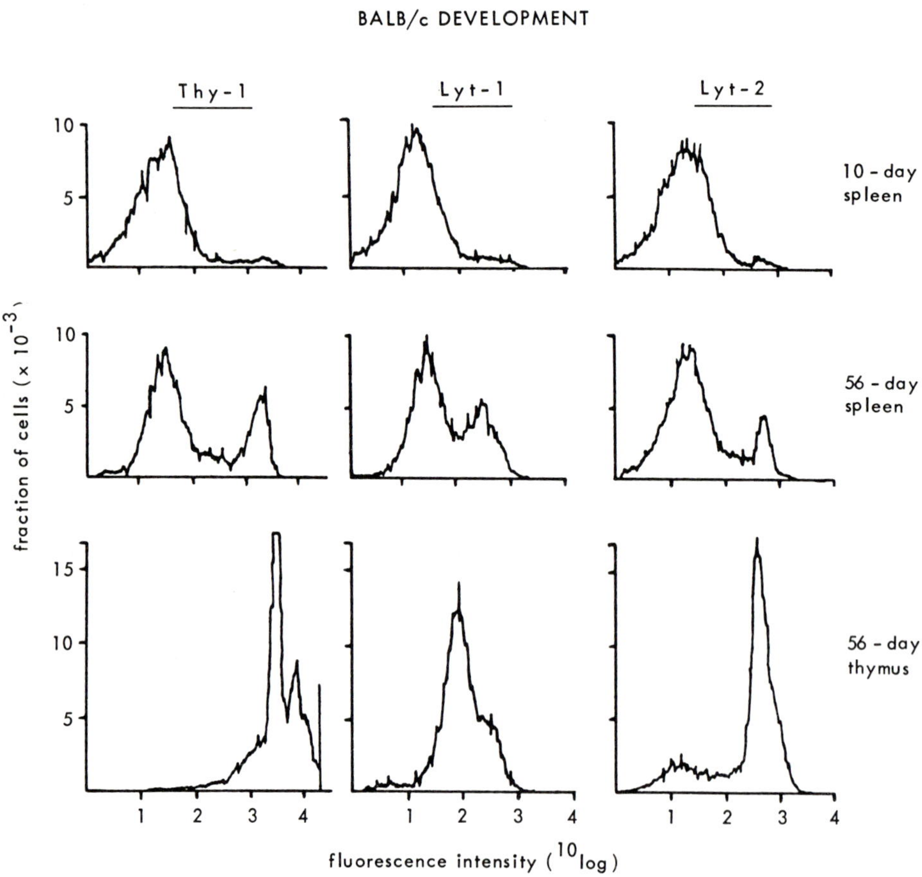

Fig. 8.5. T-cell development in the spleen. Each histogram represents the analysis of 10^4 cells. Monoclonals used: anti-Thy-1, 59-AD2.2; anti-Lyt-1, 53-7.3; and anti-Lyt-2, 53-6.7. (For details on these monoclonals, see Ledbetter and Herzenberg [12].)

differences were observed between the mean fluorescence intensity of the positive cells. This then indicates that splenic T cells in the neonate and adult are indistinguishable with regard to their division in Lyt-2 subpopulations and their maturational state as defined by their surface marker density.

8.4.2. The ontogeny of B cells

IgM and IgD are the major immunoglobulin isotypes represented on the surface of B cells. The kinetics of the appearance of these two Ig's on individual B cells is still poorly understood, although it is known that IgD appears later than IgM during development on a population basis [21]. For our experiments we felt it necessary to generate a monoclonal anti-IgM to avoid ambiguity due to possible low levels of anti-Fab activity present in conventional anti-IgM preparations. The existence, moreover, of surface forms of immunoglobulins distinct from those found in serum [17, 22] makes it difficult to assess the specificity of a given antiserum, for instance, by radioimmunoassay. Using the monoclonal rat anti-mouse IgM (see above) and a monoclonal anti-IgD [16], we confirmed the observations of others [7] that the first IgM-positive cells in the spleen carry a large amount of IgM and are negative for, or very dully stained with anti-IgD. These cells will be called IgM^{2+}/IgD^{-}. In the course of 3–6 weeks there is a gradual appearance of a population of cells with a low density of IgM and this goes hand in hand with an increase in the mean staining intensity of the IgD positive cells (Fig. 8.6). From this kind of single color analyses no conclusions can be drawn with regard to the behavior of IgM and IgD on individual cells. Two-color experiments were complicated by our inability to label the rat anti-mouse IgM sufficiently strongly for a direct technique.

Fig. 8.7 shows the results obtained with a double-sandwich technique: IgM was demonstrated with the rat anti-mouse IgM followed by fluorescein-conjugated mouse anti-rat IgG, and IgD by biotin-conjugated anti-IgD followed by rhodaminated avidin (Vector labs, lot No. 90513). Spleen of 28-day-old BALB/c mice was chosen in this example. Three populations of positive cells can be recognized: cells that are bright with anti-IgM and negative for IgD – the IgM^{2+}/IgD^{-} cells already mentioned; cells bright with IgM and dully stained with anti-IgD – IgM^{2+}/IgD^{+}; and cells which stain dully for IgM and dull to bright for IgD – IgM^{+}/IgD^{+} cells. These populations are depicted schematically in Fig. 8.8. In adult spleen and lymph node the large majority of the B cells belong to the IgM^{+}/IgD^{+} class. Within this class the densities of IgM and IgD on individual cells are positively correlated. In animals younger than 14 days of age the proportion of the IgM^{2+}/IgD^{-} cells is clearly the highest. The most logical maturational sequence for B lymphocytes would thus be: $IgM^{2+}/IgD^{-} \rightarrow IgM^{2+}/IgD^{+} \rightarrow IgM^{+}/IgD^{+}$. Taking into account the positive correlation between IgM and IgD density on "mature" B cells one might ask which cells within this population are the most fully differentiated,

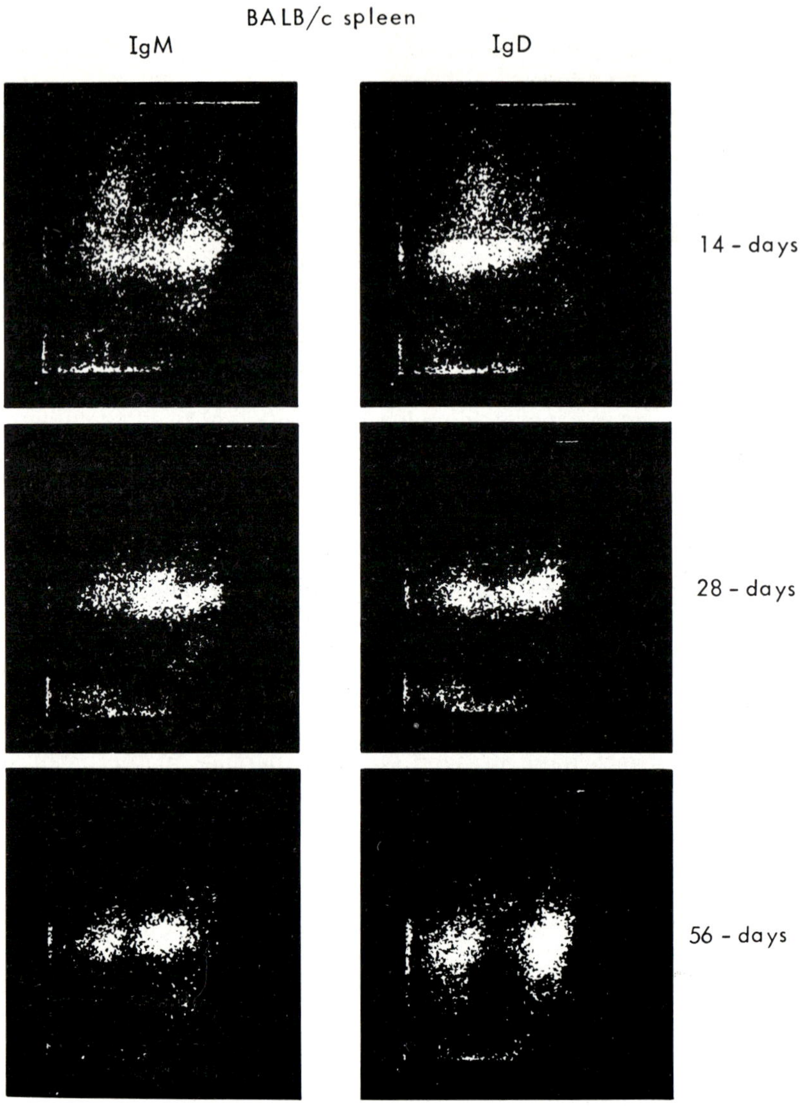

Fig. 8.6. B-cell development in spleen. Dot-plot photographs of spleen cell preparations obtained from animals of different ages stained for IgM with the 151-119 antibody followed by MARa/FITC and for IgD with FITC-conjugated mouse anti-mouse IgD of "a" allotype (antibody code: 10-4.2; see ref. 16). In the dot-plot, individual cells are represented by single dots. Vertical axis: scatter signal. Horizontal axis: log fluorescence intensity. The spleen cell suspension was treated with distilled water to remove red cells.

i.e. those with low IgM and low IgD or those which are slightly brighter for IgM and significantly brighter for IgD (population A and B in Fig. 8.8). The implied question would be whether A is derived from B or vice versa. The only clue available at the moment is the observation that lymph node B cells are enriched for population B. Lymph nodes allegedly contain proportionally more mature B and T cells than spleen. Should this prove to be true, then A is most

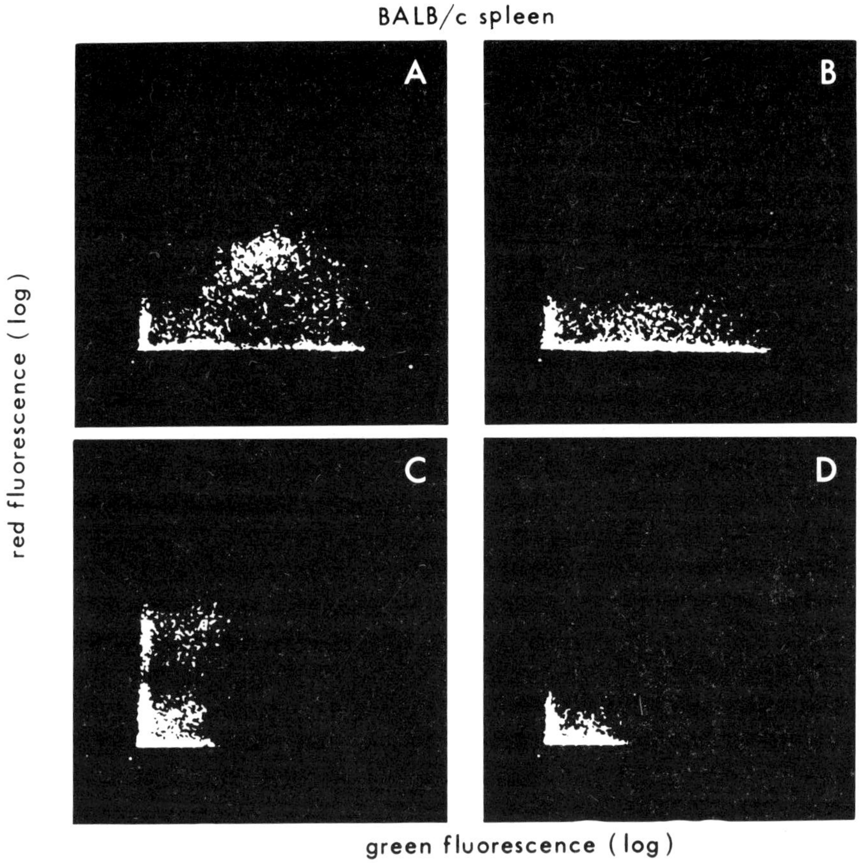

Fig. 8.7. Representation of IgM and IgD on young spleen cells. A) Spleen cells of 28-day-old BALB/c mice were incubated first with a mixture of the antibody 151-119 and biotin-conjugated anti-IgD of "a" allotype and then with a mixture of MARa/FITC- and TRITC-conjugated avidin. With the FACS only those cells giving a low-angle scatter signal characteristic of a small lymphocyte were processed. Vertical axis: logarithm of the red fluorescence (anti-IgD). Horizontal axis: logarithm of the green fluorescence (anti-IgM). B) Cells incubated for IgM only. C) Cells incubated for IgD only. D) Unstained cells. The FACS was calibrated with microspheres [18], using the compensation network reported by Loken et al. [14].

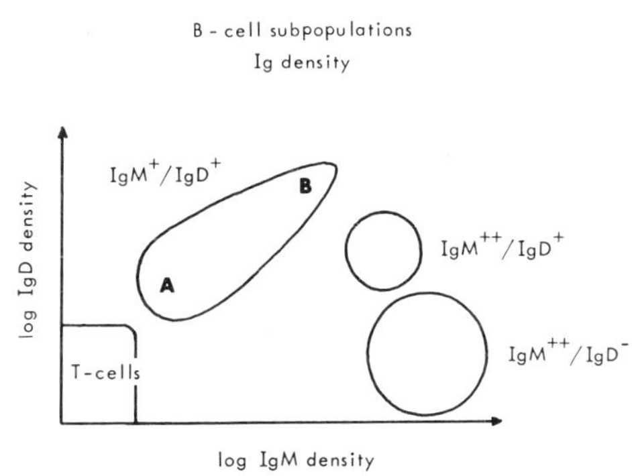

Fig. 8.8. Schematic representation of the three B-cell populations in young spleen characterized by differential surface Ig density.

likely the precursor of B. It then follows that most of the IgM is first lost from a B cell (precursor) before it acquires IgD. IgM and IgD would thereafter increase simultaneously. This model would be in line with the hypothesis suggesting a common m-RNA transcript of the μ and δ genes (for a review, see Adams [1]). Consequently, it is necessary to postulate a different transcription process for the IgM^{2+}/IgD^{-} cells. A strong argument against loss of IgM before the acquisition of IgD is the existence of the IgM^{2+}/IgD^{+} cell. The proportion of these cells is always small and it may be that they do not belong to the main B-cell differentiation pathway. Common to all models of B-cell differentiation up to now is the assumption that the IgM^{2+}/IgD^{-} cells are indeed precursor cells. This hypothesis is based only on the development type of data. To prove or disprove the hypothesis we have sorted the IgM^{2+}/IgD^{-} and IgM^{-} cells from 4-day-old BALB/c spleen and transferred them into mildly irradiated BAB/14 mice ("b" allotype congenic of BALB/c). Seven, 14 and 21 days later the peripheral blood lymphocytes were analysed for the presence of IgD^{+} cells of BALB/c origin ("a" allotype). BALB/c B-cells were found only in those animals receiving the IgM^{-} fractions. Although this result may indicate that the IgM^{2+}/IgD^{-} cells are not the precursors of IgM^{+}/IgD^{+} cells, it is very well possible that neonatal B cells are more readily irreversibly blocked by anti-IgM treatment than adult B cells [19]. The only solution to this problem would be to find a B-cell marker which changes in density together with IgM and whose occupation by an antibody would not block cellular differentiation. Such a marker has not been described to date.

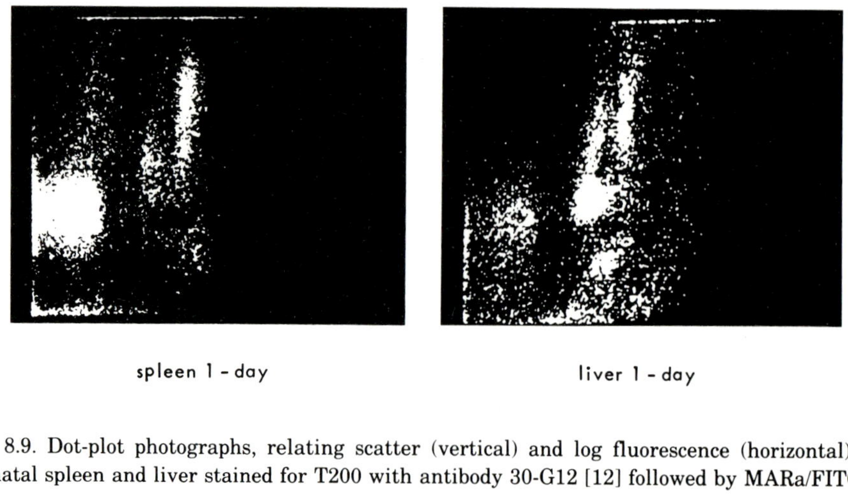

Fig. 8.9. Dot-plot photographs, relating scatter (vertical) and log fluorescence (horizontal) of neonatal spleen and liver stained for T200 with antibody 30-G12 [12] followed by MARa/FITC.

8.4.3. Markers not restricted to B or T cells

In postnatal development the spleen changes from a predominantly erythropoietic organ into a lymphopoietic organ. This change is clearly illustrated by using antibodies against markers present on cells both of the erythroid and lymphoid series. Two examples will be discussed here: the marker T200 and the antibody H11 [12]. T200 was first described by Trowbridge et al. [20] as a surface glycoprotein exclusively of T cells. Analysis using the FACS instead of cytotoxic depletion showed the antigen to be present in almost equal amounts on both B and T cells. Still, only the latter are killed if complement is added to the system. Also non-lymphoid cells carry T200 as evidenced by the staining profile of adult bone marrow. In our studies on murine development, monoclonal anti-T200 (generated and generously supplied by Dr. J.A. Ledbetter, Stanford University, CA) revealed clear subpopulations in nursling spleen and liver (Fig. 8.9). Whereas the positive lymphocyte-sized cells stain more or less homogeneously for T200, the larger cells are

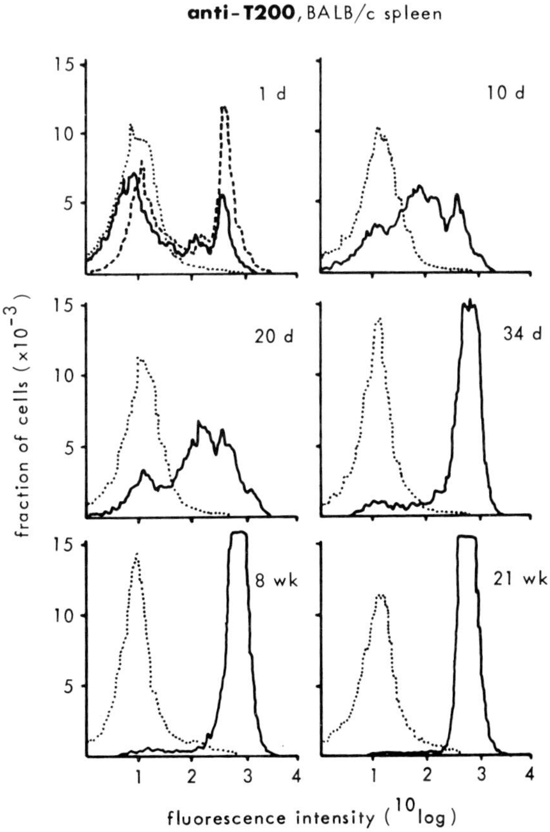

Fig. 8.10. Development of anti-T200 staining in spleen. Staining procedure as in Fig. 8.9. Each histogram represents 10^4 cells, dotted lines are MARa/FITC-negative controls, dashed lines are profiles of the large cells only. d = days; wk = weeks.

divided in two, perhaps even three subpopulations: a very dull (only in spleen), an intermediate, and a bright population. In the course of development, the larger cells disappear from the spleen. At the same time the lymphocytes acquire a high density of T200. This phenomenon results in a tightening of the fluorescence histogram (Fig. 8.10), until virtually 100% of spleen cells are T200-positive. A very small population remains, however, T200-negative. No indication as to the nature of these cells is available at the moment.

The 30-H11 antibody [12] recognizes an antigen of unknown molecular structure on: a) all thymocytes, b) all peripheral T cells, and c) large non-lymphoid cells in bone marrow and spleen. For thymus the H11-staining profile shows the same characteristics as that of anti-Lyt-1, i.e. the medullary thymocytes stain slightly brighter than the cortical thymocytes. The FACS histogram of an adult spleen is bimodal; only the T cells are positive. This pattern is observed from 4–5 weeks of age onwards. In neonatal animals the H11 pattern resembles that seen with anti-T200, viz. all lymphocyte-sized cells

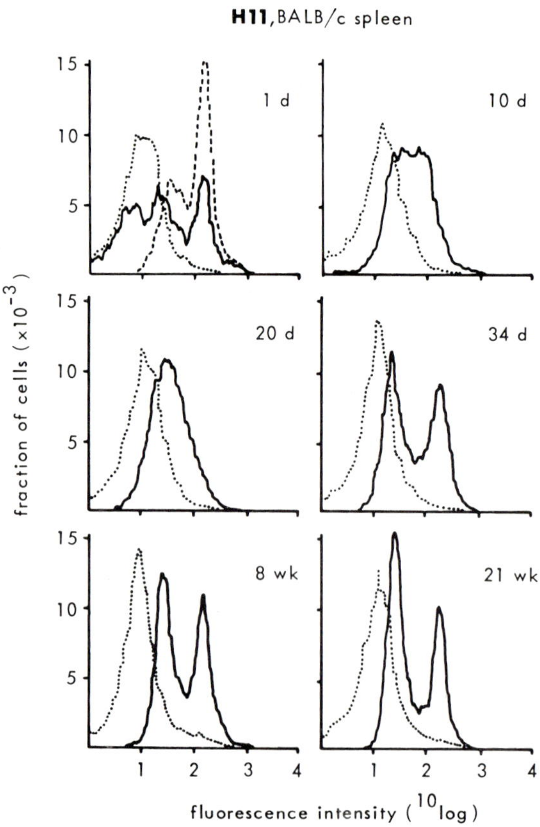

Fig. 8.11. Development of 30-H11 staining in spleen. Binding of the 30-H11 antibody [12] was demonstrated with MARa/FITC. Each histogram represents 10^4 cells. Dotted lines stand for negative control cell preparations treated with only MARa/FITC, dashed lines again represent profiles of the large cell population only. d = days; wk = weeks.

are more or less negative and the larger cells are divided into a medium bright and a very bright population. Two-color analysis using directly fluoresceinated anti-T200 and biotin-labelled H11 followed by rhodaminated avidin showed that in neonatal liver all bright and large H11 cells also carry T200. Interestingly, in neonatal spleen there are a few cells which do react with H11 but not with anti-T200. In the course of development (Fig. 8.11) the large H11-positive cells disappear from the spleen. By 10 days of age the FACS histogram is bell-shaped due to the disappearance of the large cells and the fact that the completely negative cells disappear and all cells become dully positive. This observation raises the question whether B cells are really H11-negative or whether they show only a weak expression of the recognized antigen. So far this question remains unanswered. The function of the H11- and T200-positive subpopulations of large cells in neonatal spleen and liver is obscure. Although it is clear that CFU-s (colony-forming unit-spleen) precursors are contained at least within the T200-positive cells, the frequency of these cells is too large for them to be stem cells only. Incubation with H11 obliterates all CFU-s precursors in vivo (Dr. H.S. Micklem, personal communication) which prevents further study along this line. Clearly, morphological studies have to be combined with fluorescence-activated cell sorting to reveal more characteristics of these intriguing cells.

8.5. CONCLUDING REMARKS

Monoclonal antibodies have proved to be very useful reagents in the study of cell surface antigens. Earlier, the conventional antisera recognizing some of these antigens were reserved for the happy few; now reagents of superior quality may be obtained commercially. It was proven possible to select from the antibody repertoire specificities which were hitherto "buried" in a heterogenous antibody response.

Combination of monoclonal antibodies with FACS analysis puts the study of cell surface markers on a firm quantitative basis. This is not to imply that the technique of cytotoxic depletion should or can be abandoned. The best example forms the history on the Lyt-1 and Lyt-2 antigens. The fact that the difference in Lyt-1 expression is only quantitative between T-helper cells on the one hand and suppressor and cytotoxic cells on the other does not diminish the contribution of the conventional alloantisera to cellular immunology. Of more interest in this respect is the role of the Lyt-1,2$^+$ cell. As has been stated in the results, we have not been able to offer evidence that the Lyt-1,2$^+$ cell is the precursor of the Lyt-2$^-$ cell. It thus remains possible that the thymus contains two separate series of cells: one being Lyt-2$^+$ and one being Lyt-2$^-$. Notwithstanding a large number of studies, the ontogeny of the B-cell system is far from understood. One of the reasons may be the lack of differentiation markers other than the expression of Ig and Ia. Using two-color FACS analysis with logarithmic amplification it was possible to define three distinct classes of

B cells on the basis of differential quantitative expression of IgM and IgD. The relationship between these three classes awaits further investigation, notably their behavior in hereditary immunologically compromised mice such as nude, CBA/N and NZB mice. Some restrictions to the use of monoclonal antibodies should be mentioned here. The signal to noise ratio with monoclonal antibodies is often smaller than with a good conventional antiserum because only one epitope is recognized. This may mean that several monoclonals directed against different epitopes on the same molecule will have to be combined for application in studies requiring visual examination. It is clear that this possibility increases the workload considerably, and consequently the price of commercial preparations will increase compared to the present. Another possible drawback of monoclonals is the restriction of Fc-mediated functions. Thus IgM antibodies may be very useful in cytotoxicity experiments but less optimal for radioimmunoassay. For IgG_1 antibodies the reverse may be true. Monoclonal antibodies generally perform poorly in agar precipitation systems, which are still widely used, especially for diagnostic purposes. Exceptions are IgM antibodies and those antibodies that recognize repeating epitopes. Again, for general use, a number of monoclonals will have to be combined to construct a general purpose reagent. The monoclonal antibody technique is now at such a stage that a lot of new antibodies are generated which have reactivity patterns not concordant with known subdivisions of cells. The T200 and H11 markers form examples in this respect. It will be the task in the coming years to sort out the different populations and to establish the functional relationships between them in order to obtain a better understanding of the development of the immensely complex hemopoietic system.

ACKNOWLEDGEMENTS

Most of the results and experiences related in this chapter were gained during a sabbatical stay in the laboratory of Dr. L.A. Herzenberg, Department of Genetics, Stanford University, Stanford, CA, U.S.A. I am grateful to acknowledge the collaboration with Drs. Lee Herzenberg, J.A. Ledbetter, V.T. Oi, J.W. Goding, T. Tokuhisa, D.R. Parks and H.S. Micklem. Further, I acknowledge the assistance given to me by J. Dangl and G. Filson.

REFERENCES

1 Adams, J.M. (1980) The organization and expressing of immunoglobulin genes. Immunol. Today *1*, 10–17.

2 Bayer, E.A. and Wilchek, M. (1974) Insolubilized biotin for the purification of avidin. Methods Enzymol. *34*, 265–267.

3 Cantor, H. and Boyse, E.A. (1975) Functional subclasses of T lymphocytes bearing different Ly antigens. I. The generation of functionally distinct T cell subclasses in a differentiative process independent of antigen. J. Exp. Med. *141*, 1376–1389.

4 Fazekas de St. Groth, S. and Scheidegger, D. (1980) Production of monoclonal antibodies: strategy and tactics. J. Immunol. Methods *35,* 1–22.
5 Galfré, G., Milstein, C. and Wright, R. (1979) Rat × rat hybrid myelomas and a monoclonal anti-Fd portion of mouse IgG. Nature *277,* 131–133.
6 Goding, J.W. (1976) Conjugation of antibodies with fluorochromes: Modification to the standard methods. J. Immunol. Methods *13,* 215–226.
7 Goding, J.W., Scott, D.W. and Layton, J.E. (1977) Genetics, cellular expression and function of IgD and IgM receptors. Immunol. Rev. *37,* 152–186.
8 Heitzmann, H. and Richards, F.M. (1974) Use of the avidin–biotin complex for specific staining of biological membranes in electron microscopy. Proc. Natl. Acad. Sci. U.S.A. *71,* 3537–3541.
9 Jones, P.P. (1980) Analysis of radiolabeled lymphocyte proteins by one- and two-dimensional polyacrylamide gel electrophoresis. *In* Mishell, B.B. and Shiigi, S.M. (eds.), Selected Methods in Cellular Immunology (Freeman and Co., San Francisco) pp. 398–440.
10 Köhler, G. and Milstein, C. (1975) Continuous cultures of fused cells secreting antibody of predefined specificity. Nature *256,* 495–497.
11 Lansdorp, P.M., Astaldi, G.C.B., Oosterhof, F., Janssen, M.C. and Zeijlemaker, W.P. (1980) Immunoperoxidase procedure to detect monoclonal antibodies against cell-surface antigens. Quantitation of binding and staining of individual cells. J. Immunol. Methods *39,* 393–405.
12 Ledbetter, J.A. and Herzenberg, L.A. (1979) Xenogeneic monoclonal antibodies to mouse lymphoid differentiation antigens. Immunol. Rev. *47,* 63–91.
13 Ledbetter, J.A., Rouse, R.V., Micklem, H.S. and Herzenberg, L.A. (1980) T cell subsets defined by expression of Lyt-1, 2, 3 and Thy-1 antigens. J. Exp. Med. *152,* 280–295.
14 Loken, M.R., Parks, D.R. and Herzenberg, L.A. (1977) Two-color immunofluorescence using a fluorescence activated cell sorter. J. Histochem. Cytochem. *25,* 899–907.
15 Oi, V.T. and Herzenberg, L.A. (1980) Immunoglobulin-producing hybrid cell lines. *In* Mishell, B.B. and Shiigi, S.M. (eds.), Selected Methods in Cellular Immunology (Freeman and Co., San Francisco) pp. 352–397.
16 Oi, V.T., Jones, P.P., Goding, J.W., Herzenberg, L.A. and Herzenberg, L.A. (1978) Properties of monoclonal antibodies to mouse Ig allotypes, H-2 and Ia antigens. Curr. Top. Microbiol. Immunol. *81,* 115–129.
17 Oi, V.T., Bryan, V.M., Herzenberg, L.A. and Herzenberg, L.A. (1980) Lymphocyte membrane IgG and secreted IgG are structurally and allotypically distinct. J. Exp. Med. *151,* 1260–1274.
18 Parks, D.R., Bryan, V.M., Oi, V.T. and Herzenberg, L.A. (1979) Antigen specific identification and cloning of hybridomas with a fluorescence-activated cell sorter. Proc. Nat. Acad. Sci U.S.A. *76,* 1962–1966.
19 Raff, M.C., Owen, J.J.T., Cooper M.D., Lawton, A.R., Megson, M. and Gathings, W.E. (1975) Differences in susceptibility of mature and immature mouse B-lymphocytes to anti-immunoglobulin-induced immunoglobulin suppression in vitro. J. Exp. Med. *142,* 1052–1064.
20 Trowbridge, I.S., Weissman, I. and Bevan, M.J. (1975) Mouse T-cell surface glycoprotein recognized by heterologous anti-thymocyte sera and its relationship to Thy-1 antigen. Nature *256,* 652–654.
21 Vitetta, E.S., Melcher, U., McWilliams, M., Lamm, M.E., Philips-Quagliata, J.M. and Uhr, J.W. (1975) Cell surface immunoglobulin. XI. The appearance of an IgD-like molecule on murine lymphoid cells during ontogeny. J. Exp. Med. *141,* 206–215.
22 Williams, P.B., Kubo, R.T. and Grey, H.M. (1978) μ-Chains from a non-secretor B cell line differ from secreted μ-chains at the C-terminal end. J. Immunol. *121,* 2435–2439.
23 Wofsy, L., Baker, P.C., Thompson, K., Goodman, J., Kimura, J. and Henry, C. (1974) Hapten-sandwich labeling. I. A general procedure for simultaneous labeling of multiple cell surface antigens for fluorescence and electron microscopy. J. Exp. Med. *140,* 523–537.

Wick et al. (eds) Immunofluorescence Technology. Selected Theoretical and Clinical Aspects © *Elsevier Biomedical Press, 1982*

CHAPTER 9

Immunofluorescence studies with monoclonal antibodies against pituitary and placental hormones

R. KOFLER, P. BERGER and G. WICK

Institute for General and Experimental Pathology, University of Innsbruck Medical School, Innsbruck, Austria

9.1. INTRODUCTION

The pituitary gland as a central endocrine organ produces several hormones regulating the function of nearly all peripheral endocrine glands. These hormones, although distinct entities from a biological viewpoint, frequently show broad structural similarities. During pregnancy the placenta contributes additional hormones which may be both biologically and structurally closely related to some of the pituitary hormones. The discrimination of all these hormones by means of conventional polyclonal antisera is difficult due to various cross-reactions on the basis of shared antigenic determinants. Such a discrimination is, however, in many instances required both in basic research and for diagnostic purposes.

The separation of structurally similar molecules sharing several antigenic determinants (epitopes) requires reagents specifically recognizing only epitopes that are unique for the respective compound. This criterion can be fulfilled by monoclonal antibodies (MAb) [12], the production and characterization of which have been described in more detail in the previous chapter. Monoclonal antibodies are produced by hybridoma cells resulting from fusions of cultured plasmocytoma cells with spleen cells from animals immunized with the respective antigen. Since all cells of a hybridoma cell line stem from a single progenitor cell, they will all secrete identical antibody molecules sharing identical specificity. Hybridoma lines producing MAb recognizing unique determinants on the hormones discussed above could, therefore, provide valuable tools for research and diagnostic purposes.

We have established hybridoma cell lines secreting MAb against human chorionic gonadotropin (hCG), bovine luteinizing hormone (LH) [11] and bovine prolactin. In addition, we had access to MAb against human growth hormone produced by Dr. J. Ivanyi [7]. In the first part of this chapter we will describe the applications of the immunofluorescence technique (IF) in the course of production and analysis of MAb against such hormones. In the second part the use of already characterized MAb in immunohistochemistry of the pituitary gland is discussed.

9.2. PITUITARY AND RELATED PLACENTAL HORMONES

9.2.1. General comments

The hormones of the pituitary gland and some related hormones produced by the placenta are commonly divided into four main families according to their chemical composition and site of production (Table 9.I) [21]. The listed hormones have been detected in several species including man. The presence of

TABLE 9.I

PITUITARY AND RELATED PLACENTAL HORMONES

1. Glycoprotein hormones	Luteinizing hormone (LH) Follicle-stimulating hormone (FSH) Thyroid-stimulating hormone (TSH) (Placental) chorionic gonadotropin (CG)
2. Protein hormones	Prolactin Growth hormone (GH), somatotropin Placental lactogen (PL), chorionic somatomammotropin (CS)
3. Adenopituitary peptide hormones	Adrenocorticotropic hormones (ACTH) Melanocyte-stimulating hormone (MSH) Lipotropin
4. Neuropituitary peptide hormones	Oxytocin Vasopressin

some of them, for example the placental hormone chorionic gonadotropin (CG) in the rat, is, however, still a matter of discussion. We will concentrate here on the glycoprotein and the protein hormones, since our investigations concern only members of these two groups. In the context of this chapter it is impossible to discuss the enormous body of literature on the biochemistry, function and other properties of these hormones in detail. For discussion purposes a simplified description of the structure and some antigenic properties of the respective hormones is given below. For more detailed information the reader is referred to some excellent recent reviews [15, 18].

9.2.2. The glycoprotein hormones

The glycoprotein group consists of three pituitary hormones: luteinizing (LH), follicle-stimulating (FSH) and thyroid-stimulating hormones (TSH), respectively, as well as the placental CG. They are all chemically composed of two subunits, the α and β chains. The α subunits are considered to be very similar within a given species and so far have not been immunologically distinguishable [22]. These subunits, however, show marked interspecies differences. Antibodies raised against an α subunit of such a hormone of a certain species will, therefore, react with all four glycoproteins of this species, but should not react with those of any other species. The β subunits carrying the biologically active site are hormone-specific, but are structurally similar in several species, thus explaining the biological cross-reactivity of these hormones. Antibodies against the β subunit thus recognize only the respective hormone, but in several species. The β subunits of LH and CG are an exception since, apart from a C-terminal peptide of 30 amino acids in CG, they are nearly identically composed [16] and the two hormones probably recognize the same receptor on the target cell membrane [1]. It has to be stated, however, that the above-mentioned concept [20] appears to be an oversimplification and that cross-reactions between α chains of different species or β chains of different hormones may also occur. The literature on this subject is still controversial. This may at least in part be due to the use of polyclonal antisera with a differing and, in many instances not completely known, composition of antibody populations. Obviously, monoclonal antibodies should be able to shed more light on this puzzling matter.

9.2.3. The protein hormones

Two pituitary hormones, growth hormone (GH) and prolactin, as well as the placental lactogen (PL) constitute the protein hormone family. They are pure proteins without carbohydrate moieties and have a molecular weight of about 20,000. The amino acid sequence has been described for these hormones in several species, human GH [13], bovine prolactin [14], and human PL [17] being the first. The striking similarity between these various amino acid sequences is a strong indication that they all originated from a common ancestral precursor. Consequently, antisera raised against one of them may cross-react with further protein hormones of the same as well as other species. Although the literature dealing with immunological inter- and intraspecies cross-reactions of these hormones is equivocal, the following conclusion may be drawn: within a given species GH and PL seem to be more closely related to each other than prolactin. Considering interspecies similarities, primate protein hormones differ significantly from those of most other mammals.

9.3. MONOCLONAL ANTIBODIES (MAb)

9.3.1. Principle of production

If spleen cells of appropriately immunized mice are mixed with murine plasmocytoma cells in the presence of polyethylene glycol, fusions may occur that result in the formation of hybridoma cells possessing chromosomes of both cell types. By subculturing the mixture consisting of plasmocytoma, hybridoma and spleen cells in a selective medium (containing hypoxanthine–aminopterin–thymidine = HAT) only the hybrid cells can survive. The subcultures able to produce specific antibody are ascertained by sensitive tracing techniques and from these cultures the single antibody-synthesizing cell is obtained by cloning procedures. The respective hybridoma cell is then cultured further and can be propagated in vivo and in vitro for large-scale antibody production. For further information the reader is referred to Chapter 8 where a more detailed description on this subject is given.

9.3.2. Production of MAb against hCG and bovine LH

BALB/c mice were immunized subcutaneously with either 6, 25 or 100 μg of the respective hormone in Freund's complete adjuvant. Animals revealing significant specific antibody titers in their sera were boosted intravenously 3–4 days before fusion. For each fusion the spleen of a single mouse was removed aseptically in Hanks' balanced salt solution (Seromed GmbH, München, F.R.G.), a single cell suspension made and mixed with mouse plasmocytoma cells (P3-NS1/1-Ag 4-1, kindly provided by Dr. C. Milstein, Cambridge, U.K.) at a ratio of 10/1. The cells were washed and carefully resuspended in 2 ml RPMI 1640 (Seromed GmbH, München), containing 10% diemethyl sulfoxide and 42% polyethylene glycol (Polyätylenglycoll, 1500 Merck-Schuchart, Hohenbrunn, F.R.G.). After 1 min the cells were washed again and subcultured in 24-well tissue culture plates (Nuncolon, Nunc GmbH, Wiesbaden, F.R.G.) containing tissue culture medium (RPMI 1640 supplemented with 10 mM Hepes, 2 mM glutamine, 100 I.U./ml penicillin, 100 μg/ml streptomycin and 10% fetal calf serum) supplemented with HAT (13.5 μg/ml hypoxanthine, 0.19 μg/ml aminopterin, 3.9 μg/ml thymidine). The plates were then incubated at 37°C in an atmosphere of 5% CO_2 in air. As soon

was not appropriate for the demonstration of prolactin and growth hormone. For these protein hormones we have therefore elaborated a different procedure [10]; the organs are fixed in Bouin's solution for 24 h, dehydrated in an ethanol row of increasing concentration (70% to absolute ethanol) and embedded in paraffin. Paraffin sections, 6 μm thick, are then deparaffinized by three washes in xylol (10 min each) and rehydrated in an ethanol row of decreasing concentrations (absolute to 50% ethanol). After a 10 min rinse in phosphate-buffered saline (PBS), pH 7.2, the sections are ready for use in indirect IF (IIF) tests. This fixation method also preserves the glycoprotein hormones in an antigenically active form and can therefore be applied in both instances.

The sections ready for IF testing were then incubated with the respective antibody preparation for 1 h at room temperature in a moist chamber. Excess antibody was removed by a 30 min rinse in PBS, and staining was performed with an optimally diluted commercial fluorescein isothiocyanate (FITC)-conjugated IgG fraction of a goat antiserum against mouse IgG (heavy and light chain) (Lot No. 0411-1212, Cappel Laboratories, Inc., Cochranville, PA) with a molar fluorochrome/protein (F/P) ratio of 3.3 and 32 standard precipitation units. After final washing in PBS for 90 min the sections were mounted in PBS-buffered glycerol (pH 7.2). Readings were performed on a Leitz Ortholux microscope equipped with an HBO-50 mercury vapour bulb and appropriate filters as described elsewhere [6]. For the identification of various cell types in the pituitary gland we have also applied the double staining technique using mouse MAb in combination with conventional polyclonal rabbit antisera against several hormones, in consecutive incubations. Staining in these instances was performed with the FITC-labelled anti-mouse IgG conjugate and a tetramethylrhodamine isothiocyanate (TRITC)-labelled anti-rabbit Ig swine conjugate (Lot No. R156, Dakopatts A/S, Copenhagen, Denmark) having an absorbance ratio of 2.8 and 8 standard precipitation units. Controls included incubations with normal sera, or unrelated MAb instead of specific antibodies, as well as preabsorption of the anti-hormone preparations with beads coated with the respective or unrelated hormones (Affi-Gel 10, Bio-Rad Laboratories, Richmond, CA). For this purpose 5 ml of antibody preparation in the highest dilution still resulting in clear staining were incubated under constant agitation with 1 ml packed volume of the respective beads for 1 at h room temperature, centrifuged, and the supernatant tested in IIF as described above.

9.5. IMMUNOFLUORESCENCE ANALYSIS OF MONOCLONAL ANTIBODIES

The IF technique has proved to be a valuable tool for the characterization of MAb. Although IF is not intended as a substitute for labelled antigen-binding techniques such as RIA and enzyme-linked immunosorbent assay (ELISA), it can provide additional information and, in particular instances, may even be the method of choice for specificity testing. The pituitary gland as a source of antigenic material offers a number of advantages. The hormones need not be purified and labelled which is not only laborious, but may also result in loss or destruction of antigenic determinants. The glands of most species are readily available allowing studies on interspecies cross-reactions. Paraffin-embedded organs can in addition be kept in an antigenically unaltered state for an indefinite time. Furthermore, the reaction of an antibody with virtually all pituitary hormones as well as non-hormonal antigens can be detected on a single section. In RIA or ELISA a whole series of binding or blocking experiments using a variety of hormones and other antigens would be required for similar information. If investigations on hormones of individual members of a certain species are undertaken – such as on possible allotypic variants of hormones (see Section 9.5.3) – immunohistochemistry using individual pituitaries as a source of individual hormone variants is especially useful. In the following section we describe some examples of IF studies on inter- and intraspecies cross-reactivity of MAb as well as investigations on reactions of MAb with possible allotypes of hormones.

9.5.1. Intraspecies cross-reactivity, between human luteinizing hormone and human chorionic gonadotropin

For studies on intraspecies cross-reactions of MAb raised against human CG, IIF on human pituitary glands was used as a simple screening assay for discrimination of MAb reacting specifically with human CG from those cross-reacting with human LH, FSH or TSH. Such a cross-reaction could be expected from antibodies recognizing the α chain which is nearly identical in all glycoprotein hormones. In the case of LH, which also shares determinants on the β-chain, cross-reactions will also occur with antibodies to β chain epitopes common to both LH and CG.

Out of 39 different supernatants tested, 17 showed a clear-cut reaction with human pituitary cells (Fig. 9.1). Since the aim of this study was to establish MAb specifically reacting with hCG, the respective hybridoma clones could be frozen in liquid nitrogen and tissue culture work on these lines discontinued for the present investigation. Negative reactions of supernatants, however, have to be reconfirmed by other techniques, since they may be due to low affinity or low concentration of the antibody under investigation. Alternatively, the antibodies may recognize allotypic variants of the respective hormones which are not present in the individual pituitary(ies) used for testing (see also Section 9.5.3).

9.5.2. Interspecies cross-reactivity between human, bovine and rat LH

For these studies the organ of production, in our case the pituitary, was again conveniently taken as an antigenic source. For studies on the function of LH in pregnant rats we have looked for MAb originally directed against bovine LH or human CG and cross-reacting with rat LH. Using the IF method on

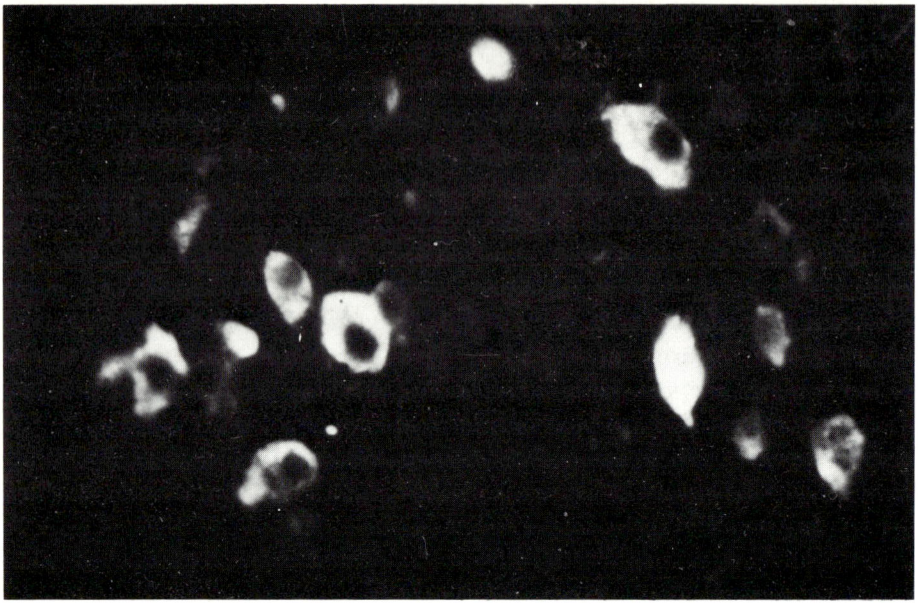

Fig. 9.1. Intraspecies cross-reaction of MAb against hCG with glycoprotein hormone-producing cells in a paraffin section of human pituitary gland as shown in IIF. Original ×400.

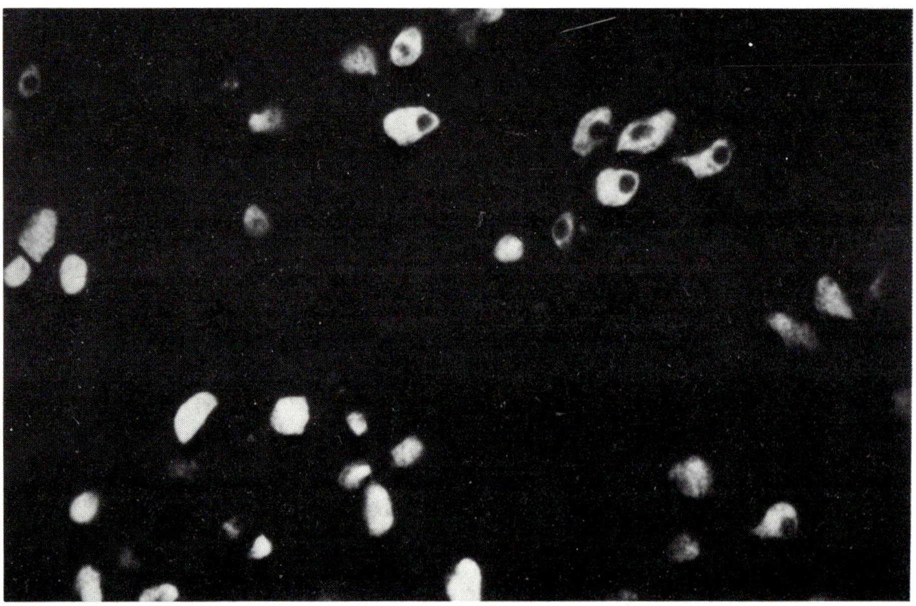

Fig. 9.2. Interspecies cross-reaction of MAb against bovine LH with rat LH in a paraffin section of rat pituitary gland as shown in IIF. Original ×250.

paraffin sections of rat pituitary glands three of five MAb against bovine LH (Fig. 9.2) and four of 39 MAb against human CG were found to stain rat pituitary cells. It is worth mentioning that in two instances the reaction with the rat hormone could only be detected in IIF but not in RIA using ^{125}I-labelled rat hormones. This suggests a loss or destruction of the respective determinants in the course of purification and labelling of the tracer.

9.5.3. Studies on possible allotypes of human GH

The exclusive reaction of a MAb with a single determinant on a hormone molecule could entail problems suggesting that the recognized epitope was not present on the hormone of all individuals of the respective species, but only in a genetically related group thereof. This phenomenon, called allotypy, is well known for, e.g., immunoglobulin molecules. In the case of bovine GH evidence for the existence of allelic forms has been presented [4]. In order to investigate the possibility that MAb against human GH may react with such allotypic epitopes, the respective reagents have been tested in IIF on pituitary glands of 14 individuals taken at autopsy. For control purposes double staining using a conventional polyclonal rabbit antiserum against human GH was applied.

Whereas three of four MAb tested reacted with all pituitaries equally well and stained only cells also recognized by the polyclonal antiserum (Fig. 9.3), one MAb behaved differently staining two different cell types. One cell type

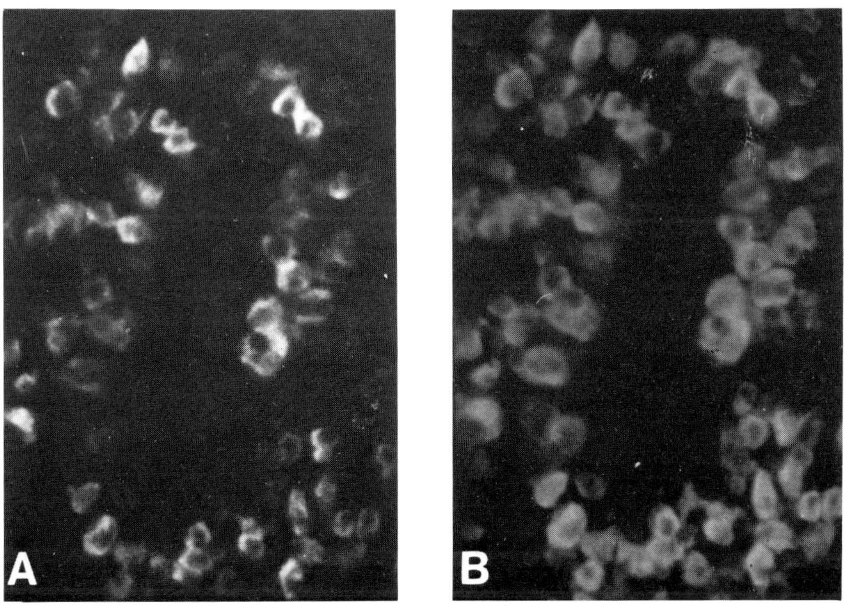

Fig. 9.3. Double staining IIF of GH-producing cells in a paraffin section of human pituitary gland using a MAb against human GH stained with a FITC-labelled anti-mouse Ig conjugate (A) and a rabbit antiserum against human GH stained with a TRITC-labelled anti-rabbit Ig conjugate (B). Note that the same cells react with both reagents. Original ×250.

was also stained with the polyclonal antiserum; the second cell type, however, reacted only with the respective MAb, but not with the polyclonal antiserum. Blocking experiments intended to identify this second cell type revealed that this cell may produce adrenocorticotropic hormone (ACTH) or a related cross-reacting hormone. This finding suggests that the respective "MAb" was not monoclonal, but contained a second antibody directed against this latter hormone. Further cloning of the respective cell line resulted in a hybridoma line the product of which was free of this contaminating antibody and consequently reacted in the same fashion as the other three MAb. This study thus far revealed no evidence for allotypic variants of human GH, but rather disclosed a contamination in one of the MAb which was not detected in RIA characterization where ACTH was originally not included.

9.6. IMMUNOHISTOCHEMISTRY WITH MONOCLONAL ANTIBODIES

The monospecificity of MAb and their suitability for methods such as IF make them excellent tools for immunohistochemical investigations. We have applied MAb for studies on the localization of the site of production of the glycoprotein hormones LH, FSH and TSH in rat pituitaries [8]. The literature in this respect is equivocal, especially regarding the question of whether production of LH and FSH occurs in the same [5] or in two different cell types [19]. We have investigated this issue by means of the double staining IF technique using a MAb specifically reacting with rat LH, but not cross-reacting with rat FSH or TSH as detected in RIA, and highly specific polyclonal rabbit antisera against rat FSH and rat TSH (kindly provided by the National Institute of Arthritis, Metabolism and Digestive Diseases, Bethesda, MD).

It could be shown that the rabbit antiserum against rat FSH reacts with exactly the same cells as did the MAb against LH. Only double stained cells could be observed. Fig. 9.4a shows the reaction of the MAb, revealed with a FITC-labelled anti-mouse IgG conjugate, with LH-producing cells in a section of a rat pituitary gland. In Fig. 9.4b the same area is photographed with a filter combination allowing for the recognition of the polyclonal antiserum against rat FSH stained with a TRITC-labelled anti-rabbit Ig conjugate. In Fig. 9.4c the pictures have been superimposed resulting in an orange colour of the double staining cells. It is evident that only such double stained cells could be found. Affinity chromatography absorption of rabbit anti-rat FSH serum with beads coated with ovine FSH led to complete disappearance of staining, whereas control absorptions using beads coated with either prolactin or LH had no effect. The cross-reacting ovine and bovine hormones had to be taken instead of the respective rat hormones, since the latter are not available in sufficient amounts for this type of experiment. These findings clearly indicate that rat LH and FSH are produced within the same cell.

Double staining experiments using rabbit anti-rat TSH serum in combina-

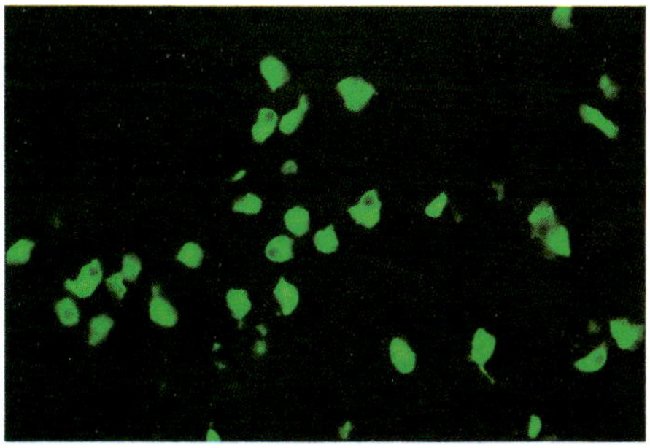

4a

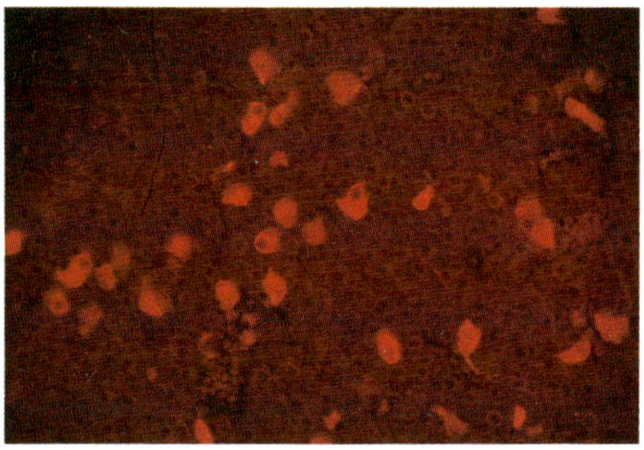

4b

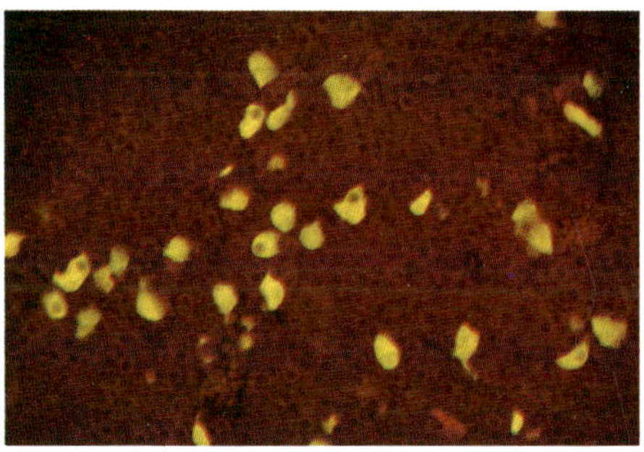

4c

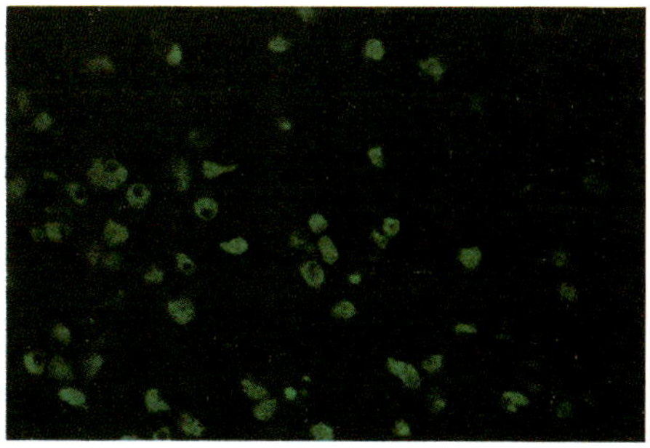

5a

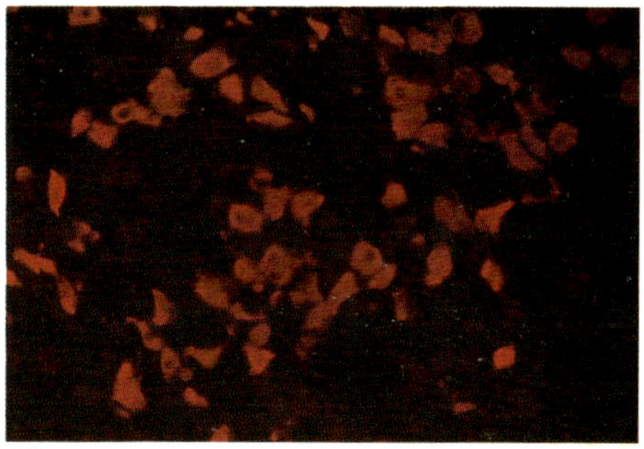

5b

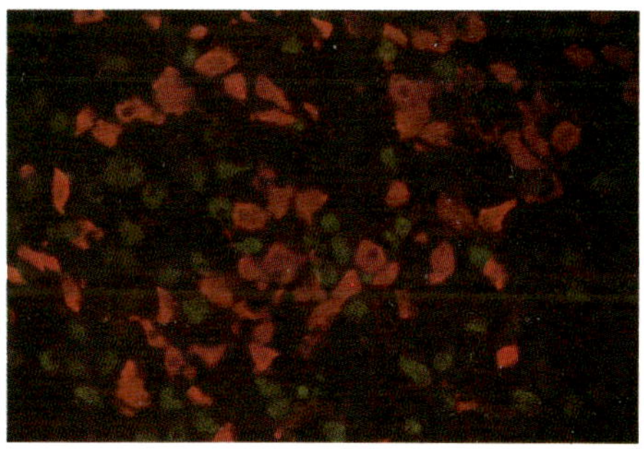

5c

Fig. 9.4. Identification of the site of production of LH and FSH in a paraffin section of rat pituitary gland by IIF double staining technique. The reaction of identical cells with MAb against LH (a) and the polyclonal antiserum to rat FSH (b) is proven by superimposition of the two pictures (c). Original ×250.

Fig. 9.5. Identification of the site of production of LH and TSH in a paraffin section of rat pituitary gland by IIF double staining technique. The MAb against LH stains different cells (a) than does the polyclonal antiserum against rat TSH (b). This is verified by superimposition of the two pictures (c). Original ×250.

tion with the same MAb against LH revealed a completely different picture. As shown in Fig. 9.5 the cells stained by the MAb (Fig. 9.5a) are not identical to those stained with the polyclonal antiserum (Fig. 9.5b). If the two pictures were again superimposed (Fig. 9.5c) it became evident that only single stained cells were present, proving that rat LH and TSH are synthesized by two different cell types.

ACKNOWLEDGEMENTS

This work was supported by a grant from the "Kamillo-Eisner-Foundation". The gift of pituitary hormones as well as the rabbit antisera against rat FSH and rat TSH by Dr. A.F. Parlow from the National Institute of Arthritis, Metabolism and Digestive Diseases, Bethesda, MD, U.S.A. is gratefully acknowledged. The authors also thank Miss Elisabeth Kalchschmid for her excellent technical assistance.

REFERENCES

1 Catt, K.J., Dufan, M.L. and Tsuruhara, T. (1971) Studies on a radioligand–receptor assay system for luteinizing hormone and chorionic gonadotropin. J. Clin. Endocrinol. Metab. *32,* 860–863.

2 Forsgren, A. and Sjöquist, J. (1966) "Protein A" from *Staphylococcus aureus.* I. Pseudo-immune reaction with human γ-globulin. J. Immunol. *97,* 882-887.

3 Galfré, G., Howe, S.C., Milstein, C., Butcher, G.W. and Howard, J.C. (1977) Antibodies to major histocompatibility antigens produced by hybrid cell lines. Nature *266,* 550–558.

4 Geschwind, I.I. (1971) Bovine growth hormone: evidence for two allelic forms. Biochem. Biophys. Res. Commun. *43,* 189–195.

5 Herbert, D.C. (1975) Localization of antisera to LH β and FSH β in the rat pituitary gland. Am. J. Anat. *144,* 379–385.

6 Herzog, F., Albini, B. and Wick, G. (1973) Comparison of filters used in immunofluorescent staining procedures with fluorescein-isothiocyanate (FITC) conjugates. J. Immunol. Methods *3,* 211–220.

7 Ivanyi, J. and Davies, P. (1980) Preliminary communication. Monoclonal antibodies against human growth hormone. Mol. Immunol. *17,* 287–290.

8 Kofler, R. (1982) Immunofluorescence localization of glycoprotein hormones in the rat anterior pituitary gland using monoclonal antibodies and polyclonal antisera. Submitted for publication. J. Histochem. Cytochem. (in press).

9 Kofler, R., Wick, G. and Loewit, K. (1977) Immunological dissection of rat pregnancy: Study of the mode of action of antisera to luteinizing hormone. Clin. Exp. Immunol. *29,* 326–333.

10 Kofler, R., Tabarelli, M., Schwarz, S., Wolf, H., Loewit, K. and Wick, G. (1980) Characterization of antisera against bovine prolactin for in vivo studies on prolactin function in the rat. Clin. Exp. Immunol. *41,* 55–62.

11 Kofler, R., Kalchschmid, E., Berger, P. and Wick, G. (1981) Production and characterization of monoclonal antibodies against bovine luteinizing hormone. Immunobiology *160,* 196–207.

12 Köhler, G. and Milstein, C. (1975) Continuous culture of fused cells secreting antibody of predefined specificity. Nature *256,* 495–497.

13 Li, C.H., Dixon, J.S. and Liu, W.K. (1969) Human pituitary growth hormone. XIX. The primary structure of the hormone. Arch. Biochem. Biophys. *133,* 70–91.

14 Li, C.H., Dixon, J.S., Lo, T.B., Schmidt, K.D. and Pankov, Y.A. (1970) Studies on pituitary lactogenic hormone. XXX. The primary structure of the sheep hormone. Arch. Biochem. Biophys. *141,* 705–737.
15 McKerns, K.W. (ed.) (1978) Structure and Function of the Gonadotropin (Plenum Press, New York).
16 Morgan, F.J., Birken, S. and Canfield, R.E. (1973) Human chorionic gonadotropin: a proposal for the amino sequence. Mol. Cell. Biochem. *2,* 97–99.
17 Niall, H.D., Hogan, M.L., Tregear, G.W., Segre, G.V., Hwan, G.P. and Friesen, H. (1973) The chemistry of growth hormone and the lactogenic hormones. Recent Prog. Horm. Res. *29,* 387–416.
18 Parson, J.A. (ed.) (1976) Peptide Hormones (The Macmillan Press Ltd., London).
19 Purandare, T., Sar, M. and Stumpf, W.E. (1978) Immunohistochemical localization of FSH and LH in rat pituitary. Mol. Cell. Endocrinol. *10,* 57–62.
20 Vaitukaitis, J.L., Ross, G.T., Reichert, L.E.Jr. and Ward, D.N. (1972) Immunological basis for within and between species cross-reactivity of LH. Endocrinology *91,* 1337–1342.
21 Wallis, M. (1975) The molecular evolution of pituitary hormones. Biol. Rev. *50,* 35–98.
22 Walsh, P.R., Wang, M.C. and Gittermann, M.L. (1980) Development and validation of a choriogonadotropin beta-subunit radioimmunoassay for serum choriogonadotropin using commercially available components. Clin. Biochem. *13,* 69–72.

Wick et al. (eds) Immunofluorescence Technology. Selected Theoretical and Clinical Aspects © Elsevier Biomedical Press, 1982

CHAPTER 10

Immunofluorescence studies of mucous membranes and exocrine glands

P. BRANDTZAEG

Histochemical Laboratory, Institute of Pathology, The National Hospital, Rikshospitalet, Oslo, Norway

10.1. FIELDS OF APPLICATION

Four biological aspects of mucous membranes and their glands have recently been in the focus of interest: a) the expression of local humoral immunity; b) the endocrine function of the gut; c) the glandular production of various important enzymes; and d) the mucosal distribution of particular tissue or organ antigens, such as oncodevelopmental proteins. Since certain functional markers of lymphoid and epithelial cells can be identified by their antigenic properties in tissue sections, immunohistochemical methods have contributed significantly to our present knowledge of the physiological role of mucous membranes and glandular products, and provided new information about functional alterations associated with mucosal pathology, including neoplastic processes. The power of the immunohistochemical methods is clearly the bridging of function and morphology.

10.1.1. Components of the humoral immune system

In quantitative terms the major humoral immune system of man consists of immunoglobulin (Ig)-producing cells present in the stroma of exocrine glands and in the lamina propria of gland-containing mucous membranes such as the gut mucosa. Most of these local immunocytes, including mature plasma cells and their immediate precursors (immunoblasts), have the ability to synthesize dimeric IgA, which is transported into the exocrine fluids through serous secretory epithelial cells. This transport apparently depends on the presence of a polypeptide called the J chain in the IgA dimers as well as on an epithelial glycoprotein, the secretory component (SC), present in the plasma membranes of the gland cells. SC seems to act as an epithelial cell surface receptor for dimeric IgA; the SC–IgA complexes formed in the plasma membrane are transported in vesicles through the cytoplasm of the epithelial cell to the gland lumen and extruded as highly stabilized secretory IgA. Pentameric IgM is transported into the secretions in a similar way. The lymphoid and epithelial cells participating in this secretory immune system, and various aspects of the external Ig translocation, have been extensively characterized by means of immunohistochemical methods [10, 11, 18, 20, 22, 31, 32].

In addition to the local IgA and IgM immunocytes of the secretory immune system, varying proportions of IgG- and IgD-producing cells are also found in mucous membranes and exocrine glands [30]. The composition of the local immunocyte populations shows marked alterations in association with inflammatory and neoplastic processes, and such pathological features have been quantified by immunohistochemical methods [20, 25, 69, 105]. There is considerable disagreement with regard to the occurrence of IgE-producing cells in normal and pathological mucous membranes; these controversies emphasize the pitfalls involved in the immunohistochemical localization of such a rare cell type present in the connective tissue along with a variety of other cellular elements, particularly eosinophilic granulocytes and mast cells [21].

The mucous membranes also contain Ig-bearing B lymphocytes, especially accumulated in solitary follicles or aggregates of such, as exemplified by the tonsils and Peyer's patches. Immunohistochemical localization of B lymphocytes by their relatively small amounts of surface IgD and IgM is feasible, though technically much more difficult than the identification of Ig-producing immunocytes, which contain comparably high concentrations of cytoplasmic immunoglobulin [25, 27, 42, 90]. By means of antisera raised against monkey or human thymus lymphocytes, even T cells can now be localized immunohistochemically, and their distribution in mucosal lesions has been described [88].

An important aspect of local immunity is the extravascular distribution of serum immunoglobulins and complement factors. Nevertheless, relatively little attention has been paid to the presence of extracellular immune components in immunohistochemical studies of mucous membranes, probably because the methods used have been devised for the characterization of lymphoid cells. The major serum immunoglobulin, IgG, normally occurs in particularly high concentrations extravascularly in the lamina propria [10, 20]. Its immunohistochemical demonstration depends on a tissue fixation method that gives fairly complete retention of diffusible proteins without undue denaturation and masking of antigenic determinants. Also complement, evidenced by C3, is detectable extravascularly with a similar fixation method; this should be kept in mind when attempts are made to distinguish between C3 bound locally in immune complexes and C3 merely present non-specifically in the tissue along with other plasma proteins [1].

Local B cells may at any stage of their differentiation turn into cancer cells and give rise to monoclonal neoplastic processes. The malignant lymphomas most commonly developing in the mucous membranes are of the immunoblastic variety [75]. In addition, most extramedullary plasma cell tumours (plasmacytomas) originate in mucous membranes, especially in the upper respiratory tract. It is important to distinguish such malignant processes from inflammatory pseudotumours, and an unequivocal distinction can sometimes be made only by immunohistochemical characterization of the cytoplasmic Ig product of the tumour cells [77].

Any B cell, with the exception of normal B lymphocytes bearing both IgM and IgD, usually shows phenotypic restriction in that at a given time it expresses only one of the five classes of Ig heavy chains (γ, α, μ, δ or ϵ) and only one Ig light chain (κ or λ). Gland-associated immune responses are dominated by IgA-producing cells with an average $\kappa : \lambda$ ratio of about 65 : 35 [23, 89]. Immunocyte populations developing in association with chronic mucosal inflammation likewise show a κ-type predominance although IgG-producing cells are the most common class [20, 24]. All these normal immune responses can be characterized immunohistochemically as polyclonal on the basis of the spectrum of cytoplasmic Ig products revealed. Conversely, all neoplastic Ig-producing cells of a malignant process usually, if not always, express a monotypic product (one heavy and one light chain); malignant immunoblasts and plasma cells can hence be characterized immunohistochemically as monoclonal.

10.1.2. Endocrine cells of the gut

During the last decade it has become apparent that the gastrointestinal glands are not only part of the secretory immune system but also constitute a major endocrine organ. The discovery and especially the specific functional identification of the individual endocrine gut cells have depended largely on the development of immunohistochemical methods for the localization of the peptide hormones present in their cytoplasm [46, 86, 98]. Many attempts have been made to classify hyperplasias and benign or malignant tumours originating from these cell populations [46]. Immunohistochemical methods represent a powerful tool in this work, and much confusion can be avoided when the morphology is evaluated, literally speaking, in the light of immunocytochemical features.

Recent studies in several laboratories have in addition tested the possibility of quantifying by immunohistochemical methods the endocrine gut cells to see whether their functional mass shows any association with common gastrointestinal disorders. Relationships have especially been sought between the population of gastrin-producing cells (G cells) in the pyloric antrum, plasma gastrin levels, and peptic ulcer disease [40, 108, 113, 115, 117]. Great difficulties have been encountered in the enumeration of these cells because of their uneven distribution and patchy fluctuations according to histopathological alterations of the mucosa [39, 113, 116, 118].

10.1.3. Enzyme-producing cells

Enzyme-producing cells can be localized by their cytoplasmic activity when a specific substrate suitable for enzyme histochemistry is available. However, a simpler and more precise identification of such cells may be achieved by immunohistochemistry based on the antigenic properties of the enzyme in question. It is often easier to preserve antigenicity than enzyme activity, and the tissue preparation method may hence be simplified by the use of fixation and paraffin embedding. Various digestive enzymes or pro-enzymes such as amylase [74] and pepsinogens [129] have been localized by immunohistochemical methods. The mysterious Paneth cell has had light thrown upon it by the immunohistochemical verification that it produces the bacteriolytic enzyme lysozyme or muramidase [111]. This enzyme is present not only in glandular epithelial cells but also in granulocytes and macrophages; its cellular distribution in the mucosa of the gastrointestinal and respiratory tracts and in the salivary glands has been the subject of several immunohistochemical studies [67, 81, 102].

Glandular kallikreins are serine proteinases that are not thought to have any significant digestive or antibacterial activity but rather mediate their function through the release of kinins, which are potent vasodilators, affect membrane permeability and stimulate the formation of prostaglandins. Indirectly, then, the glandular kallikreins may be very important in regulating the water–electrolyte balance and the local blood flow. Several recent immunohistochemical studies have been made to elucidate the function of kallikreins by clarifying their distribution in exocrine glands and renal tubuli of animals and man [28, 92, 94, 95].

10.1.4. Distribution of tissue or organ antigens, including oncodevelopmental proteins

Immunohistochemistry has also been used to study the mucosal and glandular distribution of a variety of epithelial antigens whose function is as yet unknown. Examples are blood group substances [6, 56, 110, 120], the parietal-cell autoantigen [114, 122, 129], the goblet cell antigen [129], and the so-called carcinoembryonic antigen (CEA) [34, 35]. The latter represents one of the oncodevelopmental or oncofoetal antigens, which have been evaluated in numerous recent studies with regard to their usefulness as tumour markers. Immunofluorescence studies in our laboratory have not revealed any association between the amount of CEA in large bowel carcinomas and their histological grade or Duke's stage. Conversely, SC has been found to show significant relationships with these two parameters and may hence be a better cytochemical tumour marker [106]. Further immunohistochemical studies are needed, however, to see whether loss of SC and secretory IgA (see Fig. 20b,c) can be of any specific value in the diagnosis of intestinal neoplasia. Thus, loss of epithelial blood group substances has been noted not only in carcinomas of the larynx and oral cavity [43, 45] but also during wound healing in the oral mucosa [44].

10.2. CHOICE OF IMMUNOHISTOCHEMICAL METHOD

During the last decade immunoperoxidase methods have become increasingly popular [47, 119, 121]. These methods have four major advantages over immunofluorescence: 1) economy of reagents in that very high dilutions can be used, especially with the peroxidase–antiperoxidase (PAP) modification; 2) specialized microscopy is not required for the examination of tissue sections; 3) antigen localization and morphological details can be evaluated concurrently in the same section; and 4) the methods can be adapted for electron microscopical studies. The latter fact has been of great importance, for example, in the investigation of the mucosal immune system [63].

Other advantages, such as the possibility of using fixed material and paraffin sections, permanent section preparations, and a higher sensitivity are often mentioned in favour of the immunoperoxidase methods; but in my opinion these arguments are not necessarily valid, as will become apparent below. Moreover, the immunofluorescence technique has likewise some definite advantages: a) it is less time-consuming than the immunoperoxidase methods; b) owing to its simplicity, the direct immunofluorescence technique is easy to standardize and to control; c) immunofluorescence currently lends itself better to quantitation; and d) the direct technique can easily be adapted for paired staining of two antigens in the same tissue section. The latter fact is perhaps at present the major advantage of immunofluorescence. Standardized and simple procedures are now available for the production of fluorochrome conjugates of contrasting colours, namely with fluorescein isothiocyanate (FITC) and tetramethylrhodamine isothiocyanate (TRITC), respectively. Using the Ploem-type epi-illuminator [73] a sensitive and clear-cut differentiation between green and red tissue elements is obtained conveniently on the basis of interference filtration of fluorescence excitation and emission light. The various immunoenzyme methods proposed for concurrent staining of two or three antigens are much more cumbersome and do not permit sensitive distinction between mixed colours in double-stained structures [80, 82, 91].

Biological problems requiring a distinct differential localization of two antigens in the same section, and especially evaluation of the occurrence of two antigens in the same cell, are therefore best studied by means of paired immunofluorescence staining. Adequate FITC and TRITC conjugates can be mixed and applied in a one-step direct technique. We have used this approach to characterize mucosal immunocytes with regard to their cytoplasmic content of Ig polymers and J chain [12, 15, 70] and to study epithelial Ig and its translocation in association with SC [10, 11, 20, 22]. Moreover, at present paired immunofluorescence staining is the best and simplest method to study immunocytes with regard to Ig class and concomitant antibody specificity, using a combination of direct and "sandwich" technique [10, 16, 20].

In our laboratory paired immunofluorescence staining is used routinely since we appreciate the fact that the localization of one antigen in this way always serves as a built-in control for the localization of another and perhaps less well-known antigen. This procedure gives a better warning against methodological artifacts and lack of reagent specificity. We have found that all of the antigens discussed above in Section 10.1 can be studied by immunofluorescence in fixed and paraffin-embedded material. Morphological details can be evaluated conveniently in adjacent sections which are easily cut serially from the paraffin blocks. Moreover, since mounting media are available for prolonged storage of fluorescence preparations, some of the advantages inherent in immunoperoxidase methods can also be achieved with immunofluorescence. It should be stressed, however, that a prerequisite is the use of optimal and well-characterized fluorochrome conjugates which by performance testing have been found to show both immunological specificity and binding specificity [8, 13]. Such conjugates give negligible non-specific background staining, and with the Ploem-type epi-illuminator autofluorescence is minimal, especially under green excitation for rhodamine staining. The signal–noise ratio of adequately performed immunofluorescence is therefore high, and its sensitivity has been found to compare favourably with the PAP method for the detection of small amounts of antigen [42, 49, 68].

Immunofluorescence and immunoperoxidase methods are based on the same immunological principle, and many pitfalls are common to both methods. The requirements for reagent specificity, for controls that can reveal both false-negative and false-positive results, and for adequate tissue preparation methods are similar. In this respect warnings have recently been issued against uncritical use of immunoperoxidase methods [47]. Although the following sections will focus on immunofluorescence, part of the information given is equally relevant to immunoperoxidase studies.

10.3. PREPARATION OF FLUOROCHROME CONJUGATES SUITABLE FOR STUDIES OF MUCOUS MEMBRANES

10.3.1. Purification of IgG from antisera

Most of the antibody activity in sera of hyperimmunized animals is found in the IgG fraction. Rabbit IgG is easily purified by batch anionic-exchange chromatography (DEAE-Sephadex A-50, Pharmacia) combined with ammonium sulphate precipitation [7]. We originally used two stirring periods with the gel, each of 1 h duration at 4°C, but these can be reduced to 15 min. Goat and sheep antisera contain "fast" and "slow" IgG which both show antibody activity. The two fractions are purified as follows. The sera are diluted 1 : 2 with phosphate-buffered saline (PBS, pH 7.5) and precipitated with ammonium sulphate of 50% saturation at 4°C. The sediment is dissolved and dialyzed against 0.01 M phosphate buffer, pH 7.6, followed by fractionation on a column of Whatman DE52 cellulose (about 0.2 ml column volume/mg protein). "Slow" IgG is eluted with the starting buffer and the "fast" fraction with a step of 0.04 M NaCl. Further purification and concentration are achieved by ammonium sulphate precipitation of the eluates. All protein solutions are finally dialyzed against large volumes of 0.01 M phosphate buffer for 24–48 h at 4°C, cleared by centrifugation, and the concentration is determined assuming an $E^{1\%}_{1\,\mathrm{cm},\,280\,\mathrm{mm}} = 14$. If the original antisera are turbid, a prolonged dialysis is useful to precipitate lipoproteins.

10.3.2. Conjugation of IgG with fluorochromes

We routinely use FITC, crystalline isomer I, and amorphous TRITC, both purchased from Baltimore Biological Laboratory. Between 7 and 10 μg FITC or 20–40 μg TRITC per mg IgG are used. Immediately before conjugation the fluorochromes are suspended in a few drops of saline and added with stirring to the protein solution which beforehand has been adjusted to 5–20 g/l with 0.1 M Tris-HCl buffer, pH 8, to obtain a convenient volume for conjugation. Thereafter, the pH of the IgG–fluorochrome mixture is raised to 9.5 by slow addition of 1 N NaOH and maintained at this level with stirring for 1 h at room temperature [7]. The solubility of TRITC is usually poor in buffer but very good in dimethyl sulphoxide (DMSO) [4]. The efficiency of the conjugation can therefore be significantly enhanced by dissolving this fluorochrome in the smallest possible volume of DMSO before adding it slowly to the protein solution. With this modification the amount of TRITC should be reduced to 20 μg/mg IgG or less; an even better control of pH is required, and the yield of conjugate is somewhat reduced owing to an increased fraction of overlabelled protein.

10.3.3. Purification of fluorochrome conjugates

Immediately after coupling, TRITC conjugates are filtered through columns of Sephadex G-50 (coarse) equilibrated with 0.01 M phosphate buffer. This is absolutely necessary in order to avoid that unreacted dye is partially eluted with the fall-through fraction on subsequent anionic-exchange chromatography. Conversely, FITC conjugates are simply dialyzed for 3–18 h against 0.01 M phosphate buffer before application on columns of Whatman DE23 or DE52 cellulose and elution with steps of NaCl (about 0.2 ml column volume/mg original IgG).

A marked heterogeneity of the conjugated IgG is always revealed by anionic-exchange chromatography. This is illustrated for a rabbit FITC conjugate in Fig. 10.1. The protein peaks are characterized by their absorbance (*A*) ratios, that is, *A* at 280 nm divided by *A* measured at the absorption maximum of the bound fluorochrome, which for FITC is 495 nm. A high absorbance ratio indicates a low degree of conjugation, and this ratio can, for FITC conjugates, be converted to the actual molar fluorochrome/protein (F/P) ratio [7]. In Fig. 10.1 an absorbance ratio of 6.3 indicates a molar F/P ratio of less than 0.5, so this fraction is "underlabelled" and not useful for immunofluorescence. An absorbance ratio of 2.3 indicates an F/P ratio between 1.5 and 2.0, and an absorbance ratio of 1.6 indicates an F/P ratio between 2.5 and 3. These two fractions are "moderately labelled", and we usually elute them from the column in a single step with 0.1 M NaCl. An absorbance ratio of 1.2 indicates an F/P ratio of about 3.5 and is therefore "highly labelled". This fraction can, if required, be relatively increased by raising the amount of FITC for conjugation to at least 10 μg/mg IgG.

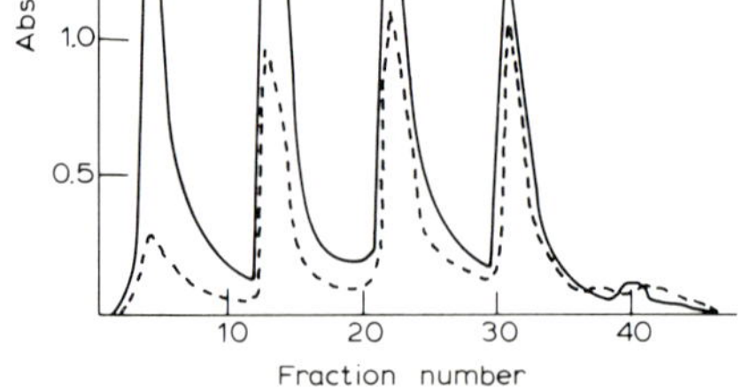

Fig. 10.1. Anionic-exchange chromatography on DE 23 cellulose (1.4 × 5 cm) of 40 mg rabbit IgG conjugated with 7 μg FITC/mg followed by dialysis against starting buffer (0.01 M phosphate buffer, pH 7.6) overnight at 4°C. Fractions (3.4 ml) were eluted with steps of NaCl as indicated. Absorbance ratios of protein peaks appear in adjacent circles: $A_{280\ nm}$, ——. $A_{495\ nm}$, -----.

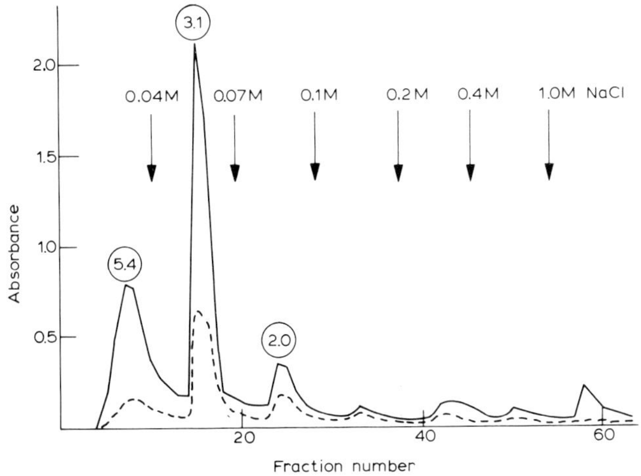

Fig. 10.2. Anionic-exchange chromatography of 28 mg rabbit IgG conjugated with 40 μg TRITC/mg followed by gel filtration to separate excess of free dye and to equilibrate the sample against the starting buffer. Column and elution conditions as in Fig. 1: $A_{280\ \mathrm{nm}}$, ——. $A_{515\ \mathrm{nm}}$, -----.

Rabbit TRITC conjugates exhibit less heterogeneity, and a typical chromatography pattern is shown in Fig. 10.2. The protein peaks are again characterized by their absorbance ratios, which for TRITC conjugates is A at 280 nm divided by A at 515 nm. At present there is no way to convert these ratios to actual F/P ratios, since an adequate TRITC standard is not available [4, 7]. We have observed great variations in the conjugation properties of various TRITC batches, and the absorbance ratios of the two major elution peaks have sometimes reached 7 and 4, respectively. Nevertheless, due to the high sensitivity of the rhodamine fluorescence, even the fall-through fraction of the conjugates is usable if the original antiserum is of a good titre. Moreover, goat and sheep IgG show a much better affinity for the fluorochromes than rabbit IgG, and a good conjugation result is always obtained. For these species a very highly labelled fraction can be collected by applying a 0.2 M NaCl step directly after the 0.04 M step.

The conjugate fractions are concentrated by Amicon filtration on Diaflo-membrane PM-10, dialyzed against PBS overnight at 4°C, passed through a 0.8 μm Millipore filter, and the final absorbance ratio and content of IgG are determined. The protein concentration is estimated by the following equations [36]:

$$\text{FITC-conjugated IgG (g/l)} = \frac{A_{280\ \mathrm{nm}} - 0.35 \times A_{495\ \mathrm{nm}}}{1.4}$$

$$\text{TRITC-conjugated IgG (g/l)} = \frac{A_{280\ \mathrm{nm}} - 0.56 \times A_{515\ \mathrm{nm}}}{1.4}$$

10.3.4. Specific and non-specific staining properties of fluorescein and rhodamine conjugates

Lack of *binding specificity* of the fluorochrome conjugate with resultant non-specific staining and lack of *immunological specificity* are the two principal causes of unwanted fluorescence. It is now generally accepted that the immunological specificity must be ascertained by performance testing on appropriate biological or artificial antigen substrates, since double diffusion techniques are not sensitive enough to show contaminating antibody activities [8, 13]. The binding specificity of a conjugate may be jeopardized due to the reduced isoelectric point of the labelled IgG. Moreover, fluorescent immune complexes show a relatively high net negative charge and are especially prone to producing non-specific staining. Therefore, when antisera have to be absorbed in order to obtain a desired immunological specificity, insoluble immunosorbents should be used to avoid the formation of soluble complexes.

The immunofluorescence sensitivity level of a conjugate is expressed as the endpoint of *specific staining*; it is determined from titrations as the lowest conjugate concentration producing barely visible staining of an appropriate antigen substrate [8, 13]. The endpoint of *non-specific staining* is taken as the lowest conjugate concentration that results in detectable fluorescence either when the antibody activity is blocked by the addition of antigen in excess or when the conjugate is tested on a comparable substrate lacking the relevant antigen. In studies of mucosal immunoglobulins, for example, it is very useful to have biopsy specimens from patients with an immunodeficiency for such reagent controls. The range of protein concentrations that produce fluores-

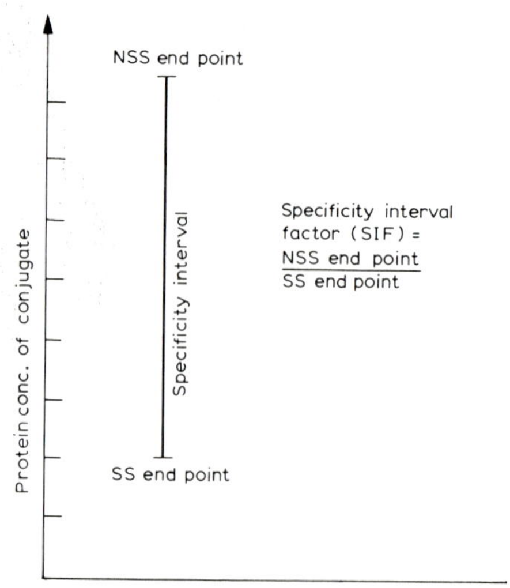

Fig. 10.3. The specific binding properties of a fluorescent conjugate depend on the magnitude of its specificity interval factor (SIF). The specificity interval represents the range of concentrations that can be expected to produce only immunologic binding with the substrate. NSS, non-specific staining; SS, specific staining.

cence depending only on immunological binding to the substrate is called the *specificity interval* of the conjugate; it is defined by the *specificity interval factor* (Fig. 10.3).

Characteristics of various anionic-exchange fractions of conjugates prepared from a rabbit antiserum specific for human IgG are exemplified in Table 10.I. Specific staining was evaluated on a plasma cell substrate, and non-specific staining on smears of rabbit leukocytes. The best sensitivity (lowest endpoint of specific staining) was obtained for the TRITC conjugate fraction eluted with 0.04 M NaCl. This fraction moreover had a wide specificity interval, as indicated by a relatively high specificity interval factor. The "fall-through" fraction of the same conjugate showed slightly less sensitivity but a wider specificity interval. A similar sensitivity could be obtained with the FITC conjugate, but only for the highly labelled fraction that showed a very narrow specificity interval [8]. These comparisons were made with an HBO 200 W lamp, whereas we now use an XBO 150 W lamp for FITC and thereby increase the sensitivity of this fluorochrome approximately twofold.

Information about non-specific staining is therefore quite irrelevant without taking the sensitivity of specific staining into consideration in parallel. A conjugate of good quality gives rise to non-specific staining only at a relatively high protein concentration but still produces specific staining at a low concentration, as indicated by a high specificity interval factor. This factor may be increased in several ways: a) the endpoint of non-specific staining can be raised by using a limited amount of fluorochrome for conjugation and by subsequent removal of both highly labelled protein and free and loosely bound dye molecules from the conjugate; b) the endpoint of specific staining can be lowered by removal of underlabelled protein from the conjugate, the use of high-titred antiserum for conjugation, the use of $F(ab')_2$ fragments of the IgG fraction, or by isolating the actual antibodies from the IgG fraction with immunosorbent technique before or after conjugation; c) by prolonging the incubation of the substrate with the conjugate, from for example 30 min to 20

TABLE 10.I

ENDPOINT OF SPECIFIC STAINING (SS) AND THE SPECIFICITY INTERVAL FACTOR (SIF) FOR VARIOUS ANIONIC-EXCHANGE FRACTIONS OF CONJUGATED RABBIT IgG PREPARED FROM THE SAME ANTISERUM

Fluorochrome		Properties of conjugate fractions			
Type	Addition (μg/mg IgG)	Elution molarity	*A* ratio	SS endpoint (g/l)	SIF
FITC	10	0.04–0.07	2.1	0.053	53
FITC	12	0.2 –0.4	1.5	0.046	24
FITC	25	0.2 –0.4	1.0	0.030	6
TRITC	20	0.01	7.7	0.028	130
TRITC	20	0.04	3.6	0.017	96

h, its working concentration can be reduced by a factor of about 10 which favours specific over non-specific staining; and d) selection of a fluorochrome that affords maximum sensitivity under the available optical conditions likewise favours specific staining since the working concentration of the conjugate can be reduced.

With the Ploem-type epi-illuminator and green excitation light from an HBO 200 W lamp we have found that TRITC usually is the better choice of fluorochrome in the above respect. Another advantage of TRITC over FITC is the virtual lack of fluorescence fading. In practical microscopy TRITC conjugates are therefore more advantageous than is indicated from the comparisons made in Table 10.I. Reproducible repeat observations by the same or different observers are made possible, and mounted preparations can be stored for many years in the dark with unaltered properties. There is one pitfall, however, namely that yellow autofluorescent granules, such as lipofuscin present in glandular duct cells [70] and in some macrophages and hepatocytes, give the impression of specific staining with conditions for rhodamine fluorescence; but these granules are easily identified by switching to microscopy conditions for FITC with blue excitation which reveals their yellow colour.

It should be pointed out that the commercial batches of amorphous TRITC contain varying amounts of impurities that apparently bind to IgG during the conjugation by low-affinity reactions without decreasing its isoelectric point [8]. Exchange of these dye molecules between IgG and the tissue section may produce diffuse non-specific staining. This can be eliminated by absorbing the conjugate with a tissue powder, such as acetone-dried mouse liver powder, or by addition of high concentrations of bovine serum albumin (BSA) [8]. Dialysis for 2–3 days against PBS containing 1% DMSO has likewise been recommended for removal of loosely bound TRITC from IgG [57]. These measures are not an alternative but an adjunct to anionic-exchange chromatography of the conjugates.

Absence of non-specific staining must be ascertained by controls that can reveal lack of binding specificity at the working concentration of the conjugate, which always should be chosen as low as possible. Absorption with the relevant, soluble antigen in excess is a highly reliable test, since non-specific staining is intensified by the formation of fluorescent, soluble immune complexes [8]. Elements in the substrate that are particularly prone to give non-specific binding of labelled IgG can thus be identified (Fig. 10.4). If the immunological specificity of the conjugate has been firmly established by performance tests on appropriate substrates, it is not necessary, although preferable [99], to use a highly purified antigen for this absorption control; a parallel test with the addition of a similar amount of irrelevant protein should be included.

In immunohistochemical studies of mucous membranes three tissue elements are particularly prone to give non-specific staining, namely eosinophilic granulocytes, squamous epithelium and columnar epithelium, in

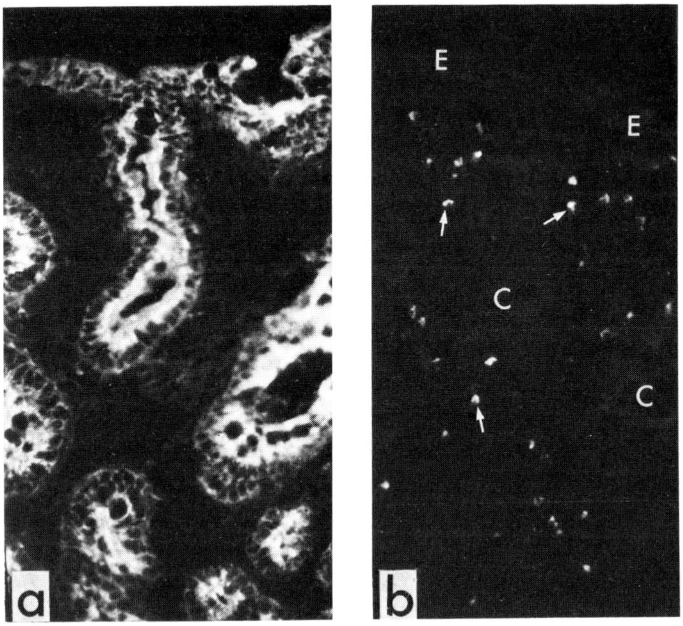

Fig. 10.4. Control of binding specificity by antigen absorption in excess. TRITC-conjugated rabbit IgG (*A* ratio = 3) specific for human SC was tested at 0.9 g/l after absorption with mouse liver powder (a), and at 1.5 g/l after absorption with 0.4 g SC/l. The test substrate was adjacent sections (comparable fields shown) of intestinal mucosa from a patient with coeliac disease preincubated with BSA at 250 g/l. Note that antigen absorption inhibited completely specific fluorescence of crypt (C) and surface epithelium (E), which was bright in (a), whereas the formation of soluble immune complexes contributed to intensification of non-specific staining of eosinophilic granulocytes (arrows) scattered in the lamina propria (b). ×235.

that order [8]. Since the morphological features of fluorescent eosinophilic granulocytes commonly mimic those of immunocytes, this type of non-specific staining should be considered a major pitfall in immunofluorescence studies of immunoglobulin- and antibody-producing cells [21]. When rhodamine conjugates are used, it is possible to identify the eosinophilic granulocytes by excitation with blue light, because their yellow-grey autofluorescence is prominent, especially after storage of mounted sections [13]. When FITC conjugates are used, however, this autofluorescence may be masked by green non-specific staining, which makes cell identification extremely difficult. Blocking of non-specific conjugate binding to these cells by prior treatment of the tissue sections with Lendrum's stain has been reported [65], but the authors rightly cautioned against the possibility of antigenic alteration with this procedure. Anyhow, non-specific staining can be rendered negligible when conjugates are made and applied according to the principles outlined above.

Although the non-specific staining endpoint of columnar epithelial cells is generally about eightfold higher than that of eosinophilic granulocytes and squamous epithelium, the goblet cells may represent a particular problem. This is illustrated by the conflicting information that has appeared about the cellular origin of SC. Mucous-type cells, including goblet cells, were originally

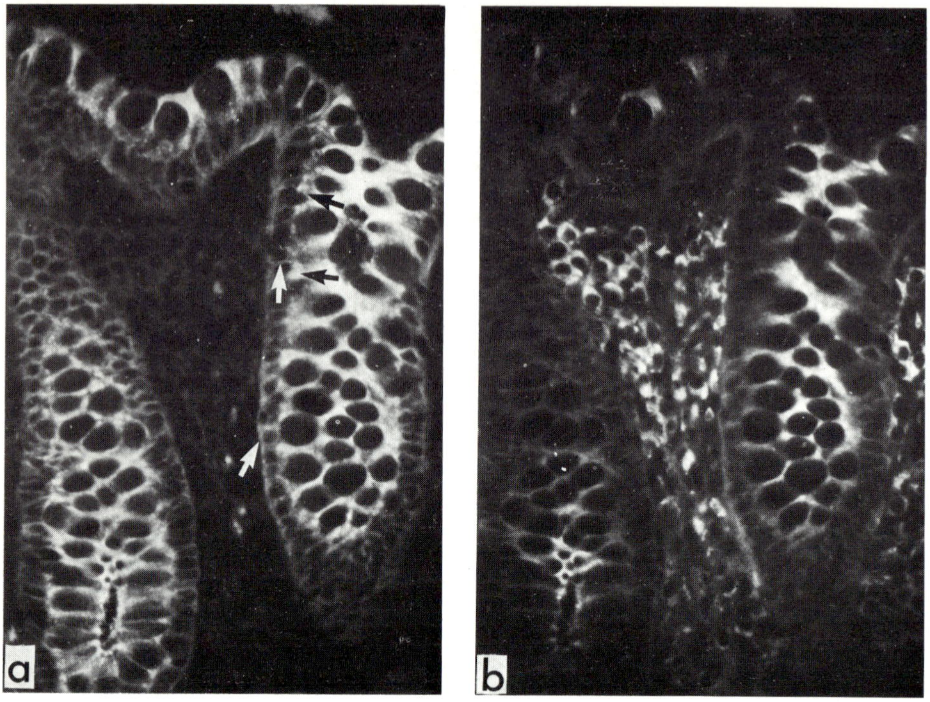

Fig. 10.5. Paired immunofluorescence staining (same field) for a) SC (red), and b) IgA (green) in directly ethanol-fixed normal human colon mucosa. SC is abundantly present in columnar cells of crypt and surface epithelium (at the top), and also appear at the basal and lateral borders of these cells (white arrows). Cytoplasmic SC is concentrated in granules adjacent to the nuclei (black arrows), indicating accumulation of free component in Golgi complexes. IgA shows an epithelial distribution corresponding to that of SC, except that the concentration seems lower, especially in the surface epithelium, and Golgi-related accumulations are lacking. The goblet cells are negative. ×310.

claimed to be the main glandular source of this epithelial product [124], and the same finding has been reported by many subsequent investigators. Conversely, in our immunofluorescence studies SC has been localized chiefly to the serous secretory cell (Fig. 10.5). Only one of our apparently SC-specific conjugates gives rise to staining of intestinal goblet cells, but this unwanted fluorescence seems to be explained by lack of immunological specificity rather than by lack of binding specificity [18]. On the other hand, some mucus-producing adenocarcinomas, such as the signet ring cells of linitis plastica, may show SC-synthesizing capacity which probably explains why they accumulate selectively IgA and IgM (see Fig. 10.15).

10.4. IMMUNOFLUORESCENCE STAINING PROCEDURES

10.4.1. Direct method

We prefer the direct immunofluorescence technique for most immunohistochemical studies of mucous membranes and exocrine glands, since it affords sufficient sensitivity for this purpose, is safer with regard to specificity controls, and can easily be adapted for paired staining of two antigens (Fig. 10.5, 10.15 and 10.20 b,c). Most of our conjugates used in these studies show absorbance ratios of 1.3–4.5 and have been applied at an IgG concentration of 0.1–1.0 g/l, corresponding to 1/10–1 precipitating unit, with an incubation period of 30 min at room temperature [17]. This sort of information should be available for every published immunohistochemical study so that at least the experienced reader may have some possibility to evaluate the basis for the reported results.

It is often preferable to prolong the incubation time to for example 20 h, with the conjugate concentration reduced to about 10% of that indicated above. This modification does not only improve reagent economy but also favours specific over unwanted staining. Besides, a better discrimination between tissue elements with a slightly different antigen concentration may be obtained. Thus, IgG-producing cells, which are often difficult to visualize because of diffusely distributed IgG in the connective tissue, stand out more clearly against the background after prolonged incubation with diluted conjugate. Using the PAP method we have found that a similar prolongation of the primary antiserum incubation permits a further reagent dilution of about 100 times. It should be noted, however, that while prolonged exposure to the antibody reagent always seems to be of advantage with formaldehyde-fixed material, some antigens such as lysozyme may be subjected to diffusion artifacts in ethanol-fixed material and to some extent go into solution during section incubation; the result is then staining of poor quality and immune complexes are sometimes smeared over the substrate.

10.4.2. Indirect methods

If there is a shortage of specific antiserum to be used for localizing antigens by immunofluorescence, an indirect method has to be carried out for the sake of economy; besides, this approach enhances the sensitivity of antigen detection, at least in theory. A better sensitivity may be masked by a tendency towards higher non-specific background staining caused by adherence of IgG in the primary antiserum (usually rabbit) to elements of the tissue section (see Fig. 10.24). This can be significantly reduced by diluting the antiserum in PBS containing BSA (100 g/l) and 0.25% Triton X-100, and in addition by including 1% Triton X-100 in the PBS used to wash the tissue sections after the primary incubation [58].

Another cause of backgound staining, which often is neglected when the indirect technique is used, is the fact that the secondary reagent (the conjugate) may show some reactivity with the substrate. Thus we have found that all goat and sheep anti-rabbit IgG conjugates, commercially obtained or prepared in our laboratory, cross-react with human IgG present in plasma cells or diffusely distributed in sections of human tissue specimens. This reactivity as macroscopically visible hybridoma colonies appeared the respective supernatants were tested in radioimmunoassay (RIA) for the binding of ^{125}I-labelled hormone. Positive colonies were transferred to wells of flat-bottom microtiter plates (Nunc) until grown to monolayer. From there the cells were transferred via 24-well Nunc plates first to 50 ml and finally to 250 ml culture bottles (Falcon F3013 and F3024 respectively, LS-Labor-Service, München, F.R.G.). The cells were kept in HAT-containing medium for the first 14 days after fusion, then transferred to HT medium (excluding aminopterin) for another week, and then passed to regular tissue culture medium (see above). All hybrid lines were cloned at least twice by limiting dilution and in many instances also by the soft agarose technique [3]. A limiting dilution was carried out as early as possible using Nunc microtiter plates containing 200 μl conditioned medium (culture medium already used by NS 1 cells) plus 1×10^4 mouse peritoneal macrophages per well. Soft agarose cloning was performed in 12-well Linbro culture plates (Linbro Scientific, Inc., Hamden, CT) filled with 5 ml 0.5% agarose (Behringwerke AG, Marburg, F.R.G.) in culture medium per well. For large-scale production of MAb 1×10^7 cells were injected intraperitoneally into BALB/c recipients pretreated with 0.5 ml 2,4,6,10-tetramethylpentadecane (Ega-Chemie, Steinheim, F.R.G.) 1–10 days before injection. The antibodies were then separated from the ascites by means of a staphylococcus protein A [2] column and concentrated to 5 mg IgG/ml in an ultrafiltration cell (Amicon cell, model 202, Amicon Corporation, Lexington, MA) equipped with a molecular filter, PM 10.

9.3.3. Production of MAb against human growth hormone

The MAb against GH have been produced by Dr. J. Ivanyi (Wellcome Research Laboratories, Beckenham, U.K.) as described in detail elsewhere [7].

9.4. IMMUNOFLUORESCENCE METHODOLOGY

IF analysis of antibodies against hormones required both a sufficient amount of the specific antibody to be tested and a properly prepared organ in which the respective hormone is present in an antigenically intact state. The first point reflects the sensitivity of the method. We have observed that crude culture supernatants usually provide sufficient amounts of antibody to be detected even in diluted form. For the tracing of low affinity antibodies, however, the use of ascites fluid or otherwise enriched and purified antibodies may be necessary.

A much more serious problem is the processing of the antigenic material, i.e. the pituitary gland. In a previous paper [9] we described a method for preserving LH in an antigenically active form in frozen sections by fixation with 5% formaldehyde in 96% ethanol. Although this quick and simple technique leads to perfect staining of glycoprotein hormone-producing cells, it can be removed by absorption of the conjugate with polymerized human serum or IgG. Similar problems have been encountered by others using the indirect technique [54], although cross-reactivity was not offered as an explanation for the unwanted staining. This source of error is apparently smaller when swine anti-rabbit IgG conjugates are used, and in our hands the cross-reactivity shown by such reagents is easily removed.

An indirect "sandwich" technique is the most reliable approach to identify cytoplasmic antibody specificity of Ig-producing cells, but only few attempts have been made to characterize mucosal and glandular immunocyte populations of man in this respect [16, 20, 24, 37]. In our studies we have combined the "sandwich" method with direct identification of concomitant Ig class by paired staining. It is important to use an adequate antigen concentration in the first incubation step. We have found that sections of inoculation granulomas or of the spleen of rabbits immunized with the actual antigen may serve as excellent substrates to establish by performance testing the working concentrations of the "sandwich" reagents. A concentration of 0.05–0.3 g/l with 30 min incubation has been found to be optimal for various solutions of bacterial and dietary antigens, the variation probably depending largely on their purity.

A combined indirect–direct immunofluorescence method has also been used to demonstrate the dimeric or polymeric nature of the Ig product of mucosal and glandular IgA and IgM immunocytes by testing for cytoplasmic SC affinity [9, 12, 23]. This in vitro SC-binding test is based on the fact that only J chain-containing IgA and IgM show a non-covalent affinity for free SC. Serial sections are first incubated with unlabelled purified colostral SC at 10 μg/ml in a 0.5% (w/v) solution of rabbit IgG for 1 h at room temperature. Control

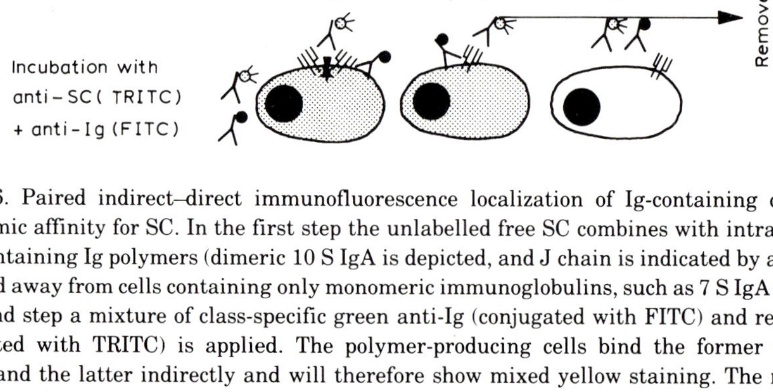

Fig. 10.6. Paired indirect–direct immunofluorescence localization of Ig-containing cells with cytoplasmic affinity for SC. In the first step the unlabelled free SC combines with intracellular J chain-containing Ig polymers (dimeric 10 S IgA is depicted, and J chain is indicated by a star). SC is washed away from cells containing only monomeric immunoglobulins, such as 7 S IgA or IgG. In the second step a mixture of class-specific green anti-Ig (conjugated with FITC) and red anti-SC (conjugated with TRITC) is applied. The polymer-producing cells bind the former conjugate directly and the latter indirectly and will therefore show mixed yellow staining. The monomer-producing cells will have a pure green colour. The figure illustrates differentiation between dimer- and purely monomer-producing IgA immunocytes.

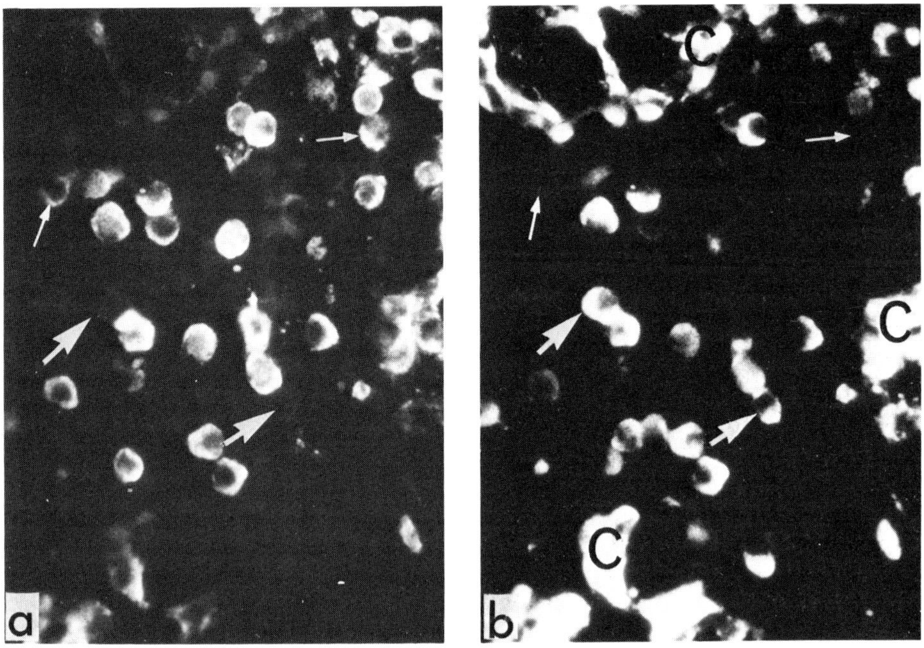

Fig. 10.7. Immunofluorescence SC-affinity test performed on IgA immunocytes in a section of saline-extracted and ethanol-fixed human intestinal mucosa. Green staining (a) represents IgA. Red staining (b) in the same field signifies positive SC-binding when related to immunocytes but innate SC when related to epithelial crypt cells (C). Small arrows indicate two negative IgA cells; large arrows indicate positive immunocytes of another Ig class, which by inference is IgM. ×540.

sections are incubated with rabbit IgG alone. After a 20 min saline wash, all sections are treated with a TRITC-labelled anti-SC conjugate mixed with an FITC-labelled class-specific anti-Ig conjugate. Dimer- and polymer-producing cells bind the latter conjugate directly and the former indirectly, and will therefore be double-stained, whereas monomer-producing IgA cells will show a pure green colour (Figs. 10.6 and 10.7). If the first incubation step is prolonged overnight in this test, which is performed on ethanol-fixed tissue sections, it may be difficult to obtain a negative control, since innate SC may diffuse from glandular structures and combine with the cytoplasm of adjacent immunocytes.

10.4.3. Exposure of hidden antigenic determinants

The J chain present in dimeric IgA and pentameric IgM is partially hidden, and even more so in secretory IgA; but the J chain determinants become exposed when the Ig polymers are unfolded by denaturation [14]. Most gland-associated IgA immunocytes produce J chain that is bound and partially concealed at the intracellular stage; during the passage of dimeric IgA through glandular epithelial cells the J chain determinants become still more hidden due to masking by incorporated SC (Figs. 10.8 and 10.9). A distinct localization

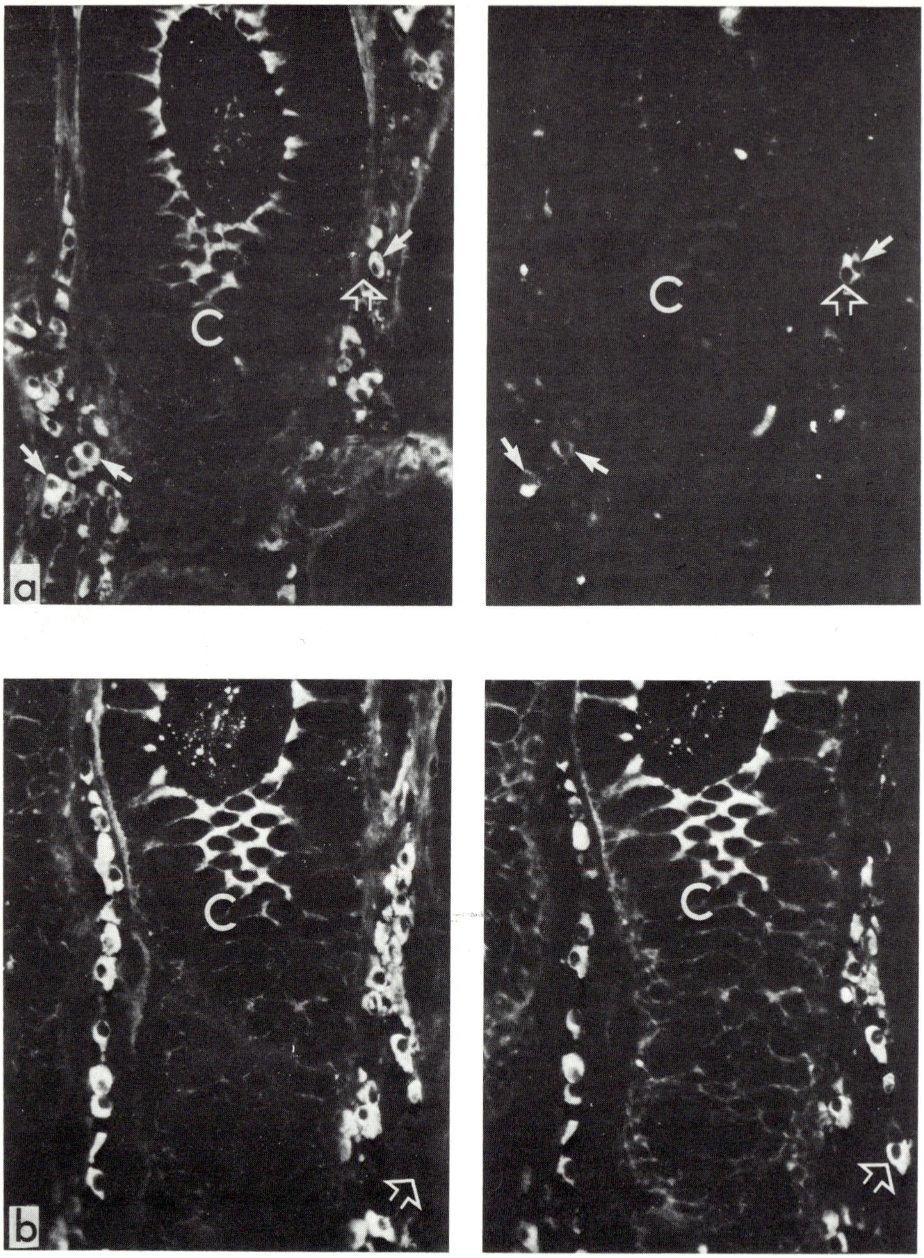

Fig. 10.8. Paired immunofluorescence staining for IgA (green to the left) and J chain (red to the right) in comparable fields from two adjacent sections of directly ethanol-fixed human colon mucosa. a) IgA is present in numerous immunocytes and diffusely in the connective tissue, as well as in the crypt epithelium (C), whereas J chain is detectable in only some of the IgA cells (small arrows) and in one immunocyte of another class (large arrows). b) This section has been denatured in acid urea; there is brisk staining for J chain in all IgA cells and in one immunocyte of another class (arrows) as well as in the epithelium, whereas diffusely distributed IgA shows negligible J-chain reactivity and hence represents chiefly monomeric IgA. ×310.

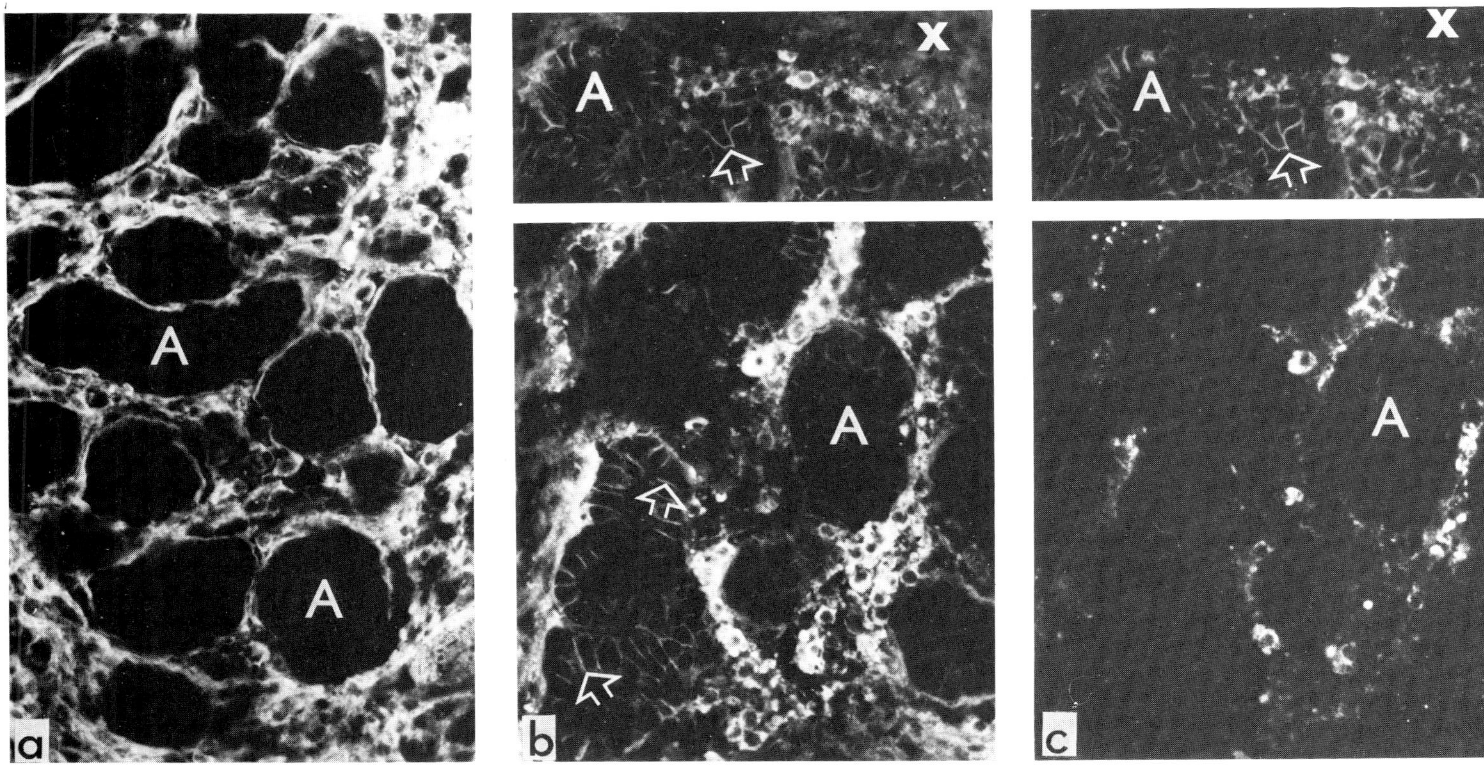

Fig. 10.9. Immunofluorescence staining for IgG (a) and IgA (b) in comparable fields from adjacent sections of directly ethanol-fixed human nasal mucosa. Paired staining for J chain in the same field as (b) is shown in (c). Insets at the top in (b) and (c) demonstrate IgA and J chain in adjacent section denatured in acid urea. IgG is abundantly present in the connective tissue, and the bright background staining obscures visualization of IgG immunocytes. Note that IgG is not taken up by the glandular acini (A). Smaller amounts of IgA are diffusely present in the stroma, and IgA immunocytes therefore stand out more clearly. Note acinar uptake of IgA related to the lateral borders of the epithelial cells (arrows). Without urea denaturation there is some cytoplasmic J-chain reactivity of IgA immunocytes, but not of interstitial and epithelial IgA. After urea denaturation a bright J-chain staining of epithelial IgA (arrows) reveals its dimeric nature, whereas interstitial IgA (X) remains virtually negative, indicating that it is chiefly monomeric. ×385.

of J chain in dimer-producing IgA immunocytes, and even more so in secretory epithelial cells, therefore, depends on preincubation of the tissue section in a denaturing solution [17, 90]. We routinely use 0.1 M glycine-HCl buffer, pH 3.2, containing 6 M urea, for 1 h at 4°C. It is important to rinse the sections thoroughly after this treatment to avoid inhibition of the reaction with the subsequently applied conjugates. Urea treatment may likewise be useful to intensify the staining of other antigens [94], but it also tends to increase non-specific background staining, especially of squamous epithelium.

10.4.4. Mounting and storage of immunofluorescence preparations

A so-called semi-permanent mounting medium [104] containing the polyvinyl alcohol Elvanol grade 51-05 (DuPont de Nemours E.I. and Co.) has been used routinely in our laboratory with excellent result. Immunofluorescence preparations have been stored in the dark at 4°C for more than 8 years with no apparent decrease in the intensity of fluorescein or rhodamine staining and no increase in autofluorescence. We prepare this medium from Elvanol, PBS, and glycerol in the proportions 1 : 4 : 3 (w/v/v), and adjust the pH to 8–8.5 to enhance the fluorescence of FITC. Elvanol grade 51–05 is no longer produced, and we are currently trying out other ways of preparing a satisfactory mountant with Elvanol grade 90–50 or Sigma Type II polyvinyl alcohol based on various proposed modifications [59, 76]. In our experience, the xylol-miscible, commercially available mountants are not satisfactory for fluorescein preparations but preserve rhodamine fluorescence well.

10.4.5. Fluorescence microscopy and photography

The microscope used in our laboratory is a Leitz Orthoplan equipped with an Osram HBO 200 W lamp for rhodamine (red) and an XBO 150 W lamp for fluorescein (green) excitation. A Ploem-type epi-illuminator is used for narrow-band excitation and selective filtration of the fluorescence colours. Dichroic mirrors and appropriate filters can be switched synchronously by a single handling, thus facilitating repeat observations of individual tissue elements with regard to mixed fluorescence features. Our findings were previously recorded on "Anscochrome" 200 daylight film but we now use Kodak Ektachrome 400 daylight film for colour slides. The exposure times vary between 2 and 15 s and are determined manually based on experience. The phototube is constructed so that 100% of the emission light reaches the film, which is contained in a Leica body. Green, red and mixed colours can be evaluated simultaneously by double exposures (see Fig. 10.15). Micrographs for cell enumerations are taken with a $\times 10/0.45$ Leitz immersion objective and a $\times 10$ ocular. Counting of cells by direct microscopy is carried out through a $\times 25/0.75$ Leitz immersion objective and an ocular grid (Leitz code No. 519902) representing a tissue section area of 0.08 mm^2.

10.4.6. Enumeration of cells by fluorescence microscopy

Various methods have been proposed to quantitate mucosal Ig-producing cells [38, 112]. We base immunocyte counts in the intestinal mucosa on an individually defined "mucosal tissue unit", constituting a 500 μm wide block of the mucosa at full height from the muscularis mucosae in properly oriented sections cut at 6 μm (Fig. 10.10). In this way we aim at a comparative quantification of the total mucosal mass of Ig-producing cells of the various classes, and do not limit the registration to cell densities in a selected area, as has been the case in previous studies. Heterogeneity in cell densities and mucosal morphology may severely jeopardize the reliability of cell enumerations based on selected areas when evaluation of disease-associated alterations is attempted (Fig. 10.11).

In each tissue unit the various immunocyte classes are recorded, usually on double-exposed colour film, after paired immunohistochemical staining with different combinations of FITC and TRITC conjugates [20]. This is done to substantiate the immunological specificity of the reagents (cells show a pure green or red colour) and to obtain reliable differential cell counts by always relating the number of one immunocyte class to that of another in the same tissue unit.

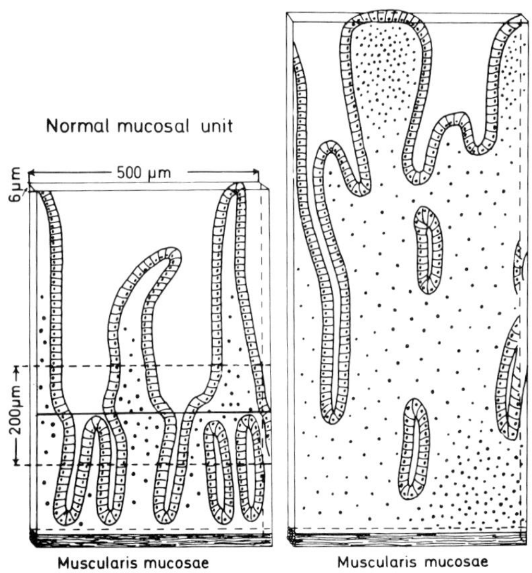

Fig. 10.10. Schematic representation of a "mucosal tissue unit" in sections cut at 6 μm from a normal small intestine (left) and from a diseased small intestine (right). The unit area is an individual characteristic which is obtained correctly only in sections oriented perpendicular to the muscularis mucosae. The total number of Ig-producing cells per tissue unit depends on variations in the unit area and on variations in cell density. The distribution of dots indicates heterogeneity in cell density that may occur within the two units. The highest density is normally found at the base of the villi. The orientation of a corresponding 200 μm zone, which may be used for quantitative comparisons within or between units [2], is shown by horizontal broken lines. (Reproduced from Brandtzaeg and Baklien [20], with kind permission of the publisher.)

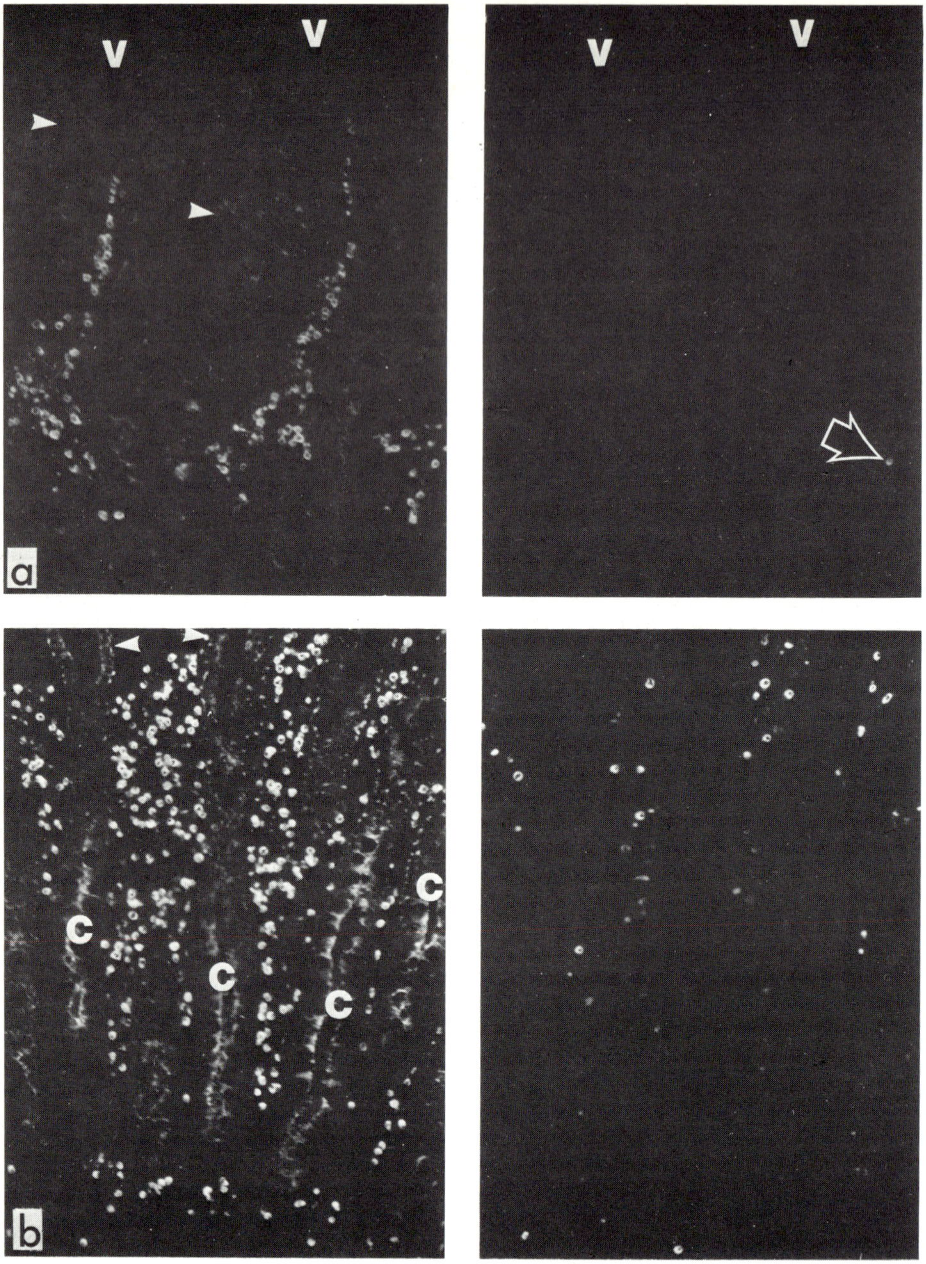

Fig. 10.11. Paired immunofluorescence for IgA (green to the left) and IgG (red to the right) in saline-extracted and ethanol-fixed specimens of a) normal duodenal mucosa and b) duodenal mucosa from a patient with coeliac disease. In the normal mucosa the IgA immunocyte population is located around the level of the crypt openings and extends for some length into the villi (V); only one IgG-producing cell is present in this field (arrow). In the coeliac mucosa there is a marked increase of the IgA-cell population and relatively more so of the IgG-cell population; intense staining of columnar crypt cells (C) indicates external transport of IgA. The tissue extraction procedure has led to some distortion of the epithelium (arrowheads) covering the villi (a) and at the opening of the crypts (b). Measurement of immunocyte density in a selected area of the lamina propria may not reveal any difference between the two specimens, whereas cell enumerations based on an individually defined tissue unit (Fig. 10.10) demonstrate marked disease-associated alterations of the intestinal IgA- and IgG-cell populations. $\times 120$.

For each case our final result gives the absolute immunocyte counts as well as the class ratios in an average unit from a particular intestinal segment; in addition, the average density of such cells in the lamina propria of the whole unit may be estimated by morphometry [2, 105]. The absolute counts vary considerably among specimens of the same category, especially in disease. A great variation may likewise be seen among different specimens from the same individual and sometimes even within the same specimen. Group calculations based on absolute counts are obviously more influenced by specimens with many cells than by those with few. Therefore, to obtain an idea about the true average shifts in local immune-response patterns associated with a disease, group calculations should in addition be based on immunocyte ratios from individual samples, which all have the same statistical weight. Such ratios are preferable when individual observations are evaluated with regard to the principal alterations in the intestinal immunocyte populations, and when results of different investigators are compared.

In other mucosal and glandular sites, such as the tonsils and salivary glands, the Ig-producing cells are even more heterogeneously distributed than in the intestinal mucosa, and we have used a modification of the above quantification method [27, 70, 71]. In these sites immunocyte enumerations should be based on counts in a defined tissue unit area repeated systematically throughout the section (Fig. 10.12). It should be determined for each tissue

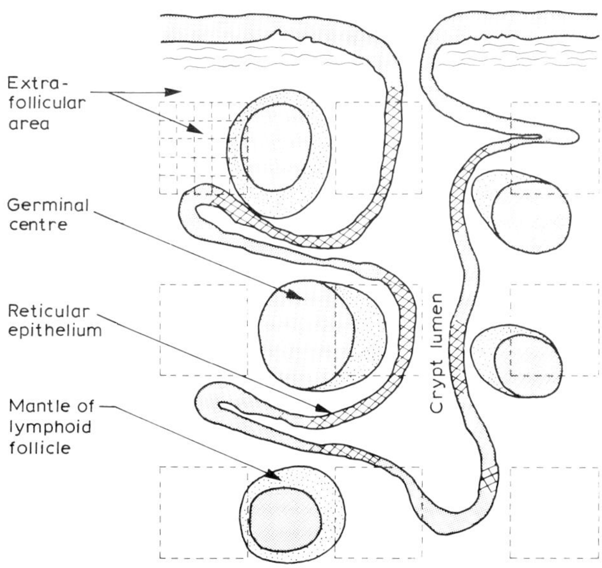

Fig. 10.12. Schematic representation of a section cut at 6 μm through a human palatine tonsil. Immunocyte enumerations are based on counts of Ig-producing cells in a defined tissue unit area which, as indicated, is evaluated repeatedly in a systematic manner throughout the section to include at random parts of four morphological compartments: the extrafollicular area (excluding the faucial epithelium at the top and the adjacent dense connective tissue), the germinal centres of the lymphoid follicles, their mantle zones, and the reticular parts of the crypt epithelium. (Reproduced from Brandtzaeg et al. [27], with kind permission of the publisher.)

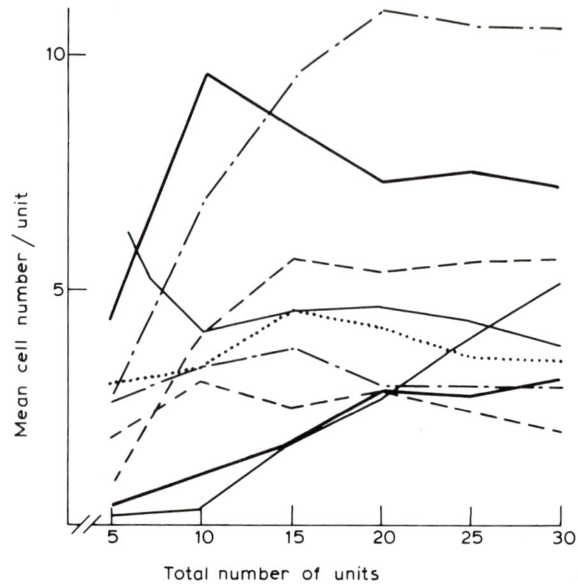

Fig. 10.13. Enumeration of IgA immunocytes in nine specimens of human salivary glands based on systematic evaluation of a defined tissue unit area (0.08 mm^2) as indicated in Fig. 10.12. The individual accumulative means (cell number/unit) show that the data are generally representative for each specimen after evaluation of about 20 tissue units. (Reproduced from Korsrud and Brandtzaeg [71], with kind permission of the publisher).

type how many units the actual observer has to evaluate to obtain a stable and hence true estimate for an individual specimen (Fig. 10.13).

Similar problems are encountered in attempts to quantify the endocrine cells of the gut, such as the antral gastrin-producing cells. The G cells are present mainly in the middle third of the pyloric glands (see Fig. 10.24); it is therefore of great importance also in these quantitative studies to orient the tissue specimens so that sections can be cut perpendicular to the muscularis mucosae. Again, we base our cell counts on a defined "mucosal tissue unit" constituted by a block of the mucosa from the muscularis mucosae to the surface epithelium [113]. Even a specimen large enough to include several such units may not be representative, however, because of the uneven distribution of G cells within the antrum and variations in cell density associated with patchy pathological alterations [115, 116, 118].

It should be stressed that these quantitative methods do not purport to give absolute values in terms of cells per tissue unit volume. We agree with Skinner and Whitehead [112] that it is almost impossible to meet the requirements for absolute measurements, including precise knowledge of variables such as section thickness and tissue shrinkage. It is therefore preferable, in comparative studies, to use non-absolute methods based on a standardized tissue unit area. The importance of a reproducible section thickness cannot be discounted, however. We use a Jung Rotary Microtome 1130, which according to the manufacturers cuts sections with a reproducibility within ± 0.5 μm of that indicated by the micrometer feed.

In all kinds of immunocytochemical cell enumerations it is difficult to decide which cells are to be included, and the observer has to define certain criteria with regard to cell size and staining intensity. Anyhow, the final count does not express the dynamic process of the cells in question. It is possible that a method measuring the amount of antigen per cell in addition to the number of cells would be more quantitative in this respect. Such studies have been carried out on endocrine cells of the gut by means of an Automatically Computed Image Analyser [100].

10.5. TISSUE PREPARATION METHODS

10.5.1. Handling of the tissue

In most laboratories, including ours, a satisfactory morphology is more easily achieved with fixed material than with cryostat sections of fresh-frozen tissue. In addition, paraffin-embedded specimens are easy to store and lend themselves better to the preparation of serial sections, which often is a prerequisite for comparisons to be made with antibody reagents of different specificities as well as between immunological localization and special histochemical staining features. Nevertheless, for several decades the notion has survived that paraffin sections cannot be used successfully for the immunofluorescence technique – a view still maintained without reservation by some authors advocating the advantages of the immunoperoxidase technique. We fully agree with Curran and Gregory [42] that there is no reason to expect some mysterious immunohistochemical difference between the two methods. Moreover, the problem of disturbing autofluorescence in formaldehyde-fixed sections exposed to ultraviolet light has been eliminated after the introduction of narrow-band epi-illumination in fluorescence microscopy [73].

Sainte-Marie [109], in a study of rabbit lymphoid tissue, apparently was the first to use paraffin sections based on a cold-ethanol fixation method to localize immunoglobulins. This approach, with the addition of a prefixation washing step to remove diffusible immunoglobulins, was next successfully applied to investigate humoral immune components present in human oral mucosa [19]. Eidelman and Berschauer [52] subsequently reported that the antigenicity of immunoglobulins was preserved after formaldehyde fixation followed by cryostat sectioning. More recently, several studies have shown that a variety of fixatives based on formaldehyde and followed by paraffin embedding can be used for immunofluorescence localization of intracellular immunoglobulins and other protein antigens [48, 51, 62, 128].

Ethanol acts as a fixative by protein precipitation, whereas formaldehyde immobilizes the antigens by the formation of cross-links, mainly methylene bridges [96]. Immobilization of small antigens, such as peptide hormones, can only be obtained safely with some kind of cross-bridging fixative, and their antigenicity is well preserved by this procedure. The antigenicity of protein antigens, on the other hand, does not depend on the primary structure alone but also on conformational features, which may be altered by the fixation process. In our laboratory we have found that the reactivity of most protein antigens tested is best preserved by ethanol fixation (see Fig. 10.15).

Due to extensive formation of cross-links, the formaldehyde fixatives may, in addition to denaturation, cause masking of antigens by steric hindrance, especially when the actual antigen is mixed with high concentrations of other proteins, such as in interstitial connective tissue fluid and in secretory epithelial cells (Fig. 10.14). This artifact is of some advantage in the immunohistochemical demonstration of Ig-producing cells because the immunoglobulins present extracellularly are relatively more masked than those

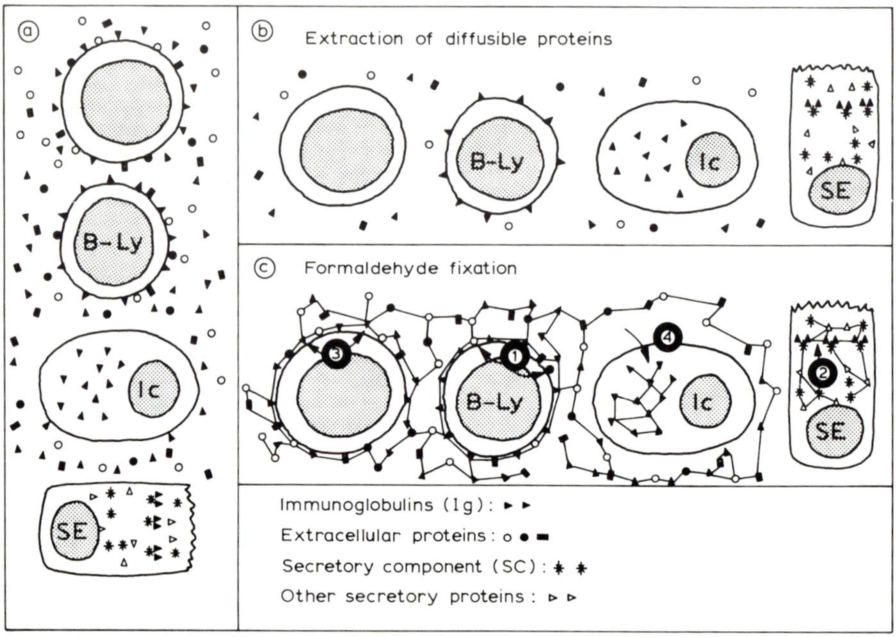

Fig. 10.14. Schematic representation of mucosal Ig distribution as shown by immunohistochemical staining in differently processed specimens containing secretory epithelium (SE), Ig-producing immunocytes (Ic), Ig-bearing B lymphocytes (B-Ly) and other mononuclear cells. a) Direct ethanol fixation: false negatives of B-Ly and Ic may occur as cellular details are obscured by background staining of interstitial Ig whose preservation is enhanced due to co-precipitation with other extracellular proteins; intracellular epithelial components are likewise well preserved. b) Saline extraction for 48 h followed by ethanol fixation: background staining is negligible and surface membrane Ig of B-Ly and cytoplasmic Ig of Ic are clearly visualized. c) Formaldehyde fixation: extracellular and intraepithelial Ig (and SC) are cross-linked with a variety of other proteins and therefore extensively masked, whereas the cytoplasmic antigenicity of Ic – whose intracellular product may be composed of more than 50% Ig – is better preserved; false negatives of Ic may nevertheless occur, and false negatives of B-Ly (1) and of epithelial Ig and SC (2) are common due to antigenic denaturation and masking; false positives mimicking B-Ly staining may occur due to condensation of interstitial Ig around a variety of cells (3); and false positives of cytoplasmic staining may occur, especially in routine pathological material, due to leakage of interstitial Ig into cells (4) before adequate fixation has been obtained.

present in the cytoplasm of the immunocytes (Fig. 10.15d), where the Ig product represents a major protein fraction. Besides, the cytoplasmic Ig is partly in a state of unconnected polypeptide chains whose antigenic determinants may be less liable to denaturation. Conversely, antigens mixed with high concentrations of other proteins are not masked by ethanol fixation but rather subjected to better immobilization than when fixed alone and consequently show intensified immunohistochemical staining [26]. Studying formaldehyde-fixed material it is necessary to be aware of the differential antigen masking that takes place according to location (Fig. 10.15c,d) in order to interpret immunohistochemical findings in a meaningful way, e.g. when a comparison is made between the staining obtained for intracellular immunoglobulins in immunocytes and in secretory epithelium, respectively [107].

The number of induced methylene bridges depends on the concentration of formaldehyde, temperature, pH, and time of exposure [96]. The bridges are not irreversible, and simple washing of fixed material before dehydration and embedding may result in significant restitution of antigenicity. Treatment of sections with proteolytic enzymes, such as pronase and trypsin, likewise unmasks antigenic determinants (Fig. 10.15c), although the underlying mechanism with possible effects on protein cross-bridging is unknown [33, 48, 50, 61, 87]. Such treatment may also reduce diffuse non-specific staining caused by lack of binding specificity of highly labelled conjugates, a problem that is more marked with formaldehyde-fixed than with ethanol-fixed sections; the enzyme treatment apparently renders the tissue elements less positively charged.

Recently many studies have been published in which immunohistochemical localization of antigens, especially immunoglobulins, was based on formalin-fixed pathological routine material. In addition to the problems caused by formaldehyde-induced denaturation and protein cross-linking, such material may present artifacts that have developed before fixation, namely leakage of interstitial proteins into cells. Rough treatment of the tissue specimen and a large specimen size with retarded fixation contribute to these artifacts. Kent [66] showed that diffusion of plasma proteins into injured cells occurs according to the size of the proteins and the degree of injury. In studies of lymphoid cells we take cytoplasmic albumin as a good indicator of cell membrane damage, even in washed tissue specimens, since intracellularly accumulated plasma proteins are not readily removed from the injured cells [66].

A still better indicator of the reliability of immunocyte studies is the demonstration that each cell contains an Ig product monotypic with regard to heavy and light chains. Since a mixture of κ- and λ-type IgG is present in high concentrations in the interstitial fluid (Fig. 10.15a), diffusion of IgG into cells may mask a monotypic product or give rise to false-positive cells with a polytypic content. This possibility can best be examined by means of paired immunofluorescence with conjugates of contrasting colours (Fig. 10.15). Such artifacts may of course also develop in vivo in dying cells. In squamous epithelia, for example, superficial cells commonly contain plasma proteins in quantitative proportions corresponding to the content found in the underlying connective tissue [19, 24, 27]. It should not be necessary to point out that the same sources of error jeopardize immunoperoxidase staining, and that the results of this technique cannot be so easily controlled with regard to false positives of individual cells.

The importance of properly oriented tissue specimens was discussed above in relation to quantitative studies of mucosal cell populations. The specimens should immediately after excision be mounted on a dry filter paper before they are placed in the processing fluid; this aids correct embedding so that sections can be cut perpendicular to the muscularis mucosae.

Fig. 10.15. Effects of various tissue preparation methods on immunohistochemical localization of IgA, IgM, IgG, SC, and CEA (standard conditions, cf. Table 10.III) in proximate samples taken from a gastric carcinoma of the linitis plastica variety. The diffusely infiltrating carcinoma cells, which produce CEA and SC, take up IgA and IgM, probably by the same receptor mechanism as that of normal secretory epithelium. The various components were revealed by paired immunofluorescence staining; the exposure times (s) for green and red in each photograph are indicated on the dark tissue areas, which represent reactive lymphoid follicles. Horizontal rows: a) sample fixed directly in ethanol; b) sample extracted in saline for 48 h prior to ethanol fixation; c) routine formalin fixation, and pronase treatment of sections; d) fixation in Lillie's AAF. Vertical rows: 1) green IgA and red IgM (double exposures); 2) comparable fields in adjacent sections, green IgA and red IgG (double exposures); 3) same fields with red filtration for IgG; 4) comparable fields in adjacent sections, green IgA and red SC (double exposures), except d4 which shows CEA; 5) same or comparable (d5) fields with red filtration for SC. Comments: a1) the carcinoma cells, which contain IgA and IgM, are distinctly visualized by their mixed yellow colour, whereas green IgA immunocytes are poorly discernible due to interstitial background staining, except in the lymphoid follicle; b1) since interstitial IgA has been removed, immunocytes of both classes are distinctly visualized by pure contrasting colours among the yellow carcinoma cells; c1) cytoplasmic IgM of carcinoma cells has been preserved poorly so that many of them appear green rather than yellow, thereby making differentiation of IgA immunocytes difficult; d1) immunocytes of both classes are relatively faint but well discernible as there is almost complete masking of interstitial IgA and cytoplasmic IgM in carcinoma cells; a2,3) due to strong interstitial staining, IgG immunocytes are obscured except in the lymphoid follicle, whereas IgA immunocytes and cancer cells appear purely green against the yellow background; b2,3) extraction of interstitial immunoglobulins markedly enhances visualization of immunocytes of both the IgG and IgA classes, but the latter type is difficult to differentiate from the purely green carcinoma cells; c2,3) the result is similar to that in (b2,3) but cytoplasmic fluorescence is somewhat less bright and the background staining for IgG, which here is reduced due to antigenic masking instead of protein extraction, is slightly intenser; d2,3) especially IgG immunocytes are faintly stained, but both classes nevertheless appear distinct due to extensive masking of background reactivity, including cytoplasmic IgA of carcinoma cells; a4,5) carcinoma cells are easily identified as they contain both IgA and SC and therefore appear yellow in double exposure; b4,5) staining for SC is somewhat fainter after tissue extraction, but the purely green IgA immunocytes are now distinctly visualized; c4,5) the result is quite comparable; d4) there is brisk staining for CEA in the carcinoma cells despite formaldehyde fixation; d5) in contrast, SC of tumour cells has been masked by the fixation and a faint cytoplasmic staining cannot be clearly distinguished from a general non-specific fluorescence. ×40.

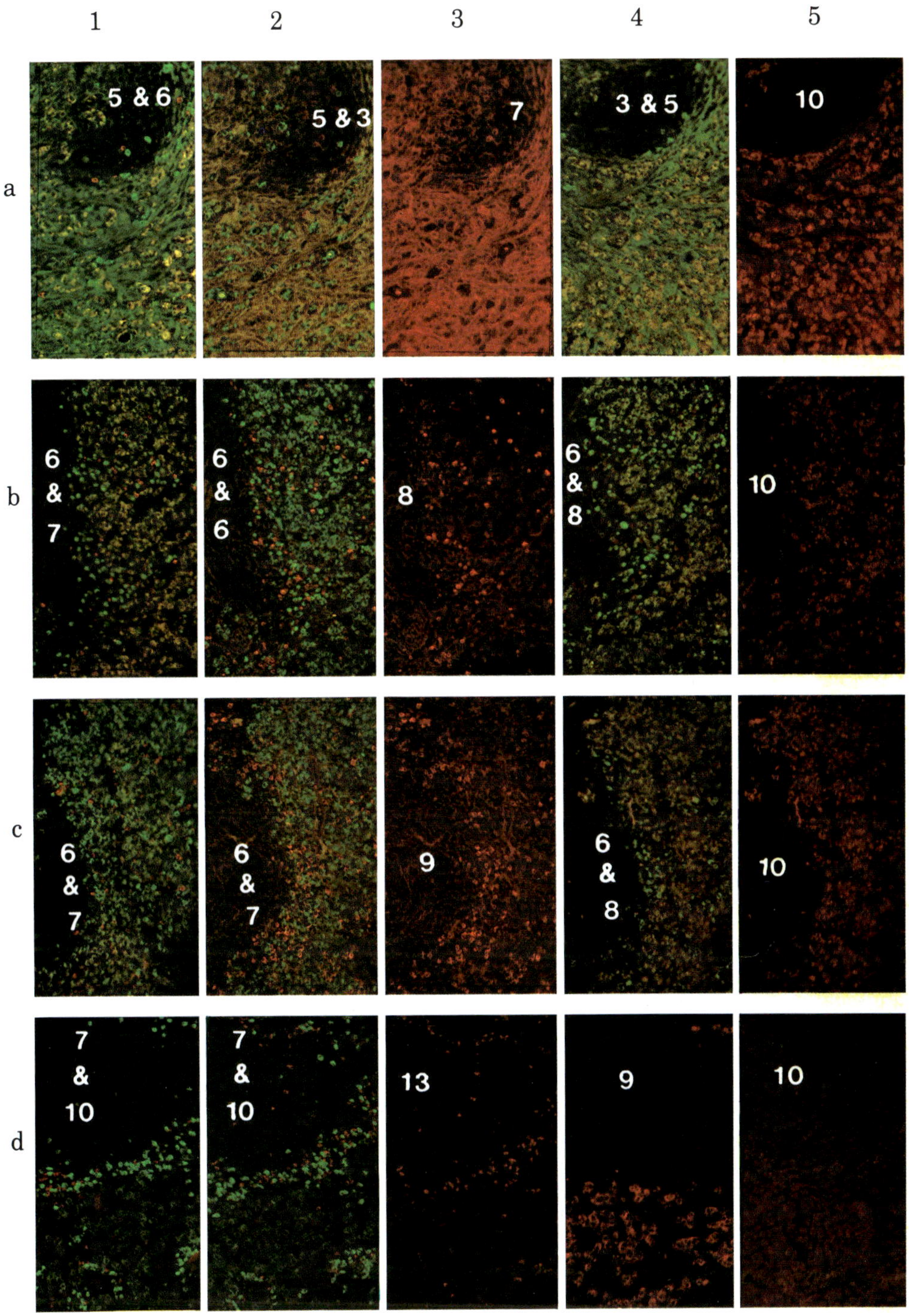

1
2
3
4
5
a
5 & 6
5 & 3
7
3 & 5
10
b
6 & 7
6 & 6
8
6 & 8
10
c
6 & 7
6 & 7
9
6 & 8
10
d
7 & 10
7 & 10
13
9
10

TABLE 10.II

SOME TISSUE PROCESSING METHODS USED IN IMMUNOFLUORESCENCE STUDIES OF MUCOUS MEMBRANES AND EXOCRINE GLANDS

Method	Comments
Extraction of diffusible components [10]	Avoid unnecessary trauma to specimen, which immediately should be placed in isotonic saline or tissue culture medium at 0–4°C and transported to the laboratory within 1–2 h. Representative portions with very small size of at least one dimension (about 2 mm) are trimmed as carefully as possible. The pieces of tissue are placed in perforated chambers or bags of cheese cloth and extracted by washing for 48 h at 4°C with slow motion in PBS (isotonic phosphate-buffered saline, pH 7.5). Thereafter the pieces are fixed in 96% alcohol at 4°C for 18–24 h, dehydrated in cold absolute alcohol for about 4 h, cleared in cold xylol for 20 h, and finally embedded in paraffin for 3–4 h at 56°C. If necessary, the specimens may be stored for several days in 70% alcohol before dehydration, or the xylol period may be prolonged.
Direct ethanol fixation [109]	Avoid sqeezing, tearing, warming or drying of the specimen, which immediately should be placed in 96% alcohol at 4°C, preferably as small pieces. If the antigens to be studied are not too easily diffusible, a better morphology is obtained by placing the pieces of tissue for 3–4 h in 96% alcohol diluted 2 : 3 with PBS before the final fixation. For easily diffusible antigens the speed of fixation may be enhanced by stirring [60]. If the specimen is thicker than 2–4 mm, it should be trimmed as soon as it has hardened. After final fixation in 96% alcohol overnight at 4°C, dehydration, clearing and embedding are performed as above.
Lillie's AAF [3]	This fixative is prepared by mixing 10 ml of 30% neutral formaldehyde, 5 ml concentrated (glacial) acetic acid, and 85 ml absolute alcohol. Small pieces of tissue are placed in this fixative at room temperature for 4 h. The specimens are thereafter left in 96% alcohol overnight and processed as above.
Methanol-free neutral formaldehyde [101]	Paraformaldehyde is dissolved in ion-free water at 60°C to 80–160 g/l. The solution is cleared by addition of 1 N NaOH and the pH adjusted to 7.5. The fixative is diluted 1 : 2 with PBS, and stored at 4°C. The fixation time may vary (3–6 days at 4°C). The specimens are taken through cold alcohol and xylol and embedded in paraffin for 4–8 h at 56°C.
Helly's and Bouin's fixatives [3]	These formaldehyde fixatives contain varying proportions of mercuric chloride, potassium dichromate, acetic acid and picric acid, reagents that are supposed to enhance fixation by fast penetration and stabilization of intracellular organelles. After fixation for 1–2 days, the specimens are rinsed thoroughly in running tap water or 50% alcohol, respectively, before further processing.
Water-soluble carbodiimide fixative	Fixation is carried out at 4°C for 24 h in a 20 g/l solution of 1-ethyl-3 (3-dimethyl-amino-propyl) carbodiimide-HCl.
Benzoquinone bifunctional liquid phase fixative [97]	Fixation is carried out at 4°C for about 3 h in a 4 g/l solution of 1,2-benzoquinone in isotonic saline.

Method	Comments
Processing through the routine pathology laboratory [107]	Fixation at room temperature for about 24 h in 10% formalin stabilized at pH 7.4 with hexamethylenetetramine, followed by post-fixation (0.5–8 h) in AAF.

Sections of ethanol-fixed material adhere well to acetone-cleaned glass slides without the use of adhesives and after only 30 min at 37°C. Formaldehyde-fixed sections are dried for 30 min at 56°C and overnight at 37°C; in addition, they require adhesives, especially when subjected to enzyme treatment. We use gelatine (10 g/l) dissolved in water by heating and stabilized by mixing with an equal volume of potassium chromium sulphate (10 g/l) immediately before the coating of the slides.

10.5.2. Extracellular protein antigens

From the above considerations it follows that proteins present in interstitial connective tissue can be adequately demonstrated only after fixation with a procedure that gives minimal denaturation and masking. We have found that direct ethanol fixation (Table 10.II) affords localization of interstitial IgG, IgA and IgM with relative intensities that accord with the established extravascular distribution of these immunoglobulins (Figs. 10.9a,b and 10.15a). It has been calculated that while most serum IgM (76%) remains in the vascular space, IgG and IgA are to a large extent (52–58%) distributed in the interstitial fluid [125]. Extravascular albumin is likewise satisfactorily preserved by ethanol fixation [123].

The staining intensities of extracellular antigens are in our hands always much lower in formaldehyde-fixed tissue, even after enzyme treatment (Fig. 10.15c and Table 10.III). Direct ethanol fixation is therefore the method of choice when the mucosal distribution of immunoglobulins in patients with immunodeficiency is to be investigated [10]. Since ethanol-precipitated proteins can go into solution, prolonged conjugate incubation may produce diffusion artifacts in ethanol-fixed sections; in our experience this is a problem with diffusely distributed interstitial antigens and some epithelial components. The adverse effect can be ascribed both to loss of antigen and to partial neutralization of the reagent during the prolonged incubation period.

10.5.3. Ig-bearing and Ig-producing cells

Immunoglobulin is the most useful functional marker of the B-cell system (Fig. 10.16). Whether a B lymphocyte is "virgin" (B_1) or belongs to the memory pool (B_2), it expresses Ig of one light-chain type on its surface – most commonly IgM or IgD or both these classes concomitantly. Immunoblasts and plasma cells express relatively much higher concentrations of cytoplasmic Ig, which is produced for secretion and generally restricted to one class and one light-chain type. Although surface membrane Ig of B lymphocytes may be demonstrated in

TABLE 10.III

RELATIVE IMMUNOFLUORESCENCE INTENSITIES OF MUCOSAL ELEMENTS IN PARAFFIN SECTIONS AFTER VARIOUS TISSUE PREPARATION METHODS

Evaluation based on staining conditions employing the same conjugate concentrations for each type of tissue substrate and incubation for 30 min at room temperature.

Processing method	Connective tissue ground substance			Ig-producing immunocytes			Secretory epithelial cells				
	IgG	IgA	IgM	IgG	IgA	IgM	IgG	IgA	IgM	SC	CEA[a]
96% Cold ethanol [109]	+++(+)[b]	+(++)	−(++)	+++[c]	+++[c]	+++[c]	−	+++	+(++)	+++	+++
48-h Saline extraction followed by 96% ethanol [10]	−(++)	−(+)	−	+++	+++	+++	−	++	+	++	+++
Lillie's AAF (4 h)	−(+)	−	−	+[d]	++	+	−	+(−)	−	−(+)	+++
Routine processing: buffered formalin (24 h) followed by AAF (0.5–8 h)	−(+)	−	−	−(+)	++(+)	+(−)	−	−(+)	−	−(+)	++
Same as above followed by pronase treatment	−(++)	−(+)	−	++(+)	++(+)	++	−	++(+)	+	++	+++

[a] CEA evaluated in dysplastic or neoplastic epithelium.
[b] Grades given in parentheses represent lesser common finding.
[c] IgM and often also IgA immunocytes may be visualized in directly ethanol-fixed tissue, whereas IgG immunocytes are usually obscured due to bright connective tissue background staining.
[d] Such faint staining of immunocytes was best revealed with rhodamine conjugate.

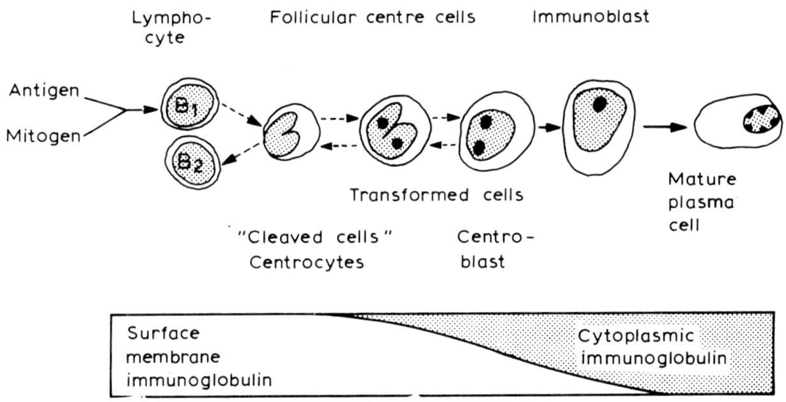

Fig. 10.16. Schematic representation of differentiation in the B-cell system from antigen- or mitogen-stimulated "virgin" (B_1) lymphocytes to production of memory (B_2) lymphocytes (clonal expansion) and maturation to end cells (far right). The terminology is adopted from Lennert [75] and Lukes and Parker [79]. The name "follicular centre cells" implies that B-cell differentiation occurs chiefly in germinal centers of activated lymphoid follicles, but transformed B cells may likewise be found in other immunologically active sites, such as inflammatory processes. Broken arrows indicate that the positions of the various morphological expressions in the differentiation pathway from B_1 to B_2 lymphocytes, and from lymphocytes to immunoblasts, have not been conclusively determined. Moreover, it should be noted that formation of plasma cells takes place especially after stimulation of B_2 lymphocytes (not depicted in the figure). The relative amounts of surface-membrane Ig and cytoplasmic Ig expressed by the various cell types are indicated at the bottom, but on different scales since membrane-incorporated Ig is of low concentration and slowly shed compared to the large concentrations of cytoplasmic Ig produced for active secretion by immunoblasts and plasma cells (cf. Fig. 10.17a).

tissue sections, it is often difficult, if not impossible, to distinguish this feature from lightly stained cytoplasmic Ig of transformed B cells (Fig. 10.16) – a problem that has also been encountered in immunofluorescence studies of fixed smears of lymphoid cells [17, 84].

In directly ethanol-fixed tissue, surface Ig may be difficult to visualize due to background staining. Surface IgD makes an exception since interstitial tissue fluid normally contains very little of this immunoglobulin (Fig. 10.17). With formaldehyde fixation, surface Ig is usually completely masked or the interpretation of the staining results is difficult due to false positive features (Fig. 10.14 and Table 10.IV). In the poorly vascularized mantle zones of lymphoid follicles, however, and also in dense infiltrates of lymphocytic B-cell lymphomas, membrane staining for IgM may stand out quite distinctly in formaldehyde-fixed enzyme-treated sections. But determination of the concomitant light-chain type is nevertheless jeopardized by polyclonal extracellular IgG. In our hands, therefore, immunofluorescence identification of Ig-bearing B cells is best obtained in tissue from which diffusible proteins have been extracted before ethanol fixation (Fig. 10.14 and Table 10.II). Others have adhered to cryostat sections of fresh-frozen tissue for similar identification [41, 42, 78, 126].

The demonstration of cytoplasmic Ig of mature B cells poses a smaller

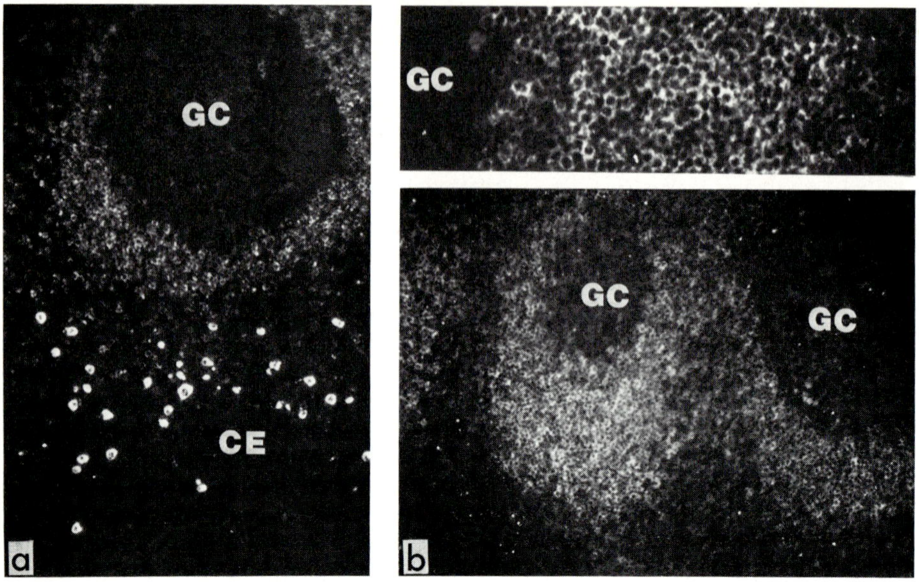

Fig. 10.17. Immunofluorescence staining (rhodamine conjugate) of IgD-bearing B lymphocytes in the mantle zones around germinal centers (GC) of tonsillar lymphoid follicles. a) Saline-extracted and ethanol-fixed clinically normal specimen; between the crypt epithelium (CE) and the follicle there is a high number of IgD-producing cells, whose cytoplasm shows much brighter staining than the lymphocyte membranes. b) Directly ethanol-fixed specimen from a subject whose serum concentration of IgD was below 0.004 g/l; since there was no background staining, the B lymphocytes are clearly visualized. ×100. The inset shows marked variability of membrane staining. ×255.

problem, and our experience with various tissue-processing methods is summarized in Table 10.III. These results were obtained with an incubation time of 30 min; a better distinction between extracellular and cytoplasmic Ig is obtained by prolonged incubation with more diluted conjugates. Using this modification we are able to visualize even IgG-producing cells after direct ethanol fixation in tissue with minimal extravascular Ig. Nevertheless, the best signal–noise ratio with regard to IgG immunocytes is obtained in saline-extracted specimens from which most diffusible IgG has been removed (Fig. 10.15b).

Owing to the relatively extensive masking of extracellular proteins, Ig-producing cells can also be visualized in formaldehyde-fixed tissue with a fairly good signal–noise ratio, despite the markedly decreased cytoplasmic antigenicity that prevails without enzyme treatment (Fig. 10.15d and Table 10.III). The reduced intracellular reactivity, that chiefly afflicts IgG and IgD cells, may to some degree be compensated for by prolonging the time of conjugate incubation or otherwise increase the sensitivity of detection. Thus, Lillie's AAF (Table 10.II) and a sublimate-formaldehyde fixative afforded good preservation of IgG-, IgA- and IgM-producing cells as revealed by the immunoperoxidase method [5, 64], and similar success seemed to have been obtained in an investigation based on Bouin's fixative (Table 10.II) and unspecified commercial FITC conjugates [51], all three studies omitting enzyme treatment of the sections. However, with the exception of Lillie's AAF fixative, which in our hands does not stabilize the immunoglobulins sufficiently to resist enzyme treatment, there is no doubt that the staining of Ig-producing cells in formaldehyde-fixed sections generally is significantly intensified after treatment with pronase or trypsin [50, 62, 87]. We have used pronase (1 g/l) for 15 min at 37°C, and find that the result (Table 10.III) is similar to that obtained with trypsin (0.25–0.5 g/l) for 2 h at 37°C [107].

Among the three major immunocyte classes, most problems are encountered in the visualization of IgG-producing cells, as indicated in Table 10.III. These immunocytes are most prone to become obscured by background staining (Figs. 10.9a,b and 10.15a) and, moreover, show a relatively poor reactivity, especially after formaldehyde fixation (Fig. 10.15c,d). The latter feature may be partially ascribed to a low content of cytoplasmic IgG. Thus, Gitlin and Sasaki [55] estimated that the Ig content per immunocyte was decreased in the order IgA : IgM : IgG by the proportions 5.6 : 3.7 : 1. Although enzyme treatment enhances significantly the staining of IgG-producing cells (Fig. 10.15c), it also increases extracellular staining where there are relatively high concentrations of interstitial IgG; in such areas the signal–noise ratio is only slightly improved. In addition, the enzyme treatment necessary to intensify IgG cells has sometimes a deteriorating effect on IgA cells. Altogether it seems to be difficult to predict variations in the results obtained after enzyme treatment [87]. Additional problems encountered in the use of formalin-fixed pathological routine material are summarized in Table 10.IV.

TABLE 10.IV

POSSIBLE PITFALLS IN THE CHARACTERIZATION OF B CELLS BY THEIR SURFACE AND CYTOPLASMIC Ig IN FORMALIN-FIXED, PARAFFIN-EMBEDDED PATHOLOGICAL ROUTINE MATERIAL

1. Masking of cells by *background staining* due to high concentrations of Ig in interstitial tissue fluid (connective tissue ground substance). This is a much smaller problem than with directly ethanol-fixed tissue.

2. Condensation of interstitial Ig around cells may give rise to *false-positive membrane staining* and mask monoclonality of surface Ig.

3. Leakage of interstitial Ig into cells may give rise to *false-positive cytoplasmic staining* and mask monoclonality of intracellular Ig.

4. Masking of Ig antigenicity due to protein cross-linking mainly via formaldehyde-induced methylene bridges may result in *false negatives*. Depends on the amount of other proteins with which the Ig is mixed, the concentration of formaldehyde, temperature, pH, and fixation time. May be counteracted before paraffin-embedding by extensive washing, which leads to partial rupture of hydroxymethyl combinations. Enhancement of cytoplasmic Ig reactivity may be obtained by treatment of tissue sections with proteolytic enzyme but unmasking of antigenic determinants may at the same time increase interstitial Ig staining.

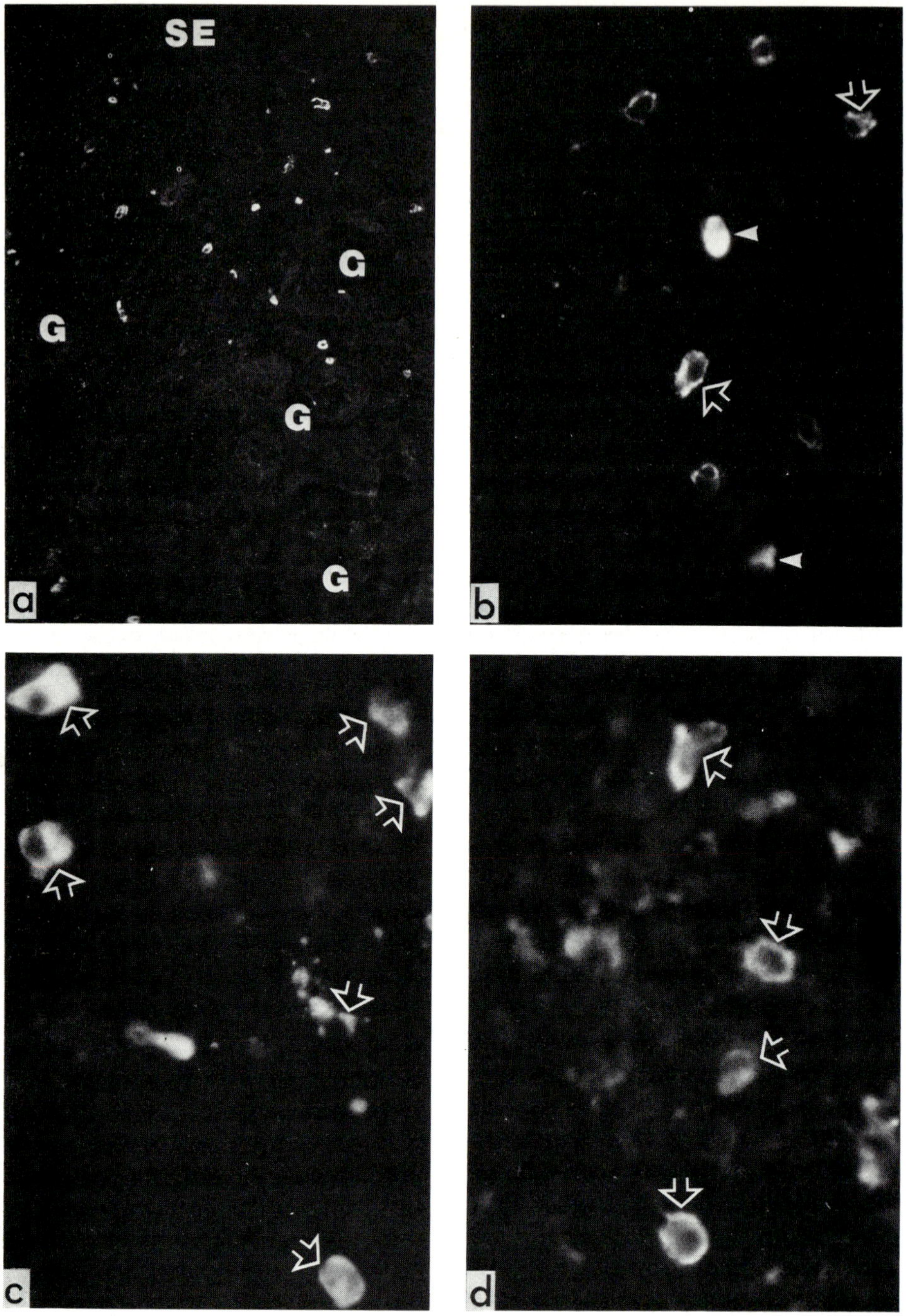

Fig. 10.18. Immunofluorescence staining of IgE-bearing mast cells and IgE-producing immunocytes. a) Nasal mucosa from an IgA-deficient atopic patient with allergic rhinitis and nasal allergy contained numerous IgE-positive mast cells, mainly scattered in the connective tissue between the surface epithelium (SE) and the glands (G. × 150. b) Examination of the same section at higher magnification shows that the staining is generally related to the surface membrane of the cells; some cells appear like plasma cells (arrows) but the fluorescence was less intense than that of IgE-

Mucosal localization of IgE immunocytes has been a subject of much controversy [21]. Even with a 1000-fold increase of the serum IgE level, the extravascular concentration of IgE should be only in the range of 0.01–0.2 g/l, while that of IgG is normally about 6 g/l. Background staining for IgE, therefore, does not interfere with the demonstration of immunocytes in directly ethanol-fixed tissue. Reports describing extracellular or epithelial IgE fluorescence should be considered with scepticism, since these staining features are most likely non-specific and suggest poor conjugate quality or too high a working concentration of the reagent. Our rabbit anti-IgE conjugates reveal very few immunocytes in normal and diseased intestinal and nasal mucosa [20]. The same holds true for tonsils and adenoids [27, 71]. The largest number of IgE-producing cells observed in our laboratory (10–15 per section) was seen in a conjunctival biopsy from an atopic patient with vernal conjunctivitis (Fig. 10.18c). According to the experiments of Mayrhofer et al. [85], IgE responses take place mainly in regional lymph nodes rather than in mucosal sites. IgE-bearing mast cells, however, which are a common immunohistochemical finding in mucous membranes of atopic subjects [53], are sometimes so brightly stained that they may be erroneously taken as IgE-producing immunocytes (Fig. 10.18). The fluorescent features are unaffected by saline extraction of the tissue specimen prior to fixation. Mayrhofer et al. [85] indeed suggested that mucosal mast cells may contain cytoplasmic IgE. As pointed out elsewhere, other sources of error in identifying IgE immunocytes in human mucosae are eosinophilic granulocytes and plasma cells producing antibodies to the animal IgG in the immunohistochemical reagent [21].

Ethanol fixation does not expose cytoplasmic J chains incorporated into dimeric IgA and pentameric IgM. Distinct staining of dimer-producing IgA immunocytes therefore generally depends on urea denaturation of ethanol-fixed sections (Fig. 10.19b,c), especially in studies of specimens from sites like the tonsils where most such cells contain only a small fraction of dimers [9, 15, 17, 70, 72]. Conversely, most IgM-producing cells show fairly bright J-chain staining without urea denaturation (Fig. 10.19a), probably because these cells contain an excess of free J chain [83]. In addition, a considerable proportion of gland-associated and tonsillar IgG and IgD immunocytes produce J chains which are demonstrated in their cytoplasm in a free form [30, 70, 72].

Free cytoplasmic J chain is also well preserved in formaldehyde-fixed tissue, and Ig-associated J chain is more exposed in such material than in

---

producing immunocytes, which were virtually lacking in this specimen; and by careful focussing up and down under the microscope the impression of surface-related staining was strengthened (arrowheads indicate two yellow autofluorescent eosinophilic granulocytes). ×450. c) Conjunctiva of a severely atopic patient with vernal conjunctivitis contained several IgE-producing immunocytes with distinct cytoplasmic staining (arrows). ×645. d) More superficially in the conjunctiva (same section) numerous scattered mast cells showed IgE staining related to the surface membrane (arrows), although in this slightly overexposed picture the cells appear like immunocytes. A distinction may be difficult when the mast-cell staining is unusually bright. ×645.

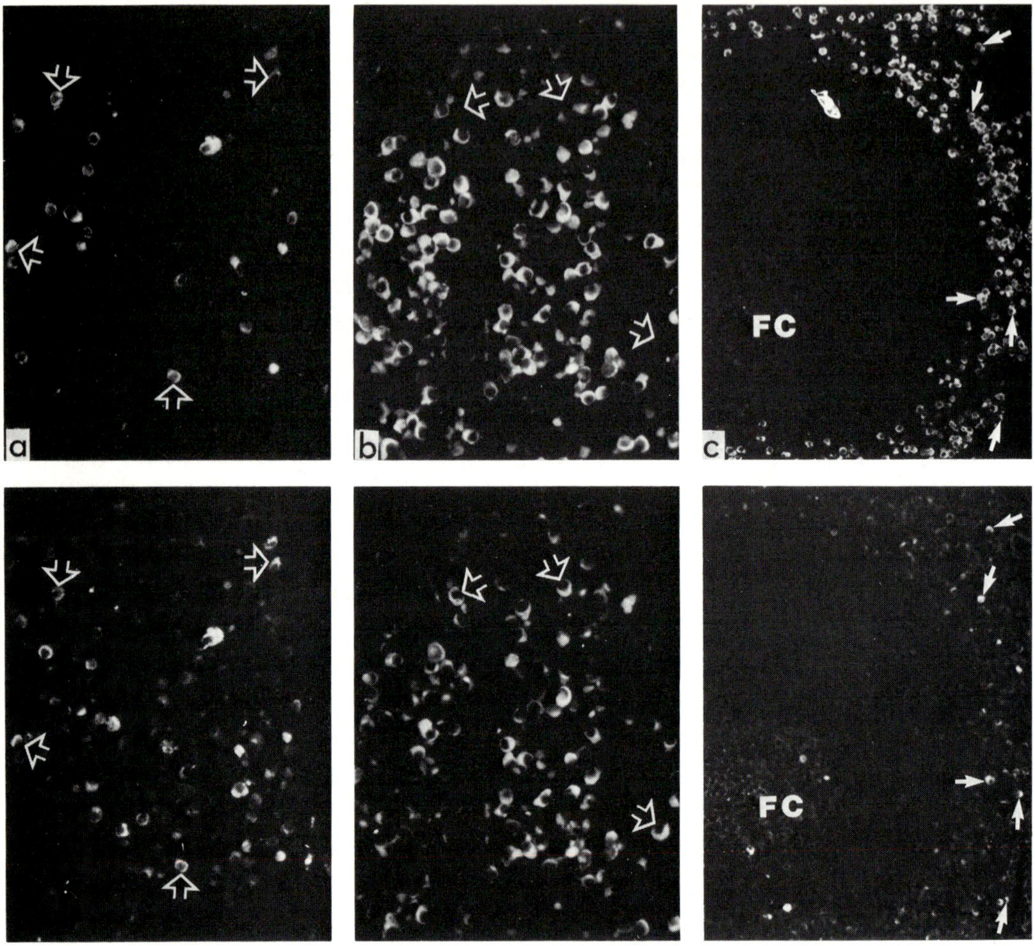

Fig. 10.19. Immunocytes of the IgM (a) and IgA (b,c) classes identified by FITC fluorescence and examined for cytoplasmic content of J chain by paired staining (bottom row shows TRITC fluorescence in the same three fields); saline-extracted ethanol-fixed tissue specimens. a) Jejunal mucosa from a patient with coeliac disease (gut lumen at the top); most of the IgM immunocytes are stained brightly for J chain (some marked with arrows), whereas the majority of other cells appearing in the lower picture represent IgA immunocytes, most of which are only faintly stained. ×245. b) Comparable field in adjacent section denatured in acid urea; most of the IgA immunocytes are now intensely stained for J chain, and some additional J chain-positive cells of other classes also appear in the lower picture (arrows) ×245. c) Urea-denatured section of palatine tonsil; only a few of the extrafollicular IgA immunocytes are distinctly stained for J chain (arrows); in the follicle center (FC) there are four J chain-positive immunocytes of other classes. ×100.

ethanol-fixed tissue, probably due to conformational alterations of the polymers. The J chain is extremely susceptible to proteolytic enzymes, and we have observed reduced J-chain staining in pronase-treated formaldehyde-fixed sections. Curran and Gregory [42] have reported a similar detrimental effect on IgD – which is also very susceptible to proteolytic degradation – and this is likewise our experience.

10.5.4. Binding properties of Ig-producing cells

When immunocytes were first studied in ethanol-fixed tissue [109], they were located by their antibody activity. With this "sandwich" approach there is a good signal–noise ratio, even in directly fixed tissue, since the interstitial fluid contains relatively low concentrations of the relevant antibody. When concomitant Ig class identification is attempted, however, one runs into problems with background staining as discussed above. With our modified method based on extraction of diffusible proteins before ethanol fixation (Table 10.II), the antibody activity of the immunocytes is well preserved [10]. A good signal–noise ratio may thus be obtained for both Ig class and specificity. We have successfully used the same tissue processing method for concurrent localization of Ig class and SC affinity of cytoplasmic polymers (Figs. 10.6 and 10.7). I am not aware of immunohistochemical localization of antibody activity or other affinity studies of immunocytes carried out with formaldehyde-fixed tissue; the possibility of preserving the conformation of binding sites after cross-linking of proteins is relatively small.

10.5.5. Epithelial components

The masking effect of formaldehyde fixation is as pronounced for some epithelial components as for proteins present in the connective tissue ground substance (Fig. 10.14). Thus, secretory IgA, secretory IgM and SC show only faint or no staining after Lillie's AAF or routine formalin fixation, compared with the brisk epithelial fluorescence seen in directly ethanol-fixed material (Fig. 10.15 and Table 10.III). The masking seems to affect both free and IgA-associated SC. Epithelial staining for J chain in contrast is faint also in ethanol-fixed sections without denaturation in acid urea (Figs. 10.8 and 10.9), which is in accordance with the fact that the J chain is about 15 times more concealed in secretory IgA than in native dimeric IgA [14, 15].

By means of pronase or trypsin treatment of formaldehyde-fixed sections, the demonstration of secretory IgA, secretory IgM and SC can be significantly restored (Fig. 10.15c). This does not apply to CEA which, however, is subjected to less masking by the cross-bridging fixatives (Fig. 10.15d and Table 10.III). In a comparative study of a variety of intestinal biopsy specimens we found that the epithelial staining for secretory IgA, SC and CEA, as revealed in enzyme-treated routine sections, was correlated with that obtained in ethanol-fixed sections from the same specimens – although generally given lower

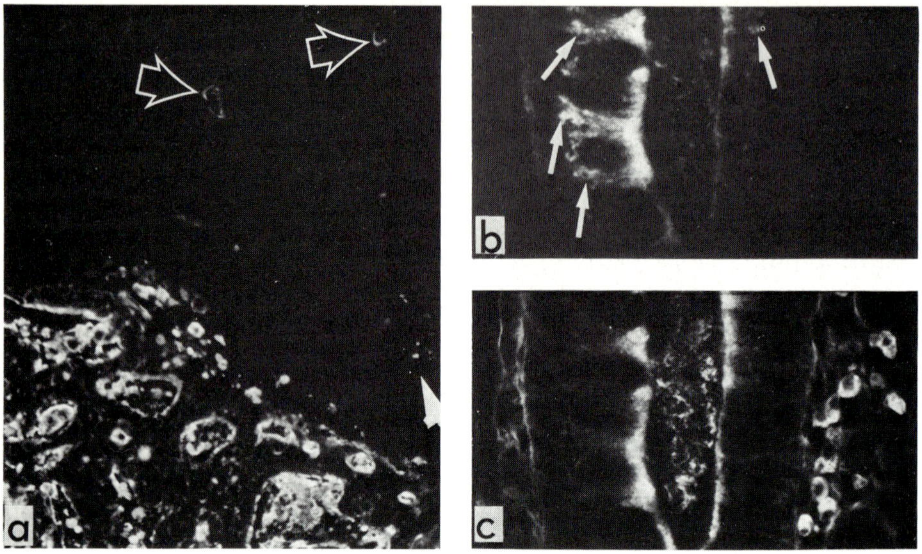

Fig. 10.20. Immunofluorescence staining for CEA, SC and IgA in directly ethanol-fixed specimens of adenocarcinomas from the large bowel. a) CEA is abundantly present in the tumour which is growing below the mucosa, whereas the apparently normal crypt epithelium at the top shows only faint luminal staining (arrows). ×120. b) Crypt epithelium is the "transitional mucosa" adjacent to a tumour shows apparently normal staining for SC in columnar cells on the left side, whereas on the right the production of SC is markedly decreased, and free SC, which normally is accumulated in the Golgi zone (arrows), is strikingly reduced. ×470. c) Paired staining for IgA in the same field shows that despite numerous nearby IgA immunocytes, the IgA transport is decreased through the dysplastic part of the crypt epithelium where the production of SC is defective. ×470.

intensity scores [107]. Thus, ethanol-fixed material is more reliable for the localization of small amounts of these epithelial antigens, including CEA (Fig. 10.20). In normal colon mucosa, for example, the latter antigen is often undetectable in formalin-fixed routine pathology specimens [107].

The masking of immunoglobulins by formaldehyde fixation is of advantage in studies based on an indirect immunohistochemical technique with human sections as the antigen substrate and human serum as the primary reagent. Thus, human autoantibodies can be used for the localization of parietal cells in gastric body mucosa after both paraformaldehyde (Fig. 10.21) and carbodiimide fixation (Table 10.II); the latter fixative gives the better preservation of the parietal-cell autoantigens but there is a disturbing background staining of plasma cells. Carbodiimide apparently preserves the mucosal immunoglobulins relatively well, and the anti-human $(F(ab')_2$ conjugate used in the second layer can therefore react directly with the tissue section [114].

The antigenicity of glandular kallikreins is best preserved by ethanol fixation. The demonstration of small amounts, such as in the rat kidney, in addition has depended on fixation in situ by perfusion [93, 94]. Excised human specimens must be immediately placed in cold ethanol; however, despite this precaution, we have been unable to localize human renal kallikrein [95]. The

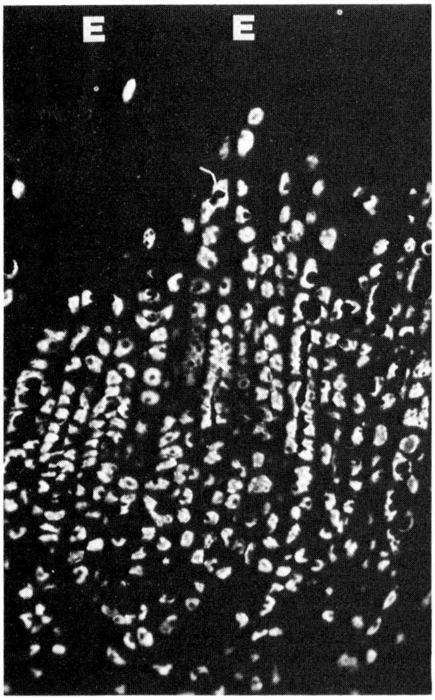

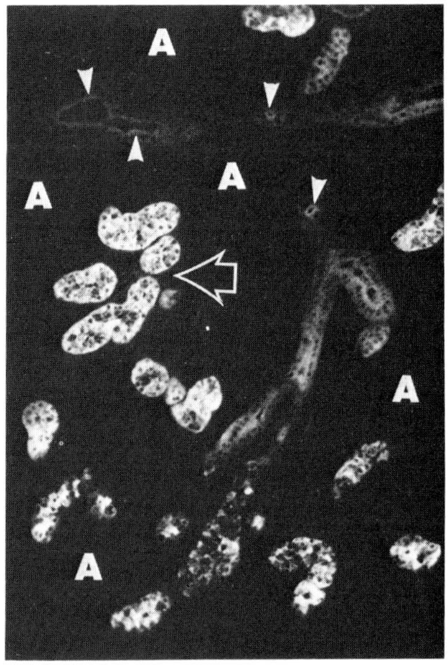

Fig. 10.21. Parietal cells in the body mucosa from paraformaldehyde-fixed human stomach stained by indirect immunofluorescence technique. The section was first incubated for 30 min with human serum (1 : 6) containing parietal-cell autoantibodies, and then with rabbit FITC conjugate specific for human $F(ab')_2$ (anti-Ig light-chain reagent). Owing to masking of intra- and extracellular Ig by the cross-linking fixative, there was no background staining of the connective tissue elements beneath the surface epithelium (E) or between the parietal cell-containing gastric glands. ×110.

Fig. 10.22. Immunofluorescence staining for glandular kallikrein in directly ethanol-fixed rat submandibular salivary gland. There is bright diffuse cytoplasmic fluorescence of granular tubules (arrow), whereas striated ducts show much fainter straining with an intensified luminal rim (arrowheads). Acini (A) are completely negative. Granular tubules are present in only some species (e.g. rodents and bats), and in man salivary kallikrein can be detected only in striated ducts. ×110.

granular intracellular distribution of kallikrein is lost after ethanol fixation (Fig. 10.22) but can be preserved by Helly's fluid (Table 10.II). The latter fixative, however, reduces the sensitivity of detection by decreasing the antigenicity and increasing the non-specific background staining [93].

A precise epithelial localization of other enzymes, such as amylase and lysozyme, also depends on a rapid fixation to avoid diffusion artifacts. Ethanol preserves well the antigenicity of both these enzymes; with this fixative we have obtained distinct localization of amylase in salivary gland acini and of lysozyme in intercalated salivary ducts and in duodenal Brunner's glands and Paneth cells (Fig. 10.23a–c) as well as in phagocytes (Fig. 10.23d). Both antigens can also be demonstrated in formaldehyde-fixed and pronase-treated sections, and a better localization of this relatively small protein molecule is indeed obtained by the latter procedure.

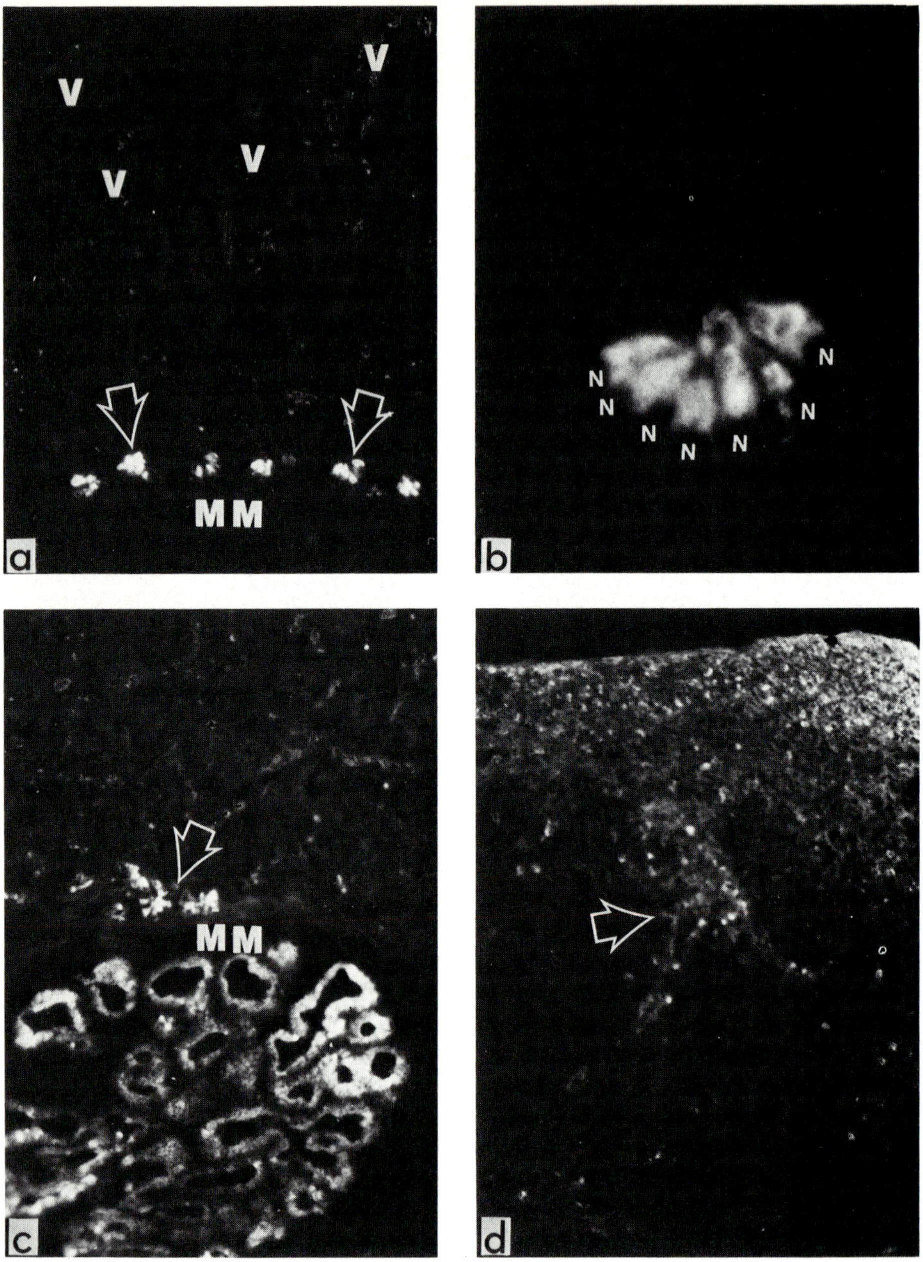

Fig. 10.23. Immunofluorescence staining of lysozyme-producing cells in directly ethanol-fixed mucosal specimens. a) Normal duodenal mucosa with slender villi (V) contains regular groups of positive Paneth cells (arrows) at the base of the crypts above the muscularis mucosae (MM). ×120. b) Larger magnification shows the characteristic pyramidal or columnar shape of the Paneth cells with the nucleus (N) near the cell base ×840. c) Duodenal mucosa from a patient with coeliac disease; only some of the hyperplastic crypts contain positive Paneth cells (arrow), whereas the epithelium of the Brunner's glands located below the muscularis mucosae (MM) is stained throughout, although with varying intensity. ×120. d) Colon mucosa from a patient with ulcerative colitis; a dense infiltrate of lysozyme-positive inflammatory cells, mainly granulocytes, are present superficially in the mucosa and partly contained in a crypt abscess (arrow). Diffuse staining indicates that lysozyme is released into the inflammatory exudate. ×150.

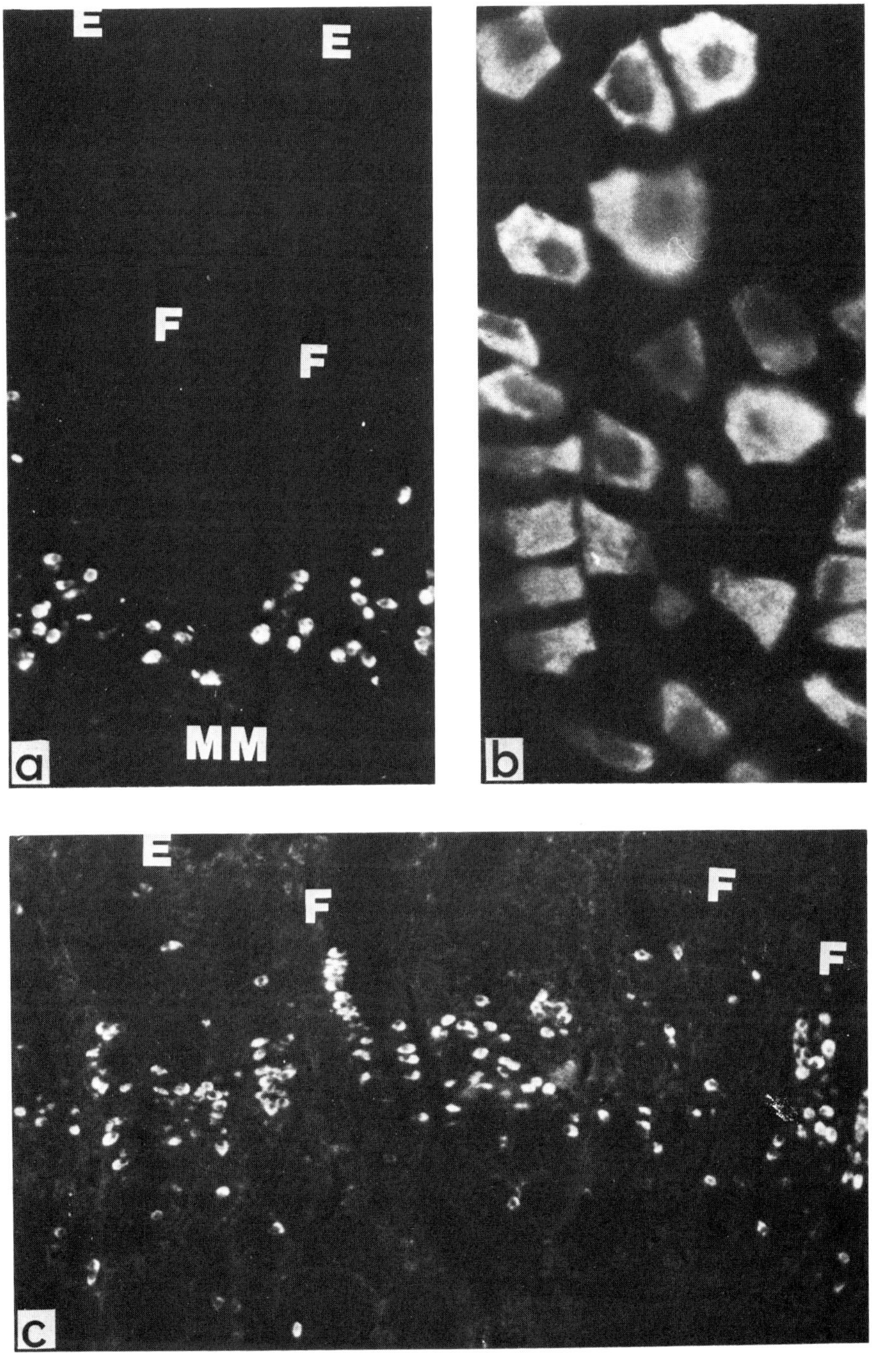

Fig. 10.24. Immunofluorescence staining of antral G cells in human gastric mucosa fixed in paraformaldehyde (a,c) and dog gastric mucosa fixed in Bouin's fluid (b). The cells are located mainly in the basal and middle parts of the pyloric glands and are absent from the surface epithelium (E), including the foveolar parts (F). There is less background staining with the direct (a,b) than with the indirect immunofluorescence method (c). Note highly variable morphology of the endocrine cells (b). MM = muscularis mucosae. a,c) ×150; b) ×970.

The peptide hormones of the gut can only be precisely localized after tissue preparation with a cross-linking reagent. Gastrin and somatostatin seem to be well preserved with several types of formaldehyde fixatives, such as paraformaldehyde solutions (Fig. 10.24b), buffered formaldehyde, and Bouin's fluid as well as with carbodiimide [101, 103, 114, 127], whereas secretin is best preserved by benzoquinone (Table 10.II). The latter bifunctional fixative has been used successfully also for gastrin, motilin and gastric inhibitory peptide [97].

10.5.6. Conclusions

One sees only what there is to see. However refined the immunohistochemical method may be, the result of antigen localization will in the end depend on the handling of the specimen. There is at present no way of tissue preparation that is ideal for all purposes; the method must be chosen according to the questions asked.

The best morphology is obtained with the cross-linking fixatives; but, due to extensive masking of certain protein antigens present in the extracellular tissue fluid and intracellularly in secretory epithelia, formaldehyde fixation is not always reliable in immunohistochemistry. Such antigen masking is avoided when ethanol fixation is used, although this procedure may render the detection of Ig-bearing and Ig-producing cells impossible due to intense background staining. Moreover, all protein antigens are not sufficiently immobilized by ethanol fixation to permit immunohistochemical staining methods that require prolonged incubation of the sections. Extraction of diffusible immunoglobulins before fixation enhances the signal–noise ratio for the localization of Ig-bearing and Ig-producing cells, but the tissue morphology suffers. An important advantage of ethanol fixation is the fact that it preserves the activity of the non-specific esterase α-naphthylbutyrase [29]. This enzyme is a good marker of macrophages and cells forming truly histiocytic lymphomas, but the erroneous consensus has prevailed that it can only be demonstrated in tissue imprints or fresh-frozen tissue [75, 79].

Some extracellular Ig is usually retained even after extensive tissue washing; a distinction between a) Ig bound immunologically to cells or basement membranes or present in immune complexes, and b) Ig trapped non-specifically in the tissue is often difficult, if not impossible, especially in inflammatory sites. Conversely, soluble immune complexes are probably lost during extraction of the tissue specimen. Thus, various methods are available for immunohistochemical investigations of components of mucosal immune responses, whereas immunological effector mechanisms involved in mucosal disease can hardly be visualized in situ, except for the demonstration of local effector cells such as macrophages, granulocytes, and mast cells.

In general, immunohistochemical studies of the immune system pose many methodological problems not encountered in studies of antigens that occur in serum and tissue fluids only in low concentrations. Experience with the localization of epithelial enzymes and peptide hormones cannot be uncritically transferred to the field of immunobiology. In other words, the relative simplicity of demonstrating certain epithelial components by immunohistochemistry should not detract the attention from the special difficulties related to studies of the immune system – both with regard to methodology and interpretation.

Some disagreement will probably prevail among various laboratories when it comes to preference of tissue preparation method for the localization of certain antigens. It should be kept in mind that various opinions may be partly based on differences between antisera of seemingly identical specificity. Such antisera may nevertheless react with different determinants of the antigen in question – a fact that may be reflected in apparent variations in antigenicity after similar tissue fixation.

ACKNOWLEDGMENTS

The studies in the author's laboratory were supported by grants from The Norwegian Research Council for Science and the Humanities, The Norwegian Cancer Society, The Norwegian Society for Fighting Cancer, Anders Jahre's Foundation, Helga Semb's Fund, and Norske Folks Forsknings Fond. I thank Liv Støttum, Kirsten Grønneberg, and Elsa Johansen for excellent secretarial assistance in the preparation of this paper.

REFERENCES

1 Baklien, K. and Brandtzaeg, P. (1974) Immunohistochemical localization of complement in intestinal mucosa. Lancet *2*, 1087–1088.

2 Baklien, K. and Brandtzaeg, P. (1976) Immunohistochemical characterization of local immunoglobulin formation in Crohn's disease of the ileum. Scand. J. Gastroenterol. *11*, 447–457.

3 Bancroft, J.D. and Stevens, A. (1975) Histopathological Stains and their Diagnostic Uses (Churchill Livingstone, London) pp. 134–138.

4 Bergquist, N.R. and Nilsson, P. (1974) The conjugation of immunoglobulins with tetramethylrhodamine isothiocyanate by utilization of dimethylsulfoxide (DMSO) as a solvent. J. Immunol. Methods *5*, 189–198.

5 Bosman, F.T., Lindemann, V., Kuiper, G., van der Wal, A. and Kreuing, J. (1977) The influence of fixation on immunoperoxidase staining of plasma cells in paraffin sections of intestinal biopsy specimens. Histochemistry *53*, 57–62.

6 Brandtzaeg, P. (1965) Localization of blood-group substances A and B in alcohol-fixed human gingivae by indirect immunofluorescence technique. Acta Odontol. Scand. *23*, 335–345.

7 Brandtzaeg, P. (1973) Conjugates of immunoglobulin G with different fluorochromes. I. Characterization by anionic-exchange chromatography. Scand. J. Immunol. *2*, 273–290.

8 Brandtzaeg, P. (1973) Conjugates of immunoglobulin G with different fluorochromes. II. Specific and non-specific binding properties. Scand. J. Immunol. *2*, 333–348.

9 Brandtzaeg, P. (1973) Two types of IgA immunocytes in man. Nature New Biol. *243*, 142–143.

10 Brandtzaeg, P. (1974) Mucosal and glandular distribution of immunoglobulin components. Immunohistochemistry with a cold ethanol-fixation technique. Immunology *26*, 1101–1114.

treated material. Acta histochem. *63,* 251–260.

34 Burtin, P. (1978) The carcinoembryonic antigen of the digestive system (CEA) and the antigens cross-reacting with it. Ann. Immunol. (Paris) *129C,* 185–198.

35 Burtin, P., Von Kleist, S., Sabine, M.C. and King, M. (1973) Immunohistological localization of carcinoembryonic antigen and nonspecific cross-reacting antigen in gastrointestinal normal and tumoral tissue. Cancer Res. *33,* 3299–3305.

36 Cebra, J.J. and Goldstein, G. (1965) Chromatographic purification of tetramethylrhodamine-immune globulin conjugates and their use in the cellular localization of rabbit γ-globulin polypeptide chains. J. Immunol. *95,* 230–245.

37 Crabbé, P.A. and Heremans, J.F. (1966) Presence of antibodies against egg-white antigens in human lymphoid tissues. Int. Arch. Allergy *30,* 597–603.

38 Crabbé, P.A., Carbonara, A.O. and Heremans, J.F. (1965) The normal human intestinal mucosa as a major source of plasma cells containing γ-immunoglobulin. Lab. Invest. *14,* 235–248.

39 Creutzfeldt, W., Arnold, R., Creutzfeldt, C. and Track, N.S. (1976) Mucosal gastrin concentration, molecular forms of gastrin, number and ultrastructure of G-cells in patients with duodenal ulcer. Gut *17,* 745–754.

40 Crivelli, O., Pera, A., Ferrari, A., Rizzetto, M., Lombardo, L., Babando, G. and Verme, G. (1977) G-cell counts in antral endoscopic biopsies by immunofluorescence. Scand. J. Gastroenterol. *12,* 721–726.

41 Curran, R.C. and Jones, E.L. (1978) Hodgkin's disease: an immunohistochemical and histological study. J. Pathol. *125,* 39–51.

42 Curran, R.C. and Gregory, J. (1978) Demonstration of immunoglobulin in crytostat and paraffin sections of human tonsils by immunofluorescence and immunoperoxidase techniques. Effects of processing on immunohistochemical performance of tissues and on the use of proteolytic enzymes to unmask antigens in sections. J. Clin. Pathol. (London) *31,* 974–983.

43 Dabelsteen, E. and Pindborg, J.J. (1973) Loss of epithelial blood group substance A in oral carcinomas. Acta Pathol. Microbiol. Scand., Section A, Pathol. *81,* 435–444.

44 Dabelsteen, E. and Fejerskov, O. (1974) Loss of epithelial blood group antigen-A during wound healing in oral mucous membrane. Acta Pathol. Microbiol. Scand., Section A, Pathol. *82,* 431–434.

45 Dabelsteen, E., Mygind, N. and Henriksen, B. (1974) Blood group substance A in carcinomas of the larynx. Acta Oto-Laryngol. *77,* 360–367.

46 Dawson, I.M.P. (1976) The endocrine cells of gastro-intestinal tract and neoplasms which arise from them. *In* Morson, B.C. (ed.), Pathology of the Gastro-Intestinal Tract. Current Topics in Pathology *63* (Springer Verlag, Berlin) pp. 221–258.

47 DeLellis, R.A., Sternberger, L.A., Mann, R.B., Banks, P.M. and Nakane, P.K. (1979) Immunoperoxidase technics in diagnostic pathology. Report on a workshop sponsored by the National Cancer Institute. Am. J. Clin. Pathol. *71,* 483–488.

48 Denk, H., Radaszkiewicz, T. and Witting, C. (1976) Immunofluorescence studies on pathologic routine material: application to malignant lymphomas. Beitr. Pathol. *159,* 219–225.

49 Denk, H., Syré, G. and Weirich, E. (1977) Immunomorphologic methods in routine pathology. Application of immunofluorescence and the unlabeled antibody-enzyme (peroxidase–antiperoxidase) technique to formalin fixed paraffin embedded kidney biopsies. Beitr. Pathol. *160,* 187–194.

50 Denk, H., Radaszkiewicz, T. and Weirich, E. (1977) Pronase pretreatment of tissue sections enhances sensitivity of the unlabelled antibody-enzyme (PAP) technique. J. immunol. Methods *15,* 163–167.

51 Dorsett, B.H. and Ioachim, H.L. (1978) A method for the use of immunofluorescence on paraffin-embedded tissues. Am. J. Clin. Pathol. *69,* 66–72.

52 Eidelman, S. and Berschauer, J.A. (1969) A method for immunocytochemical study of human gastrointestinal suction biopsies. Stain Technol. *44,* 43–44.

53 Feltkamp-Vroom, T.M., Stallman, P.J., Aalberse, R.C. and Reerink-Brongers, E.E. (1975) Immunofluorescence studies on renal tissue, tonsils, adenoids, nasal polyps, and skin of atopic

and nonatopic patients, with special reference to IgE. Clin. Immunol. Immunopathol. *4,* 392–404.

54 Galbraith, G.M.P., Galbraith, R.M. and Fault, W.P. (1978) Removal of unwanted staining in fluorescence microscopy. J. Clin. Lab. Immunol. *1,* 163–167.

55 Gitlin, D. and Sasaki, T. (1969) Immunoglobulins G, A, and M determined in single cells from human tonsils. Science *164,* 1532–1534.

56 Glynn, L.E., Holborow, H.J. and Johnson, G.D. (1957) The distribution of blood-group substances in human gastric and duodenal mucosa. Lancet *2,* 1083–1088.

57 Goding, J.W. (1976) Conjugation of antibodies with fluorochromes: modification to standard methods. J. Immunol. Methods *13,* 215–226.

58 Hartman, B.K. (1973) Immunofluorescence of dopamine-β-hydroxylase. Application of improved methodology to the localization of the peripheral and central noradrenergic nervous system. J. Histochem. Cytochem. *21,* 312–332.

59 Heimer, G.V. and Taylor, C.E.D. (1974) Improved mountant for immunofluorescence preparations. J. Clin. Pathol. *27,* 254–256.

60 Horikawa, M., Chisaka, N., Yokoyama, S. and Onoé, T. (1976) Effect of stirring during fixation upon immunofluorescence. Results with distribution of albumin-producing cells in liver. J. Histochem. Cytochem. *24,* 926–932.

61 Huang, S.-N. (1975) Immunohistochemical demonstration of hepatitis B core and surface antigens in paraffin sections. Lab. Invest. *33,* 88–95.

62 Huang, S.-N., Minassian, H. and More, J.D. (1976) Application of immunofluorescent staining on paraffin sections improved by trypsin digestion. Lab. Invest. *35,* 383–390.

63 Isobe, Y., Chen, S.-T., Nakane, P.K. and Brown, W.R. (1977) Studies on translocation of immunoglobulins across intestinal epithelium. I. Improvements in the peroxidase-labeled antibody method for application to study of human intestinal mucosa. Acta Histochem. Cytochem. *10,* 161–171.

64 Jacobsen, M., Clausen, P.P. and Smidth, S. (1980) The effect of fixation and trypsinization on the immunohistochemical demonstration of intracellular immunoglobulin in paraffin embedded material. Acta Pathol. Microbiol. Scand. Sect. A 88, 369–376.

65 Johnston, N.W. and Bienenstock, J. (1974) Abolition of nonspecific fluorescent staining of eosinophils. J. Immunol. Methods *4,* 189–194.

66 Kent, S.P. (1967) Diffusion of plasma proteins into cells: a manifestation of cell injury in human myocardial ischemia. Am. J. Pathol. *50,* 623–637.

67 Klockars, M. and Reitano, S. (1977) Tissue distribution of lysozyme in man. J. Histochem. Cytochem. *23,* 932–940.

68 Knowles, D.M., Winchester, R.J. and Kunkel, H.G. (1977) A comparison of peroxidase- and fluorochrome-conjugated antisera for the demonstration of surface and intercellular antigens. Clin. Immunol. Immunopathol. *7,* 410–425.

69 Korsrud, F.R. and Brandtzaeg, P. (1979) Immunohistochemical studies on the epithelial and lymphoid components of Warthin's tumour. Acta Oto-Laryngol., Suppl. *360,* 221–224.

70 Korsrud, F.R. and Brandtzaeg, P. (1980) Quantitative immunohistochemistry of immunoglobulin- and J-chain-producing cells in human parotid and submandibular salivary glands. Immunology *39,* 129–140.

71 Korsrud, F.R. and Brandtzaeg, P. (1980) Immune systems of human nasopharyngeal and palatine tonsils. Histomorphometry of lymphoid components and quantification of immunoglobulin producing cells in health and disease. Clin. Exp. Immunol. (in press).

72 Korsrud, F.R. and Brandtzaeg, P. (1980) Immunohistochemical evaluation of J-chain expression by intra- and extra-follicular immunoglobulin-producing human tonsillar cells. Scand. J. Immunol. 13, 271–280.

73 Kraft, W. (1975) The technology of new fluorescence illumination systems. Mikroskopie *31,* 129–146.

74 Kraus, F.W. and Mestecky, J. (1971) Immunohistochemical localization of amylase, lysozyme and immunoglobulins in the human parotid gland. Arch. Oral Biol. *16,* 781–789.

75 Lennert, K. (1978) Malignant Lymphomas Other than Hodgkin's Disease (Springer Verlag,

Berlin).

76 Lennette, D. A. (1978) An improved mounting medium for immunofluorescence microscopy. Am. J. Clin. Pathol. *69,* 647–648.

77 Leonardo, E., Palestro, G. and Stramignoni, A. (1979) Identification of rhinopharyngeal plasmocytic tumours by immunofluorescence on paraffin-embedded sections. Oncology *36,* 89–93.

78 Levy, R., Warnke, R., Dorfman, R.F. and Haimovich, J. (1977) The monoclonality of human B-cell lymphomas. J. Exp. Med. *145,* 1014–1028.

79 Lukes, R.L. and Parker, J.W. (1978) The pathology of lymphoreticular neoplasms. *In* Twomey, J.J. and Good, R.A. (eds.), Immunopathology of Lymphoreticular Neoplasms. Comprehensive Immunology *4* (Plenum Medical Book Company, London), pp. 239–279.

80 Martin-Comin, I. and Robyn, C. (1976) Comparative immunoenzymatic localization of prolactin and growth hormone in human and rat pituitaries. J. Histochem. Cytochem. *24,* 1012–1016.

81 Mason, D.Y. and Taylor, C.R. (1975) The distribution of muramidase (lysozyme) in human tissues. J. Clin. Pathol. *28,* 124–132.

82 Mason, D.Y. and Sammons, R. (1978) Alkaline phosphatase and peroxidase for double immunoenzymatic labelling of cellular constituents. J. Clin. Pathol. *31,* 454–460.

83 Mather, E.L. and Koshland, M.E. (1977) The role of J chain in B cell activation. *In* Sercartz, E.G., Herzenberg, L.A. and Fox, C.F. (eds.), Immune System: Genetics and Regulation. Symp. Molec. Cell. Biol. *6,* 727–733.

84 Mayrhofer, G. (1979) A method for specifically detecting internal immunoglobulin by immunofluorescence. J. Immunol. Methods *27,* 319–325.

85 Mayrhofer, G., Bazin, H. and Gowans, J.L. (1976) Nature of cells binding anti-IgE in rats immunized with *Nippostrongylus brasiliensis:* IgE synthesis in regional nodes and concentration in mucosal mast cells. Eur. J. Immunol. *6,* 537–545.

86 McGuigan, J.E. (1968) Gastric mucosal intracellular localization of gastrin by immunofluorescence. Gastroenterology *55,* 315–327.

87 Mepham, B.L., Frater, W. and Mitchell, B.S. (1979) The use of proteolytic enzymes to improve immunoglobulin staining by the PAP technique. Histochem. J. *11,* 345–357.

88 Meuwissen, S.G.M., Feltkamp-Vroom, T.M., Brutel de la Rivière, A., von dem Borne, A.E.G.K. and Tytgat, G. N. (1976) Analysis of the lympho-plasmacytic infiltrate in Crohn's disease with special reference to identification of lymphocyte-subpopulations. Gut *17,* 770–780.

89 Mul, N.A.J., De Boer, L.E.M., Taminiau, J.A. and Ballieux, R.E. (1975) Light chain type ratio of IgA-producing cells in human jejunal biopsies. Eur. J. Clin. Invest. *5,* 63–67.

90 Nagura, H., Brandtzaeg, P., Nakane, P.K. and Brown, W.R. (1979) Ultrastructural localization of J chain in human intestinal mucosa. J. Immunol. 123, 1044–1050.

91 Nakane, P.K. (1968) Simultaneous localization of multiple tissue antigens using the peroxidase-labelled antibody method: a study on pituitary glands of the rat. J. Histochem. Cytochem. *16,* 557–560.

92 Ørstavik, T.B. (1978) The distribution and secretion of kallikrein in some exocrine organs of the rat. Acta Physiol. Scand. *104,* 431–442.

93 Ørstavik, T.B., Brandtzaeg, P., Nustad, K. and Halvorsen, R.M. (1975) Cellular localization of kallikreins in rat submandibular and sublingual salivary glands. Acta Histochem. *54,* 183–192.

94 Ørstavik, T.B., Nustad, K., Brandtzaeg, P. and Pierce, J.V. (1976) Cellular origin of urinary kallikreins. J. Histochem. Cytochem. *24,* 1037–1039.

95 Ørstavik, T.B., Brandtzaeg, P., Nustad, K. and Pierce, J.V. (1980) Immunohistochemical localization of kallikrein in human pancreas and salivary glands. J. Histochem. Cytochem. 28, 557–562.

96 Pearse, A.G.E. (1968) Histochemistry. Theoretical and Applied *1,* 3rd ed. (Churchill Livingstone, London) pp. 70–105.

97 Pearse, A.G.E. and Polak, J.M. (1975) Bifunctional reagents as vapour- and liquid-phase

fixatives for immunohistochemistry. Histochem. J. 7, 179–186.

98 Pearse, A.G.E., Polak, J.M. and Bloom, S.R. (1977) The newer gut hormones. Cellular sources, physiology, pathology and clinical aspects. Gastroenterology *72,* 746–761.

99 Petrusz, P., Sar, M., Ordronneau, P. and DiMeo, P. (1976) Specificity in immunocytochemical staining. J. Histochem. Cytochem. *24,* 1110–1115.

100 Polak, J.M. and Bloom, S.R. (1978) Peptide hormones of the alimentary tract. *In* Vilardell, F. and Pérez-Mota, A. (eds.), Sixth World Congress of Gastroenterology, Rev. Esp. Ap. Digest. Quadriennal Reviews, pp. 107–134.

101 Polak, J.M., Hoffbrand, A.V., Reed, P.I., Bloom, S.R. and Pearse, A.G.E. (1973) Qualitative and quantitative studies of antral and fundic G cells in pernicious anaemia. Scand. J. Gastroenterol. *8,* 361–367.

102 Reitamo, S., Klockars, M. and Raeste, A.M. (1977) Immunohistochemical identification of lysozyme in the minor salivary glands of man. Arch. Oral Biol. *22,* 515–519.

103 Robinson, G. and Dawson, I. (1979) A formalin fixative for immunochemical and ultrastructural studies on gastrointestinal endocrine cells. J. Clin. Pathol. *32,* 40–45.

104 Rodriguez, J. and Deinhardt, F. (1960) Preparation of a semipermanent mounting medium for fluorescent antibody studies. Virology *12,* 316–317.

105 Rognum, T.O., Brandtzaeg, P., Baklien, K. and Hognestad, J. (1979) Immunoglobulin-producing cells in the "transitional" mucosa adjacent to adenocarcinomas of the human large bowel. Int. J. Cancer *25,* 165–173.

106 Rognum, T.O., Brandtzaeg, P., Ørjasaeter, H., Elgjo, K. and Hognestad, J. (1980) Immunohistochemical study of secretory component, secretory IgA, and carcinoembryonic antigen in large bowel carcinomas. Pathol. Res. Pract. 170, 126–145.

107 Rognum, T.O., Brandtzaeg, P., Ørjasaeter, H. and Fausa, O. (1980) Immunohistochemistry of epithelial cell markers in normal and pathological colon mucosa. Comparison of results based on routine formalin- and cold ethanol-fixation methods. Histochemistry 67, 7–21.

108 Royston, C.M.S., Polak, J.M., Bloom, S.R., Cooke, W.M., Russell, R.C.G., Pearse, A.G.E., Spencer, J., Welbourn, R.B. and Baron, J.H. (1978) G cell population of the gastric antrum, plasma gastrin, and gastric acid secretion in patients with and without duodenal ulcer. Gut *19,* 689–698.

109 Sainte-Marie, G. (1962) A paraffin embedding technique for studies employing immunofluorescence. J. Histochem. Cytochem. *10,* 250–256.

110 Sanders, E.M. and Kent, S.P. (1970) The distribution of water-soluble blood group A antigen in the human large intestine. A mosaic pattern. Lab. Invest. *23*, 74–78.

111 Sandow, M.J. and Whitehead, R. (1979) Progress report. The Paneth cell. Gut *20,* 420–431.

112 Skinner, J.M. and Whitehead, R. (1976) Immunological aspects of gastro-intestinal pathology. *In* Morson, B.C. (ed.), Pathology of the Gastro-Intestinal Tract, Current Topics in Pathology *63,* (Springer Verlag, Berlin) pp. 259–288.

113 Stave, R. and Brandtzaeg, P. (1976) Immunohistochemical investigation of gastrin-producing cells (G cells). The distribution of G cells in resected human stomachs. Scand. J. Gastroenterol. *11,* 705–712.

114 Stave, R. and Brandtzaeg, P. (1977) Fluorescence staining of the gastric mucosa. A study with special reference to parietal cells. Scand. J. Gastroenterol. *12,* 885–891.

115 Stave, R. and Brandtzaeg, P. (1978) Immunohistochemical investigation of gastrin-producing cells (G cells). Estimation of antral density, mucosal distribution and total mass of G cells in resected stomachs from patients with peptic ulcer disease. Scand. J. Gastroenterol. *13,* 199–203.

116 Stave, R., Elgjo, K. and Brandtzaeg, P. (1978) Quantification of gastrin cells (G cells) and parietal cells in relation to histopathological alterations in resected stomachs from patients with peptic ulcer disease. Scand. J. Gastroenterol. *13,* 747–757.

117 Stave, R., Gedde-Dahl, D. and Gjone, E. (1978) Fasting and food-stimulated serum gastrin-concentrations in relation to the antral G-cell population. Study in patients with peptic ulcer disease. Scand. J. Gastroenterol. *13,* 845–849.

118 Stave, R., Brandtzaeg, P., Nygaard, K. and Fausa, O. (1978) The transitional body-antrum

zone in resected human stomachs. Anatomical outline and parietal-cell and gastrin-cell characteristics in peptic ulcer disease. Scand. J. Gastroenterol. *13,* 685–691.

119 Sternberger, L.A. (1974) Immunocytochemistry, 2nd ed. (John Wiley, New York) pp. 82–169.

120 Szulman, A.E. (1960) The histological distribution of blood group substances A and B in man. J. Exp. Med. *111,* 785–800.

121 Taylor, C.R. (1978) Immunoperoxidase techniques. Arch. Pathol. Lab. Med. *102,* 113–121.

122 Taylor, C.R., Roitt, I.M. Doniach, D., Couchman, K.G. and Shapland, C. (1962) Autoimmune phenomena in pernicious anaemia: gastric antibodies. Br. Med. J. *24,* 1347–1352.

123 Tolo, K., Brandtzaeg, P. and Jonsen, J. (1977) Mucosal penetration of antigen in the presence or absence of serum-derived antibody. Immunology *33,* 733–743.

124 Tourville, D.R., Adler, R.H., Bienenstock, J. and Tomasi, T.B. (1969) The human secretory immunoglobulin system: immunohistochemical localization of γ A secretory "piece", and lactoferrin in normal human tissues. J. Exp. Med. *129,* 411–429.

125 Waldmann, T.A. and Strober, W. (1969) Metabolism of immunoglobulins. Prog. Allergy *13,* 1–110.

126 Warnke, R., Pederson, M., Williams, C. and Levy, R. (1978) A study of lymphoproliferative diseases comparing immunofluorescence with immunohistochemistry. Am. J. Clin. Pathol. *70,* 867–875.

127 Weinstein, W.M. and Lechago, J. (1977) Gastrin cell immunofluorescence in conventionally fixed and stained tissue sections. Gastroenterology *73,* 765–767.

128 Witting, C. (1977) Immunofluorescence studies on formalin-fixed and paraffin-embedded material. Beitr. Pathol. *161,* 288–291.

129 Wurster, K., Kuhlmann, W.D. and Rapp, W. (1978) Immunohistochemical studies on human gastric mucosa. Virchows Arch. A, Pathol. Anat. Histol. *378,* 213–228.

Wick et al. (eds) Immunofluorescence Technology. Selected Theoretical and Clinical Aspects

CHAPTER 11

Immunofluorescence in the diagnosis of autoimmune disease

G. WICK

Institute for General and Experimental Pathology, University of Innsbruck Medical School, Innsbruck, Austria

11.1. CONCEPTS OF AUTOIMMUNITY

Autoimmunity is the immunological reaction against the body's own antigenic material, the so-called "self" determinants. Autoimmune reactions have long been considered to be purely pathologic, an opinion that has been summarized by the term "horror autotoxicus" [21]. Later, Grabar [25] and

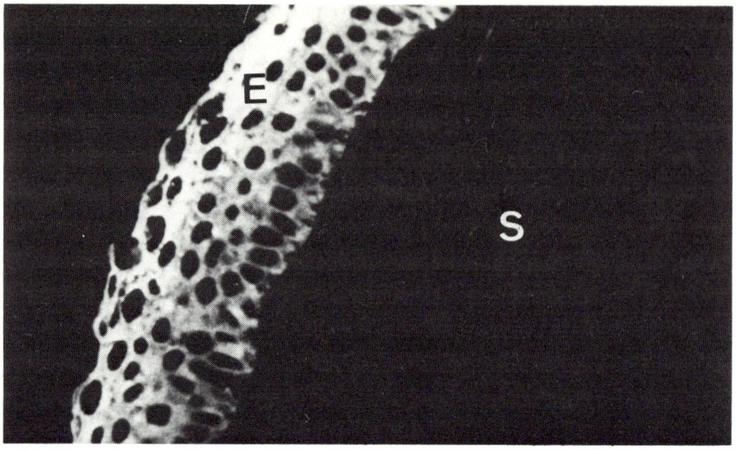

Fig. 11.1. Indirect immunofluorescence test on a frozen, unfixed section of the cornea of a human eye treated with a 1 : 10 dilution of normal human serum and an anti-Ig FITC conjugate. A similar phenomenon to that described in the text for sections of skin is observed, namely the strong "non-specific" staining of the epithelium (E) while the corneal stroma (S) remains negative. Original ×250.

others put forward the idea that autoimmunity may also serve a physiological role and that autoantibodies (AAb) can, e.g., play a role as "transporteurs" of altered or aged autologous material. This concept has been supported by Beutner et al. [8,9], who have studied in detail the well-known phenomenon that most normal human sera give indirect immunofluorescence staining of the stratum corneum of the skin which has usually been considered to be non-specific. These authors, however, showed that this reaction is due to the presence of specific antibodies which seem to have the above-mentioned "pitting" function, in this case for aged stratum corneum cells (Fig. 11.1). By the same token they also clearly demonstrated that fluent transitions exist between this "physiological" autoimmunity and the pathological reaction against stratum corneum cells in patients with psoriasis vulgaris [27].

More recently, "physiological" autoimmunity has experienced a surge of renewed interest after Jerne [28] put forward his concept of the idiotype–antiidiotype network where autoantibodies to idiotypic epitopes serve regulatory functions for immune reactions. The observation that mononuclear cells capable of killing virus-infected target cells can only do so if the latter share certain histocompatibility determinants with the former [70] is a good example for the interrelationship of physiological and pathological autoimmunity. It is obvious that these considerations must be kept in mind when discussing immunofluorescence data with regard to the diagnosis of autoimmune disease. Cellular and humoral autoimmune phenomena which are not commonly found in normal individuals can thus be considered pathological. The mere presence of autoantibodies or autoreactive lymphoid cells alone is, however, not yet synonymous with the presence of an "autoimmune disease". The latter diseases are characterized by organ-specific or systemic lesions which will finally manifest themselves by altered function. Milgrom and Witebsky [32] have summarized the requirements for calling a disease "autoimmune" in the following five postulates: 1) demonstration of antibodies or lymphoid cells which specifically react with autologous material of the tissue or organ in question (e.g. obtained during an operation); 2) the autoantigen in question should be exactly defined (e.g. thyroglobulin); 3) the immunogenicity of this antigen has to be proven by immunization of another organism of the same or a different species; 4) following appropriate immunization with this antigen (e.g. with adjuvants) tissue lesions should be produced in the recipient which correspond with the distribution of the antigen in the immunized individual (e.g. production of thyroiditis after immunization with thyroid antigens, but no development of encephalomyelitis); and 5) passive transfer of the disease by serum or cells.

For obvious reasons the last postulate cannot be fulfilled in humans. Taking the first four postulates as a guideline, however, there are several human autoimmune diseases which rightly deserve this classification, such as Hashimoto's thyroiditis, Graves' disease, systemic lupus erythematosus, etc. Many others, such as rheumatoid arthritis and multiple sclerosis, are good candidates, but cannot yet be listed under this heading without reservations.

The state of immunological tolerance towards "self-antigens" normally experienced by an organism seems to be kept in operation by several mechanisms.

a) Autoreactive B cells are present, but kept in tolerant condition by either relatively high available concentrations of the autoantigens in question or by the lack of cooperating T cells, the latter being in a state of low zone tolerance [16].

b) Suppressor cells, which will be discussed later, exert an active regulatory function.

c) Clonal deletion, which may take place in the thymus [14], is a further possibility. In this respect the recent description of so-called nurse cells [59] in the normal thymus which seem to have a purgatory function may be of importance. Some authors claim that lymphoid cells capable of binding autoantigens (e.g. thyroglobulin-binding cells) can be demonstrated, albeit in low numbers, also in peripheral blood of normal individuals [6, 43], while others, including ourselves, challenge this view [41]. The question that arises is how the state of immunological homeostasis gets out of control and possibly even leads to the development of autoimmune disease.

Table 11.I lists some of the more generally cited answers to this question and some comments on these points. The "forbidden" clone theory now seems to be obsolete and three arguments in support of this statement are listed. In most instances the "sequestered" antigen theory is also not completely valid, e.g. because of the demonstration in the circulation of many autoantigens previously considered to be sequestered from the immune system, such as thyroglobulin [55]. On the other hand, the occurrence of autoantibodies to spermatozoal antigens in about 65% of men after vasectomy [5] or in patients

TABLE 11.I

THEORIES FOR AUTOIMMUNITY

(1) Forbidden clone
autoantigen-binding cells in normals
autoantibodies in normals
polyclonal B-cell activation
(2) Sequestered antigens
no experimental evidence in most cases
(3) Autoantibodies are physiological
autoantibodies as "transporteurs" of cell debris
(4) Cross-reactive antigens
T-cell bypass
virus-induced antigen modifications
(5) Disordered immunological regulation
imbalance of helper and suppressor T cells
Ir genes
idiotype network

with traumatic lesions of the testes to my mind gives credence to the existence of the sequestration phenomenon at least in this case; spermatozoa mature rather late in the development and their antigens could therefore not pass the control of immunological "self-recognition". Any later contact with the immune system will thus entail formation of autoantibodies.

The confrontation of the immune system with antigens cross-reactive with autoantigenic determinants may also be a major basis for the development of autoimmune diseases. The cross-reaction of streptococci A_{12} and human heart muscle antigens is a good example that also has important implications for immunofluorescence studies in this field and will be discussed later [30]. Furthermore, viral infections have been incriminated as causative processes for the initiation of autoimmune diseases in animals and men [38]. Bacterial and viral infections as well as the use of certain adjuvants (and the allogeneic effect) are all able to allow for a direct activation of autoreactive B cells bypassing the requirement of T cells [17]. Ample experimental and clinical evidence also exists for disordered immunologic regulation underlying the development of autoimmune disease. Many examples for an imbalance of helper and suppressor T cells have been described; among these, e.g. the Obese strain (OS) of chickens which are afflicted with an hereditary spontaneous autoimmune thyroiditis characterized by autoreactive B cells and cytotoxic T cells which escaped the regulation by suppressor T cells [13]. In human systemic lupus erythematosus (SLE) the deficiency of T suppressor cells has been well documented [47].

TABLE 11.II

FACTORS INFLUENCING AUTOIMMUNITY

(1) Genetic
- familial aggregation
- association with MHC
  - A) B and D locus
  - B) DR or "Ia-like" B-cell antigens
- spontaneous animal models

(2) Environmental
- drug-induced AAb
  - A) drug-induced LE
  - B) heparin-induced thrombocytopenia
  - C) penicillamine-induced myasthenia gravis
- infections
  - A) chronic bacterial, viral, parasitic
  - B) polyclonal B-cell activation (LPS)
  - C) acute viral (EBV)

(3) Thymus
- suppression
- thymic hormones

(4) Aging
- AAb without disease

(5) Immunodeficiency
- cellular immune deficiency
- selective IgA deficiency
- complement deficiency (C2)

(6) Hormonal
- female/male ratio
- Klinefelter's syndrome

That Ir genes influence the susceptibility of animals to the elicitation of experimental autoimmune diseases has been elegantly demonstrated by Vladutiu and Rose [57] for murine experimental autoimmune thyroiditis. The same is true for man where the development of several autoimmune diseases has been shown to be associated with certain histocompatibility antigens [18]. The role of the idiotypic network in immune regulations has already been briefly alluded to above. Anti-idiotypic humoral and cellular immune reactions are, however, also conceivable as initiating mechanisms for autoimmune disease and, conversely, possible means for specific therapeutic intervention [10].

Some of the factors influencing autoimmune diseases are summarized in Table 11. II.

11.2. EFFECTOR AND SUPPRESSOR MECHANISMS

The effector mechanisms operative in the development of autoimmune disease can be humoral or cellular immune reactions or both. It is obvious that appropriate therapeutic measures for this group of diseases can only be introduced if accurate diagnostic data are first available. In experimental work the emergence of a spontaneously occurring or an artificially (with adjuvants) induced autoimmune disease can be monitored from the beginning. In contrast, when patients are seen by a physician they already have symptoms of the disease, i.e. a condition where several types of effector mechanisms may simultaneously contribute to the histological and clinical characteristics. While the experimental situation thus allows for a therapeutic intervention already in the initial phases the diagnostic tests performed in human patients will most often reveal a leading immunological phenomenon which does not necessarily contribute significantly to the underlying pathogenetic mechanisms.

Fig. 11.2 summarizes our current concept of pathogenetic immunologic effector mechanisms which may be responsible for the development of autoimmune disease. This emerged from our work with the above-mentioned animal model of the OS chicken with spontaneous hereditary autoimmune

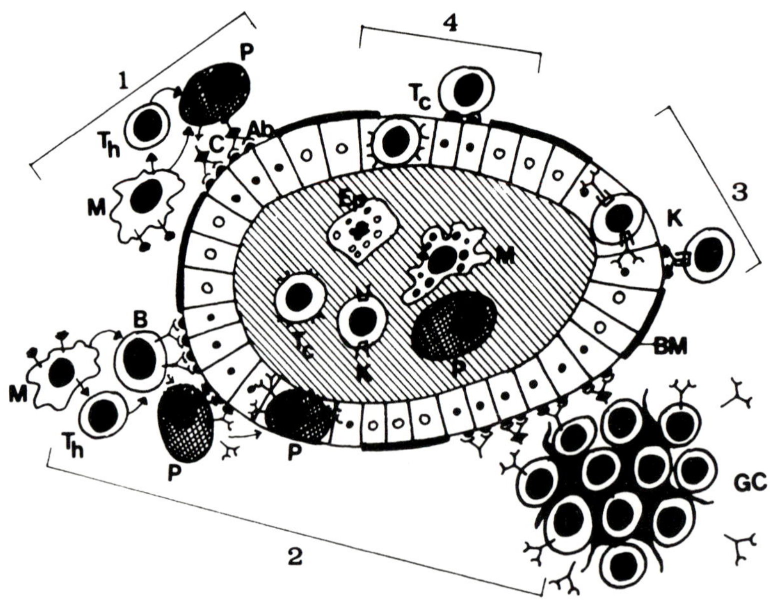

Fig. 11.2. Representation of possible effector mechanisms in autoimmune thyroiditis. For detailed explanations see text. Mechanism 1: cytotoxic antibodies need T-cell help for production and complement for induction of damage; mechanism 2: periopolesis by plasma cells that produce autoantibodies in situ; mechanism 3: direct cytotoxicity by sensitized T cells; mechanism 4: antibody-dependent cellular cytotoxicity (ADCC) by K cells. P, plasma cell; T_h, T helper cell; T_c, cytotoxic T cell; M, macrophage; B, B cell; GC, germinal center; Ab, antibody; C, complement; Ep, thyroid epithelial cell; BM, follicular basement membrane; K, killer cell. (Reproduced from Wick et al. [68] with kind permission of the publisher.)

thyroiditis [63, 68]. Humoral immunity (e.g. autoantibodies to thyroglobulin either produced systemically or in situ) play a central role either via direct complement-mediated cytotoxicity (mechanism 1) or via antibody-dependent cellular cytotoxicity (ADCC, mechanism 3). In addition, a humorally mediated mechanism that seems to be rather peculiar for this model and its human counterpart, i.e. Hashimoto's disease, is a possible cytotoxic action of autoantibody producing plasma cells in situ (mechanism 2), which can be found between the thyroid epithelial cells (a phenomenon called "periopolesis"); these antibodies can either act as shown in (1) or (3). Finally, T cell-mediated cellular cytotoxicity is also involved in the natural history of this disease (mechanism 4). So far we have suggestive data, but not definitive proof, speaking in favour of humorally mediated immunity as being of prime relevance in the initiation of spontaneous autoimmune thyroiditis, while T cell-mediated direct cellular cytotoxicity merges later into this process [67]. In certain forms of human autoimmune disease, such as lupus erythematosus, immune complexes, and thus complement, are certainly the main mediators while in another group, i.e. experimental allergic encephalitis or human allergic encephalitis, cytotoxic T cells seem to constitute the first line of immunological attack. The reasons for these differences are still hypothetical and will not be discussed in the present context.

In the last few years defects in number or function of suppressor cells became a very fashionable way to explain the abnormal autoreactivity of B and/or T cells in experimental animals and humans with autoimmune disease [24]. The most common approach to analyze this problem has been evaluation of the suppressive potential of syngeneic or autologous suspensions of lymphoid cells (peripheral blood, spleen, etc.) on the response of effector cells (i.e. peripheral blood lymphocytes) to stimulation with non-specific mitogens [47]. The clinical relevance of such an approach should be considered with scrutiny, since these mitogens will lead to blast transformation of certain subpopulations of mononuclear cells, but not specifically those responding to the autoantigen(s) in question. Assays for suppression of specific immune reactions, such as direct cellular cytotoxicity to thyroglobulin-coated target cells, would therefore seem to be more indicative for the actual situation in vivo [13].

This finally leads us to the role of immunofluorescence as a diagnostic procedure in the field of autoimmunity; most methods routinely available for the analysis of autoimmune diseases concern the recognition of autoantibodies and only a few deal with cellular immune reactions. Among the former group all serological tests, such as passive hemagglutination, precipitation, complement fixation, radioimmunoassays and enzyme-linked immunosorbent assays, are used, but immunofluorescence (and more recently also other immunohistological procedures) is the most valuable of these tests because it allows the demonstration of both circulating and in vivo bound autoantibodies. From the comments made earlier in this chapter it is clear that the demonstration of autoantibodies does not yet prove the existence of an autoimmune disease and

– if other clinical parameters are in favour of this diagnosis – such autoantibodies cannot automatically be considered to be of pathogenetic significance; in many instances autoantibodies have only diagnostic value and their occurrence may be secondary to the underlying disease.

11.3. HUMAN AUTOIMMUNE DISEASES

It is most probably a correct statement that experimental autoimmune diseases in animals can be produced in any tissue or organ if one "tries hard enough". Also in humans, diseases with a clearcut autoimmune etiology fulfilling the criteria of Milgrom and Witebsky and diseases with a secondary or suspicious relationship to autoimmunization can afflict nearly every organ or tissue. While in the former group of diseases the demonstration of humoral or cellular autoimmune phenomena may be of pathogenetic importance, they are only of diagnostic relevance in the latter.

Table 11.III lists various, but not all, human diseases with clearcut autoimmune facets. Roughly, autoimmune diseases can be divided into organ-specific and systemic forms. This chapter will deal with the methodological aspects of immunofluorescence tests for the diagnosis of human autoimmune diseases and their clinical significance only. It is, of course, beyond the scope of this contribution to discuss further details of each of these diseases, such as clinical and histological aspects.

TABLE 11.III

HUMAN AUTOIMMUNE DISEASES

1. Organ-specific autoimmune diseases
   - 1.1. Endocrine system
     - thyroid: Hashimoto's disease
       - Graves' disease (thyrotoxicosis, Basedow's disease)
       - primary myxedema
     - parathyroid: autoimmune parathyroiditis
     - adrenal: Addison's disease
     - pancreas: juvenile, insulin-dependent diabetes
     - gonads: autoimmune aspermatogenesis
   - 1.2. Hematopoietic system
     - autoimmune hemolytic anemia
     - pernicious anemia
     - autoimmune (idiopathic) thrombocytopenic purpura
     - autoimmune agranulocytemia
     - cold hemagglutinin disease
     - paroxysmal cold hemoglobinuria
     - pancytopenia
     - autoimmune hemophilia
   - 1.3. Muscular system
     - myasthenia gravis

1.4. Gastrointestinal system
    pernicious anemia
    primary biliary cirrhosis
    chronic aggressive hepatitis
    lupoid hepatitis
    coeliac disease
    ulcerative colitis
    regional enteritis
    pancreatitis

1.5. Nervous system
    Myasthenia gravis
    acute demyelinating encephalitis
    multiple sclerosis
    Guillain–Barré syndrome
    peripheral neuritis

1.6. Skin
    pemphigus vulgaris
    bullous pemphigoid
    psoriasis vulgaris
    dermatitis herpetiformis (Duhring's disease)
    exfoliative dermatitis
    vitiligo

1.7. Eye
    sympathetic ophthalmia
    phacoanaphylactic endolphthalmus
    uveitis

1.8. Vascular system
    postcardiotomy syndrome
    postinfarction syndrome
    endocarditis–rheumatoid fever

1.9. Kidney
    glomerulonephritis
    Goodpasture's syndrome

1.10. Lung
    Goodpasture's syndrome
    idiopathic lung fibrosis

2. Systemic autoimmune diseases
    systemic lupus erythematosus
    dermatomyositis
    scleroderma
    Sjögren's disease
    rheumatoid fever
    polyarteritis nodosa
    erythema nodosum

11.4. THE RELEVANCE OF IMMUNOFLUORESCENCE AS A TOOL FOR THE DIAGNOSIS OF AUTOIMMUNE DISEASE

11.4.1. Basic requirements

As for all immunofluorescence tests the basic methodological requirements consist of standardized optical equipment, reagents and test procedures [64]. Elsewhere in this volume and in extensive earlier publications [8, 34] these aspects have been dealt with in detail.

11.4.2. Optical equipment

In our laboratory microscopes equipped for incident light illumination and observation by phase contrast in transmitted light are employed. Among the many objectives available we prefer water-immersion objectives with high numerical aperture. Although low magnification oculars should be preferred on the basis of the Stokes law (fluorescence intensity decreases with square root of eyepiece magnification) we generally select wide angle $\times 10$ oculars, since reading for several hours can get rather tiresome and these are easier on the eye. Optimal filter combinations are available from most microscope manufacturers and their main characteristics are described in detail elsewhere [64]. Due to the way of production, individual filters with identical specifications obtained from the same supplier may still show considerable variation. This is especially true for interference filters. The customers of fluorescence microscopes are therefore well advised to compare several filter sets from the same origin for optimal fulfillment of their special requirements.

Photographic documentation of results may be essential in many instances of immunofluorescence tests for the diagnosis of autoimmune diseases. Although any simple camera will suffice and provide excellent pictures, automatic types of equipment are recommended to facilitate work without distraction from the task of microscope reading. For the selection of correct exposure times it is important to distinguish between integrated (for immunofluorescence on sections) or point measurements (e.g. for membrane immunofluorescence).

Well-characterized conjugates of any desired specificity labelled with various fluorochromes (generally fluorescein isothiocyanate; FITC), or tetramethylrhodamine isothiocyanate, TRITC) can be purchased. Most commercial companies provide appropriate information about their products, such as total protein concentration, antibody content, molar fluorochrome/protein (F/P) ratio or F/Ab ratio, the addition of preservatives, etc. A recently issued manual lists all worldwide commercially available immunologic reagents including conjugates (Lincotts Catalogue of Immunological and Biological Reagents, Second Edition, 1982. Glen Drive, Mill Valley, CA 94941). For most diagnostic purposes polyvalent conjugates will first be used with a later selection of monospecific preparations, if necessary. In order to avoid non-specific staining by adherence to Fc receptors of isolated cells, and also of tissue sections, Fab (or $F(ab')_2$) conjugates should be routinely employed. As mentioned by Holborow et al. in Chapter 1 of this volume, the optimal working dilution of each conjugate should be determined by means of chessboard titrations for a given system.

Finally, care should be taken that the test procedure is rigorously standardized, including the preparation of antigenic material, incubation times and temperatures, reagent dilutions and washing buffers, reading habits, etc.

Table 11.IV lists the profile and incidence of autoantibodies in various autoimmune diseases and the antigenic substrates used for their demonstration in indirect immunofluorescence. Only those conditions will be dealt with in more detail in the present chapter the diagnoses of which centrally depend on the use of immunofluorescence. It should be understood, however, that a variety of other autoimmune diseases can also be diagnosed by immunofluorescence in addition to the routinely employed standard procedures, e.g. immunofluorescence instead of hemagglutination tests for the diagnosis of autoimmune hemolytic anemia.

11.5. DISCUSSION OF SPECIFIC METHODOLOGICAL ASPECTS OF IMMUNOFLUORESCENCE TESTS IN HUMAN AUTOIMMUNITY

11.5.1. Autoimmune diseases of the thyroid gland

As in all other instances cited in this chapter immunofluorescence is only one (albeit of high diagnostic significance) of the immunological and non-immunological tests which help to discriminate autoimmune disorders of the thyroid gland. Table 11.V gives a broad classification of autoimmune thyroid diseases.

Interestingly, diseases of the thyroid are often clustered together with disorders of an autoimmune nature affecting other organs, such as pernicious anemia (Fig. 11.3). Approximately 30% of patients with thyroiditis also display autoantibodies to parietal cells of the stomach mucosa and approximately 50% of the patients with pernicious anemia also have thyroid antibodies.

11.5.1.1. Indirect immunofluorescence tests for autoantibodies to thyroid antigens

11.5.1.1.1. Antibodies to thyroglobulin. The antigenic substrate for these tests consists of 4 μm thick, frozen sections of fresh human colloid goiter or normal monkey thyroid gland. Thyroglobulin has a molecular weight of about 660,000 and is water-soluble. Therefore, tissue sections have to be fixed in absolute methanol for 15 min in a Coplin jar at 56°C. After air drying with a fan the

11 Brandtzaeg, P. (1974) Mucosal and glandular distribution of immunoglobulin components: differential localization of free and bound SC in secretory epithelial cells. J. Immunol. *112,* 1553–1559.

12 Brandtzaeg, P. (1974) Characteristics of SC–Ig complexes formed in vitro. Adv. Exp. Med. Biol. *45,* 87–97.

13 Brandtzaeg, P. (1975) Rhodamine conjugates: specific and nonspecific binding properties in immunohistochemistry. Ann. N.Y. Acad. Sci. *254,* 35–54.

14 Brandtzaeg, P. (1975) Immunochemical studies on free and bound J chain of human IgA and IgM. Scand. J. Immunol. *4,* 439–450.

15 Brandtzaeg, P. (1976) Structural, functional and cellular studies of human J chain. Ricerca Clin. Lab. *6* (Suppl. 3), 15–38.

16 Brandtzaeg, P. (1976) Synthesis and secretion of secretory immunoglobulins: with special reference to dental diseases. J. Dent. Res. *55,* C102–C114.

17 Brandtzaeg, P. (1976) Studies of J chain and binding site for secretory component in circulating human B cells. I. The surface membrane. Clin. Exp. Immunol. *25,* 50–58.

18 Brandtzaeg, P. (1977) Immunohistochemical studies on various aspects of glandular immunoglobulin transport in man. Histochem. J. *9,* 553–572.

19 Brandtzaeg, P. and Kraus, F. W. (1965) Autoimmunity and periodontal disease. Odont. Tidskr. (Scand. Dent. J.) *73,* 281–393.

20 Brandtzaeg, P. and Baklien, K. (1976) Immunohistochemical studies of the formation and epithelial transport of immunoglobulins in normal and diseased human intestinal mucosa. Scand. J. Gastroenterol. 11 (Suppl. 36), 1–45.

21 Brandtzaeg, P. and Baklien, K. (1976) Inconclusive immunohistochemistry of human IgE in mucosal pathology. Lancet *1,* 1297–1298.

22 Brandtzaeg, P. and Baklien, K. (1977) Intestinal secretion of IgA and IgM: a hypothetical model. *In* Immunology of the Gut. Ciba Found. Symp. 46 (Elsevier/Excerpta Medica/ North-Holland, Amsterdam) pp. 77–108.

23 Brandtzaeg, P. and Baklien, K. (1977) Characterization of the IgA immunocyte population and its product in a patient with excessive intestinal formation of IgA. Clin. Exp. Immunol. *30,* 77–88.

24 Brandtzaeg, P. and Tolo, K. (1977) Immunoglobulin systems of the gingiva. *In* T. Lehner, (ed.), The Borderland between Caries and Periodontal Disease (Academic Press, London) pp. 145–183.

25 Brandtzaeg, P. and Baklien, K. (1980) Immunohistochemical studies of the immunoglobulin-producing cell systems of the human intestinal mucosa. Acta Histochem. Suppl. *12*, 105–119.

26 Brandtzaeg, P. and Rognum, T.O. (1982) Evaluation of nine different fixatives. 2. Preservation of IgG, IgA, and secretory component in artificial substrates. Submitted for publication.

27 Brandtzaeg, P., Surjan, L. and Berdal, P. (1978) Immunoglobulin systems of human tonsils. I. Control subjects of various ages: quantification of Ig-producing cells, tonsillar morphometry and serum Ig concentrations. Clin. Exp. Immunol. *31,* 367–381.

28 Brandtzaeg, P., Gautvik, K.M., Nustad, K. and Pierce, J.V. (1976) Rat submandibular gland kallikreins: purification and cellular localization. Br. J. Pharmacol. *56,* 155–167.

29 Brandtzaeg, P., Gjeruldsen, S.T., Elgjo, K. and Hörven, I. (1979) Histiocytic lymphoma of the orbita characterized by functional macrophage markers. XIX. Scandinavian Congress of Pathology and Microbiology, Program and Abstracts, p. 34.

30 Brandtzaeg, P., Gjeruldsen, S.T., Korsrud, F., Baklien, K., Berdal, P. and Ek, J. (1979) The human secretory immune system shows striking heterogeneity with regard to involvement of J chain-positive IgD immunocytes. J. Immunol. *122,* 503–510.

31 Brown, W.R. (1978) Relationships between immunoglobulins and the intestinal epithelium. Gastroenterology *75,* 129–138.

32 Brown, W.R., Iosobe, Y. and Nakane, P.K. (1976) Studies on translocation of immunoglobulins across intestinal epithelium. II. Immunoelectron-microscopic localization of immunoglobulins and secretory component in human intestinal mucosa. Gastroenterology *71,* 985–995.

33 Brozman, M. (1978) Immunohistochemical analysis of formaldehyde- and trypsin- or pepsin-

TABLE 11.IV

INCIDENCE OF AUTOANTIBODIES IN VARIOUS AUTOIMMUNE DISEASES

Autoimmune disease	Sections of organs used as antigenic substrate for IIF tests	Prevalence of autoantibodies (%)
Hashimoto's thyroiditis	Human colloid goiter (fixed)	Thyroglobulin and thyroid epithelial cells (95%)
Thyrotoxicosis	Human thyrotoxic goiter (unfixed)	Thyroid epithelial cells and thyroglobulin (85%)
Pernicious anemia	Human gastric fundus mucosa (unfixed)	Gastric parietal cells (90%)
Prim. Addison's disease	Monkey or human adrenal glands, preferentially from Cushing's disease (unfixed)	Adrenal cortical cells (70%)
Insulin dependent diabetes mellitus (juvenile or rec. diagnosed)	Monkey or human (blood group O) pancreas (unfixed)	Pancreatic islet cells (70%)
Hypoparathyroidism	Monkey or human parathyroid gland (unfixed)	Parathyroid chief cells (40%)
Myasthenia gravis	Human, monkey or rat striated muscle (e.g. diaphragm) or thymus myoid cells (unfixed)	Muscular striations – I and A bands (50%, in patients with thymoma 95%)
	Inhibition of binding of fluorochrome-labelled α-bungarotoxin to motoric endplates in striated muscle (unfixed)	Acetylcholine receptors (90%)
Sjögren's disease	Monkey or human (blood group O) parotid gland (unfixed)	Salivary duct epithelial cells (70%)
Idiopathic male infertility	Autologous native or trypsinized (swollen sperm heads) spermatozoa (unfixed)	Head, intermediate piece or tail of sperm (40%) (post-vasectomy: 70%)
Postcardiotomy syndrome and postmyocarditis syndrome	Human or rat heart muscle (unfixed)	Z bands (50%)
Idiopathic thrombocytopenic purpura	Platelets (autologous or allogeneic, blood group O; unfixed)	Thrombocyte plasma membrane (60%)
Pemphigus vulgaris	Human gingiva or skin, monkey or rabbit esophagus	Intercellular space of squamous epithelial cells (80%)

Autoimmune disease	Sections of organs used as antigenic substrate for IIF tests	Prevalence of autoantibodies (%)
Bullous pemphigoid	As for pemphigus vulgaris, or guinea pig lip (unfixed)	Basement membrane zone (80%)
Goodpasture's syndrome	Human kidney, basement membrane-producing mouse tumor (EHS sarcoma; unfixed)	Glomerular basement membrane (70%). Tumor basement membrane (70%)
"Collagen diseases"	Rat liver (acetone fixed); chicken erythrocyte nuclei (for screening only); baby hamster kidney cell monolayers (for screening) Hemoflagellate Crithidia luciliae (unfixed)	Nuclear IF SLE: 100% Mixed conn. tissue syndrome: 70% Scleroderma: 60% Sjögren's disease: 70% Native DNA in kinetoplast (SLE 100%)
Primary biliary cirrhosis	Rat kidney	Mitochondria in tubuli (95%)
Chronic active hepatitis	Rat stomach	Smooth muscle layers (80–90%)

TABLE 11.V

THYROID DISORDERS WITH AUTOIMMUNE MANIFESTATIONS

1. Diffuse goitrous lymphocytic thyroiditis
   1.1. Hashimoto's thyroiditis (struma lymphomatosa)
   1.2. Juvenile lymphocytic thyroiditis
2. Diffuse non-goitrous thyroiditis
   2.1. Myxedema (atrophic)
   2.2. Asymptomatic, mild form
3. Multifocal lymphocytic thyroiditis in
   3.1. Goiters with adenoma
   3.2. Goiters with primary thyrotoxicosis (Graves' disease)
   3.3. Carcinoma

sections are ready for use in indirect immunofluorescence. An example of the characteristic "cloudy" positive staining with accentuation at the acinar border is shown in Fig. 11.4.

11.5.1.1.2. Antibodies to the second colloid antigen (CA_2). In rare instances, patients with Hashimoto's disease fail to show thyroglobulin autoantibodies in complement fixation or passive hemagglutination, but still show a "flat",

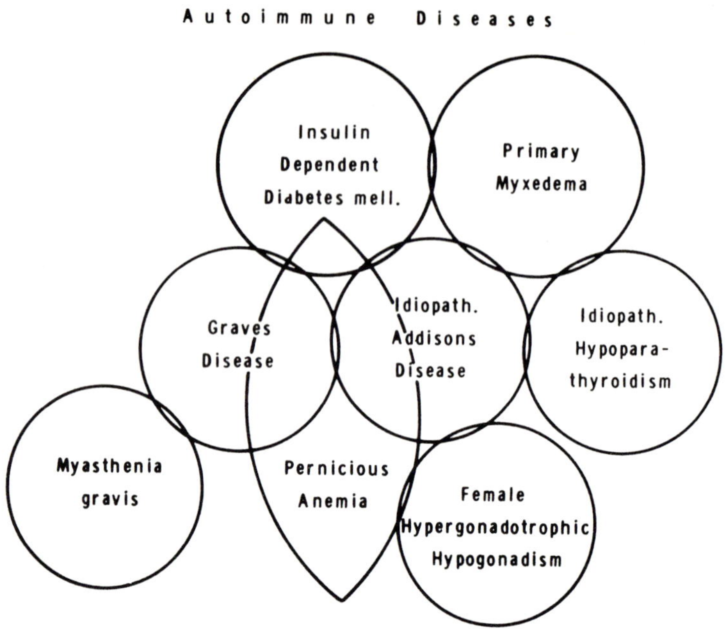

Fig. 11.3. Schematic representation of interrelationships among autoimmune endocrinopathies. (Reproduced from Wick and Albini [62] with kind permission of the publisher.)

uniform indirect immunofluorescence staining of the colloid. These antibodies are indirected against an antigen distinct from thyroglobulin which therefore cannot be removed from a given serum by absorption with thyroglobulin. Their diagnostic significance is questionable since they also occur in autoimmune diseases not involving the thyroid and in approximately 10% of the normal population (Fig. 11.5).

11.5.1.1.3. Autoantibodies to microsomal antigens. In contrast to the chemically well-defined antigen thyroglobulin, microsomal antigens are sensitive to fixation and therefore demonstrable on unfixed material only. The high columnar follicular epithelium of thyrotoxic goiters is very rich in these antigens and thus best suited as antigenic substrate for indirect immunofluorescence tests. Unfixed frozen sections (4 μm thick) of thyrotoxic goiter can be mounted on the same slide, but at the opposite end, as the colloid goiter. The latter can be immersed into the fixative amounting to only 1/3 of the volume of the narrow part of the Coplin jar, thus leaving the former section unfixed for a demonstration of microsomal antibodies. The characteristic staining pattern of cytoplasmic thyroid fluorescence is depicted in Fig. 11.6. It is important to avoid misinterpretation due to the presence of mitochondrial autoantibodies which give similar staining patterns. The presence of these antibodies can, however, be controlled by a parallel performance of the test on kidney sections and/or absorption of the patient's serum with kidney homogenate which should remove the reactivity of mitochondrial antibodies but not affect the activity of microsomal antibodies.

Indirect immunofluorescence tests are valuable screening procedures for the detection of thyroid autoantibodies; in positive instances, passive haemagglutination and/or complement fixation should be performed, these being approximately 10 times more sensitive than immunofluorescence.

11.5.1.1.4. Antibodies to thyroid epithelial cells. Autoantibodies to the thyroid epithelial cell membrane have been demonstrated by membrane immunofluorescence of living or paraldehyde-fixed epithelial cells [22]. However, it later turned out that this staining pattern actually is obtained by antibodies to microsomal antigens, the latter representing internalized cell surface membrane components [20]. This type of staining is shown in Fig. 11.7.

11.5.1.2. Interpretation of results from indirect immunofluorescence tests

The lack of autoantibodies to thyroglobulin and microsomal antigens practically excludes the diagnosis of Hashimoto's disease and of primary myxoedema, thereby allowing the differentiation of these conditions from other non-toxic types of goiters and thyroid carcinoma. In patients with long standing – "burned out" – Hashimoto's thyroiditis, autoantibodies may gradually disappear from the circulation. The temporary disappearance of thyroid autoantibodies in women with Hashimoto's thyroiditis during pregnancy is presumably due to in vivo absorption by the foetal thyroid gland. The antibodies are of both the IgG and, albeit in lower titer, the IgM class. Positive

Fig. 11.4. Indirect immunofluorescence test with the serum from a human Hashimoto patient on a frozen, methanol-fixed section of a human colloid goiter. Note characteristic cloudy staining of colloid with accentuation at the acinar border. Original ×250.

Fig. 11.5. Demonstration of the second colloid antigen (CA_2) in an indirect immunofluorescence test on a frozen, methanol-fixed section of a human colloid goiter using a thyroglobulin-absorbed serum from a patient with Hashimoto's thyroiditis. Note "flat" appearance of colloid staining. Original ×250.

Fig. 11.6. Indirect immunofluorescence test on a frozen, unfixed section of human thyrotoxic goiter using a serum from a patient with Graves' disease. Note cytoplasmic staining of epithelial cells. Original ×250.

Fig. 11.7. Human thyroid monolayer culture stained by indirect immunofluorescence with the serum of a patient with Hashimoto's thyroiditis. Granular type of surface staining of epithelial cells and no reaction with stroma. Original ×700. (Kindly provided by Drs. E. Khoury and G.F. Bottazzo, London.)

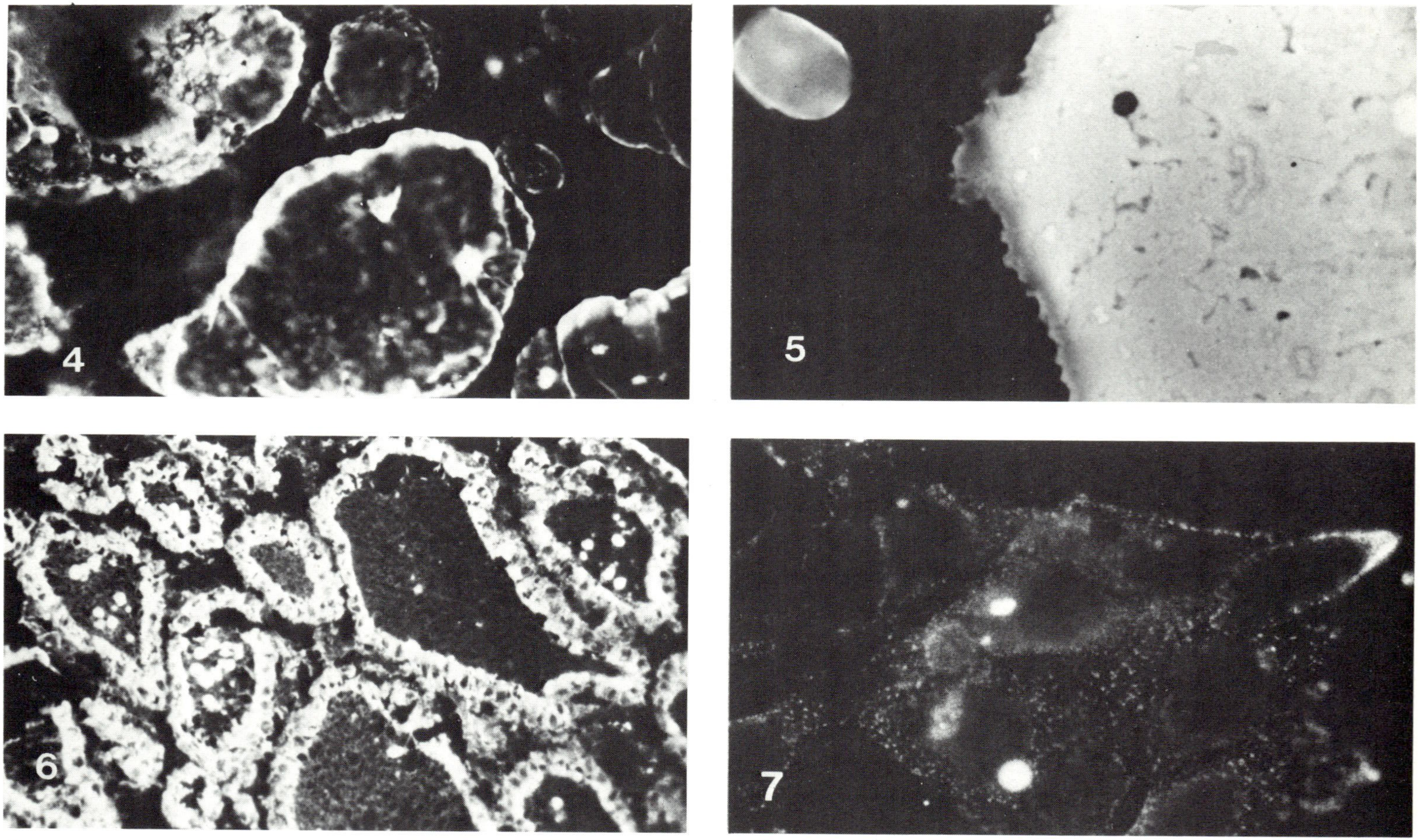

(For legends, see previous page)

results are obtained in patients with Hashimoto's disease, thyrotoxicosis and a variety of other autoimmune disorders with an overlapping pattern, such as pernicious anemia, rheumatoid arthritis and systemic lupus erythematosus. Occasionally low titers (1 : 10) of thyroid antibodies are also observed in apparently normal persons without any clinical symptoms. The frequency of these autoantibodies is significantly higher in females than in males and increases with age.

The analysis of needle biopsies from thyroid glands of patients with Hashimoto's disease revealed in vivo bound IgG class thyroglobulin autoantibodies which apparently do not bind complement. In the light of recent experimental data in OS chickens this observation supports our hypothesis that antibody-dependent cellular cytotoxicity may play a major role as an initial pathogenic mechanism in Hashimoto's disease.

Graves' disease (Basedow's disease or thyrotoxicosis) which is characterized by goiter, hyperthyroidism, often focal mononuclear cell infiltration of the thyroid gland and proptosis, is also associated with thyroid antibodies especially thyroid-stimulating Ig (TSI). As the demonstration of the latter is routinely done by methods other than immunofluorescence they will not be discussed within the framework of this article. A significant number (approximately 50%) of these patients have thyroglobulin and microsomal autoantibodies, but in lower titers than in Hashimoto's disease. While Hashimoto's thyroiditis is much more frequent (20 : 1) in females than in males, Graves' disease shows no sex predilection. The overlap of thyroid autoantibodies with non-thyroid autoantibodies, such as parietal cell autoantibodies and adrenal autoantibodies, can also be found in this condition.

11.5.2. Autoimmunity of the parathyroid gland

Patients with idiopathic hypoparathyroidism frequently also display autoimmune adrenalitis, thyroiditis and pernicious anemia. Likewise, the latter diseases are often associated with idiopathic hypoparathyroidism. In addition to the histological signs of lymphocytic infiltration and destruction of parathyroid parenchyma, rare reports in the literature describe organ-specific parathyroid autoantibodies in the sera of such patients [12, 26], but this observation is not undisputed. In indirect immunofluorescence tests, Blizzard et al. [11] found parathyroid autoantibodies in 38% of 74 patients with idiopathic hypothyroidism, 26% of 92 patients with idiopathic Addison's disease, and 12% of Hashimoto patients. Only 6% of controls contained such antibodies. Fresh, unfixed postmortem parathyroid tissue seems to be superior to parathyroid adenomas as antigenic substrate for indirect immunofluorescence, the latter differing widely in reactivity. Both oxyphil and chief cells are stained in these instances. It should be stressed that organ specificity has to be verified in every case, especially with respect to the concomitant occurrence of antimitochondrial antibodies.

11.5.3. Autoimmune diseases of the adrenal gland

As antigenic substrate for the demonstration of adrenal antibodies we use human surgical specimens from patients operated for Cushing's syndrome or metastatic carcinoma as well as normal adrenals obtained at autopsy, not later than 4 h after death. However, human fetal (last trimester) or newborn adrenals and especially glands from rhesus monkeys are probably most suited for routine tests. We always use 4 μm thick, unfixed frozen sections, but 30 s fixation in acetone (for lipoprotein antigens) is also recommended. The antigen(s) detected in indirect immunofluorescence most probably are lipoproteins associated with carbohydrates. They are localized in the microsomes of cortical cells and seem to be present also in mitochondria. The species specificity of these antigens is restricted, since human autoantibodies react only with monkey, bovine, pig, rabbit, guinea pig, canine and feline material, but not with adrenals from rat or mouse. Human adrenocortical neoplasms do not react, and tissue from patients under steroid therapy is often deficient in these antigens. In order to obtain reproducible results, careful selection of an appropriate antigenic substrate and positive and negative control sera is of crucial importance.

These autoantibodies are usually of IgG class and occur in low titers, generally below 1 : 100, and we start titration usually with a dilution of 1 : 5. In most cases the titers persist also under therapy. Young subjects with short duration of the disease display autoantibodies more frequently, but the titers are similar to those of older patients. The reported frequency of adrenal autoantibodies in Addison's disease ranges from 38% to 64% with a female

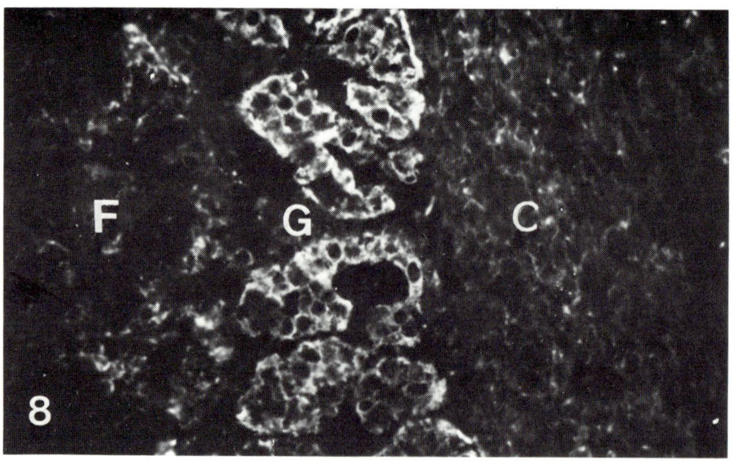

Fig. 11.8. Indirect immunofluorescence test on an unfixed, frozen section of a normal human adrenal gland from a young adult incubated with serum from a patient with Addison's disease. Strong fluorescence of the zona glomerulosa (G), weak fluorescence of the zona fasciculata (F). C = capsule. Original ×500 (Reproduced from Wick and Albini [62] with kind permission of the publisher.)

preponderance. In patients with tuberculosis of the adrenal gland the incidence is 18%, and less than 1% of normal sera show such antibodies.

Several staining patterns can be observed, ranging from fluorescence of the whole cortex to reaction of the zona fasciculata and glomerulosa only (Fig. 11.8) or a combination of the zona fasciculata and reticularis [36]. In addition to the presence of circulating autoantibodies to still unidentified cytoplasmic antigens of adrenocortical cells, patients with Addison's disease may – although rarely – show autoantibodies to steroid producing cells of the theca interna and the corpus luteum of the ovary, with interstitial cells of the testes and the trophoblast in the placenta. In the case of adrenal tissue these autoantibodies to steroid-producing cells all react with the zona fasciculata.

11.5.4. Diabetes mellitus

Indirect immunofluorescence tests for islet cell antibodies (ICA) with sera from patients with diabetes mellitus may be performed on postmortem human blood group O pancreas or monkey pancreas. Due to the secretion of blood group substances by secretory glands, tissues from donors with blood groups A or B are unsuitable antigenic substrates. Recently, a method for the demonstration of ICA on Bouins-fixed, paraffin-embedded human pancreas has been described [35]. These sections were treated with trypsin before use (see also Chapter 12).

The antigenic structures reactive with ICA seem to be constituents of cytoplasmic organelles within islets and not, however, insulin itself. ICA are generally of the IgG class and complement-binding. They are organ-, but not species-specific (binding to rat and guinea pig islets has been described), but the reactivity with human or monkey material is strongest. Fig. 11.9 shows

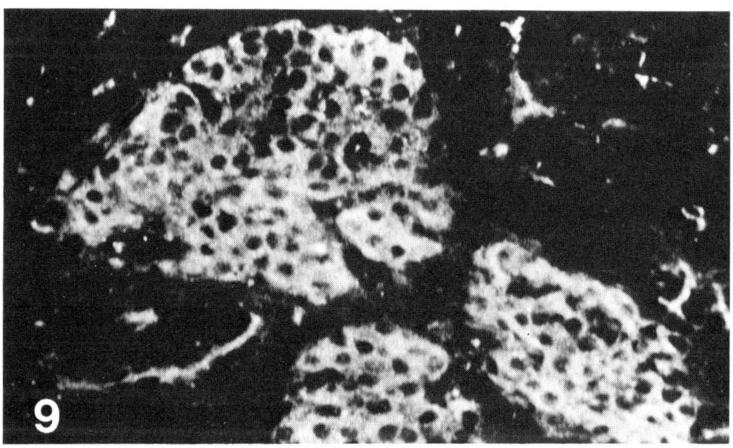

Fig. 11.9. Indirect immunofluorescence test on an unfixed, frozen section of human pancreas incubated with the serum from a patient with diabetes mellitus. Fluorescence of *all* endocrinologically active islet cells can be observed. Nuclei and epithelial cells are unstained. Original ×500. (Kindly supplied by Dr. H. Ludwig, Vienna.)

the appearance of islet immunofluorescence with ICA; the reaction of all islet cells can be appreciated. In this particular instance we start titrations with undiluted and 1 : 5 diluted patient's sera and, of course, also include appropriately diluted negative controls. ICA can be demonstrated in 60–85% of patients with juvenile insulin-dependent diabetes mellitus, 20% of patients with late-onset insulin-dependent diabetes but only rarely (1–2%) in the sera of non-insulin-dependent patients who acquire the disease later in life. The latter value approximately corresponds to the frequency of ICA in non-diabetic controls except the relatives of diabetic patients. Here the incidence is about 9%. The appearance of ICA may herald diabetes mellitus long before clinically manifested symptoms appear and they are observed more constantly in cases with short duration, the titers declining later in the process. There is a considerable overlap with autoantibodies to other endocrine organs, notably 48% of patients with Addison's disease also reveal ICA (see Fig. 11.3).

11.5.5. Autoimmune aspermatogenesis

Human spermatozoa possess several auto- and isoantigens, the former obviously being of importance in cases of male infertility, the latter for the possible production of anti-spermatozoal antibodies in women. Such antibodies can be detected by a variety of techniques such as immobilization, agglutination, cytotoxicity and immunofluorescence tests. Only the immunofluorescence techniques will be considered in the present context; the relative diagnostic impact of the various methods of analysis has been discussed in detail by others, e.g. by Rose et al. [44]. In general, antigenic material for indirect immunofluorescence tests, using both male and female sera, is prepared from the fresh ejaculate. Briefly, the test procedure is as follows:

1. Spermatozoa in 0.2 ml of ejaculate are first washed at least five times in saline by centrifugation at 650 $\times$ g for 5 min at room temperature. Extensive washing is crucial to minimize the adherence of antigenic components from the seminal plasma.

2. The washed spermatozoa are resuspended in saline to a final concentration of 1 $\times$ 10^7 ml; 0.025 ml drops of this suspension are then deposited onto Teflon-coated slides with an appropriate number of holes and gently air-dried under a *cool* fan.

3. The dried preparations are then fixed in absolute methanol for 10–30 min and washed free of the fixative with PBS (pH 7.2) for another 15 min.

4. Serum dilutions are applied for 60 min in a moist chamber at room temperature followed by 30 min washing in PBS with changes of the buffer every 10 min.

5. An anti-total human Ig-conjugate in an appropriate working dilution determined by chessboard titrations is then added for 30 min followed by a final wash of 90 min.

6. The mounting of the test is done in buffered glycerol.

As methanol fixation, albeit more suited than ethanol or acetone, may lead to destruction of some, especially midpiece, antigenic determinants, 0.1% buffered formaldehyde (in PBS) for 3–5 min can also be tried. The rather high degree of non-specific staining and the heterogeneity of the staining pattern (only approximately 30% of the spermatozoa afford the predominant pattern) require a) careful inclusion of strict controls, b) disregarding positive results with serum dilutions below 1 : 16 (this will also exclude weak reactions due to antibodies to blood group antigens or HLA), and c) optimal microscopic facilities. As the preparation of Fab fragments from patients' sera is not feasible in routine tests for practical reasons, we have overcome the problem of Fc-receptor binding by only using sera and conjugates which have been ultracentrifuged (100,000 × g for 20 min in a Beckman Airfuge) immediately before application.

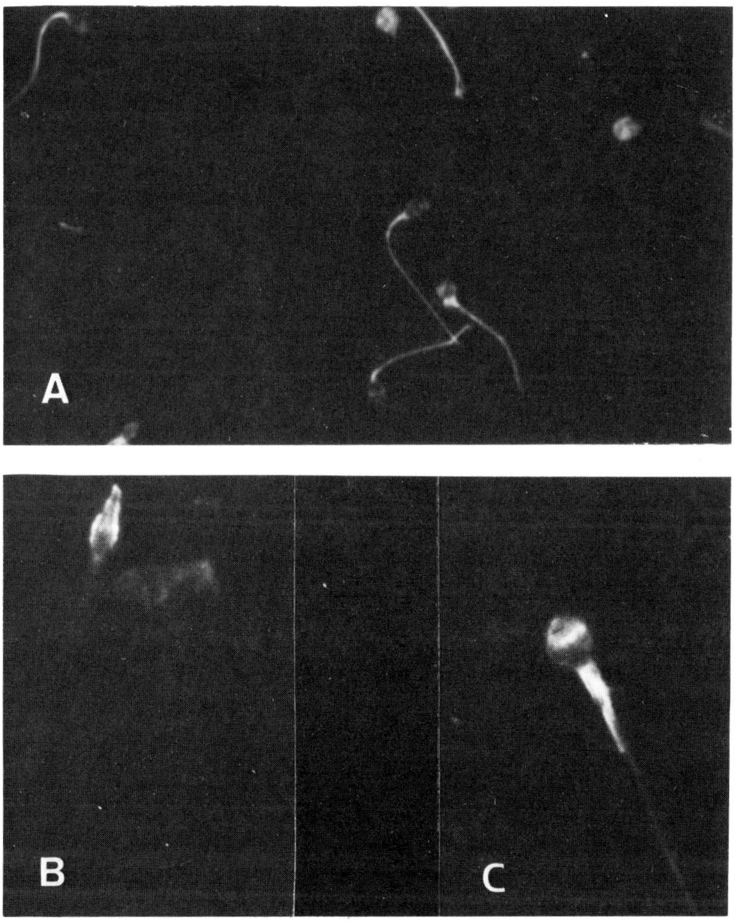

Fig. 11.10. Indirect immunofluorescence test on air-dried spermatozoa treated with sera from male patients with unexplained infertility. Staining of the tail and mid-piece (A), sperm head (B) or the mid-piece and acrosome (C). Note that not all spermatozoa in a visual field afford the characteristic staining pattern. Original ×500.

The use of monospecific conjugates reveals anti-sperm antibodies belonging mainly to the IgG, less frequently to the IgM, and occasionally also to the IgA class.

Fluorescence patterns can consist in the reaction with the sperm head, midpiece and/or tail (Fig. 11.10). The head seems to contain separate antigens on the anterior acrosome and the equatorial fragment. The sera of some infertile male patients may also contain antibodies which react with antigens on swollen spermheads. Briefly, the swelling procedure is as follows.

1. Centrifugation of fresh semen for 15 min at 1400 $\times$ g at 4°C.

2. Three times washing of the pellet in PBS and resuspension in solution containing 50 mM Tris-HCl at pH 9.0 and 0.4 mM dithiothreitol.

3. After 2–5 min a fresh trypsin solution in 1 mM HCl is added to a final concentration of 10 mg/ml.

4. The reaction is left to proceed for 1–30 min (dependent on reagents this incubation period should be first established for each laboratory in model experiments by control under phase contrast).

5. Now the suspension is diluted to 2 $\times$ 10^6 spermatozoa/ml deposited in 0.025 ml droplets on Teflon-coated slides, air-dried, fixed in absolute methanol for 30 min, dried and stored below –20°C if necessary.

6. The indirect immunofluorescence test is performed as described above for native spermatozoa.

A correlation has been found between high titers in the gelatine-agglutination test, immunofluorescence of head and midpiece and the reaction with swollen spermheads. The occurrence of antibodies to the anterior acrosome, the equatorial segment and the postnuclear cap cannot be correlated with any of the agglutinating antibodies. The sensitivity of immunofluorescence tests is higher than that of immobilization and cytotoxicity techniques, but less sensitive than the tray agglutination test.

Among infertile couples 3–4% of men reveal circulating spermatozoal autoantibodies [46] in titers $\geqslant 1:64$. In our patients spermatozoal autoantibodies can also frequently – however, in lower titers than in the circulation – be demonstrated in the seminal plasma (mainly IgG and anti-IgA, but rarely IgM). In men who underwent vasectomy the incidence of circulating spermatozoal antibodies rose to 30–40% [4]. Isoantibodies to sperm antigens have been reported [48] in up to 30% of women with unexplained infertility values, although in our own experience this seems far too high a percentage. Finally, isoantibodies can also be found in cervical mucus which, however, poses considerable problems due to a) the usually low amount of fluid that can be collected, b) problems in sampling on the right day of the menstrual cycle for optimal yield, c) the poor availability of appropriate controls, and d) difficulties in extracting or solubilizing the mucous material. The experience involving immunofluorescence analysis of cervical mucous for isoantibody to spermatozoa reported in the literature is rather limited and we also do not allot too much significance to positive results in this system due to the rather high incidence of non-specific staining.

11.5.6. Pernicious anemia

Autoantibodies to gastric parietal cells are seen in about 90% of patients with pernicious anemia, and this greatly facilitates differential diagnosis in the field of macrocytic anemias. In addition, anti-parietal cell autoantibodies occur in the majority of cases with atrophic gastritis and also take a significant share in those instances where we observe an overlap of various autoantibodies, even if the primary disease apparently does not involve the stomach, such as iron deficiency, Addison's disease, thyroid diseases, and juvenile insulin-dependent diabetes mellitus. Among the latter group, 30% of patients with Hashimoto's thyroiditis and Graves' disease possess anti-parietal cell autoantibodies. Autoantibodies to intrinsic factor which can be demonstrated in 15% of pernicious anemia patients by radioimmunoassays [56] can generally not be found in the absence of pernicious anemia. These antibodies are mainly of the IgG class.

In the young normal population parietal cell autoantibodies can only rarely be seen, but the incidence increases with age, both in females and in males, reflecting the higher frequency of atrophic gastritis in this age group.

As an antigenic substrate, human blood group O stomach fundus mucosa (which can be obtained from surgical specimens) or monkey tissue is superior to gastric mucosa from rodents. In our laboratory we employ unfixed, frozen sections only, but fixed and paraffin-embedded material has also been recommended recently [39]. Fig. 11.11 exemplifies the appearance of parietal cell indirect immunofluorescence on rat tissue.

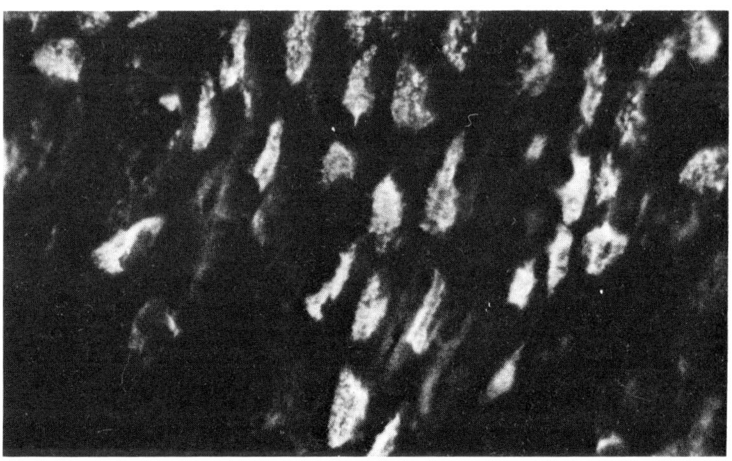

Fig. 11.11. Indirect immunofluorescence test on a frozen, unfixed section of rat stomach using a serum from a patient with pernicious anemia. Bright cytoplasmic fluorescence of parietal cells. Original ×500.

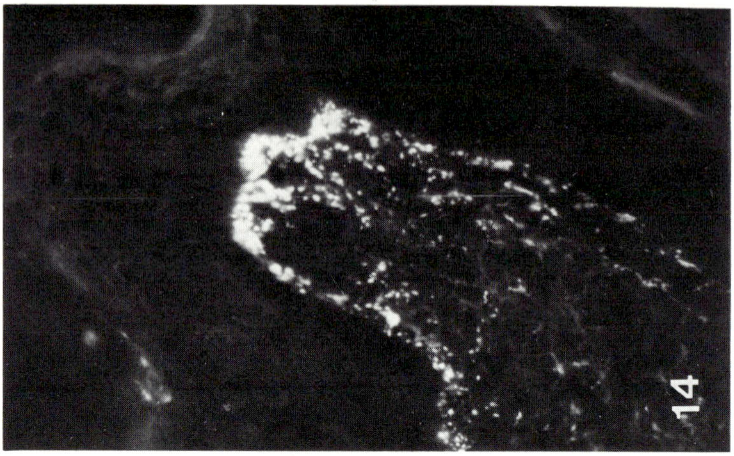
14

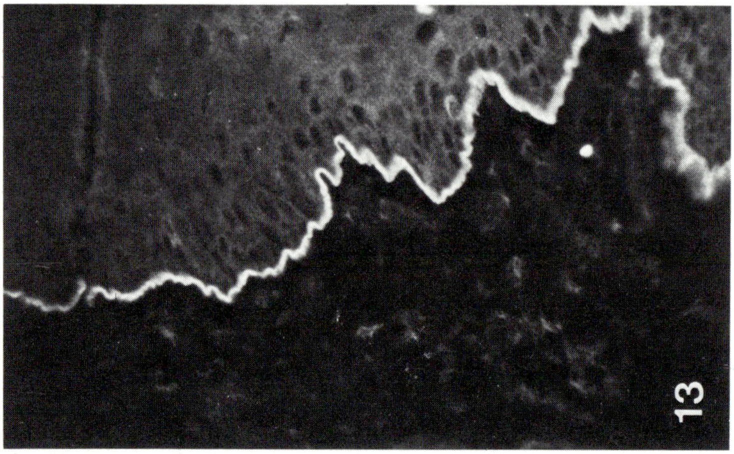
13

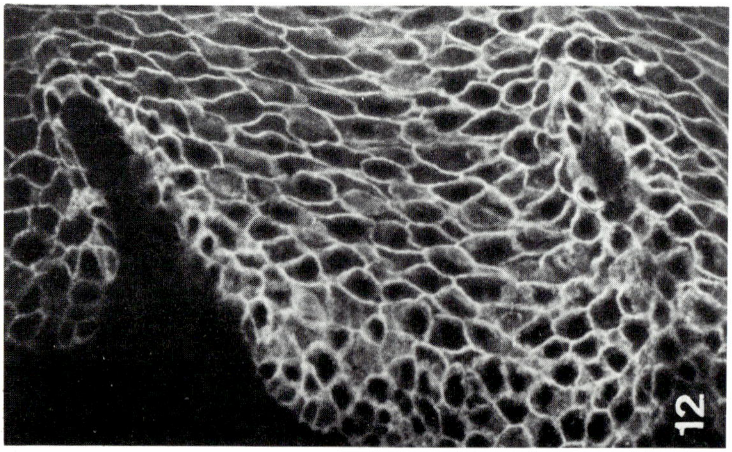
12

11.5.7. Autoimmune skin diseases

Only those instances which are primarily manifested in the skin and external mucosa will be considered under this heading, excluding generalized autoimmune diseases with skin involvement, such as SLE. The main candidates thus are pemphigus vulgaris, bullous pemphigoid (including cicatricial pemphigoid) and dermatitis herpetiformis [8]. Autoantibodies in patients with *pemphigus vulgaris* are directed against the intercellular substance of epithelial cells (prickle cell layer) and those with *bullous pemphigoid* against components on the basement membrane of squamous epithelia (Figs 11.12 and 11.13). In both instances the autoantibodies are not species-specific, but show a limited tissue specificity; they do, e.g., not react with the intercellular substance of columnar epithelia or the basement membrane of lung and kidney, respectively. In both instances the antibodies are of the IgG class and fix complement. IgA and IgM autoantibodies of this kind have been described in rare instances at low titers. Also, autoantibodies can be demonstrated in the blister fluid and bound to the above-mentioned structures in sections of biopsies from involved skin (not yet showing blisters) in vivo. For the visualization of in vivo bound Ig deposits and complement in direct immunofluorescence, frozen sections of biopsies can be used either unfixed or fixed. For fixation, various possibilities exist, such as equal parts of 96% ethanol and ether for 15 min at room temperature, absolute ethanol for 15 min at room temperature or 4% acetic in 96% ethanol for 15 min at –20°C. With appropriate conjugates both Ig (IgG, IgA, IgM) and complement (C3) can be demonstrated in these sections.

For *indirect immunofluorescence* tests we usually use guinea pig lip or human gingiva (which can be obtained easily from dental surgery departments). In addition to the easy availability and low background staining, guinea pig lip has the advantage of providing both epidermis and oral mucosa for evaluation. This is important since different parts of the same tissue have been found to afford different titers of autoantibodies on the same preparations [60]. Monkey skin and monkey esophagus can also be successfully used for the demonstration of these antibodies. Although acetone fixation is sometimes

---

Fig. 11.12. Indirect immunofluorescence test on a frozen, unfixed section of guinea pig lip treated with the serum from a patient with pemphigus vulgaris. Staining of the intracellular space of the mucosal epithelium. Original ×250.

Fig. 11.13. Indirect immunofluorescence test on a frozen, unfixed section of guinea pig lip treated with the serum from a patient with bullous pemphigoid. Bright staining of the epithelial basement membrane zone. Original ×250.

Fig. 11.14. Direct immunofluorescence test on a frozen, methanol-fixed section from a biopsy of lesioned skin from a patient with dermatitis herpetiformis demonstrating subepithelial granular IgA-positive staining. Original ×250. (Kindly provided by Dr. K. Holubar, Vienna.)

recommended for indirect immunofluorescence tests, we rather prefer unfixed tissue as antigenic substrate. Sera should not be tested in dilutions less than 1 : 10.

In *dermatitis herpetiformis* granular deposits of IgA (Fig. 11.14) and – less frequently IgG – and complement (C3), but not earlier components of the classical pathway (C1, C4, C2) have been shown at the dermal–epidermal junction in biopsies of lesioned skin. No skin-reactive autoantibodies can be found in the sera of patients with dermatitis herpetiformis. A close association exists between dermatitis herpetiformis and gluten-sensitive enteropathy (adult coeliac disease). Approximately 20% of patients with dermatitis herpetiformis show circulating antibodies to wheat proteins (gluten) and – interestingly – to reticulin fibers. The significance of these latter two kinds of antibodies in the natural history of dermatitis herpetiformis still remains to be clarified. The demonstration of reticulin autoantibodies will be dealt with later in this chapter.

11.5.8. Myasthenia gravis

Clinical and experimental observations lend credence to an important role of autoantibodies to striated muscle cell antigens and acetylcholine receptors in myasthenia gravis. We have recently reviewed some of this evidence, such as the pathology of the neuromuscular lesion, the presence of thymic changes, the good correlation between high titers of anti-muscular autoantibodies and low complement levels with disease activity, and the presence of other autoantibodies, notably to adrenal and thyroid components as well as gastric parietal cells [3]. On the other hand, destruction of muscular or nervous tissue on the basis of other causes does not lead to myasthenia-like symptoms.

Indirect immunofluorescence has become instrumental for the diagnosis of myasthenia gravis. Screening for autoantibodies to antigens of striated muscle is performed on unfixed, frozen sections of human or rat muscle (e.g. rat diaphragm) and the actual appearance of a positive immunofluorescence test is depicted in Fig. 11.15.

The myoid cells on frozen sections of thymus from mammals or even lower vertebrates can also be used as apt substrates for the evaluation of these autoantibodies. The relevant antigens are situated in the I-band of the sarcomere and often antibodies are also present which bind to the A-I junction. Among possible non-specific and undesired specific staining which may interfere with the classical staining pattern are the presence of heterophile antibodies and the binding of IgG to Fc receptors of the I-bands. The use of single glycerinated fibers of striated muscle has also been recommended for the demonstration of these antibodies. Our own experience with this preparation is limited, since we do not find it superior to the use of frozen muscle sections. The preparation of glycerinated fibers does, however, not require a microtome.

Autoantibodies to striated muscle are generally of the IgG class and occur in about 40% of all myasthenia gravis patients; in patients with myasthenia gravis and concomitant thymoma this percentage amounts to 90–100%, in cases with thymoma without myasthenia gravis this figure is 25%.

Autoantibodies to acetylcholine receptors are of proven and crucial clinical importance. They are also IgG antibodies, fix complement and lead to blockade and finally destruction of the motoric endplate resulting in muscular weakness. These antibodies are usually demonstrated by competitive radioimmunoassays where the antigen is solubilized from the electric organ of fish, such as the electric eel or torpedo. An inhibition of 10–20% binding by the patient's serum is considered significant. However, a snake venom, α-bungartoxin (α-BT), also binds to acetylcholine receptors, and radiolabelled α-BT is therefore now routinely used as a tracer in radioimmunoassays for acetylcholine receptor autoantibodies.

Up to 70% of myasthenia gravis patients have been described in various reports to possess such acetylcholine receptor autoantibodies. Recently, a sensitive immunofluorescence test has been described for the visualization of motoric endplates [49]. The principal process consists in treating frozen unfixed sections of a striated muscle with a patient's serum suspected to contain acetylcholine receptor autoantibodies and a FITC anti-human Ig conjugate, followed by α-BT and a TRITC anti-α-BT conjugate. Inhibition of the red fluorescence by the patients' serum indicates the presence of antibodies competing for α-BT binding sites. Fig. 11.16 is an example of the demonstration of the binding of α-BT to acetylcholine receptors as visualized by fluorescent α-BT (see also front page of Nature 292/No. 5826, 1981).

11.5.9. Postcardiotomy and postmyocarditis syndrome

The heart can both be a non-specific target for immunological reactions manifested, e.g. by the deposition of antibodies to streptococcal antigens cross-reactive with antigenic components of this organ [30] and represent the site for triggering specific autoantibodies after traumatic lesions, such as following surgical operations (postcardiotomy syndrome), heart infarctions, inflammatory processes (postmyocarditis syndrome). Such antibodies can be demonstrated by different serological procedures, but most conveniently by indirect immunofluorescence on human or rat heart sections [31]. Taking advantage of lower background we prefer frozen, unfixed sections of rat heart for these tests (Fig. 11.17). A high percentage of the sera of such patients display strong granular staining of cardiac myofibrils with high titers shortly (from 1 to 2 weeks to 1–2 months) after the disabling event and these eventually later subside. The percentages of positive sera amount to 70–90% in patients with cardiotomy to about 50% after myocardial infarction. Although the nature and clinical relevance of these autoantibodies are still not elucidated, their presence may be of diagnostic value, especially since they are not absorbed out by streptococci, in contrast to the above-mentioned situation in rheumatoid

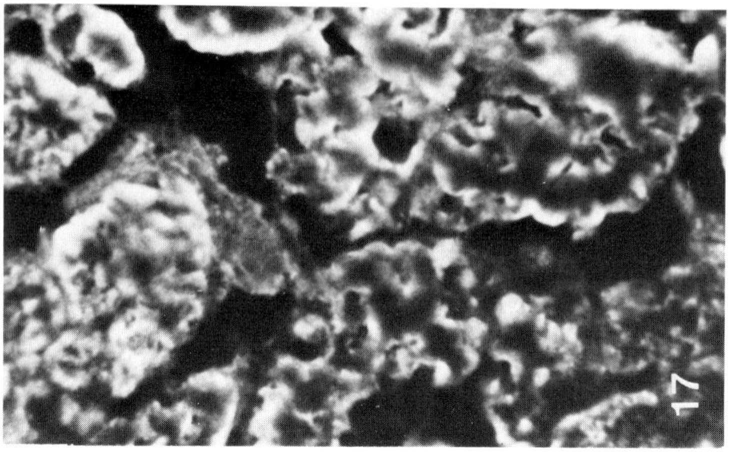
17

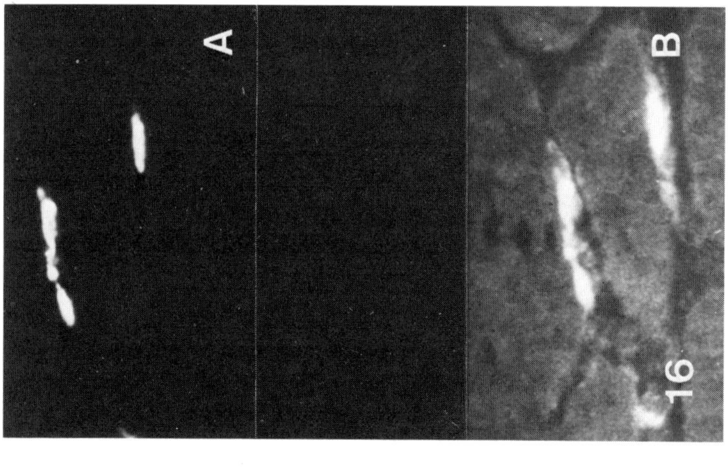
A
B
16

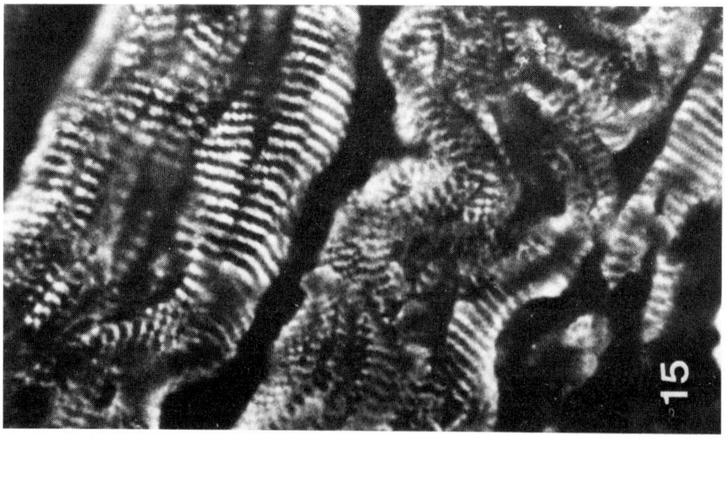
15

fever. Heart autoantibodies have also been observed after mild, unnoticed cardiac lesions and do not persist in quiescent intervals, e.g. between heart attacks. They also react with striated, but not with smooth muscle. Interestingly, autoantibodies to cardiac conducting tissue can also be demonstrated by indirect immunofluorescence in the sera of about 9% of patients with idiopathic heart block. Ox heart false tendons were used as antigenic substrate in these tests [23].

11.5.10. Idiopathic thrombocytopenic purpura (ITP)

As mentioned at the beginning of this chapter, I intend to deal only with those conditions where immunofluorescence is a routinely used and often indispensable diagnostic tool. ITP is a disease where autoantibodies to platelets can be demonstrated by variety of techniques, immunofluorescence being rather seldomly used. Appropriately equipped for immunofluorescence techniques we have, however, found this method to be the most useful and easy to perform. Direct immunofluorescence using the patient's own antibody-coated platelets and a conjugate to total human Ig gives about 60% positive results. This percentage can still be increased by employing the more sensitive indirect techniques where normal thrombocytes are first incubated with the patient's serum followed by an anti-rabbit Ig conjugate as the second layer. Anti-platelet antibodies can also be demonstrated using normal blood group O platelets, incubated with various dilutions of the patients' sera and normal controls (e.g. 1 : 10 and 1 : 100 for screening purposes) followed by the appropriate conjugate as mentioned above. The incidence of autoantibodies demonstrated by immunofluorescence in the sera of patients' with ITP comes to about 80 – 90% using the indirect method. For all these tests two requirements have to be exactly evaluated: a) an optimal platelet preparation, and b) the use of specific conjugates in subagglutinating dilutions.

As for the first point we now always use the method described in detail by Rossi [45]. The suspension is adjusted to a cell concentration of 3×10^8/ml and the test performed in siliconized tubes. To 0.1 ml of the suspension 0.1 ml of serum dilution is added, the mixture incubated for 90 min at room tempera-

---

Fig. 11.15. Indirect immunofluorescence test on a frozen, unfixed section of human striated muscle incubated with a serum from a patient with myasthenia gravis. Fluorescence of cross striations. Original ×250. (Reproduced from Albini and Wick [63] with kind permission of the publisher.)

Fig. 11.16. Double immunofluorescent staining of motoric endplate in frozen, unfixed section of human striated muscle using a FITC anti-human IgG conjugate (A) and TRITC-labelled α-bungarotoxin (B). Original ×500. (Kindly provided by T.E.W. Feltkamp, Amsterdam.)

Fig. 11.17. Indirect immunofluorescence test on frozen, unfixed section of rat heart treated with a serum from patients with postcardiotomy syndrome. Strong staining of cardiac muscle fibers. Original ×250.

ture with occasional gentle stirring. After three washings in buffer* the sediment is resuspended to 0.5 ml in appropriately diluted anti-human Ig conjugate and incubated for another 30 min. After three final washings the test must be read *immediately*, putting 25 μl drops of only one tube at a time on a slide under a cover slip. This is best done next to the immunofluorescence microscope.

The second point can be clarified by chessboard titrations using a known control serum and conjugate. This will also allow for a selection of a dilution including a safety margin which will make it applicable for a broad range of platelet autoantibodies. Agglutinates of platelets (and also other cells) always bear the risk of false-positive results because of the non-specific adherence of serum proteins to these. Singly lying cells also permit quantitation of platelet immunofluorescence by microfluorimetric methods [19].

Finally, we have recently also used indirect immunofluorescence to identify antibodies in patients with thrombocytopenia after treatment with heparin on glycosaminoglycan polysulfate (GAGPS) [69]. In this case we isolate blood group O normal platelets, adjust the concentration of the suspension to 3×10^8 ml, as mentioned above and incubate these with heparin or GAGPS (12.5 mg/ml, 1 I.U. $= 7.7 \times 10^{-3}$ mg) for 30 min at room temperature. The platelets are then washed three times in PBS and used for indirect immunofluorescence tests as outlined above. Using this technique it could be shown that a) patients with these conditions had antibodies to heparin or GAGPS-coated platelets, b) antibodies to heparin-coated platelets cross-react with GAGPS-treated cells and vice versa, and c) they cannot be absorbed out by either platelets alone or heparin and/or GAGPS alone and were thus directed against determinants formed by both the drug and the platelet surface or a cryptogenic platelet membrane structure not accessible on normal thrombocytes.

11.5.11. Goodpasture's syndrome

A detailed recollection of the role of immunofluorescence in the diagnosis of renal disease is given elsewhere in this volume. I will therefore only concentrate on Goodpasture's syndrome (GPS) which deserves special mention in view of advances made in this laboratory for the demonstration of autoantibodies to basement membranes of glomeruli and lung alveoli characteristic for this condition.

---

* Buffer consists of: 150 mM NaCl, 5 mM KCl, 5 mM glucose, in 5% sodium citrate solution (3.2 g/100 ml H_2O) and + 5 mg/ml BSA. This buffer is prepared immediately before use, heated to 35°C and adjusted to pH 6.5 with 0.1 N HCl.

GPS is the prototype of a renal disease developing on the basis of autoantibodies to glomerular basement membrane associated with pulmonary haemorrhage. Analyses of renal and pulmonary biopsies of such patients show linear, smooth fluorescence of the glomerular (Fig. 11.18) and alveolar basement membranes, respectively, in direct immunofluorescence using conjugates reacting with IgG or C3; the exact nature of the basement membrane antigen(s) which are the targets of these autoantibodies is not yet known. They must, however, be specific for renal glomerular and tubular as well as lung alveolar basement membranes, since sera from GPS patients do not react with basement membranes in other tissues, such as skin. The identification of these antigens would not only be of theoretical interest, but also bear practical relevance, since the now widely used procedure of plasmapheresis could be combined with selective depletion of basement membrane autoantibodies from the serum of patients by affinity chromatography.

Basement membranes have been known for some time to consist mainly of collagenous and non-collagenous glycoproteins. The progress made in this area has been reviewed in detail recently [52]. While the isolation of various basement membrane components has been rather tedious and technically difficult in the past (using renal glomerular preparations, basement membrane of the cornea or amniotic membranes), we have used a transplantable basement membrane-producing mouse tumour (the EHS sarcoma) for the isolation and characterization of these materials, especially an almost unaltered form of type IV collagen [54] and a non-collagenous glycoprotein named laminin [40]. In addition, we were left with a remaining mixture of non-collagenous basement membrane specific glycoproteins which still need further discrimination [65]. Rabbit antibodies to type IV collagen react with all basement membranes of a variety of tissues in mouse, man and other species (Figs. 11.19 and 11.20). We then used frozen sections of the EHS tumour as antigenic substrate for indirect immunofluorescence tests of sera from patients with GPS and bullous pemphigoid. Surprisingly, GPS sera strongly reacted with the basement membrane matrix on tumor sections (Fig. 11.21), while sera from bullous pemphigoid remained negative [66]. After examination of a great number of sera from patients with GPS we now always include sections of the EHS tumor in addition to the conventional tissues, i.e. lung and kidney, when testing for basement membrane autoantibodies. So far, no discrepancy has been observed with these two types of antigenic substrates. Further attempts to identify the antigen(s) reacting with antibodies in the sera of patients with GPS included radioimmunoassays with type IV collagen and laminin. As expected, none of these proved to be the target for these antibodies. The antigen(s) in question will rather be found among the glycoproteins in the above-mentioned still undefined mixture of non-collagenous material [61].

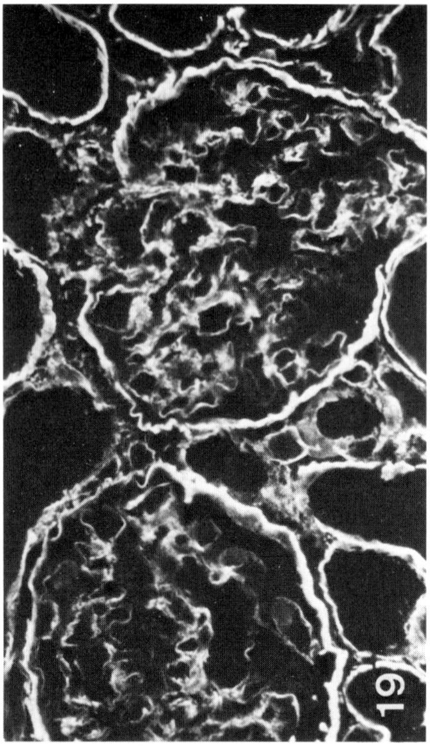
19

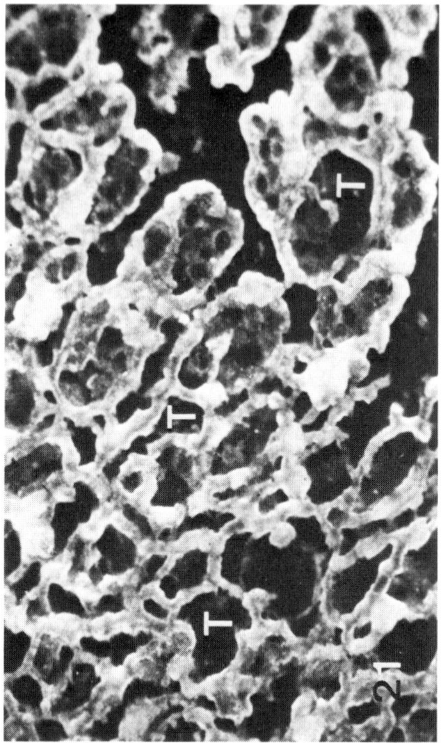
T
T
T
21

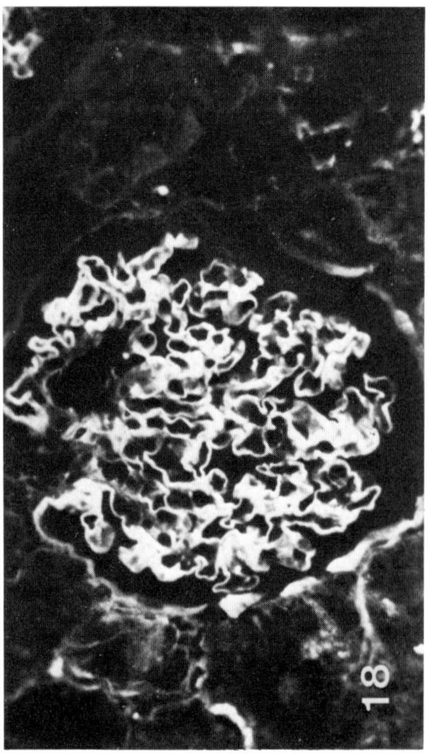
18

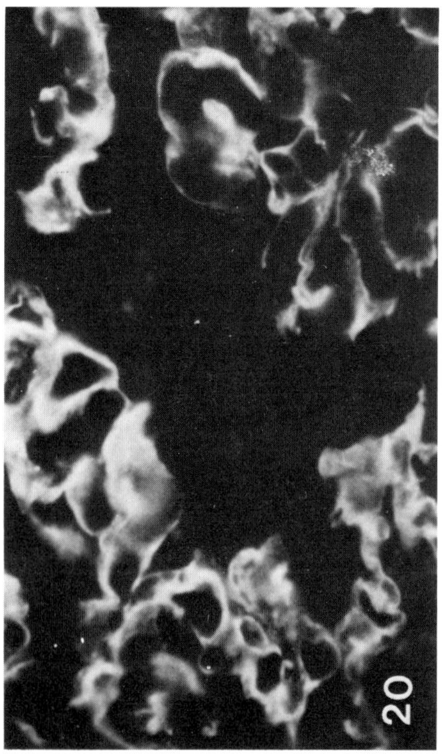
20

11.5.12. Reticulin autoantibodies

This type of non-organ-specific autoantibodies occurs in the sera of patients with different autoimmune diseases and can essentially be demonstrated on any tissue. Rat liver is, however, chosen most frequently for this purpose. Similar to what has been mentioned for basement membranes, reticulin fibers consist of type III collagen and non-collagenous constituents. Anti-reticulin autoantibodies can be found in approximately 40% of patients with adult coeliac disease and 60% of childhood coeliac disease, 28% of patients with dermatitis herpetiformis and 25% of patients with Crohn's disease. In sera of normal patients reticulin autoantibodies occur only very rarely (approximately 1%).

Similar to the situation in GPS the reticular components representing the antigen(s) reacting with reticulin autoantibodies in patients with coeliac disease are not yet exactly identified. We have put forward evidence that type III collagen is *not* the antigen in question, but that it should rather be sought in the reticulin-specific non-collagenous fraction of glycoproteins [53], thus supporting earlier data by Pras and Glynn [37]. The pathological role of reticulin autoantibodies in the disease is not yet clear, nor is the significance of the various staining patterns summarized by Rizzetto and Doniach [42]. Some of the latter are exemplified in Fig. 11.22A–D.

11.5.13. Sjögren's syndrome

Sjögren's syndrome is principally characterized by a triad consisting of keratoconjunctivitis sicca, xerostomia and rheumatoid arthritis. It has become evident, however, that this is a complex disease occurring in several variants which will not be detailed here [33]. For the diagnosis of Sjögren's syndrome immunofluorescence is an important laboratory tool. The most characteristic organ-specific feature is the occurrence of autoantibodies to salivary gland

---

Fig. 11.18. Direct immunofluorescence test on a 6 μm thick paraffin section of a formaldehyde-fixed renal biopsy from a patient with GPS. Before application of the FITC anti-IgG the section was treated with pronase as described in Chapter 13 of this volume. Smooth linear staining of the glomerular basement membrane and interrupted linear fluorescence of tubular basement membrane. Original ×250.

Figs. 11.19 and 11.20. Indirect immunofluorescence tests on frozen, unfixed sections of human kidney (19) and lung (20) treated with purified rabbit antibodies to murine type IV collagen. Note linear fluorescence of *all* basement membranes including the glomerular and alveolar basement membranes. Originals ×250.

Fig. 11.21. Indirect immunofluorescence test on a frozen, unfixed section of the basement membrane producing EHS mouse sarcoma treated with the serum from a patient with GPS. Note strong fluorescence of broad bands of basement membrane matrix material. The tumor cells themselves (T) appear unstained. Original ×250.

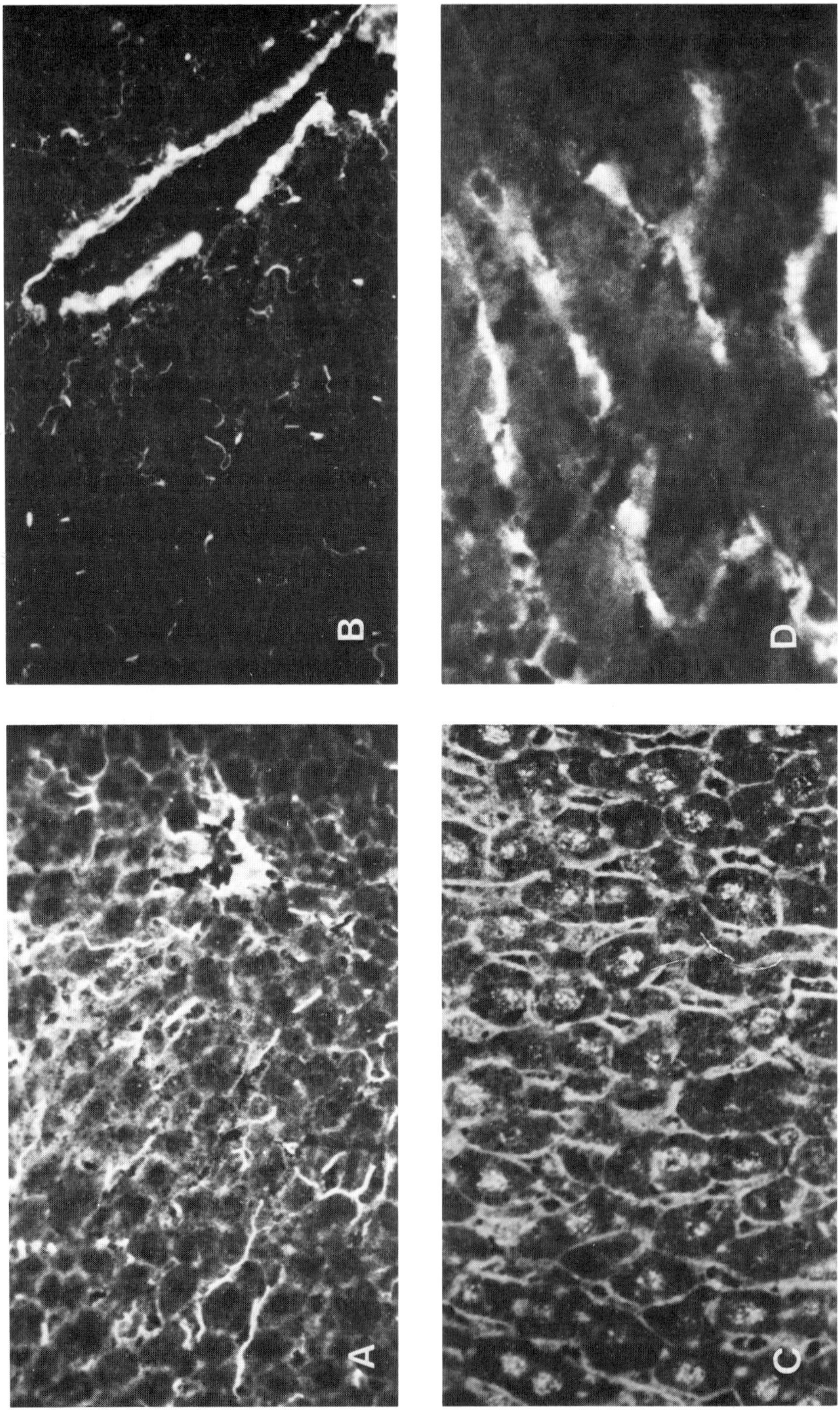
A
B
C
D

excretory ducts [7]. For this purpose, frozen, unfixed sections of human blood group O salivary gland tissue (most conveniently obtained as normal portions of the tissue in surgical material from patients with tumors of the parotid gland) are used. As the blood group of the donor of a tissue used as an antigenic substrate is crucial in the case of an excretory gland the provision of this material may meet with great difficulties in many instances. Monkey salivary glands are equally well suited and may be obtained commercially (e.g. from Pel-Freez Biologicals, Rogers, AR), and thus obviate the necessity to wait for appropriate human tissue. Fig. 11.23 exemplifies the characteristic staining pattern on parotid excretory ducts.

Antinuclear antibodies are found in patients with Sjögren's syndrome with high frequency, the homogenous pattern appearing most consistently. However, cases with ring-like, speckled and nucleolar patterns have also been described. Antibodies to native DNA are not present in most instances. In addition, several types of overlapping autoantibodies have been found in this disease, notably thyroglobulin antibodies. Since Sjögren's syndrome is observed mainly in females over 40 years of age, the latter finding is of questionable significance in the light of the known high incidence of various autoantibodies in women of this age group (Table 11.VI).

TABLE 11.VI.

INCIDENCE OF ANA, ANTI-SALIVARY DUCT ANTIBODIES AND Tg-AUTOANTIBODIES IN SICCA SYNDROME WITH AND WITHOUT RHEUMATOID ARTHRITIS

SS, Sjögren's syndrome; RA, rheumatoid arthritis; ANA, antinuclear autoantibodies; Tg-AAbs, thyroglobulin autoantibodies. (Data from ref. 71).

Specificity	SS with RA (% positive cases)	Sicca syndrome alone (% positive cases)
ANA	56	88
Antisalivary duct-AAbs	65	16
Tg-AAbs	33	38

Fig. 11.22. Various types of anti-reticulin autoantibodies demonstrated in indirect immunofluorescence tests on frozen, unfixed sections of rat liver. A) Staining pattern obtained with serum containing antibodies reacting with structures lining the hepatic sinusoids, but not the intrasinusoidal reticuloendothelial cells. B) Interrupted pattern of reticulin staining and fluorescence of the endothelium of a central vein. C) Fine reticular continuous network with concomitant occurrence of antinuclear antibodies giving a speckled staining pattern. D) Reaction with reticuloendothelial cells. A,B) originals ×250; C) original ×300; and D) original ×500.

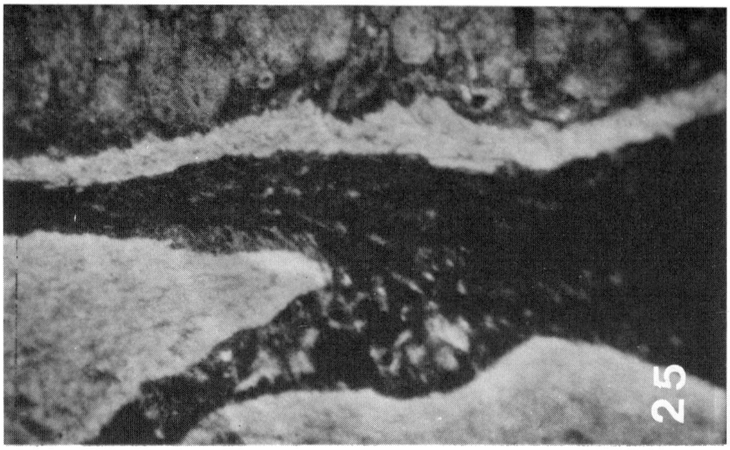
25

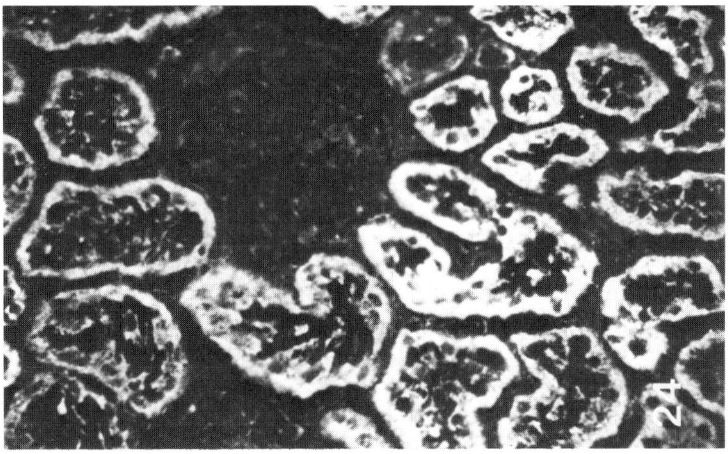
24

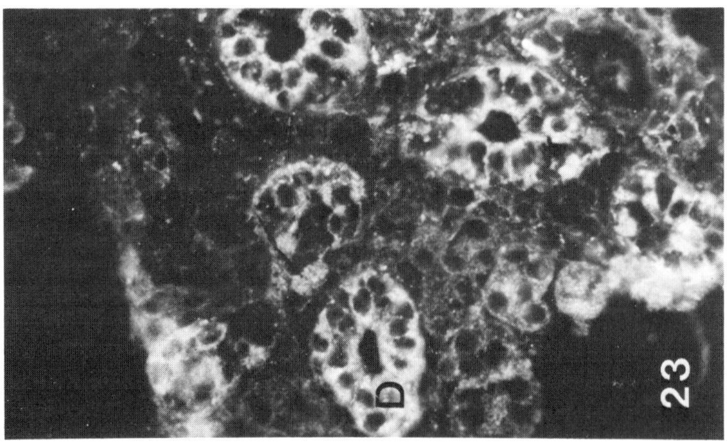
D
23

11.5.14. Liver diseases with autoimmune characteristics

Two forms of liver diseases are mainly associated with autoimmune features: primary biliary cirrhosis and chronic aggressive hepatitis (so-called lupoid hepatitis). In all these instances, the non-organ specific autoantibodies occurring in the circulation of these patients have so far been considered rather a sequel than causative to the disease.

Primary biliary cirrhosis (PBC) is a progressive disease that first occurs mainly in young women. High titers of non-organ specific anti-mitochondrial autoantibodies (AMA) are pathognomonic for PBC [58], but titers may vary from ten to several thousand. These antibodies are of all Ig classes (IgG, IgA, IgM) and bind complement. They are directed against antigens of the inner membrane of mitochondria which are lipoproteins and can be demonstrated on sections of unfixed tissue. A recent report, however, also claims preservation of mitochondrial antigens in fixed and paraffin-embedded tissue [39]. In addition, about a quarter of all patients with chronic aggressive hepatitis and cryptogenic cirrhosis possess such antibodies. In all these instances, there is no clear-cut correlation between the presence and titer of AMA and the severity and activity of the disease. Since AMA cannot be found in the sera of patients with extrahepatic obstructive jaundice, viral hepatitis and drug-induced or alcohol-dependent liver damage, their determination is of great differential diagnostic value. Furthermore, only about 1% of "normal" individuals show AMA and these only in low titer.

As an antigenic substrate for AMA any tissue can be used, but rat kidney has proven to be the best source. Patients' control sera are first diluted 1 : 10 for screening purposes. In indirect immunofluorescence tests on 4 μm thick *unfixed* frozen sections, a granular staining is observed in the entire cytoplasm of proximal tubular cells (Fig. 11.24). Care should therefore be taken to section rat kidney in its whole thickness in order to be sure to include those inner cortical areas rich in proximal tubular structures. This pattern has been distinguished from several others with similar reactivity, such as anti-ribosomal antibodies reactive with liver and kidney and the cardiolipin antibodies found in secondary syphilis. The former are found in rare instances in various liver disorders, including some cases of chronic aggressive hepatitis,

---

Fig. 11.23. Indirect immunofluorescence test on unfixed, frozen section of monkey parotid gland treated with the serum from a patient with Sjögren's syndrome. Cytoplasmic fluorescence of excretory ducts (D). Original ×250.

Fig. 11.24. Indirect immunofluorescence test on a frozen, unfixed section of rat kidney treated with the serum of a patient with primary biliary cirrhosis. Strong cytoplasmic staining of proximal tubular epithelial cells. Original ×250.

Fig. 11.25. Indirect immunofluorescence test on a frozen, unfixed section of rat stomach treated with the serum of a patient with chronic aggressive hepatitis. Staining of smooth muscle layers. Original ×250.

drug-induced and viral hepatitis. They are not directed against ribosomal RNA, but rather against determinants in the microsomal membranes. The staining pattern is finer as compared to the coarse mitochondrial staining. The cardiolipin antibodies on the other hand can be absorbed out with cardiolipin antigens.

In addition to AMA antibodies to bile duct, epithelia can be found in 80–90% of the sera of patients with chronic aggressive hepatitis, and antibodies to bile canaliculi occur in about 70% of these cases.

Chronic aggressive hepatitis (or active chronic hepatitis) is also mainly afflicting young women; it is often associated with antinuclear factors and is then called "lupoid hepatitis". Anti-smooth muscle autoantibodies (SMA) are found in about 50% of these patients [29] and are mostly directed against actin and myosin. They are of the IgG and IgM classes and do not fix complement. 90% of sera from patients with lupoid hepatitis also show SMA. However, SLE patients lack these antibodies. SMA also appear in over 80% of patients with infectious hepatitis and infectious mononucleosis, the latter mainly being of the IgM class. Furthermore, a high incidence of SMA has been reported in patients with malignancies. Low titer antibodies of this type can be found in only 2% of apparently normal individuals.

As SMA are again tissue-specific, but not organ- or species-specific, various tissues from different species can be used as antigenic substrate. Preferentially, unfixed frozen sections of human uterus blood group O, rat stomach or even mussel are employed. Patients' sera are tested in dilutions of 1 : 10 and above. Fig. 11.25 shows the characteristic staining pattern obtained with SMA on the longitudinal and circular smooth muscle layers of rat stomach. Often the first hint of the presence of SMA in patients' sera tested for other reasons is fluorescence of smooth muscle in vessel walls. Table 11.VII summarizes the occurrence and a clinical significance of autoantibodies in liver disease.

TABLE 11.VII

NON-ORGAN SPECIFIC AUTOANTIBODIES IN LIVER DISEASES

Antibody	Primary biliary cirrhosis	Chronic aggressive hepatitis	Drug-induced liver disease	Viral hepatitis	Extra hepatic biliary obstruction
ANA	< 50%	> 50%	n.o.[a]	n.o.	n.o.
AMA	> 50%	< 50%	> 50%[b]	n.o.	n.o.
SMA	< 50%	> 50%	n.o.	< 50%	n.o.

[a] n.o., not observed.

[b] Halothane-induced hepatitis.

11.5.15. Collagen diseases

The main, but not the only hallmark of this group of diseases is the occurrence of antinuclear antibodies (ANA). Among these one can now differentiate antibodies with different specificities and most of these can be demonstrated by immunofluorescence methods.

1. Autoantibodies to native, double-stranded DNA, the specificity of which is determined by the structural arrangement of the double helical DNA molecule.

2. Autoantibodies to native single-stranded DNA which are directed against antigenic determinants of the deoxyribose, purines and pyrimidines.

3. Autoantibodies to single-stranded DNA directed against purines and pyrimidines.

4. Autoantibodies to basic nuclear protein (histones).

5. Autoantibodies to a histone–DNA complex (= soluble nucleoprotein, sNP).

6. Autoantibodies to acidic nuclear proteins: Sm antigen, a glycoprotein; ribonucleoprotein antigen (RNP), a complex of nuclear RNA and protein.

7. Autoantibodies to nucleolar RNA.

ANA can be demonstrated by many different methods such as precipitation, agglutination, complement fixation or labelled antibody techniques, such as radioimmunoassays, immunofluorescence and enzyme-labelled antibody procedures. Of these immunofluorescence enjoys the highest degree of practicability in most laboratories. Since ANA are again neither organ- nor species-specific, all nuclei-containing tissues of different species can be taken as antigenic substrate for indirect immunofluorescence tests. Frozen sections of rat liver are used by most laboratories. Acetone fixation must be used in order to avoid dissolution of water-soluble nuclear antigens, such as Sm. No major diagnostic importance should be given to ANA titers below 1 : 10, especially in older persons who are known to have a significantly elevated incidence of autoantibodies in general. The different patterns of the nuclear fluorescence depicted in Fig. 11.26A–D to a certain extent may reflect the specificity of the various types of ANA [15, 50].

Membraneous or peripheral: antibodies to DNA.

Homogenous: different nuclear proteins.

Speckled: Sm antigen and acidic nucleoproteins.

Shaggy: Sm (not shown).

Nucleolar: RNA.

Table 11.VIII shows the association of the various ANA patterns with the collagen diseases. The approximate percentages of ANA in the various diseases are given in Table 11.IX. The incidence of nucleolar autoantibodies is listed for various diseases in Table 11.X. While tissue sections, such as rat liver, afford all of the above-mentioned reactions, some of the other antigenic substrates are good for initial screening purposes but not for final titration and detection of staining patterns. Among the latter are chicken erythrocyte

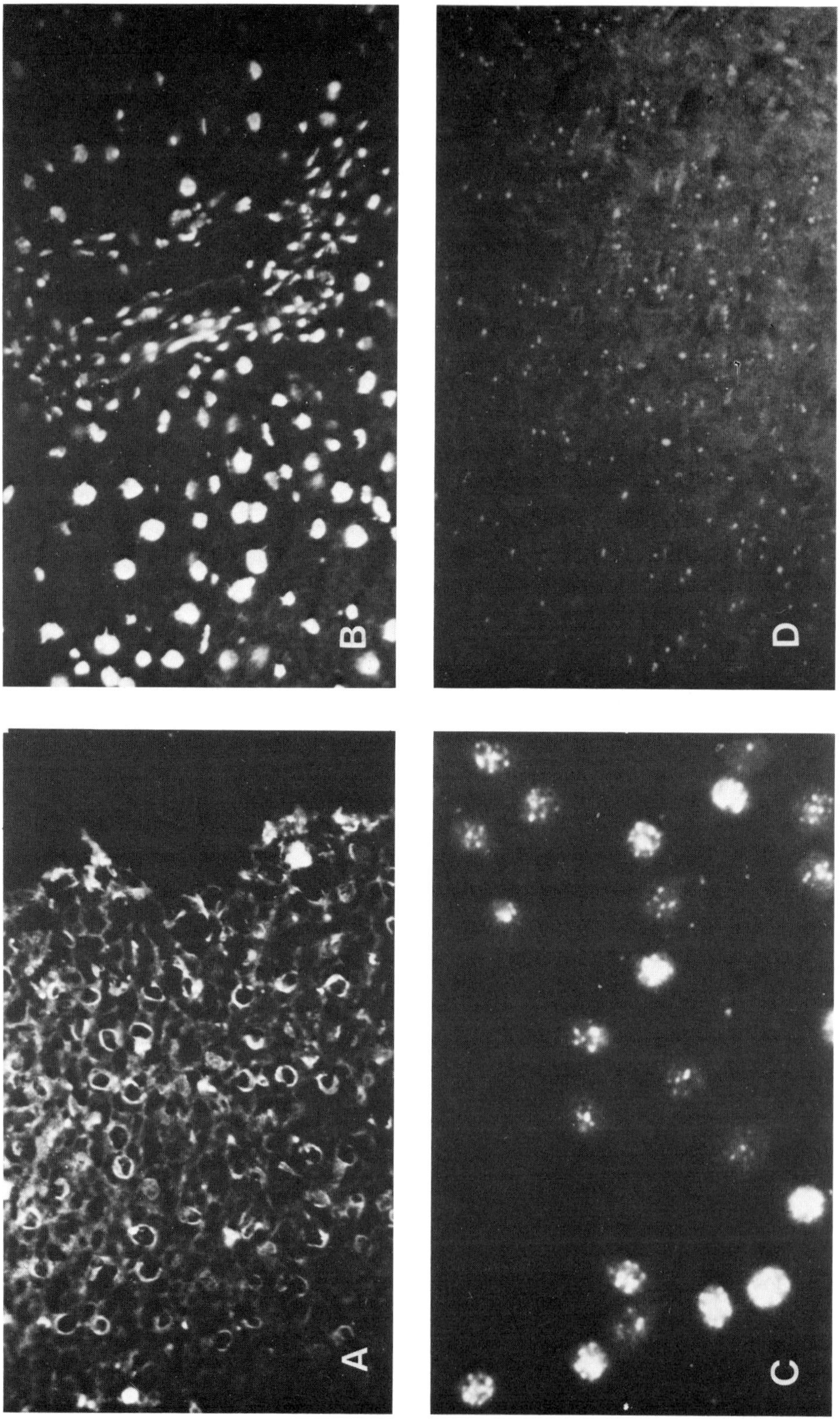
B
D
A
C

TABLE 11.VIII

ANA STAINING PATTERNS IN COLLAGEN DISEASES

ANA staining pattern	Disease association
Homogeneous	
high titer	SLE
low titer	Rheumatoid arthritis and other diseases mentioned above
Peripheral	SLE
Speckled	Scleroderma Sjögren's syndrome Raynaud's syndrome Mixed connective tissue disease (Sharp syndrome) SLE
Nucleolar	Scleroderma
Shaggy	SLE

TABLE 11.IX

INCIDENCE OF ANA IN VARIOUS DISEASES

Disease	% Incidence of ANA
SLE	~100
Sjögren's syndrome	70
Scleroderma	40
Rheumatoid arthritis	25
Mixed connective tissue disease	70

nuclei, tissue culture cells (e.g. baby hamster kidney cells, BHK) and human leucocytes. The use of human tissues harbours the risk of false-positive results due to blood group and isoantibody interference. Erythrocyte nuclei have the advantage of being antigenically stable for many months at room temperature. Their preparation, storage and use have been described in detail [2, 51]. Briefly, chicken red blood cells are lysed either by saponin or distilled water and subsequently stored in diluted formaldehyde.

Fig. 11.26. Different staining patterns obtained with antinuclear antibodies in indirect immunofluorescence tests on acetone fixed, frozen sections of rat liver (A, B, D) or formaldehyde-fixed chicken erythrocyte nuclei (C). Nuclear staining is peripheral (A), homogeneous (B), speckled (C) or nucleolar (D). The speckled fluorescence observed on chicken erythrocyte nuclei is a very rare finding, since this antigenic substrate – in contrast to tissue sections – generally does not allow the discrimination of different patterns. A, B and D) Original ×250; C) original ×400.

TABLE 11.X

INCIDENCE OF NUCLEOLAR AAbs IN VARIOUS DISEASES

Disease	% Incidence of nucleolar AAbs
SLE	25
Systemic sclerosis	50–60
Rheumatoid arthritis	10

A promising new development in this area is the so-called FIAX™ system which represents an instrumentation for semi-automated performance and computerized evaluation for ANA determinations and other immunofluorescence tests (IDT Europe, Division of Boehringer Ingelheim Diagnostica GmbH, F.R.G.). The principle of the FIAX system lies in the use of plastic sticks which carry at one end a round, flat area to which a non-fluorescent support is glued which is covered by a layer of BHK cells. For indirect immunofluorescence tests these sticks are immersed into appropriate dilutions of patients' sera and controls, diluted conjugates and washing buffer. Finally, the fluorescence is evaluated by inserting these sticks into an especially designed fluorometer which is linked to a minicomputer that calculates the titers on the basis of a standard curve constructed from values obtained with standard sera included in every single test kit. The FIAX system is also available for other purposes and may be adapted to a variety of other autoantibody determinations, such as immune complex analyses, etc.

The lack of ANA practically rules out the diagnosis of SLE. Also ANA titers are usually higher in patients with SLE, although a low titer can occasionally be observed. In any case, additional tests are required for confirmation or exclusion of the diagnosis. Some of these consist in the differentiation of the specificity of ANA.

Antibodies to DNA are indicative of SLE; while most other autoantibodies are only of diagnostic value the antibodies to DNA are those which form immune complexes and thus they are responsible for the clinical symptoms of SLE due to the immune complex deposition in kidneys, in skin, choroid plexus, etc. Furthermore, antibodies to the Sm antigens are observed in about one-third of SLE patients and only very rarely in other diseases of this group. RNP antibodies, on the other hand, are a characteristic feature of mixed connective tissue disease (MCTD, Sharp syndrome) in very high titers (>2000–4000), and present in lower frequency and lower titers in SLE. Finally, the assessment of fluorescence patterns is useful for the differentiation of a drug-induced lupus-like syndrome which usually lacks Sm and RNP autoantibodies.

In order to be able to properly assess the nuclear staining patterns, sera found positive in screening tests have to be titrated, since certain types of reactivity may be obscured, e.g. by strong homogeneous fluorescence in high serum concentrations. Antibodies to nDNA are most frequently determined by non-immunofluorescence methods, such as the Farr technique. However, the use of a hemoflagellate, *Crithidia luciliae,* has proven to give results which are in good agreement with these other methods [1]. *Crithidia* organisms have a kinetoplast (i.e. an organelle – a mitochondrium – to which the flagellum is anchored) that consists of nDNA easily accessible to specific antibodies. Multiwell slides, coated with dried unfixed *Crithidia* can be obtained commercially and should be used unfixed in the same way as regular frozen sections. The appearance of the positive test of *C. luciliae* demonstrating antibodies to nDNA is shown in Fig. 11.27.

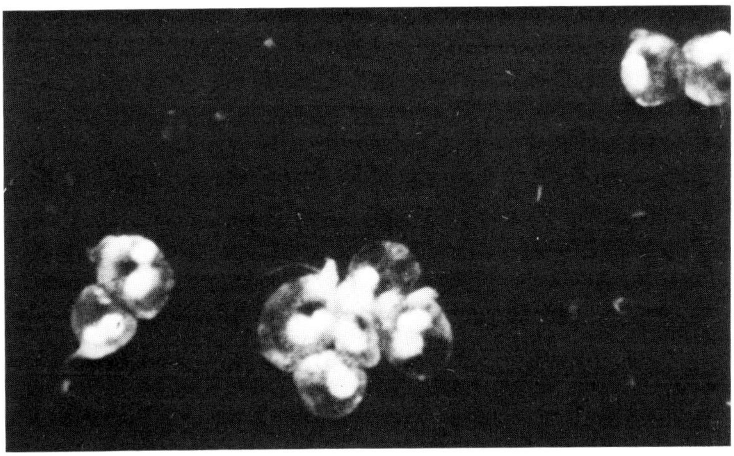

Fig. 11.27. Indirect immunofluorescence test on an airdried unfixed preparation of *Crithidia luciliae* treated with the serum from a patient containing antibodies to nDNA. The bright fluorescence of the kinetoplast is evident. Original ×500.

11.6. SUMMARY

In this chapter I have mainly discussed those diseases the diagnosis of which critically relies on immunofluorescence tests. There are, of course, many other instances which could not be mentioned in detail, such as autoantibodies to myelin, lymphocytotoxic autoantibodies, autoantibodies to the stratum corneum of skin, etc. In all of the above-mentioned instances and certainly in many more in the future, immunofluorescence has become an indispensable diagnostic tool.

ACKNOWLEDGEMENTS

Part of our own work cited in this chapter was supported by the Austrian Research Council (project No. 4114). I wish to thank Ms. Christa Oschinski for her help in performing immunofluorescence tests and Ms. Margit Geir for excellent secretarial work in preparing this manuscript. We acknowledge the permission by the publishers to reproduce Figs. 11.2, 11.3, 11.8, and 11.15 from the original papers cited in the legends.

REFERENCES

1 Aarden, L.A., De Groot, E.R. and Feltkamp, T.E.W. (1975) Immunology of DNA III. Crithidia luciliae, a simple substrate for the determination of anti-dsDNA with the immunofluorescence technique. Ann. N.Y. Acad. Sci. *254,* 505–515.

2 Albini, B. and Wick, G. (1972) Hühnererythrozytenkerne als Dauerpräparation für den Nachweis antinukleärer Faktoren im indirekten Immunfluoreszenztest. Wien. Klin. Wochenschr. *84,* 416–417.

3 Albini, B. and Wick, G. (1981) Myasthenia gravis. *In* Milgrom, F., Abeyounis, J.C. and Kano, K. (eds.), Principles of Immunodiagnosis in Medicine (Lea and Febiger, Philadelphia) pp. 372–374.

4 Alexander, N.J. and Anderson, D.J. (1978) Vasectomy: consequences of autoimmunity to sperm antigens. Fertil. Steril. *32,* 253–260.

5 Ansbacher, R. (1973) Vasectomy: sperm antibodies. Fertil. Steril. *24,* 788–792.

6 Bankhurst, A.D., Torrigiani, G. and Allison, A.C. (1973) Lymphocytes binding human thyroglobulin in healthy people and its relevance to tolerance for autoantigens. Lancet *1,* 226–230.

7 Bertram, K. and Halberg, P. (1964) A specific antibody against the epithelium of the salivary ducts in sera from patients with Sjögren's syndrome. Acta Allergol. *19,* 458–466.

8 Beutner, E.H., Chorzelski, T.P. and Bean, S.F. (eds.) 1978) Immunopathology of the Skin, 2nd ed. (John Wiley, New York–Chichester–Brisbane–Toronto).

9 Beutner, E.H., Jablonska, S., Chorzelski, T.P. and Binder, W.L. (1978) A unified concept of autoimmunity and the nature of stratum corneum antigen (SCAg) conversion phenomenon. *In* Milgrom, F. and Albini, B. (eds.), Immunopathology. 6th Int. Convocation on Immunology, Niagara Falls, NY (Karger, Basel) pp. 142–147.

10 Binz, H. and Wigzell, H. (1979) Induction of specific transplantation tolerance in adult animals. Transplant Proc. *11,* 914–918.

11 Blizzard, R.M., Chee, D. and Davis, W. (1966) The incidence of parathyroid and other antibodies in the sera of patients with idiopathic hypoparathyroidism. Clin. Exp. Immunol. *1,* 119–128.

12 Blizzard, R.M., Chee, D. and Davis, W. (1967) The incidence of adrenal and other antibodies in the sera of patients with idiopathic adrenal insufficiency. Clin. Exp. Immunol. *2,* 19–30.

13 Boyd, R. and Wick, G. (1980) Effector mechanisms in spontaneous autoimmune thyroiditis of Obese strain chickens. *In* Pinchera, A., Doniach, D., Fenzi, G.F. and Baschieri, L. (eds.), Serono Symposia, *Vol. 33.* Autoimmune Aspects of Endocrine Disorders (Academic Press, London–New York) pp. 199–206.

14 Burnet, F.M. (1959) The Clonal Selection Theory of Acquired Immunity (Vanderbilt University Press, Nashville).

15 Burnham, T.K. (1973) Antinuclear antibodies. II. The prognostic significance of nuclear immunofluorescent patterns in lupus erythematosus. Arch. Dermatol. *111,* 203–207.

16 Chiller, J.M., Habicht, G.S. and Weigle, W.O. (1970) Cellular sites of immunologic unresponsiveness. Proc. Natl. Acad. Sci. U.S.A. *65,* 551–556.
17 Clagett, J.H. and Weigle, W.O. (1974) Roles of T and B lymphocytes in the termination of unresponsiveness to autologous thyroglobulin in mice. J. Exp. Med. *139,* 643–660.
18 Dausset, J. and Svejgaard, A. (eds.) (1977) HLA and Disease (Munksgaard, Copenhagen).
19 Denk, H., Fischer, M., Pilgersdorfer, H.W. and Schnack, H. (1969) Immunfluoreszenzmikroskopie zur quantitativen Erfassung antithrombozytärer Autoantikörper. Thromb. Diath. Haemorrh. (Stuttgart) *21,* 387–396.
20 Doniach, D., Bottazzo, F.G. and Khoury, E.L. (1980) Prospects in human autoimmune thyroiditis. *In* Pinchera, A., Doniach, D., Fenzi, G.F. and Baschieri, L. (eds.) Serono Symposia. *Vol. 33.* Autoimmune Aspects of Endocrine Disorders (Academic Press, London–New York) pp. 25–38.
21 Ehrlich, P. and Morgenroth, I. (1900) Über Haemolysine. 3. Mitteilung. Berl. Klin. Wochenschr. *37,* 453–458.
22 Fagraeus, A. and Jonsson, J. (1970) Distribution of organ antigens over the surface of thyroid cells as examined by the immunofluorescence test. Immunology *18,* 413–416.
23 Fairfax, A. and Doniach, D. (1978) Autoantibodies to cardiac conducting tissue and their characterization by immunofluorescence. Clin. Exp. Immunol. *23,* 1–8.
24 Goodwin, J.S. and Williams, R.C. (1979) Suppressor cells – a recent conceptual epidemic. J. Clin. Lab. Immunol. *2,* 89–91.
25 Grabar, P. (1975) Hypothesis. Auto-antibodies and immunological theories: an analytical review. Clin. Immunol. Immunopathol. *4,* 453–466.
26 Irvine, W.I. and Scarth, L. (1969) Antibody to the oxyphil cells of the human parathyroid in idiopathic hypoparathyroidism. Clin. Exp. Immunol. *4,* 505–510.
27 Jablonska, S., Beutner, E.M., Binder, W.L., Jarzabek-Chorzelska, M., Rzésa, G. and Chowaniek, O. (1979) Immunopathology of psoriasis. Arch. Dermatol. Res. *264,* 65–71.
28 Jerne, N.K. (1974) Towards a network theory of the immune system. Ann. Immunol. (Paris) *125C,* 373–389.
29 Johnson, S.D., Holborow, E.S. and Glynn, L.E. (1965) Antibody to smooth muscle in patients with liver disease. Lancet *2,* 878–879.
30 Kaplan, M.H. and Frengley, J.D. (1969) Autoimmunity to the heart and in cardiac disease. Current topics of the relation of autoimmunity to rheumatic fever, postcardiotomy and postinfarction syndromes and cardiomyopathies. Am. J. Cardiol. *24,* 459–473.
31 Maisch, B., Berg, P.-A. and Kochsiek, K. (1979) Clinical significance of immunopathological findings in patients with post-pericardiotomy syndrome. Clin. Exp. Immunol. *38,* 189–197.
32 Milgrom, F. and Witebsky, E. (1962) Autoantibodies and autoimmune disease. J. Am. Med. Assoc. *181,* 706–716.
33 Moutsopoulos, H.M. (1980) Sjögren's syndrome (Sicca Syndrome). Current Issues. Ann. Intern. Med. *92,* 212–226.
34 Nairn, R.C. (1976) Fluorescent Protein Tracing, 4th ed. (Churchill Livingstone, Edinburgh–London–New York).
35 Nishiyama, R.H., Torretti, B., Martin, D.B., Pek, S.B., Keren, D.F. (1980) The detection of islet-cell antibodies by immunofluorescence in Bouin's fixed paraffin-embedded human pancreas. Lab. Invest. *43,* 191–195.
36 Petri, M. and Nerup, I. (1971) Addison's adrenalitis. Acta Pathol. Microbiol. Scand. Sect. A, Pathol. *79,* 381–388.
37 Pras, M. and Glynn, L.E. (1973) Isolation of a non-collagenous reticulin component and its primary characterization. Br. J. Exp. Pathol. *54,* 449–450.
38 Proffitt, M.R., Hirsch, M.S. and Black, P.H. (1977) Viruses, autoimmunity and murine lymphoma. *In* Talal, N. (ed.), Autoimmunity. Genetic, Immunologic, Virologic and Clinical Aspects (Academic Press, London–New York), pp. 385–401.
39 Rabin, B.S. and Nakamura, R.M. (1980) Improved method for detection of anti-tissue antibody by indirect immunofluorescence using fixed tissue. J. Clin. Lab. Immunol. *4,* 119–124.

40 Rhode, H., Wick, G. and Timpl, R. (1979) Immunochemical characterization of the basement membrane glycoprotein laminin. Eur. J. Biochem. *102,* 195–201.

41 Richter, E., Wick, G., Zambelis, N., Ludwig, H. and Schernthaner, G. (1978) Demonstration and characterization of thyroglobulin binding peripheral blood cells in Hashimoto patients by fluoroimmunocytoadherence (FICA). Clin. Immunol. Immunopathol. *11,* 178–189.

42 Rizzetto, M. and Doniach, D. (1973) Types of "reticulin" antibodies detected in human sera by immunofluorescence. J. Clin. Pathol. *26,* 841–851.

43 Roberts, I.M., Whittingham, S. and McKay, I.R. (1973) Tolerance to an autoantigen-thyroglobulin. Lancet *1,* 936–940.

44 Rose, N.R., Hjort, T., Rümke, P., Harper, M.J.K. and Vyazov, O. (1976) Techniques for detection of iso- and autoantibodies to human spermatozoa. Clin. Exp. Immunol. *23,* 175–199.

45 Rossi, E.C. (1972) The effect of albumin upon the losses of enzymes from washed platelets. J. Lab. Clin. Med. *79,* 240–246.

46 Rümke, P. and Hellinga, G. (1959) Autoantibodies to spermatozoa in sterile men. Am. J. Clin. Pathol. *32,* 357–361.

47 Sakane, T., Steinberg, A.D., Reeves, P.J. and Green, I. (1979) Studies of immune functions of patients with systemic lupus erythematosus. T-cell subsets and antibodies to T-cell subsets. J. Clin. Invest. *64,* 1260–1269.

48 Schumacher, G.F.B. (1979) Immunologic factors in infertility. Antibodies against spermatozoa. J. Reprod. Med. *23,* 272–278.

49 Sondag-Tschroots, I.R.J.M., Schulz-Raateland, R.C.M., Van Walbeek, H. K. and Feltkamp, T.E.W. (1979) Antibodies to motor endplates demonstrated with the immunofluorescence technique. Clin. Exp. Immunol. *37,* 323–327.

50 Tan, E.M., Northway, I.D. and Pinnas, J.L. (1973) The clinical significance of antinuclear antibodies. Postgrad. Med. *54,* 143–150.

51 Ten Veen, J.H. and Feltkamp, T.E.W. (1969) Formalinized chicken red cell nuclei as a simple antigen for standardized antinuclear factor determination. Clin. Exp. Immunol. *5,* 673–678.

52 Timpl, R. and Martin, G.R. (1981) Components of basement membrane. *In* Furthmayr, H. (ed.), Immunochemistry of the Extracellular Matrix II (CRC Press, Boca-Raton/Fa) pp. 1–59.

53 Timpl, R., Wick, G. and Granditsch, G. (1977) Reticular autoantibodies in childhood coeliac disease not directed against type III collagen. Clin. Exp. Immunol. *28,* 546–547.

54 Timpl, R., Martin, G.R., Bruckner, P., Wick, G. and Wiedemann, H. (1978) Nature of the collagenous proteins in a tumor basement membrane. Eur. J. Biochem. *84,* 43–52.

55 Torrigiani, G., Doniach, D. and Roitt, I.M. (1969) Serum thyroglobulin levels in healthy subjects and in patients with thyroid disease. J. Clin. Endocrinol. Metabol. *29,* 305–314.

56 Ungar, B., Stocks, A.E., Martin, F.I.R., Whittingham, S. and MacKay, I.R. (1968) Intrinsic-factor antibody, parietal-cell antibody, and latent pernicious anaemia in diabetes mellitus. Lancet *2,* 415–417.

57 Vladutiu, A. and Rose, N.R. (1971) Autoimmune murine thyroiditis: relation to histocompatibility (H-2) type. Science *174,* 1137–1139.

58 Walker, I.G., Doniach, D., Roitt, I.M. and Sherlock, S. (1965) Serological tests in diagnosis of primary biliary cirrhosis. Lancet *1,* 827–831.

59 Wekerle, H., Ketelsen, U.P. and Ernst, M. (1980) Thymic nurse cells. Lymphoepithelial cell complexes in murine thymuses: morphological and serological characterization. J. Exp. Med. *151,* 925–944.

60 Wick, G. and Beutner, E.H. (1968) Quantitative studies of immunofluorescent staining. III. Comparison of different antigens in an indirect immunofluorescent staining system for human IgG using basement zone antibodies of bullous pemphigoid. Immunology *16,* 149–156.

61 Wick, G. and Timpl, R. (1980) Study on the nature of the Goodpasture antigen using a basement membrane-producing mouse tumour. Clin. Exp. Immunol. *39,* 733–738.

62 Wick, G. and Albini, B. (1981) Adrenalitis, idiopathic hypoparathyroidism and diabetes mellitus. *In* Milgrom, F., Abeyounis, J.C. and Kano, K. (eds.), Principles of Immunodiagnosis in Medicine (Lea and Febiger, Philadelphia) pp. 359–365.

63 Wick, G., Sundick, R.S. and Albini, B. (1974) Review. The Obese strain (OS) of chickens. An animal model with spontaneous autoimmune thyroiditis. Clin. Immunol. Immunopathol. *3,* 272–300.
64 Wick, G., Baudner, S. and Herzog, F. (1978) Immunofluorescence, 2nd ed. (Die Medizinische Verlagsgesellschaft, Marburg/Lahn, F.R.G.).
65 Wick, G., Glanville, R.W. and Timpl, R. (1979) Characterization of antibodies to basement membrane (type IV) collagen in immunohistological studies. Immunobiology *156,* 372–381.
66 Wick, G., Müller, P.U., Timpl, R. and Martin, G.R. (1979) Studies on the immunology of basement membrane collagens using antibody to a tumor basement membrane. Front. Matrix Biol. *7,* 120–129.
67 Wick, G., Kofler, R., Gundolf, R., Müller, P.U. and Boyd, R. (1979) The nature of effector cells in experimental and spontaneous autoimmune thyroiditis. *In* Milgrom, F. and Albini, B. (eds.), Immunopathology. 6th Int. Convocation on Immunology, Niagara Falls, NY (Karger, Basel) pp. 101–109.
68 Wick, G., Boyd, R., Hála, K., De Carvalho, L., Kofler, R., Müller, P.U. and Cole, R.K. (1981). The Obese strain (OS) of chickens with spontaneous autoimmune thyroiditis. Review of recent data. Curr. Top. Microbiol. Immunol. *91,* 109–128.
69 Wolf, H., Nowack, H. and Wick, G. (1982) Detection of antibodies against glycosaminoglycan-polysulfate (GAGPS) in patients treated with heparin or other GAGPS. Submitted for publication.
70 Zinkernagel, R.M. and Doherty, P.C. (1977) Major transplantation antigens, virus and specificity or surveillance T cells. The altered "self hypothesis". Contemp. Top. Immunobiol. 7, 179–220.
71 Hardin, J.A. and Bloch, K.J. (1978) Sjögren's Syndrome. In Samter, M. (ed.), Immunological Diseases, Vol. II (Little, Brown & Co., Inc., Boston–New York) pp. 1151-1157.

Wick et al. (eds) Immunofluorescence Technology. Selected Theoretical and Clinical Aspects © Elsevier Biomedical Press, 1982

CHAPTER 12

Immunofluorescence in the diagnosis of glomerular and interstitial nephropathies

B. ALBINI,[1], D. KERJASCHKI[2] and B. NOBLE[1]

[1]Department of Microbiology, State University of New York, Buffalo, NY; and [2]Department of Cell Biology, Yale University, New Haven, CT, U.S.A.

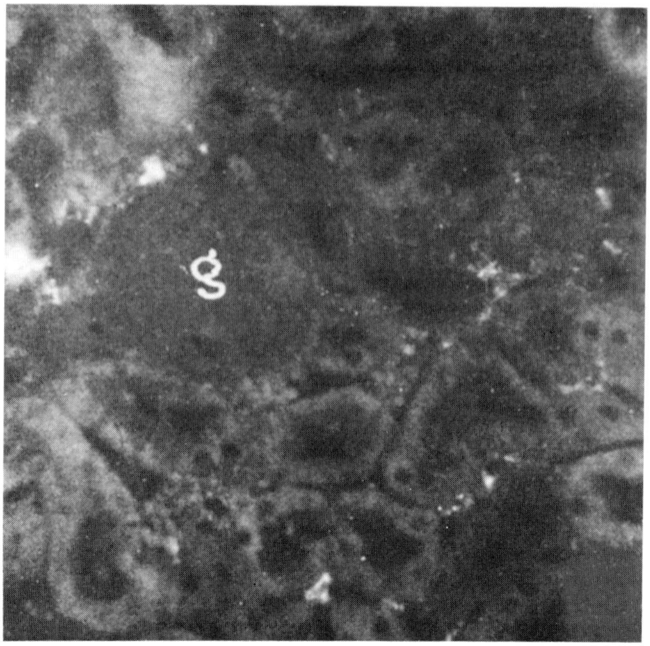

Fig. 12.1. Distribution of pneumococcal polysaccharide type III in the "capillaries around Henle's loops in the kidney"; g, glomerulus. (Reproduced from J. Exp. Med. *91*, 15, 1950, with kind permission of the authors and publisher.)

12.1. INTRODUCTION

Immunohistology was instrumental in establishing the involvement of immune mechanisms in a large number of experimental and spontaneous kidney diseases [3, 58, 74, 78, 91, 133, 134, 215]. Immunofluorescence tests and, later, other immunohistological techniques made it possible to demonstrate specific immune reactants, i.e. antigen and antibody, and inflammatory mediators, e.g. complement and fibrinogen, in kidneys in a variety of human and animal diseases [76, 77, 132, 141, 142, 158, 185, 206]. Antibodies in kidney tissue had first been demonstrated using autoradiography by Pressman et al. [167]. To our knowledge the first microphotograph of immunofluorescent staining of kidney tissue was published by Kaplan et al. [102] (Fig. 12.1). Subsequently, Cruickshank and Hill [53] demonstrated the binding of nephrotoxic serum to glomerular basement membranes (GBM) using fluorescein-labeled antibody (Fig. 12.2). In 1955-1956, Mellors et al. [141, 142, 158] used immunofluorescent staining to study experimental kidney diseases (Fig. 12.3). This method was applied also in the evaluation of human biopsy material [141, 143, 206] (Fig. 12.4). An extensive description of the immunofluorescent staining patterns in human kidney diseases was published by Seegal et al. [185]. With the establishment of percutaneous kidney biopsy as a routine clinical procedure [14, 68, 103, 126, 184, 186], immunofluorescence staining became a cornerstone in the diagnostic approach [31, 81, 85, 132, 134].

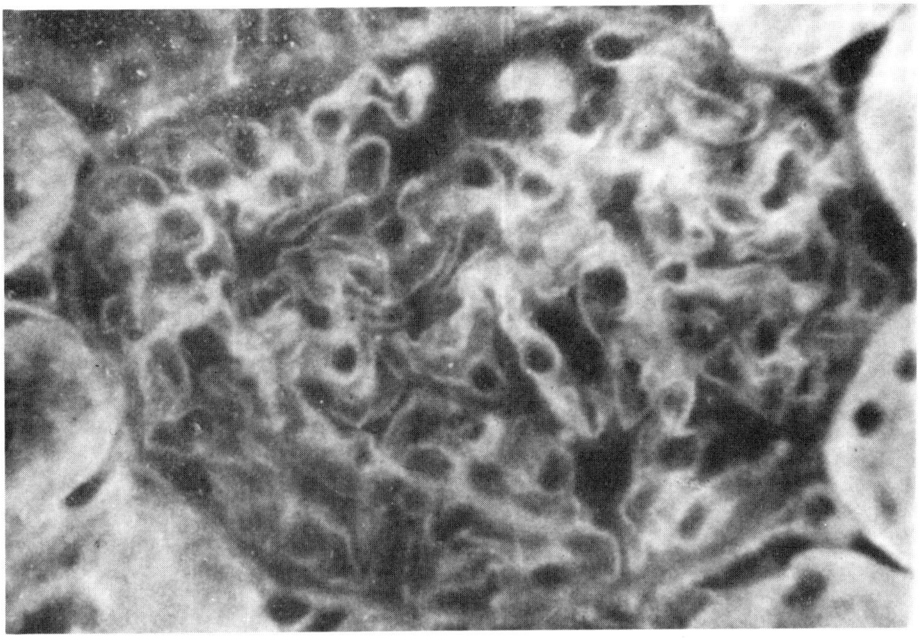

Fig. 12.2 Demonstration of binding of rabbit antiserum to glomerular basement membrane of a rat kidney. The staining is linear. (Reprinted from J. Pathol. Bacteriol. *66*, 283, 1953, with kind permission of the authors and the publisher.)

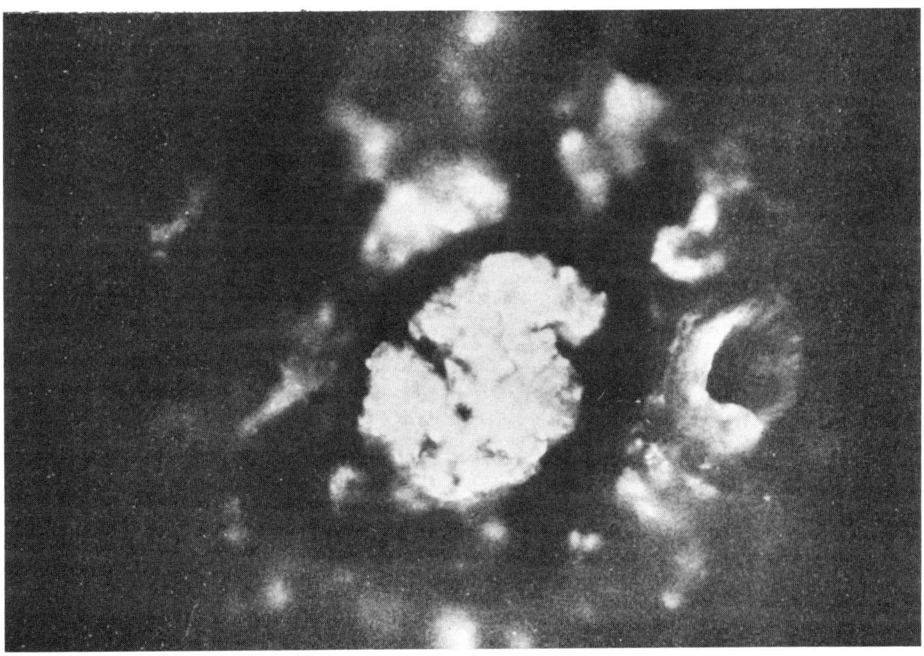

Fig. 12.3. Glomerulus from a rabbit with proliferative glomerulonephritis receiving 800 mg bovine gamma-globulin i.v. Staining for rabbit gamma-globulin. (Reproduced from Am. J. Pathol. *31*, 687, 1955, with kind permission of the authors and the publisher.)

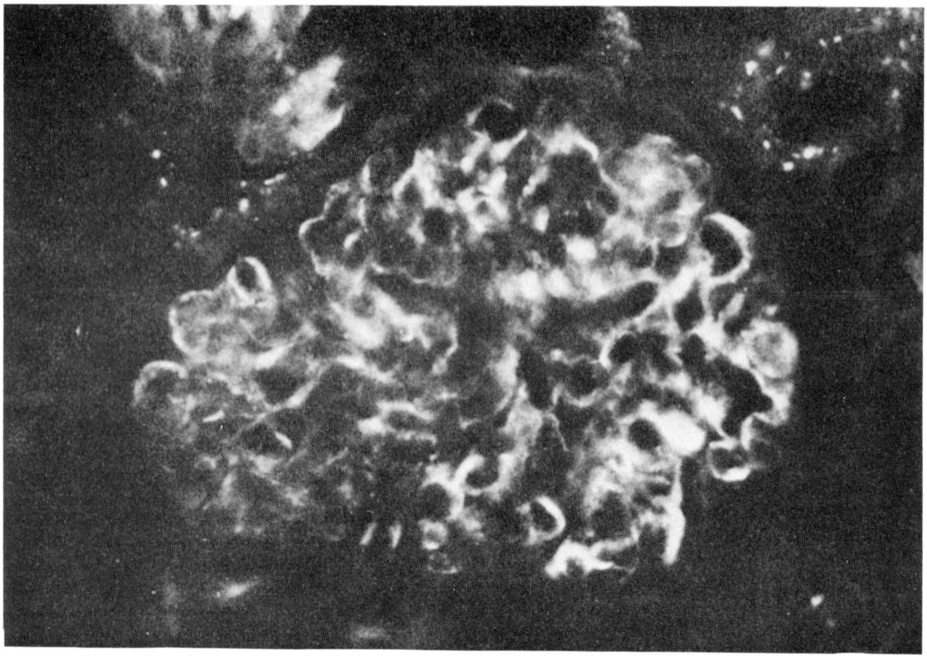

Fig. 12.4. Glomerulus from a patient with "acute diffuse membranous glomerulonephritis". Gamma globulin in glomerular capillary walls. (Reproduced from Am. J. Pathol. *32*, 455, 1956, with the kind permission of the authors and the publisher.)

To date, thorough interpretation of kidney pathology seems impossible without immunohistological procedures. This is true for glomerulonephritides (GN) and, in view of recent developments, also for tubulointerstitial (TI) diseases [5, 6, 108].

Kidney biopsy still has the risk of serious side effects. This risk is outweighed by the information obtained from study of kidney tissue when strict criteria for indication of kidney biopsy can be guaranteed (Table 12.1). Optimal interpretation of the patient's kidney tissue obtained by biopsy requires complete clinical and laboratory work-up prior to biopsy. Reliable processing of tissue for electron microscopy, equipment for, and experience with, immunofluorescence (or immunoperoxidase) staining are also required. Finally, direct communication between pathologist and clinician is indispensable. The most useful results are obtained employing all three methods of histology, i.e. immunofluorescence (IF) [3, 4, 132], electron microscopy [20, 52, 226], and light microscopy [140, 226]. Together, they allow for detection and characterization of most aspects of tissue lesions and make comparison, confirmation, and control possible. Whereas histopathology evaluated by light microscopy still provides the basis for the analysis [140], immunofluorescence tests have a special place in diagnosis [85, 132] (Table 12.II). In some cases, IF tests may allow for detection of the antigen(s) responsible for the pathology and thus contribute to the elucidation of the etiology (e.g. refs, 9, 102). More

TABLE 12.I

INDICATIONS AND CONTRAINDICATIONS FOR KIDNEY BIOPSY

A. Indications
1. Persistent proteinuria without definitive clinical diagnosis
2. Persistent nephrotic syndrome without definitive clinical diagnosis or response to therapy
3. Persistent hematuria of renal origin without definitive clinical diagnosis
4. Hypertension of unknown origin, when difficult to manage conservatively
5. Acute renal failure without definitive clinical diagnosis
6. Kidney involvement in systemic diseases, when diagnosis of systemic disease may be possible by evaluation of biopsy or when treatment regimen depends on evaluation of biopsy (e.g. SLE)
7. Familial nephropathies
8. Suspicion of renal complications of gout
9. Suspicion of diabetic glomerulosclerosis
10. Suspicion of amyloidosis
11. Nephrocalcinosis without classification demonstrated by X-rays
12. Familial nephropathies
13. Differential diagnosis glomerulonephritis versus pyelonephritis
14. Differential diagnosis of interstitial nephritides

B. Restricted indications
1. Prognostic evaluation
2. Monitoring of treatment
3. Monitoring of course of disease

C. Contraindications
1. Hemorrhagic disorders
2. Only one kidney present or functioning satisfactorily
3. Known or suspected kidney abscesses or kidney tuberculosis
4. Polycystic kidneys
5. Kidney tumors
6. Pyonephrosis
7. Perinephritis
8. Advanced renal insufficiency
9. Contracted kidneys (bilaterally)
10. Malignant hypertension
11. Patients with poor general condition and contraindications for elective surgical procedures (possibly necessary in the wake of complications arising from biopsy)
12. Inadequate possibilities to analyze biopsy specimens (no immunofluorescent staining or electron microscopy available; lack of communication between pathology and clinics; biopsy material cannot be processed adequately)
13. Academic interest without direct benefit to the patient (diagnostic or prognostic)
14. Unwilling patients

D. Relative contraindications
1. Senescence
2. Terminally diseased patients
3. Debilitated patients
4. Neurological or psychiatric disorders
5. Pregnancy
6. Recent kidney biopsy has been performed

TABLE 12.II

MAJOR CONTRIBUTIONS OF IMMUNOFLUORESCENT STAINING PROCEDURES TO DIAGNOSIS OF KIDNEY DISEASES

1. Differential diagnosis only possible by immunofluorescence:
   a) mesangial IgA-IgG deposits, i.e. diagnosis of Berger's disease and purpura Henoch-Schönlein
   b) anti-GBM or TBM antibody-mediated versus immune complex-mediated glomerulonephritis or tubulointerstitial nephritis

2. Supportive evidence for histopathological diagnosis:
   a) membranous glomerulonephritis
   b) diffuse mesangiocapillary glomerulonephritis
   c) basement membrane dense deposit disease
   d) diffuse endotheliomesangial glomerulonephritis
   e) SLE nephritis

3. Definition of pathoetiological mechanism:
   a) characterization of antigens
   b) characterization of antibodies

4. Definition of pathogenetic mechanism:
   a) involvement of soluble inflammatory mediators
   b) characterization of cells participating in inflammatory infiltrates
   c) evaluation of derangement in amounts and distribution of normal tissue components

5. Evidence for cell-mediated immunity in kidney disease: detection of effector or delayed hypersensitivity T cells

6. Exclusion of "conventional" immunological mechanisms in kidney diseases (e.g. in minimal nephropathy)

recently, availability of reagents to detect various normal tissue components of the kidney [179-181, 182, 212] as well as classes and subclasses of infiltrating cells [198] adds a fascinating new perspective to the interpretation of kidney biopsies.

Renal pathology may be classified using only clinical [195] or histopathological criteria [52, 140, 226]. Although a classification based on one class of criteria seems intellectually most satisfactory, "compromise" classifications, taking into account all the parameters available in the process of diagnosis, may be more practical. "Compromise" classifications seem to be necessary because our understanding of individual kidney diseases and the pathogenetic and pathoetiological mechanisms involved encompass a wide range of certainty and sophistication. It seems appropriate that the level of sophistication in describing distinct kidney diseases be adapted to the achieved degree of understanding. In addition, a single etiological factor may lead to a variety of distinct histopathological patterns. This is best illustrated by the experimental models of chronic serum sickness (CSS), induced by daily intravenous (i.v.) injections of bovine serum albumin (BSA) and characterized by deposits of immune complexes (IC) in the GBM). In rabbits, the glomerular pathology in CSS varies among individuals and may develop as membranous, membrano-proliferative, necrotizing, or exudative glomerulonephritis [60, 75]. In CSS of rats, subendothelial and subepithelial deposits are seen in the GBM [15]. Mice may show either one of two well-defined histopathological patterns, either mesangial IC deposition with focal or diffuse mesangial proliferation or a fulminant extracapillary (crescentic) and necrotizing glomerulonephritis (Fig. 12.5) [154]. Chickens exhibit predominantly subendothelial deposits (Fig. 12.6) with predominantly endothelial proliferation [4]. In human systemic lupus erythematosus (SLE), nephritis may take a variety of histological forms. Moreover, kidney lesions in human and animal diseases can change their appearance during the course of illness. Anti-GBM disease may develop into membranous lesions [173] and vice versa [109], and in some diseases focal injury may become diffuse and then focal again with healing. In addition, similar histopathology may be seen with a number of distinctly different diseases, e.g. focal mesangial glomerulonephritis of SLE, nephritis in Schönlein-Henoch's purpura and the glomerulonephritis of Berger's disease, or membranous nephropathy in idiopathic disease, SLE, and some forms of post-infectious nephropathies.

Diagnosis most often can be made only on the basis of data obtained with a number of different techniques. Interpretation of a kidney biopsy together with clinical data may allow the classification of a patient's renal disease as a

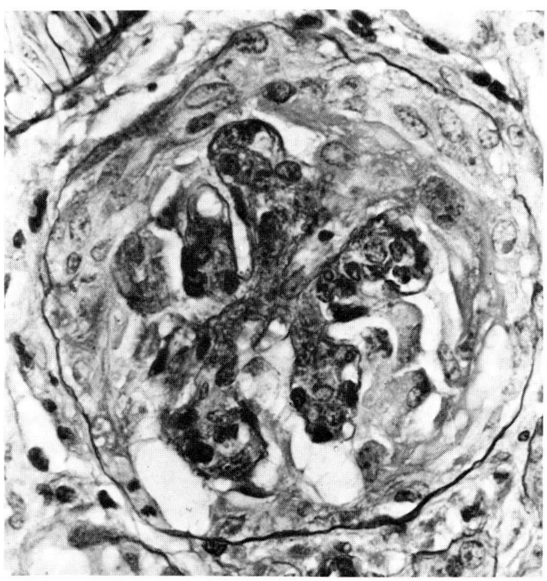

Fig. 12.5. Extracapillary proliferative (crescentic) lesions in mice with chronic serum sickness. (Reproduced from Clin. Exp. Immunol *42*, 255, 1980, with the permission of the authors and the publisher.) ×400.

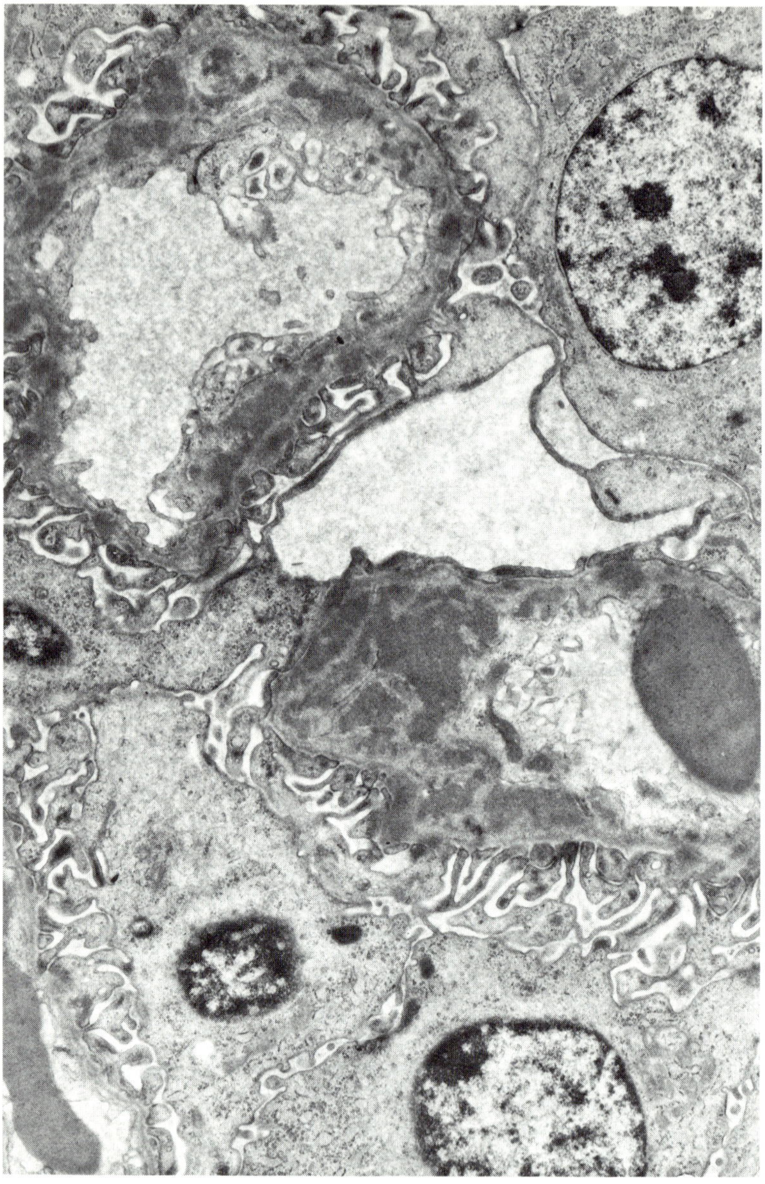

Fig. 12.6. Subendothelial electron-dense deposits with relatively well-preserved foot processes of podocytes in the glomerulus of a kidney from a chicken with chronic serum sickness ×14,400.

well-defined pathoetiological category (e.g. post-streptoccal glomerulonephritis), as a nosological entity defined by a basic immunopathogenic mechanism (e.g. anti-GBM disease) or a category defined only by descriptive histopathological findings (e.g. focal proliferative glomerulonephritis). Use of clinical data, evidence for etiological agents, association with systemic diseases, morphological and, importantly, immunopathological presentations have all to be considered in the interpretation of kidney biopsies.

Optimal results in immunofluorescence tests are ensured only with prompt and satisfactory preservation of specimens and adequate handling of tissue. With some experience, it is possible to divide the biopsy cylinder into three longitudinal parts to ensure presence of glomeruli in the specimens for immunofluorescence, light microsopy, and electron microscopy. For immunofluorescence, the specimen should be placed in OCT ("optimal controlled temperature" compound, Lab Tek Products, Naperville, IL) to prevent drying and ensure uniform freezing. The tissue should be snap-frozen in liquid nitrogen and stored either in it or at –70°C. Should liquid nitrogen not be available, freezing in acetone-dry ice is the best alternative. Thin tissue sections (2–3 μm) cut in a cryostat allow for a good resolution of the kidney structure and satisfactory localization of immunological reactants. Recently, 1 μm thick sections have been used in immunofluorescence tests [182]. Together with the use of phase contrast optics, this approach allows for exact localization of immune reactants in tissue structures. Fixation of kidney biopsy tissue in Michel's transport medium [145] seems possible but has not been tested extensively.

Fixed and paraffin-embedded tissue also may be suitable for immunofluorescence tests [178]; these preparations have to be treated with trypsin [54] or pronase [57] (see also Chapter 14, this Volume) prior to staining. Antigenic reactivity of such tissue seems to depend on the nature of antigen or antibody (e.g. IgG seems more readily demonstrable in trypsin-treated tissue sections than other immunoglobulins) and the length of the time of fixation in formalin. Still, this seems a valuable technique, especially in making old specimens accessible to evaluation with immunohistological techniques.

In our experience, immunofluorescence staining is best performed on unfixed sections. However, if plasma cells should be evaluated in biopsy tissue, methanol- or ethanol-ether fixation is advisable. The use of fluorochrome conjugates with a molar F/P ratio of 2.0-2.6 is optimal [33]. Lower F/P ratios entail a low sensitivity, and ratios higher than 3.0 may result in a significant increase of background staining [33.] As always, direct staining procedures are more specific but less sensitive than indirect ones. An increase in the sensitivity of immunofluorescence tests can be obtained by the complement-fluorescence method [80]. More recently, the introduction of the biotin-avidin system [95] and the use of indirect staining and haptenated antibodies [48, 119, 221] have increased the potential and the economy of staining procedures. Double staining methods with fluorescein isothiocyanate (FITC)- and tetramethylrhodamine isothiocyanate (TRITC)-coupled antisera may be useful in establishing the spatial relation of immune reactants and their distribution in tissue structures. Indirect immunofluorescent staining procedures with haptenated antibodies allow for double staining with two antibodies raised in the same species. Thus, they are of special value in work with monoclonal antibodies. In addition, they help circumvent undesired specific staining of tissues containing immunoglobulin as seen when using conjugates specific for

TABLE 12.III

SELECTED PATTERNS OF IMMUNOFLUORESCENT STAINING

Pattern of immune deposition			Site	Immune reactants involved	Associated pathognomonic entity
Type	Distribution	Subtype			
No deposits	—	—	—	—	MGL; MPG; FSHS: DSG; HUS; IN
Granular	Focal	Varies	Mesangium or Mesangium/GBM	IgM/C3 or IgG/Clq	FSHS; FSG
Granular	Focal	Coarse, branching	Mesangium	IgA/IgG/IgM	FG (Berger's disease, SLE)
Granular	Focal	Coarse, branching	Mesangium	IgA/IgG/IgM/FAA	FG (Henoch-Schönlein)
Granular	Diffuse/global	Fine	GBM/mesangium	κ	KG
Granular	Diffuse/global	Fine to coarse "pseudolinear"	GBM	IgG/C3	MGN
Granular	Diffuse/global	Fine to coarse	GBM	IgG/IgM/C3/IgA/IgE	SLE
Granular	Diffuse	Fine to coarse	TBM	IgG/C3/IgA/IgM	SLE
Granular	Diffuse/global	Fine to coarse "lumps"	GBM Mesangium	C3/IgG (C3/IgG/IgM/FAA)	DEPG
Granular	Diffuse/global	Coarse, lump ribbon-like	GBM Mesangium Crescents	C3/IgG/Properdin, C1q, C4 C3/IgG/Properdin FAA	DMG
Granular	Diffuse/global	Coarse, ribbon-like "double-contour"	GBM Mesangium	C3 C3/IgM	BMD
Granular	Diffuse/global or segmental	Coarse, "wire loops"	GBM	IgG/C3/IgA or IgM/IgA	SLE
Linear	Diffuse/global	—	GBM Mesangium Crescents	IgG/C3 FAA	DEG
	Focal/segmental	—	GBM	IgG	DSG (Heroin)
Linear	Diffuse	—	TBM	IgG/C3	TIN
Linear	Diffuse/global or segmental	—	GBM	IgG/IgA/IgM	Diabetes mellitus

MGL, Minimal glomerular lesion; MPG, mesangial proliferative glomerulonephritis; DSG, diffuse sclerosing glomerulonephritis; FSHS, focal and segmental hyalinosis and sclerosis; HUS, hemolytic uremic syndrome; IN, interstitial nephritis; KG, kappa-chain glomerulonephritis; MGN, membranous glomerulonephritis; SLE, nephritis in systemic lupus erythematosus; DEPG, diffuse endocapillary proliferative glomerulonephritis; DMG, diffuse mesangiocapillary glomerulonephritis; BMD, basement membrane dense deposit disease; FG, focal glomerulonephritis; DEG, diffuse extracapillary glomerulonephritis; TIN, anti-TBM interstitial nephritis.

immunoglobulin. They also are useful in immunofluorescence tests with alloantibodies. The use of monoclonal antibodies in immunofluorescence has the advantage that the reagents are homogenous and highly specific. Under certain circumstances, however, they may be less efficient than polyclonal antibodies; their restricted specificity may be of disadvantage in detecting all molecules of a specific class, e.g. "IgG" or "IgM".

In the past, immunohistological techniques have focused on the identification of immunologically reactive molecules (i.e. immunoglobulins and antigens) and inflammatory mediators (complement and fibrinogen) in tissue lesions (Table 12.III). Presently, immunohistology is also used to analyze changes in the tissues of kidneys injured by immunological mechanisms [179–182]. Attempts to associate specific patterns of derangement of basement membrane components with individual types of glomerulonephritis have been made (Table 12.IV) [182]. The availability of antisera to various types of collagen and other connective tissue components (e.g. fibronectin, laminin) has opened new approaches toward the understanding of the histopathological changs in kidney diseases and may become a valuable diagnostic tool [212]. Furthermore, the nature of the cells involved in interstitial infiltrates in kidneys may be ascertained by both tissue hemadsorption techniques [198] and immunofluorescence or immunoperoxidase methodology [34]. The availability of monoclonal antibodies to human T and B lymphocytes and subpopulations of these cell types [172] will be of great importance in clarifying the precise patterns of cellular infiltrates seen in individual kidney diseases.

Interpretation of kidney biopsy in immunofluorescence tests should follow a well-defined step-by-step protocol, evaluating separately glomerular structures (mesangium, GBM, endothelium, podocytes, Bowman's capsule, urinary space), tubules (cells, TBM), the vasculature (medium and large vessels, arterioles, peritubular capillaries), and the interstitium (ground substance, infiltrating cells.) The extent and character of lesions and of immune deposits should be recorded in as much detail as possible (Table 12.III). The intensity of

TABLE 12.IV

CHANGES IN GBM ANTIGENS IN VARIOUS GLOMERULOPATHIES[a]

	Inner GBM Ag	GPAg	Outer GBM Ag
Minimal change	n	n	n
Mesangiocapillary GN	d	n	d
BMD	d	i	d
Membranous GN	n	d	i
Diabetic glomerulopathy	i (+ +)	?	i

[a] Summary of results reported by Schiffer et al. [182]; n = normal amounts; d = decreased; i = increased amounts (or thickness on slides). Inner GBM Ag and outer GBM Ag = antigens detected by rabbit anti-human GBM serum; GPAg = antigen detected by Goodpasture's serum.

IF staining should be estimated semiquantitatively with reference to standard preparations. Specific immunofluorescence always has to be evaluated against autofluorescence of tissue structures [94]. Microphotographs make it easy to document the histology and immunohistology seen in biopsies and autopsy specimens; they facilitate the comparison and integration of results obtained with immunofluorescence, light and electron microscopy.

In the following, a brief description of the histopathological patterns seen in diseased kidneys will be given and the immune deposits associated with these patterns listed. Subsequently, a discussion about the value of immunofluorescence in the differential diagnosis of the major clinical syndromes of nephropathies will be presented. Finally, an attempt will be made to review a "compromise" classification of kidney diseases based on the integrated evaluation of morphological, immunohistological, serological, and clinical data, with emphasis on classification of kidney diseases according to the immunopathological mechanisms involved [3, 100, 134].

Changes of the kidney in allograft rejection will not be discussed here. The interested reader is referred to the reviews on this subject [10, 21, 93].

12.2. CLASSIFICATION OF GLOMERULONEPHRITIDES AND INTERSTITIAL NEPHROPATHIES BY HISTOPATHOLOGICAL CRITERIA

Classification of kidney diseases by histopathology has been attempted many times [52, 83, 84, 91, 106, 226]. A comparison of the major schemes of classification is given in the monograph of Zollinger and Mihatsch [226]. The folowing is a modification of a classification proposed by Churg and Grishman [52].

12.2.1. Glomerulonephritides

12.2.1.1. Minimal glomerular lesions (MGL)

These lesions are characterized by normal or marginally abnormal glomeruli in light microscopy; minimal mesangial hypercellularity (clusters of up to three mesangial cells) and slight broadening of the mesangial space may be seen by light microscopy. Occasional splitting and thickening of the GBM may be present in some cases. MGL has been reported in 17–43% of biopsies of the kidney [37, 45, 50, 74, 92, 148, 149, 226]. In some series of pediatric patients, this class of glomerulonephritis may account for up to 65% of all biopsies [186].

Immunofluorescence tests are usually negative in the MGL of familial glomerulopathy and idiopathic nephrosis. Scattered IgM and/or C3 deposits are seen in rare cases, but are usually within the normal range. Deposits of IgA suggest the presence of Berger's disease (see Section 12.4.2.2.) Sparse and weak deposits of various classes of immunoglobulins and C3 may be seen in early lesions of SLE. Early stages of membranous nephropathy and lesions of some patients with Henoch–Schönlein's purpura may also appear as MGLs with focal and segmental immunoglobulin or C3 deposits.

Normal or slightly abnormal glomeruli may be seen in biopsies of patients with focal glomerular lesions, in which the more characteristic lesions have not been sampled by the biopsy needle. This should always be kept in mind in interpreting MGLs in biopsies, especially when only very few glomeruli are available or when minimal immunofluorescence indicates the presence of immunoglobulins or C3 in focal and segmental distribution.

12.2.1.2. Mesangial proliferative glomerulonephritis (MPG)

There is focal or diffuse, unequivocal mesangial hypercellularity (clusters of more than four mesangial cells) and, sometimes, broadening of the mesangial space. A continuous spectrum of abnormalities ranges from MGL to MPG to mesangial sclerosis.

Immunofluorescence tests usually are negative in kidneys of patients with MPG and idiopathic nephrotic syndrome,l but IgM and/or C3 deposits may be seen. In patients with hematuria, IgA and IgG and/or C3 are frequently seen and suggest Berger's disease. Another rather ill-defined group of patients has IgG and C3 deposits.

12.2.1.3. Focal and segmental hyalinosis and sclerosis (FSHS)

Light microscopy shows collapsed capillary loops and areas occupied by amorphous eosinophilic periodic acid-Schiff (PAS)-positive material. There is no overt hypercellularity. In the earliest lesions only glomeruli in juxtamedullary position are affected [101]. The sclerotic or hyalinotic segments of the glomeruli may adhere to Bowman's capsule. Tubular atrophy and focal interstitial fibrosis are frequently found and are useful in differentiating focal sclerosis from the occasional sclerotic glomerulus seen in perfectly healthy subjects. The lesion is seen most often in patients with idiopathic nephrotic syndrome. Its diagnosis is of clinical value because patients with FSHS frequently are resistant to cortisone therapy and have, in general, a poorer prognosis than patients with MGL.

In immunofluorescence tests, frequently no staining is detectable. In some cases, IgM and C3 and, occasionally, IgG and C1q may be present in sclerotic areas and in the mesangium. Fibrin-associated antigens (FAA) are seen only infrequently.

12.2.1.4. Focal glomerulonephritis (FG)

FG in characterized by focal-segmental lesions of varying patterns, is sometimes difficult to differentiate from FSHS, and usually occurs as part of systemic (Henoch-Schönlein's purpura, periarteritis nodosa, Wegener's granulomatosis, SLE rheumatic fever) or hereditary diseases (e.g. Alport's syndrome). Only a small fraction of FG is "idiopathic". The lesions seen in association with systemic diseases heal with amelioration of the underlying disease. In the idiopathic forms spontaneous healing may occur, but recurrence is frequent. FG may be superimposed on various diffuse GN. FG is not unusual with MPG, diffuse endocapillary proliferative, mesangiocapillary, dense-deposit and membranous GN. Focal lesions may become diffuse with progression of the disease, reverting eventually to focal lesions during healing. As with the diffuse forms of GN, the focal lesions may also be classified as proliferative, crescentic, necrotizing, or sclerosing. Focal proliferative lesions usually are associated with a mild course of disease, although healing often leads to segmental scars. Necrotizing FG may be associated with thrombosis, endothelial damage, and extravasation into Bowman's space, followed by cell proliferation and crescent formation. Healing usually results in segmental scarring and adhesions. Electron microscopy may show mesangial hypercellularity and sclerosis and, in some specimens, mesangial electron dense deposits. Fibrillary fibrin may be present in Bowman's capsule and in glomerular capillaries. Occasionally, subendothelial electron-dense deposits are seen.

Immunofluorescent staining procedures often are important for the diagnosis of the underlying disease. IgA and IgG deposits accompanied by C3 are characteristic for Berger's disease and their demonstration is the only reliable method for definitive identification of this nosological entity. In the kidneys of some patients linear IgG and C3 deposits seen in the GBM together with extensive crescent formation may indicate an early stage of rapidly progressive glomerulonephritis or Goodpasture's disease (see Section 12.2.1.9)

12.2.1.5. Diffuse endocapillary proliferative glomerulonephritis (DEPG)

This condition is characterized by a uniform increase in glomerular cellularity involving both endothelial and mesangial cells. Patency of capillary lumina is always impaired and total occlusion is frequent. Leucocytic infiltration is common and often extensive. Extracapillary proliferation involving parietal epithelial cells and leading to crescent formation may be seen [226]. This type of tissue injury is often seen in conjunction with the clinical syndrome of acute glomerulonephritis.

DEPG is seen most frequently in post-streptococcal GN and in some other post-infectious GN [120, 208]. Most frequently, especially in pediatric patients, the early lesions described above resolve with little residual tissue injury persisting for up to 1–2 years. However, the disease sometimes develops further into a "chronic latent GN" or "chronic sclerosing GN". This latter condition has a grave prognosis [17, 19].

It has been attempted to define four stages of post-infectious, in particular post-streptococcal, GN [226]: 1) an exudative stage defined by leucocytosis of the glomerulus, tissue infiltration with granulocytes and monocytes, and hematuria – this stage may persist for 2–6 months; 2) a proliferative phase, ensuing some 9 weeks after infection, with proliferation and swelling first of endothelial and then of mesangial cells; no increase of mesangial matrix is detectable (DEPG); 3) a proliferative-sclerosing stage which may involve all of the mesangium ("panmesangial" variant) or single loops ("axial" variant) – in this condition, mesangial matrix is significantly increased, and the tissue lesion often presents as diffuse mesangial proliferative GN; and 4) a sclerosing GN, presenting as FSHS or as diffuse and global sclerosis, often combined with fibrotic crescents.

DEPG is seen in 2–9% of biopsies from adults [50, 74] and 17% of biopsies from children [83]. It is the most frequent (over 90%) [120, 177] histopathology encountered in patients with clinically defined acute GN. Association with infections is the entity most frequently seen with DEPG. However, a similar histopathological pattern may be seen with SLE, Henoch–Schönlein's purpura, and polyarteritis nodosa.

IF staining most frequently is positive for deposits of C3 in the GBM, alone or together with IgG, and, less frequently, IgM and IgA. The staining pattern is finely to coarsely granular. In addition, C3 and IgG/IgM are present in the mesangium. FAA may be detected in Bowman's capsule and mesangium. Properdin has also been described in the lesion. In exceptional cases, linear staining patterns may be observed in the GBM.

Authors proposing the subdivision of post-streptococcal GN into four stages point out that finely to coarsely granular IF for C3 and IgG in the GBM predominates in the first two stages, and that IgM deposits in the mesangium become a salient feature in the stage of sclerosing lesions. However, IF may be negative late in the disease [149].

In post-streptococcal GN, streptococcal antigens can be demonstrated only very early in the immune deposits [8, 203, 222, 223]. Mounting evidence suggests that antibodies to autologous immunoglobulins constitute part of immune deposits later in the disease [136, 139, 146, 160]. Streptococci may have the ability to attach to the Fc portion of immunoglobulins in a manner similar to staphylococcal protein A [49]. Thus, direct interaction of bacterial protein and immunoglobulin may induce changes in the antigenicity of the immunoglobulin; this then may elicit the production of antibodies to newly expressed antigens on the immunoglobulins. As stated above, only C3 is seen in the glomeruli of patients with poststreptococcal GN. The hypothesis has been advanced that components of streptococci may interact directly with complement and thus initiate tissue lesions [199, 200].

12.2.1.6. Diffuse mesangiocapillary glomerulonephritis (DMG)

This histopathological entity is often referred to as "membranoproliferative GN type I" or "hypocomplementemic GN" [130, 211]. There is impressive capillary wall thickening, mesangial hypercellularity, and incrase in mesangial matrix. Polymorphonuclear granulocytes are frequently seen in glomeruli. The glomeruli are enlarged and the lobular structure accentuated by nodular changes, especially in the sclerosing variety (or stage) of the disease. Often, the capillary wall shows a "double contour" in insolated segments. Electron-dense deposits are seen in the subendothelial space, more precisely in the interposed subendothelial mesangium, and in the mesangium proper. Subepithelial electron-dense deposits are seen in up to 50% of biopsies with DMG [24, 176]. Focal, small crescents are frequent [226]. Extensive crescents are seen in 10–20% of patients [84] and may be cellular or fibrotic. Various types of crescents found in the same biopsy may indicate repeated attacks of the disease. In patients with this form of GN low levels of C3 are often demonstrable. Serum C1q, C4, and C2 also may be diminished [124]. A C3-activating factor, "C3NeF" is sometimes found in the sera [157]. The profile of complement components in circulation and in tissue deposits suggests a role for both the classical and the alternative pathways of activation of complement in this disease. Patients with DMG clinically present with proteinuria, nephrotic syndrome, acute nephritic syndrome, gross hematuria, or isolated proteinuria and microscopic hematuria [226]. In patients with severe crescent formation, rapidly progressing renal failure is common [88].

A variant of DMG, "Type III", is distinguished as a separate entity by some authors. It is characterized by scattered electron-dense deposits in the lamina densa of the basement membrane of glomerular capillaries. This disease, although seen in all age groups, is found most frequently in older children and young adults.

Granular, lumpy or interrupted linear deposits of C3 in the GBM are characteristic of this disease [31, 42, 144, 165]. Less frequently, such deposits also occur in the mesangium. In addition to C3, properdin C1q, C4 and C2 may be detected in the deposits. IgG, IgM, and, infrequently, IgA may be found segmentally in a granular pattern. FAA is seen predominantly in crescents. In DMG associated with ventriculo-atrial shunt, IgM deposits seem to predominate [210].

Randall et al. [168] reported on a variant of DMG which is characterized by granular deposition of kappa chains in the GBM and mesangium. Since then, eight cases with similar immunohistopathology have been presented [71, 97, 155, 169]. Despite the presence of kappa light chains there is no histological staining for amyloid. In electron microscopy, the deposits are granular in the GBM and granular or fibrillar in the mesangium. Some patients had myeloma diagnosed prior to the occurrence of the kidney disease, but in two of the patients [71] myeloma could be suspected only on the basis of biochemical tests.

12.2.1.7. Basement membrane dense deposit disease (BMD)

This disease is often referred to as "membranoproliferative GN type II". It shares many histological characteristics as well as hypocomplementemia with DMG. There is a thickening of the glomerular capillary wall with mesangial hypercellularity and an increase in mesangial matrix. In some cases, these changes lead to accentuation of glomerular lobulation. In this type of GN however, lobulation is not as frequently observed as in DMG. Mesangial interposition may be seen, but is also less extensive than in DMG. The most characteristic lesion is the intramembranous deposition of fibrinoid osmiophilic material [70]; thus electron microscopy is the most reliable and diagnostic procedure for this disease. Intramembranous deposits, however, may also be detected with light microscopy. They are strongly PAS-positive, give a reddish color in azan-carmine staining and are luxol fast-blue-positive. There is no reaction with Sudan black B and in conventional PASM stains. Overstaining with PASM, however, may lead to a brownish or black staining. There is some evidence that deposits may consist of glycoproteins [70, 72]. The electron-dense deposits are found in the lamina densa and at low magnifications appear homogenous [89]; high resolution electron microscopy reveals fine granularity [226]. Electron-dense deposits of lower density frequently are subepithelial, forming humps, or are subendothelial (possibly in the interposed mesangium). Less frequently, the deposits are found in Bowman's capsule and in the mesangium. The extent of mesangial sclerosis is variable. Cellular proliferation may be moderate. Fibrotic or cellular crescents may occur and are associated with rapidly progressive disease and a poor prognosis [89, 226]. The basement membrane may be thickened impressively (up to 16,000 Å) [226], although in other instances the thickening may be only moderate, irregular and segmentally accentuated. The hypocomplementemia, in contrast to the decrease of complement in DMG usually is restricted to C3; C3NeF is found rather frequently [157, 205].

In immunofluorescence, staining for C3 usually is impressive [23, 148]. It appears in a ribbon-like, coarsely granular or segmental-linear, sometimes "double-contour" pattern. Isolated deposits of C3, however, may also be considered artifacts [31]. Immunoglobulins, C1q, C4 and properdin are not detectable in most cases. C3 may also occur in the mesangium, Bowman's capsule, TBM, and tubular capillaries. Sometimes IgM may be seen in the mesangium. On the whole, immunofluorescence is of little value in the diagnosis and differential diagnosis of this disease.

12.2.1.8. Membranous glomerulonephritis or nephropathy (MGN)

Bell [26] coined the name "membranous nephropathy" to describe histopathology characterized by thickening of basement membrane without impressive exudative and proliferative alterations of the glomerulus. Nevertheless, polymorphonuclear granulocytes may dominate the very early stages of this disease. The morphological and immunohistological similarities among MGN in humans, CSS in rabbits, and Heymann nephritis in rats suggest an IC-mediated pathogenesis.

A synonym frequently used for the definition of this nephropathy is "epimembranous glomerulonephritis". This term stresses the localization of electron-dense deposits on the epithelial side of the membrane [64, 226]. Habib [84] has argued that epimembranous glomerulonephritis is a histopathological entity distinct from truly "membranous" (i.e. intramembranous) disease with immune complexes in the central part of the basement membrane. However, sequential biopsies of a patient may show both epi- and intramembranous deposits [175, 226]. Thus, at least until further confirmation of exclusively intramembranous deposits in GN, both varieties of membranous nephropathy are more appropriately considered together.

With the exception of the very early lesions, all or almost all glomeruli are involved. The lesion is characterized by global thickening of capillary walls. The basement membrane of glomeruli may reach a width of 20,000-30,000 Å. Subepithelial deposits may be seen in light microscopy as slightly irregular protrusions of PAS-positive material or as reddish granules in Masson's trichrome stain on the epithelial side in the capillary wall. In the stage of most active disease, silver stain reveals spikes of basement membrane-like material around and between the deposits. Mesangial proliferation and sclerosis become prominent only in the very late stages. Capillary lumina are narrowed with progression of the usually slowly evolving disease.

The disease may occur in individuals of all ages, but the majority of patients are over 40 years of age at the time of diagnosis [1, 51, 174]. The idiopathic form of the disease occurs with the highest frequency at the age of 60–75. There is a preponderance of males over females in the patient population, 1.5 : 3.0 in adults [27, 65] and 4 : 1 in pediatric patients [86]. Up to 70% of patients with membranous glomerulonephritis have no detectable underlying disease, and 30% have "secondary" membranous glomerulonephritis [152, 226]. Among the pathognomonic entities in the latter group, SLE, infections (e.g. secondary congenital syphilis, malaria, filiariasis, schistosomiasis), malignant tumors, and drug and toxic reactions (including the effects of penicillamine, gold and mercury) are the most prominent causes. The prognosis is that of a chronic, slowly progressing disease, with some probability of spontaneous remission and healing.

Defined by histopathology, the disease has been subdivided into four [64] or six [226] stages; the latter authors arrived at six stages by adding a recovery and a recurrence stage). *Stage I.* Very early in disease, high numbers of polymorphonuclear granulocytes may be seen. Deposition of fine subepithelial electron-dense granules, presumably representing immune complexes, occurs. There is mild enlargement of foot processes of podocytes first restricted to the area above the deposits. Usually, the mesangium is inconspicuous. The interstitium is normal and shows only minimal edema. This stage may be confused with MGL. *Stage II.* Electron-dense and immune deposits become larger and basement membrane-like material forms spikes between the deposits. This argyrophilic material increases with progression of the disease. Glomeruli are moderately enlarged and GBM is homogenously thickened in light microscopy. There may be endothelial swelling and loss of fenestration of the endothelium. Mild mesangial fibrosis may be seen. *Stage III.* The basement membrane spikes, originating in the lamina densa of GBM, now envelop the electron-dense deposits, appearing as a "twisted rope" or "ladder". The density of the deposits decreases and the thickening of the basement membrane reaches its maximum. The ribbon-like deposits are predominantly intramembranous. The interstitium may show patchy fibrosis and few lymphoid cells, rarely also foam cells. *Stage IV.* There is extensive fibrosis and sclerosis of glomeruli and the immune deposits may become undetectable. The thickening of the basement membrane is irregular. The number of obsolescent glomeruli increases, tubular atrophy ensues, and interstitial fibrosis and sclerosis become diffuse.

Various stages of the disease may be seen in individual glomeruli of the same biopsy. Deposits of electron-dense material in the mesangium are rare in early stages and, when found, may suggest SLE as underlying disease. In remission, the glomerular capillary walls may be reconstructed and resemble normal tissue. Isolated synechias and crescents may be observed in MGN, and acute proliferative glomerulonephritis may be superimposed on the membranous disease. In patients with MGN, transformation to acute proliferative GN with antibodies to GBM has been reported [109].

Renal vein thrombosis may occur in the course of this disease, often accompanied by sudden deterioration of renal function [62, 165]. An interesting association has been noted between Lyell's disease (a bullous dermatitis) and idiopathic MGN [115].

Serum complement concentrations are normal in MGN. Recently, predominantly non-complement binding immune complexes have been detected in all sera tested of patients with MGN [192]. There are some indications that complement-binding complexes also appear, but only intermittently.

In early disease, immunofluorescence tests show finely granular, regularly distributed deposits of IgG and usually C3 in the GBM [56]. They even may be seen in a pseudo-linear pattern [63, 153]. IgM and IgA deposits are not frequently seen. In the mesangium, deposits are rare but may become obvious with progressive disease [166]. Complement may be absent in early lesions. C1q and C4 usually accompany C3 in deposits. FAA are infrequent.

The granular deposits become coarser later in disease, and diminish in number and size in stages III and IV. In some of the biopsies from patients with an underlying systemic disease, it has been possible to identify the antigen (e.g. DNA antigens in SLE; tumor proteins; hepatitis B antigen). In biopsies from three patients with idiopathic MGN, dispersion experiments suggested a participation of antibodies to human aggregated immunoglobulin in immune deposits [160].

12.2.1.9. Diffuse extracapillary (crescentic) glomerulonephritis (DEG)

This histopathologically defined syndrome encompasses a variety of patholletiological entities. They all have unfavorable prognoses with rapid development of kidney insufficiency ("rapidly progressive glomerulonephritis") [96].

Crescents may be seen in a variety of GN (e.g. DEPG, DMG), and clinical syndromes (SLE, Wegeners disease, and hemolytic uremic syndrome). In these instances, crescents are usually present in only a few of the glomeruli. Sometimes, however, they are present in the majority of glomeruli, and in these cases the differentiation from the entity discussed here (DEG) is difficult [191] and depends on clinical criteria.

DEG is characterized by the presence of crescents in most glomeruli (>50%) [83, 226]. According to a study by Habib [83, all patients with more than 80% of glomeruli showing crescents lose their kidney function within a few weeks or months.

Many patients have an upper respiratory illness prior to the kidney disease [196]. In patients with DEG and hemorrhagic pneumonitis (Goodpasture's syndrome), influenza A_2 virus antibodies have often been detected in serum.

In light microscopy, there is first segmental thrombosis and necrosis of glomerular capillary loops, fibrin deposition in Bowman's space, and development of cellular crescents. The crescents are derived mainly from the parietal epithelium of glomeruli. The contain monocytes or macrophages, polymorphonuclear granulocytes, and platelets. Fibrin is present between the cells of the crescents [31, 106, 147, 156, 219]. The epithelial cells may have a clear cytoplasm devoid of most cell organelles or they may have abundant organelles implying active metabolism. They crescents may be either negligible [i.e. localized adhesions) or global, embracing the glomerular capilary tufts completely and occluding Bowman's space; in consequence, the capillary tufts are compressed. They crescents often extend into the proximal tubules. In the fully developed disease, basement membrane-like material is deposited between the cells. Infrequently, foreign body-type giant cells may be seen in the crescents [116, 125]. In areas of widened intercellular space fibrin fibrils are found. Subsequently, cells resembling fibroblasts are seen, and collagen fibers are deposited between the cells of the crescents ("fibrocellular crescents"). Later, cells disappear and a fibrous crescent consisting of connective tissue surrounds the compressed glomerular capillaries or their remnants. Often, cellular, fibrocellular, and fibrous crescents are seen in the same biopsy specimen. Deposition of fibrin may be impressive and a major pathogenic factor in the mechanism of crescent formation. In the serum and urine of these patients, degradation products of fibrin may reach high concentrations. Periglomerular cell infiltration is frequently seen.

In electron microscopy there may be translucent areas in the lamina rara interna, almost always associated with fibrin deposits [107]. In few cases, subendothelial dense deposits are seen. Breaks in the capillary walls are common.

The etiology of DEG is still enigmatic except in a few cases (e.g. SLE). In roughly 25% of patients, antibodies to GBM are present [13]. In these cases, immunization with microbial antigens cross-reacting with GBM components may be involved (e.g. streptococcal or viral antigens), but there is no conclusive evidence to substantiate such a hypothesis [74, 217]. Alternatively, release of normal or abnormal basement membranes by toxins or drugs could occur in some patients [170]. This might explain the alleged association between Goodpasture's disease and inhalation of hydrocarbon compounds [25]. Antibodies to GBM and diffuse extracapillary glomerulonephritis have also been seen in patients with cortical necrosis, basement membrane damage caused by immune complexes, Alport's disease, and the nail-patella syndrome. The last two are associated with genetic defects and abnormalities of connective tissue and/or basement membranes.

Approximately 50% of patients with diffuse extracapillary glomerulonephritis may have IC deposits in the glomeruli, while over 20% have no demonstrable deposits [226]. In the latter cases, either no known immunological mechanism is involved or the immunological reactants do not remain long enough in glomeruli to be detected in biopsy. In the rare patient with remission, focal crescentic glomerulonephritis may be observed.

In the majority of patients, diffuse granular deposits of IgG, IgM, and IgA, and C3 seen in the glomerular capillaries and sometimes also in the mesangium suggest IC-mediated pathology.

In other patients, immunofluorescence tests show linear binding of IgG to glomerular capillary basement membranes [122, 132]. Elution experiments have documented the specificity of the immunoglobulin deposited for GBM [122, 218]. There is, however, cross-reactivity with other basement membranes. Over 80% of eluates from kidneys with linear deposits of IgG in the basement membrane of glomeruli also react with tubular basement membrane in vitro, even though often there is no in vivo binding to TBM [11]. Some patients show a wide variety of cross-reactive specificities, e.g. with basement membranes of the choroid plexus; frequently, these patients have lung involvement in addition to kidney disease ("Goodpasture's disease"). C3 frequently is segmental in distribution and may be deposited in a finely granular pattern [74]. Only a fraction of the antibodies eluted from the GBM with linear deposits bind complement [130]. FAA are demonstrable in Bowman's space, in the crescents and in capillary tufts in more than 70% of cases [31, 147]. Deposits of IgA and IgM may be seen in segmental patterns. Immunoglobulin deposits are almost never seen in the crescents themselves. Even in late stages of the disease with extensive destruction of the normal structures, some portion of the glomerulus may show linear deposits of IgG.

12.2.1.10. Diffuse (chronic) sclerosing glomerulonephritis (DSG)

DSG is found in the end stages of various forms of GN, e.g. FSHS, hereditary and post-infectious GN, or Berger's disease. In most cases, it is extremely difficult to diagnose the underlying disease from end-stage kidney biopsies. Diffuse sclerosing glomerulonephritis may fallow other forms of GN either in continuo or with a latency period of 2-20 years. Light microscopy shows an apparent increase in density of glomeruli because of cortical thinning; the actual number of glomeruli, however, is diminished. The "contracted" end-stage kidney may show only a few obliterated glomeruli per section. Glomeruli appear as sclerotic nodules, often mounted in a thick bracelet of fibrous tissue arising from Bowman's capsule. Besides obliterated glomeruli, a few glomeruli may be less severely damaged. The presence of fibrocellular crescents may mark relatively recent acute phases of recrudescence of the underlying disease. Even in the less advanced lesions of glomeruli, areas of fibrosis and sclerosis, hypertrophic mesangium, and adhesions to the capsules may be seen. Sometimes Bowman's space is filled with cuboidal epithelial cells forming "pseudotubules" between the sclerotic capillary tufts and thc fibrotic capsule of Bowman. Vessels usually show subintimal fibrosis or moderate to severe sclerosis. Often, there is extensive interstitial fibrosis together with a sparse lymphocytic infiltrate. Most tubules show focal atrophy while few are hypertrophic.

Electron microscopy usually does not add any additional information to that obtained by light microscopy. In some instances, however, it may reveal remnants of the original disease (e.g. electron-dense deposits in segmental distribution).

Immunofluorescence microscopy may be negative or reveal granular or patchy deposits of IgM and C3 in some tissue sections (74, 99, 207]. These deposits may well reflect "non-specific" trapping rather than specific immunological damage. IgG, IgA, "early" complement components, and FAA are seen less frequently. Faint linear deposits of IgG in the GBM and TBM have also been reported, especially in glomerulonephritides of heroin addicts [81, 101, 134]. On rare occasions, the patterns of immunofluorescence in DSG may be sufficiently characteristic to suggest the pathogenesis. Thus IgA and IgG may suggest Berger's disease or Henoch–Schönlein purpura as the original disease; granular deposits in preserved segments of glomerular capillaries may hint at a preceding MGN, and linear deposits of IgG may suggest anti-GBM disease [207].

12.2.2. Interstitial nephritides (IN)

12.2.2.1. Interstitial nephritis with destructive lesions ("pyelonephritis")

The patients usually suffer from lever, flank pain, pyuria, dysuria and pollakisuria. Acute pyelonephritis, however, may also be asymptomatic. Pyelonephritis is characterized by interstitial inflammation, and secondary tubular derangements with "destructive" foci in medulla and cortex [226]. The infiltrating cells are predominantly granulocytes and macrophages or monocytes. Later in the disease, lymphocytes and plasma cells appear; sometimes lympoid follicles may be seen. The lymphocytes are almost exclusively B cells [198].

The immunohistology varies and does not suggest a primary role for any immune reactant in pyelonephritis. Patchy and granular irregular deposits of immunoglobulin may be seen in the mesangium or segmentally in the GBM [16, 28]. Cells of the interstitium (macrophages or plasma cells) may stain with fluorochrome-conjugated antibodies to immunoglobulins [226].

12.2.2.2. Acute non-destructive interstitial nephritis

This seems to be a rather rare nosological entity, accounting for approximately 1% of biopsies in a representative series [226]. The most impressive clinical manifestation is oliguria or anuria of abrupt onset. A similar sudden onset of kidney failure is also seen in experimental tubulointerstitial nephritis of guinea pigs [194]. Other forms of acute interstitial nephritis may be dominated by increased serum creatinine and polyuria ("non-oliguric renal failure") [226]. This is frequently seen with interstitial nephritis in the wake of antibiotic nephrotoxicity. Light microscopy reveals edema and mononuclear cell infiltrates which may consist of macrophages, B cells or T cells according to the underlying pathogenesis [198].

Immunofluorescence most often is negative; infrequently, it may show linear deposition of IgG and C3 or granular deposition of immunoglobulins and complement in the TBM [11]. It should be emphasized, however, that interrupted linear deposits of C3 and IgG may occur in normal kidney tissue.

12.2.2.3. Chronic non-destructive interstitial nephritis

The onset usually is insiduous; polyuria and metabolic acidosis may develop. The interstitial cellular infiltrates may resemble those of acute interstitial nephritis, with fibrosis more prominent than edema. Immunohistology is similar to that seen in acute non-destructive interstitial nephritis, as is the pathoetiology.

In the course of Weil's disease, an interstitial nephritis with changes in the endothelium of interstitial vessels may develop. Further immunopathological studies are required to determine if immune reactants are involved [227].

12.3. CORRELATION OF CLINICAL SYNDROMES AND HISTOPATHOLOGICAL ANALYSIS OF KIDNEY TISSUE

Here, the association of the major clinical syndromes of kidney disease with patterns of histopathology is presented. This may help in defining the usefulness of histopathological and immunohistopathological interpretation of kidney biopsy specimens in various clinical syndromes.

12.3.1. Acute nephritis

This syndrome is defined by usually macroscopic hematuria of abrupt onset [40, 117, 197, 209, 226]. Often the glomerular filtration rate is decreased. Facial edema (not severe in the morning), circulatory overload, mild to moderate proteinuria (usually without nephrotic syndrome), hypertension, and oliguria may be present. The acute phase of disease is transient, resulting either in the death of the patients, in complete recovery, or in the development of nephrotic syndrome which may lead either to chronic renal failure or to healing.

Acute nephritis most often is associated with diffuse endocapillary proliferative glomerulonephritis (DEPG). Thus, it has been proposed to define acute nephritis histopathologically using the criteria for DEPG (see Section 12.2.1.5). Acute nephritis, however, is also seen in some patients with DEG, DMG, and even MGN as well as in some forms of focal glomerulonephritis (FG).

By immunofluorescence tests, granular deposits of complement and IgG are found in glomerular capillary walls in classical acute nephritis seen after infections ("acute post-infections GN"). In acute nephritis associated with

DEG, often linear deposits of IgG and linear or granular deposits of C3 may be found in the GBM and, sometimes, in the TBM.

12.3.2. Nephrotic syndrome

When urinary loss of protein results in hypoalbuminemia, nephrotic syndrome becomes manifest [40, 69, 110, 117, 209, 226], and edema is a direct consequence. In addition, there is usually hyperlipoproteinemia and lipiduria, induced by hepatic overproduction of lipoproteins and/or impaired clearance of plasma lipids. The coagulation system is profoundly disturbed; some changes favor coagulation (primarily the increase in plasma fibrinogen and platelets in circulation); other changes promote fibrinolysis and impair coagulation (e.g. increased serum concentrations of plasminogen and deficiencies of factor IX). Thrombus formation may occur anywhere in the body, but the lower extremities and renal veins are frequent sites. the nephrotic syndrome may arise in the course of a vast variety of nosological processes.

The findings in immunofluorescence tests are as varied as the underlying diseases causing nephrotic syndrome. It is obvious from Table 12.V that

TABLE 12.V

DIFFERENTIAL DIAGNOSIS OF THE NEPHROTIC SYNDROME

Clinical presentation	Histopathology	Immunofluorescence
Acute nephritis	DEPG	Scattered coarse-granular
post-streptococcal GN		staining IgG/C3 in GBM (subepithelial)
post-infectious GN	MGN, DMG	Finely to coarse-granular staining IgG/C3 in GBM (subepithelial, intramembranous)
idiopathic	Varies	Varies
Rapidly progressive GN	DEG	Global linear IgG, linear or granular C3 in GBM; or granular IgG and C3 in GBM
Chronic idiopathic GN	MGN	Finely granular IgG and C3 in GBM
	DMC	Coarsely granular C3/IgG in GBN (intermembranous)
	BMD	Nodular patchy C3 in mesangium
	KCD	Nodular granular kappa in mesangium and GBM
	DEG	Scattered coarsely granular IgG/C3 in GBM (subepithelial)
Chronic GN in systemic diseases		
SLE	Varies	Varies
Idiopathic mixed cryoglobulinemia	MGN	Finely to coarse granular IgG/IgM in GBM
Henoch–Schönlein	MPG, FG	Patchy granular IgA/IgG in mesangium

Clinical presentation	Histopathology	Immunofluorescence
polyarthritis	Varies	Fibrinogen alone or IgG, IgM, C3 granular in GBM
neoplasia	MGN	Negative or finely granular IgG/IgM/C3 in GBM
lipoid nephrosis	MGL (MPG)	Negative
heavy metals	MGN	Finely granular IgG/C3 in GBM (mesangium)
drugs	IN	Negative
(methicillin)	IN	Linear IgG/C3 in TBM
allergens	IN (with eosinophils)	IgE? or negative
Berger's disease	MPG, FG	Coarse-patchy IgA/IgG/C3 in mesangium
Focal glomerular sclerosis	FSHS	Negative or IgM/C3 coarsely granular in mesangium
purpura Moschkovitz	Varies	FAA in glomerulus
hemolytic-uremic syndrome	Varies	FAA in glomerulus, immunoglobulins variable, usually absent

Other syndromes in which IF does not contribute significantly to diagnosis:

- diabetic glomerulosclerosis
- amyloidosis
- preeclampsia
- recurrent nephrotic syndrome of pregnancy
- malignant hypertension
- congestive heart failure
- constrictive pericarditis
- renal transplant rejection
- congenital nephrotic syndrome
- sickle cell disease

TABLE 12.VI
ASSOCIATION OF NEPHROPATHIES WITH ACUTE RENAL FAILURE

A Prerenal
B Postrenal
C Parenchymal:

- *rapidly progressive* GN (DEG)[a]
- *post-streptococcal GN* (DEPG)
- *Henoch–Schönlein's purpura* (MPG, FG)
- *polyarthritis*
- *scleroderma*
- hemolytic uremic syndrome, Moschkovitz' purpura, cortical necrosis
- pyelonephritis
- *heavy metal-induced nephritis*
- *drug-induced nephritis*
- trauma, etc.

[a] Categories in which IF may contribute to diagnosis are in italics.

immunofluorescence tests are helpful in the differential diagnosis of the nephrotic syndrome.

12.3.3. Acute renal failure

This syndrome is characterized by an abrupt decrease of urine flow (oliguria, anuria) and azotemia [47, 123, 190]. The term "acute uremia" is sometimes used instead of "acute renal failure". Histopathological features and clinical presentations which may be associated with this condition are summarized in Table 12.VI.

12.3.4. Chronic renal failure

Chronic renal failure is defined as chronic reduction of the glomerular filtration rate as reflected in a reduced creatinine clearance and increased serum creatinine [45, 100]. The syndrome of chronic renal failure or "chronic uremia" is complex and of increasing importance because of the prolonged survival of patients with this condition in the wake of chronic dialysis and kidney transplantation. It is beyond the framework of this chapter to cover clinical aspects of uremia. A correlation with the underlying pathological conditions associated or leading to chronic renal failure is given in Table 12.VII. All progressive kidney diseases involving destruction of glomeruli and of vascular supply may lead to chronic renal failure. Ultimately, chronic renal failure is associated histopathologically with the "end-stage" or "contracted" kidney.

TABLE 12.VII
CORRELATION OF CHRONIC RENAL FAILURE AND NEPHROPATHIES

Chronic glomerulonephritis[a] (MGN, DMG, BMD, MPG; DSG; SLE; polyarthritis; Wegener's syndrome)
Interstitial nephritis
Hereditary renal diseases
Hypertension
Diabetes mellitus
Sickle cell disease
Multiple myeloma
Amyloidosis
Gout
Nephrocalcinosis
Tuberculosis
Unresolved acute renal failure

[a] Categories in which IF may contribute to diagnosis are in italics.

12.3.5. Interstitial nephritides (IN)

Interstitial nephritides have variable clinical manifestations. In early disease, these manifestations are rather non-specific (e.g. malaise, nausea, vomiting, fever, arthralgia, purpura, rash). Often, the disease is first detected by high serum/blood urea nitrogen (BUN), oliguria or anuria. There may be hematuria, moderate (selective) proteinuria, and glucosuria. These latter symptoms are seen more commonly with "acute" IN, especially when caused by drug allergy [115]. In methicillin-induced acute IN, linear staining for IgG, C3 and methicillin epitopes is demonstrable with immunofluorescence in the TBM [18]. Antibodies to TBM may be detected in the serum of these patients. Many biopsies from patients with acute interstitial nephritis do not show deposits of any immune reactants. If immunological mechanisms play a role in such nephritides, they would be expected to depend on cell-mediated rather than humoral reactions.

Acute pyelonephritis caused by bacteria is associated with enlarged kidneys and cellular infiltration by polymorphonuclear leucocytes of the edematous interstitium, and frank abscess formation: the "alterative glomerulonephritis" of Kimmelstiel and Wilson [105]. Immunofluorescence is not useful in the diagnosis of this disease.

Chronic IN is often diagnosed only after serum BUN and creatinine have become markedly abnormal. Again, a vast variety of pathogenetic entities are grouped as chronic IN, among them "true" bacterial chronic pyelonephritis, and immunologically mediated nephritides with antibodies to TBM. The cellular infiltrates in chronic IN are often exclusively mononuclear (lymphocytes, macrophages, plasma cells) and the kidney interstitium shows fibrosis, sclerosis and extensive scar formation [226]. As a rule, only glomeruli in the areas of interstitial pathology show marked changes. Similarly, arteries and arterioles in areas of sclerosis may show pathology. Some form of interstitial nephritis may lead to the development of Fanconi's syndrome.

12.4. CLASSIFICATION AND DIAGNOSIS OF RENAL PATHOLOGY BASED ON IMMUNOPATHOLOGICAL MECHANISMS

The classification to be discussed here distinguishes glomerular and tubulointerstitial diseases according to the underlying immunopathological mechanisms [3, 59, 132, 134, 138, 213, 220]. These main categories are subdivided based on evidence for the involvement of immunological mechanisms. The immunologically mediated diseases are further subdivided according to the probable immunopathogenetic mechanisms involved (Table 12.VIII). This classification lists pathoetiological entities (e.g. post-streptococcal GN), clinically and morphologically defined syndromes (e.g. SLE nephritis), and syndromes defined only immunohistologically or histologically (e.g. IgA/IgG nephritis) side by side. Thus it clearly lacks consistency; but with it the attempt has been made to define each disease with as much precision as present knowledge permits. Immunofluorescence has been essential in providing the data which made it possible to understand immunopathogenesis of

TABLE 12.VIII
IMMUNOPATHOLOGICAL CLASSIFICATION OF KIDNEY DISEASES

I. Diseases presumed or known to result from immunological mechanisms
  A. Mediated by antibodies to renal basement membranes
    1. Antiglomerular basement membrane glomerulonephritis
      a) some cases of rapidly progressive glomerulonephritis
      b) Goodpasture's disease
    2. Antitubular basement membrane interstitial nephritis
      a) tubulointerstitial nephritis with immune complex glomerulonephritis
      b) tubulointerstitial nephritis with antiglomerular basement membrane glomerulonephritis
      c) isolated tubulointerstitial nephritis

  B. Mediated by circulating or in situ formed immune complexes
    1. Immune complex-mediated glomerulonephritides
      a) Diseases of known etiology: post-infectious glomerulonephritides:
        i) bacterial
        ii) viral
        iii) parasitic
      b) Diseases of unknown etiology:
        i) associated with systemic diseas
          SLE-nephritis
          nephritis in anaphylactoid purpura
          nephritis in polyarthritis nodosa
          nephritis in idiopathic mixed cryoglobulinemia
        ii) primary renal diseases
          membranous glomerulonephritis
          mesangiocapillary glomerulonephritis
          basement membrane dense deposit disease
          kappa-chain disease
          Berger's disease (IgA/IgG nephropathy)
          IgM nephropathy
          some cases of rapidly progressive glomerulonephritis
          some cases of focal glomerulonephritis
          some cases of chronic sclerosing glomerulonephritis
          histologically undefined immune complex-mediated glomerulonephritis
    2. Immune complex-mediated interstitial nephritides (e.g. SLE interstitial nephritis)

  C. Reagin-mediated hypersensitivity in interstitial nephritides (eosinophilic nephritis)
  D. Cell-mediated pathology

II. Diseases without evidence of involvement of immunological pathogenesis:
  most cases of chronic sclerosing glomerulonephritis
  some cases of focal glomerulonephritis
  minimal glomerular changes (lipoid nephrosis)
  hemolytic-uremic syndrome (HUS)
  diabetic nephropathies
  amyloidosis
  dysproteinemias
  histologically and clinically undefined glomerulopathies

---

kidney diseases. In the following, the main immunopathological mechanisms seen in kidney diseases will be discussed briefly and representative examples will be given.

12.4.1. Kidney diseases involving autoantibodies to renal basement membranes

12.4.1.1. Autoantibodies to GBM

The human counterpart of nephrotoxic serum nephritis and autoantibody-mediated anti-GBM disease in animals [127, 131, 193] was described by Lerner et al. in 1976 [122]. Although only a minor fraction of GN involve autoantibodies to GBM [3, 74, 218], it is important to recognize this mode of immunopathogenesis because of the poor prognosis it entails for the patient. Immunofluorescence tests are essential to distinguish anti-GBM disease from other rapidly progressive GN. The hallmark of glomerulonephritis associated with antibodies to GBM is linear staining of GBM for IgG (Fig. 12.7).

Antibodies to GBM react with the lamina densa as shown by immunoperoxidase electron microscopy [43, 100]. More recently, improved immunofluorescence techniques made it possible to locate the GBM antigen(s) reacting with antibodies in sera from patients with Goodpasture's disease in the inner aspects of the glomerular capillary wall [66]. The moiety reactive with nephrotoxic serum antibodies in experimental anti-GBM disease probably is a glycoprotein [179, 188]; the GBM antigen involved in human anti-GBM

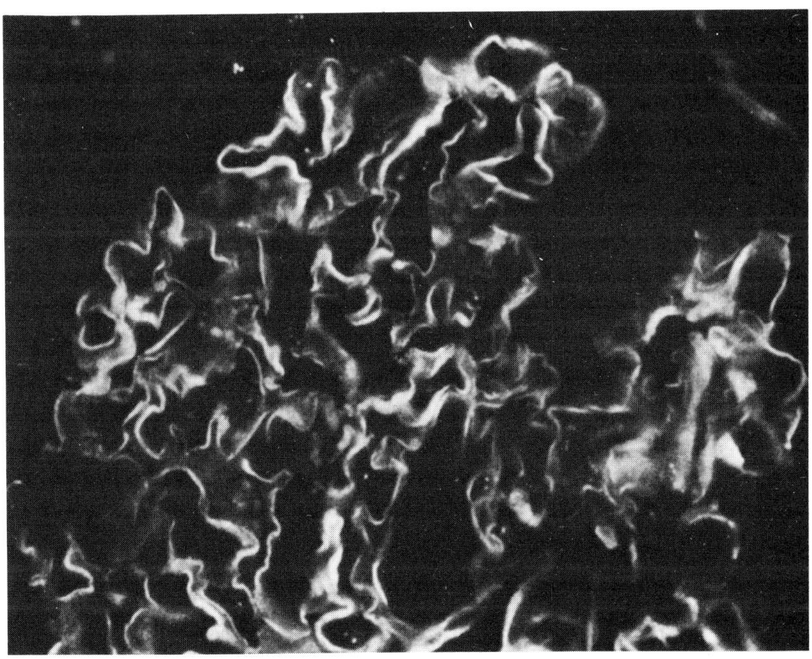

Fig. 12.7. Anti-GBM glomerulonephritis in a human. Staining for human IgG. (Reproduced from Albini et al. [4], with kind permission of the authors and the publisher.) ×400.

nephritis is not yet known. C3 may also be found in the GBM, sometimes in a more granular pattern [74]. Linear, usually rather weak, deposits of IgG may be seen also in diabetes mellitus and early SLE nephritis. In diabetes mellitus it seems well established that this IgG is not specific antibody to GBM. Therefore, elution of antibody from kidney tissue and serological studies to demonstrate circulating antibodies to GBM are sometimes necessary to establish the diagnosis of anti-GBM disease [139].

Eluates or sera may be tested for anti-GBM activity by using indirect immunofluorescence techniques or radioimmunoassays [214]. Although the latter procedure can be exquisitely sensitive, some GBM antigens may be lost during purification procedures for test antigens. In addition to demonstration of circulating and tissue-deposited antibodies to GBM, evaluation of histology is useful. Crescentic (extracapillary) proliferative GN with linear IgG deposits in GBM strongly suggest the diagnosis of anti-GBM disease.

Reactivity of sera and/or eluates with both GBM and alveolar basement membrane (ABM) is consistent with the diagnosis of "Goodpasture's disease" (pulmonary hemorrhage with anti-GBM glomerulonephritis). As pulmonary disease usually precedes, but in rare cases may also follow the kidney pathology, some cases of Goodpasture's disease may be missed on first clinical examination. It is possible that isolated lung anti-basement membrane disease also exists. Thus, a patient with lymphoid interstitial pneumonitis had IgG linear deposits in the alveolar basement membrane but not in kidney basement membranes [216]. In 25–60% of patients with circulating antibodies to GBM there is also reactivity with antigens of the TBM [7]. IgG bound *in vivo* to TBM may be associated with interstitial inflammation and tubular injury [5].

It is important to note that anti-GBM disease is not synonymous with rapidly progressive GN or Goodpasture's syndrome or DEG or crescentic glomerulonephritis. Goodpasture's syndrome may occur in association with immune complex-mediated diseases; the term "Goodpasture's disease" should be reserved for Goodpasture's syndrome associated with antibodies to GBM and ABM. Rapidly progressive GN may be seen in patients with presumably immune complex-mediated pathology, e.g. polyarthritis nodosa, SLE, or in hemolytic uremic syndrome. Alternatively, early lesions of Goodpasture's disease may be focal and segmental and may, therefore, not have the appearance of DEG.

12.4.1.2. Autoantibodies to TBM

In the TBM, linear immune deposits of IgG, often together with C3 (Fig. 12.8) are found in a majority of patients with anti-GBM disease, in some patients with immune complex-mediated glomerulonephritis, in some patients with methicillin- or diphenylhydantoin-induced interstitial nephritis, and in 10–15% of long-surviving kidney allografts [3, 5, 6, 92, 134]. A small number of patients seems to have isolated anti-TBM disease. Eluates and sera of patients with immunoglobulin deposits in TBM show antibody reactivity with TBM,

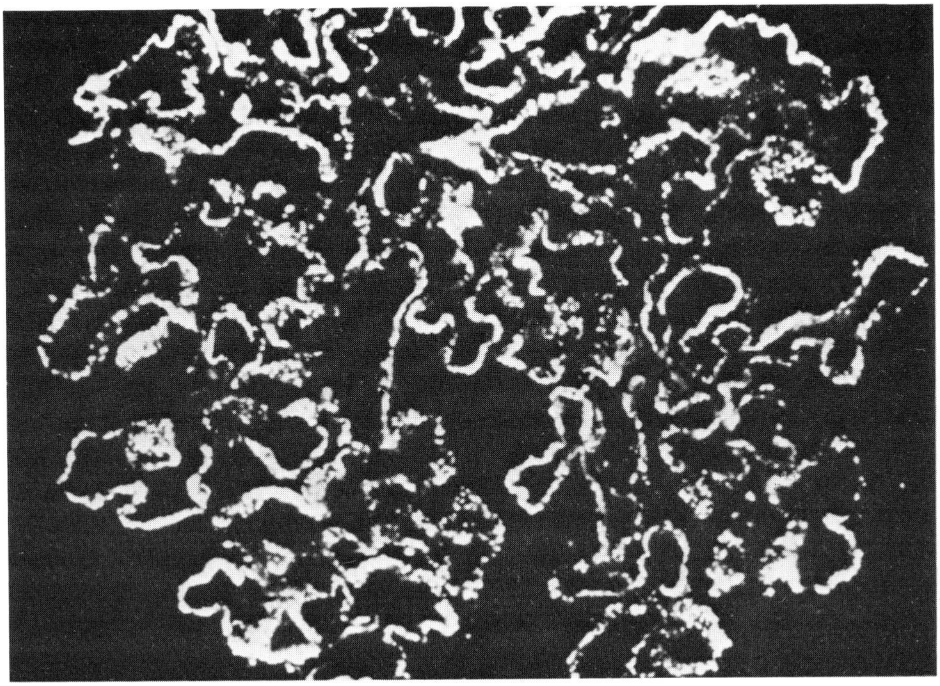

Fig. 12.8. Membranous glomerulonephritis in a human. Staining for human IgG. (Reproduced from Albini et al. [4], with kind permission of the authors and the publisher.) ×350.

usually also with glomerular (GBM) and alveolar basement membranes (ABM). The morphological changes accompanying antibody deposition include extensive infiltration with inflammatory cells of the interstitium, composed first of polymorphonuclear leucocytes but later predominantly of mononuclear cells.

Tissue hemadsorption techniques [187, 202] show predominance of macrophages; some B lymphocytes, but only negligible numbers of T cells, may be seen [198]. At first, there is interstitial edema; progression of the disease leads to fibrosis and sclerosis. Giant cells of the Langerhans type are seen occasionally. Focal proliferative tubulitis, necrotic tubular lesions, and accumulation of cell detritus in distal tubules occur. Tubular dysfunction usually is marked including selective proteinuria, glycosuria, aminoaciduria, and occasionally a full-blown Fanconi's syndrome [3, 133, 134, 159].

Antibodies to TBM seen in patients with allografts may be either autoantibodies or alloantibodies. Rejection phenomena may enhance the formation of antibodies to TBM by liberating TBM antigens.

12.4.2. Kidney diseases involving immune complex deposition of in situ formation

IC-mediated pathogenesis is assumed when immune deposits of immunoglobulin and complement, possibly also of antigen, are demonstrated in a

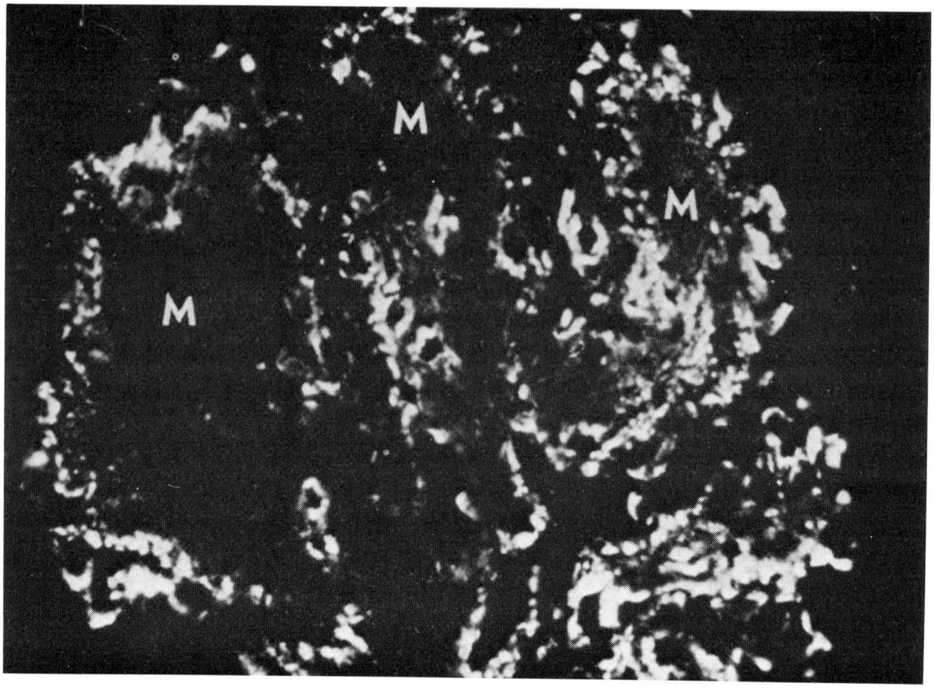

Fig. 12.9. Membranoproliferative glomerulonephritis in a human. Staining for human IgG. (Reproduced from Albini et al. [4], with kind permission of the authors and the publisher.) ×250.

finely granular (Fig. 12.9), lanceolar, interrupted-linear, or ribbon-like pattern, and when ultrastructural analysis shows electron-dense deposits in the same location (see Chapter 15, this volume). Demonstration of decreased complement concentrations in serum, circulating immune complexes, specific antigens in kidney eluates, detection of the same antigen in circulation and at the site of tissue deposition, and positive anti-antibody consumption tests with tissue sections are regarded as corroborative evidence for IC-mediated pathology (see Chapter 15). IC formation or deposition in kidney may lead to glomerulonephritis with or without tubulointerstitial disease. IC-mediated glomerulonephritis may be associated with a variety of different patterns of histopathology.

Among IC-mediated diseases, two distinct groups can be defined [5, 134]. In one, the antigen is definitely or tentatively established. In the other group, the relevant antigen is not known.

12.4.2.1. IC-mediated diseases with definitely or tentatively defined antigens

Tentative identification relies on clinical associations and serological tests (e.g. the presence or rise of concentrations of antibodies to streptolysin). Conclusive proof requires the demonstration of the antigen in the immune deposits in tissue and/or in immune complexes in circulation. Methods available for such demonstrations have been outlined in Chapter 15. Suffice it here to stress again the difficulty in demonstrating antigens as components of immune complexes; antigens may be covered by antibodies and complement, making interaction of antibodies with antigen in the immune complex impossible. In such situations attempts to disperse immune complexes using an excess of an antigen assumed to partake in the immune complex may be of value [160]. Thus, in the one-shot acute serum sickness, antigen may become undetectable as disease progresses and antibody production is intensified. Demonstration of the antigen, bovine serum albumin (BSA) becomes increasingly difficult. Still, dispersion of immune complexes with BSA in excess is possible (Penner, Albini, Andres, and Milgrom, unpublished observations). This is the case also during incipient chronic serum sickness proteinuria, when the immune complexes are formed in antibody excess.

The antigens which may be identified in immune complexes deposited or formed in kidney tissues are listed in Tables 12.IX and 12.X. It is impossible to review adequately all listed antigens here. The following brief discussion attempts to illustrate the involvement of some of the antigens. Detailed accounts are available elsewhere [3, 59, 74, 100, 133, 134, 213, 220].

In post-streptococcal glomerulonephritis, the antigen involved in immune complexes has only been identified tentatively. There is clinical association with preceding streptococcal infection and with raised titers of circulating antibodies to streptococcal products [73]. Some reports have documented streptococcal antigens in immune deposits of the kidney [8]; others were

TABLE 12.IX

EXOGENOUS ANTIGENS INVOLVED IN HUMAN IMMUNE COMPLEX-MEDIATED NEPHRITIDES

Antigen	Clinical condition
Foreign species serum proteins:	Serum sickness
staphylococcus	Infected atrioventricular shunt
pneumococcus	
enterococcus	Subacute bacterial endocarditis
streptococcus	Post-streptococcal glomerulonephritides
Treponema pallidum	Syphilitic glomerulonephritis
hepatitis B antigen	Viral hepatitis
oncornaviruses	Lymphoma, leukemia
measles	Subacute sclerosing panencephalitis
plasmodium malariae	Malaria nephropathy
Only tentatively identified:	
antigens in nephritis associated with:	
leprosy	
bacterial endocarditis	
infectious mononucleosis	
Guillain-Barré syndrome	
schistosomiasis	
filiariasis	
drug hypersensitivity	

TABLE 12.X

ENDOGENOUS (AUTO)ANTIGENS INVOLVED IN HUMAN IMMUNE COMPLEX-MEDIATED NEPHRITIDES

Nuclear components	SLE
Cytoplasmic antigens (e.g. Ro)	Scleroderma
Thyroglobulin	Hashimito's tyroiditis
Renal brush border antigen	Membranous glomerulonephritis
	Sickle cell anemia
	Renal vein thrombois
Carcinoembryonic antigen	Colonic carcinoma
Erythrocyte stromal antigen(s)	Gardner-Diamond syndrome
Immunoglobulin	Mixed cryoglobulinemia
	SLE
	Membranous glomerulonephritis (?)
	Post-streptococcal glomerulonephritis (?)
Only tentatively identified:	
tumor-specific or associated antigens	
histocompatibility antigens	

unable to confirm these observations. This discrepancy may have been caused by the presence of streptococcal antigens in kidney deposits only during the early phase of the disease.

The majority of patients with post-streptococcal glomerulonephritis (PSGN) clinically have acute nephritis with very good prognosis. Histopathology usually reveals diffuse endocapillary proliferative glomerulonephritis (DEPG); in some cases, there is mesangiocapillary glomerulonephritis, and transformation of endocapillary into mesangiocapillary forms has been described [100, 106]. The mesangiocapillary variant shows reduplication of basement membranes and subendothelial deposits. Crescents may also develop. DEG in post-streptococcal disease is associated with a rapidly progressive clinical course. The DMG variants have a less favorable prognosis than the "classical" DEPG. Infrequently, post-streptococcal GN may appear by histology to be indistinguishable from membranous glomerulonephritis.

Immune deposits in tissues are characteristically finely to coarsely granular and encompass IgG, C3 and properdin. Sometimes only C3 deposits are demonstrable [11, 59, 74, 100, 106, 133, 134, 138, 213, 220, 226]. There is mounting evidence that the immune complexes in post-streptococcal GN contain rheumatoid factor-like activity, and that the major antigen involved may be immunoglobulin [136, 137, 160]. Finally, cross-reactions of streptococcal and GBM antigens may be involved in the pathogenesis.

Other post-infectious glomerulonephritides may present focal proliferative, sclerosing, or crescentic lesions in histology. Immune complexes involving microbial or host antigens may participate in the pathogenesis. In some forms no immunoglobulin deposits are detectable.

Autoantigens are involved in the immune complex-mediated glomerulonephritis of SLE. Autoantibodies associated with this disease have a variety of specificities [171] and possibly may be directed to epitopes shared by a number of molecules. DNA and cytoplasmic antigens (e.g. Ro) have been demonstrated in IC deposits in kidneys [6, 113, 114]. Antibodies to immunoglobulin seem to be involved in renal IC deposits [2]. With the great variety of immunohistopathological patterns of glomerulonephritis seen in experimental serum sickness [60, 74], it is not surprising to find a wide variety of histopathological alterations in the kidneys of patients with SLE [3, 46, 100, 106, 134, 163, 226]. The development of specific immunohistopathological forms of SLE nephritis may depend on involvement of specific autoantibodies, characteristics of immune complexes, the status of the reticuloendothelial system, the availability of inflammatory mediators, and other genetic and constitutional factors of the host. Kidney involvement is the second most common manifestation of SLE [61]. It occurs in 50–80% of the patients with SLE [151, 189]. The incidence among glomerulonephritides seen in diagnostic laboratories varies widely with the frequency of SLE in individual patient populations (2–22%) [74, 226]. Although the disease can occur in the newborn and in the aged, its main incidence is seen in the period of 15–40 years of age. There is a marked predominance of female patients (1 : 4 to 1 : 10) [67, 189, 226]. Clinically, patients may show nephrotic syndrome, asymptomatic proteinuria, rapidly progressive renal failure, or acute nephritis syndrome. Analysis by histopathology of kidney biopsies allows for classification into four main groups [3, 46, 162].

A. Minimal SLE nephritis. This rather benign condition is seen infrequently in biopsies because the patients do not have clinical manifestations of kidney disease or have only minimal proteinuria or hematuria. Histopathologically the glomeruli are normal or have a slight increase of mesangial matrix. In immunofluorescence tests, however, granular deposits of IgG and C3 are visible in the glomerular mesangium. Less frequently, finely granular deposits of IgG and C3 may be seen in the GBM. With electron microscopy, electron-dense deposits are seen in the mesangium. In some specimens, there is linear deposition of IgG and C3 in GBM [112], possibly representing interaction of antibodies to basement membranes with kidney components; indeed, this immunological reaction could be the earliest trigger of kidney injury in SLE. The immune deposits are usually present in all glomeruli of a specimen, even in those showing only mild alteration of glomerular structure or appearing normal by light microscopy. Some authors subdivide this group of SLE nephritides into forms with morphologically normal glomeruli and those with "minimal disease" (with or without "segmental lesions").

B. Focal proliferative SLE nephritis. Less than 50% of glomeruli are affected by proliferative, exudative, necrotising, and sclerosing changes. Electron-dense deposits are found predominantly in mesangial areas. GBM may be involved segmentally. In immunofluorescence tests, immunoglobulin and C3 deposits are seen in all glomeruli despite the focal histopathology. Again, they are found predominantly in the mesangium.

C. Severe diffuse proliferative and exudative SLE nephritis (Fig. 12.10). In this condition, more than 50% of glomerular tufts are involved. The glomeruli show a variety of patterns of histopathology. Immunoglobulin and C3 deposits are also seen in a variety of patterns, from linear to granular to lumpy in the GBM, often in the TBM, and in peritubular capillaries [41, 121]. Fibrinoid necrosis, lupus erythematosus cells and hematoxylin bodies may be found, and crescent formation is seen is some patients. Immune deposits in the endothelial space may have wire-loop staining patterns. These deposits may contain a variety of plasma proteins, e.g. fibrinogen, transferrin, and albumin. Immune and electron-dense are seen between proliferating mesangial cells and in the subendothelial and subepithelial spaces in the GBM. Intracapillary precipitates – the "hyaline thrombi" – consist of plasma proteins, and contain usually IgG and IgM but no fibrinogen. Some authors subdivide this group of SLE nephritides into those with mesangiocapillary lesions and those showing endotheliomesangial glomerulonephritis [226]. Some patients with this type of SLE nephritis develop crescents in glomeruli.

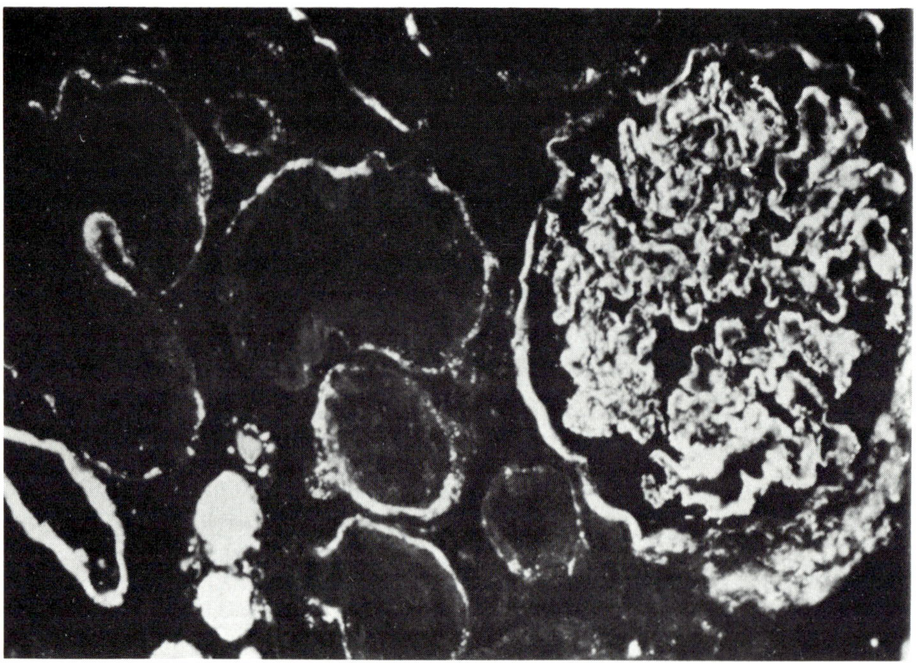

Fig. 12.10. Proliferative glomerulonephritis in a patient with systemic lupus erythematosus (SLE). Granular immune deposits of human IgG in the GBM, Bowman's capsule and in the TBM (×400). (Reproduced Albini et al. [4] with kind permission of the author and the publisher.) ×250.

D. Membranous SLE nephropathy. This category allegedly is associated with the most pronounced depression of circulating C3 in SLE. There is a global but somewhat irregular thickening of GBM. Electron microscopy reveals diffuse subepithelial deposits with little mesangial involvement. Immunofluorescence tests show diffuse granular deposits of immunoglobulins in the GBM. Wire-loop lesions are unusual in this group.

The evaluation of kidney biopsies from SLE patients should concentrate on the determination of the disease activity (Table 12.XI). Proliferative lesions have a more fulminant course and a poorer prognosis, and intensive anti-inflammatory and aggressive immunosuppressive therapy is required to stop the progress of disease [161]. Minimal change glomerulonephritis (see above) and membranous glomerulonephritis (see above), on the other hand, have a more favorable prognosis and probably should be treated much more cautiously, almost exclusively with anti-inflammatory drugs. In all types of SLE glomerulonephritis, C1q, C4, C3 and properdin deposits are present and indicate activation of both the alternative and the classical pathway of complement activation. As mentioned above, in addition to the obligatory IgG, IgA, IgM, and, rarely, IgE, DNA can be demonstrated in the immune deposits of the majority of diseased kidneys [6].

TABLE 12.XI

ASSAYS USED IN MONITORING THE IMMUNOLOGICAL ACTIVITY OF SYSTEMIC LUPUS ERYTHEMATOSUS

Kidney immunohistology: extent and pattern of immune deposits
Kidney histology: membranous versus proliferative, diffuse versus focal lesions
Serum antibodies to double-stranded DNA
Serum complement concentrations
Determination of circulating immune complexes (see Chapter 15)
Excretion of immune reactants and inflammatory mediators (immunoglobulin light chains, complement, fibrin degradation products)

Tubulointerstitial nephritis in SLE is seen in an appreciable number of patients [41, 121]. It is characterized by finely to coarsely granular deposits of immunoglobulin and complement in the TBM and in peritubular capillaries (Fig. 12.10). The extensive cellular infiltrates usually are composed of small mononuclear cells. In hemadsorption studies on renal tissue, the infiltrating cells do not react with EA, EAC, nor anti-thymocyte serum [198].

12.4.2.2. IC-mediated kidney diseases with unknown antigens

In this group of IC-mediated GN, those associated with deposition of IgA are of special interest. IgA–IgG nephritis or "Berger's disease" [29] is diagnosed only on the basis of immunofluorescence tests. IgA, IgG, and C3 are seen in the mesangium (Fig. 12.11). The GBM is involved to a much lesser degree. FAA are found only rarely. Occasionally, only IgA is detectable.

Electron microscopy shows mesangial electron-dense deposits and minor subendothelial changes. Clinically, there is an association with upper respiratory tract infections, and the major manifestation of this disease is repeated episodes of hematuria. The majority of patients have a rather benign disease. Others, however, progress to renal failure, and the disease may recur in kidney allografts [30].

The kidney lesion seen in roughly 50% of patients with Henoch–Schönlein's purpura also shows predominantly mesangial deposition of IgA, IgG, and C3. Immune deposits are found less frequently in the GBM. The disease may be focal or diffuse, with cell proliferation and splitting of GBM. Crescent formation as well as glomerulosclerosis accompany an increase in mesangial matrix and cellularity found in many patients. Fibrin can often be demonstrated in electron microscopy; mesangial FAA is the only antigen detectable by immunofluorescence tests early in the disease. Presence of properdin deposits indicates alternative pathway complement activation.

A similar histopathology and immunohistopathology may also be seen in mild cases of SLE nephritis. Although Henoch–Schönlein's purpura is more often associated with fibrin deposits than Berger's disease, differential diagnosis among the three diseases often must rely on integration of immunohistological data with clinical evaluation.

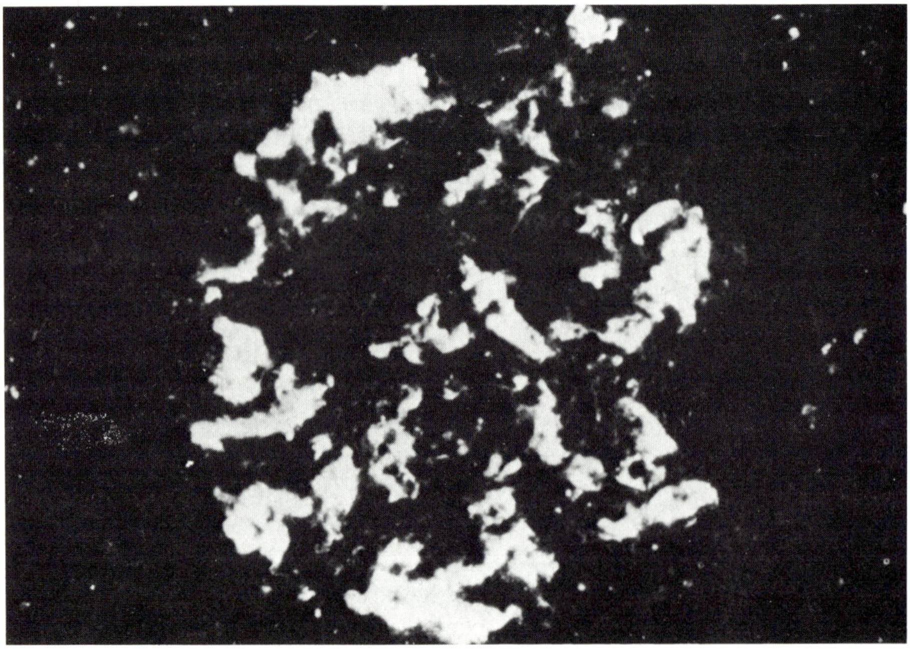

Fig. 12.11. Berger's glomerulonephritis. Mesangial IgA deposits (×400). (Reproduced from Albini et al. [4], with kind permission of the author and the publisher.) ×250.

12.4.3. Cell-mediated immunity

Cell-mediated immunity and delayed hypersensitivity have for long fascinated those doing research in kidney immunopathology [204]. Involvement of cell-mediated immunity in kidney diseases of man, however, has not been unequivocally demonstrated except in classical allograft rejection reactions.

12.4.4. Reaginic hypersensitivity

Participation of IgE-mediated hypersensitivity may be suggested in some kidney diseases by the presence of basophilic and eosinophilic granulocytes in the interstitium of the biopsy or autopsy tissue. Demonstration of IgE antibody in the lesions is severely hampered by the transitory nature of anaphylactic phenomena and by the non-specific staining of eosinophils and basophils with fluorochrome-conjugated antiserum preparations [6, 11]. Acute eosinophilic rheumatoid nephritis has been documented in a few patients with ascariasis, drug allergy, and dermatitis herpetiformia Duhring [224]. The concept of an "asthma of the nephron", although interesting, still remains a hypothesis.

12.5. SUMMARY

Immunofluorescence and other immunohistological procedures are essential for the analysis of the etiopathogenesis and classification of a vast variety of kidney diseases. In some forms of glomerulonephritis and interstitial nephritis in which immune mechanisms are involved immunofluorescence tests make it possible to identify the antibody specificity and/or antigens involved. Furthermore, documentation of the pattern of immune deposits, detection of inflammatory mediators (e.g. complement, FAA), delineation of subpopulations of mononuclear cells in infiltrates, and appreciation of changes in tissue structures in the wake of deposition of immune reactants all contribute to our understanding of pathogenetic mechanisms. Results obtained by immunofluorescence procedures may permit the definition of nosological entities according to immunopathogenesis or pathoetiology. Finally, immunofluorescence techniques are indispensable in the diagnostic interpretation of biopsy material and sometimes useful in evaluation of therapy and prognosis.

ACKNOWLEDGEMENTS

We thank Dr. G.A. Andres for helpful discussions, Miss Philippa George for excellent secretarial help, and Miss Carol Soroka and Miss Ingrid Glurich for assistance in compiling the references.

REFERENCES

1 Abrams, E., Forland, M. and Spargo, B.H. (1968) Clinical-pathologic correlations in idiopathic nephritis syndrome with glomerular membrane change. Lab. Invest. *18,* 317.

2 Agnello, V., Koffler, D., Eisenberg, J.W., Winchester, R.J. and Kunkel, H.G. (1971) C1q precipitins in the sera of patients with systemic lupus erythematosus and other lypocomplementemic states: characterization of high and low molecular weight types. J. Exp. Med. *134,* 228-241s.

3 Albini, B., Brentjens, J.R. and Andres, G.A. (1979) Immunopathology of the Kidney (Arnold, London).

4 Albini, B., Brentjens, J., Olson, K., Ossi, E. and Andres, G.A. (1979) Studies on the immune response of rabbits and chickens with chronic serum sickness (CSS). *In* Milgrom, F. and Albini, B. (eds.), Immunopathology (Karger, Basel) pp. 207-211.

5 Andres, G.A. and McCluskey, R.T. (1975) Tubular and intestinal renal diseases due to immunologic mechanisms. Kidney Int. *7,* 271–289.

6 Andres, G.A. Albini, B and Ossi, E. (1978) Interstitial renal inflammation. *In* Fogarty Intern. Center Series on Prev. Med. *Vol. 5,* pp. 251–262.

7 Andres, G.A., Elwood, C.M. and McCluskey, R.T. (1978) Rapidly progressive glomerulonephritis (RPGN). *In* McCluskey, R.T. and Andres, G.A. (eds.), Immunology Mediated Renal Disease (Dekker, New York), pp. 63–69.

8 Andres, G.A., Accinni, L., Hsu, K.C., Zabriskie, J.B. and Seegal, B.C. (1966) Electron microscopic studies of human glomerulonephritis with ferritan-conjugated antibody. Localization of antigen-antibody complexes in glomerular structures of patients with acute glomerulonephritis. J.Exp. Med. *123,* 339-412.

9 Andres, G., Accinni, L., Beiser, S., Christian, C., Cinotti, C., Erlanger, B., Hsu, K. and Seegal, B.C. (1970) Localization of fluorescence-labeled antinucleoside antibodies in glomeruli of patients with active systemic lupus erythematosus nephritis. J. Clin. Invest. *49.* 2106-2108.

10 Andres, G.A., Accinni, L., Hsu, K.C., Penn, I., Porter, K.A., Randall, J.M., Seegal, B.C. and Starzl, T.E. (1970) Human renal transplants. III. Immunopathologic studies. Lab. Invest. *22,* 588–604.

11 Andres, G.A., Albini, B., Brentjens, J., Milgrom, M., Noble, B., Ossi, E. and Szymanski, C. (1979) Immunologically mediated tubulointestinal nephritis in experimental animals and in man. *In* Milgrom, F. and Albini, B. (eds.), Immunopathology (Karger, Basel) pp. 123–126.

12 Antoine, B. and Faye, C. (1972) The clinical course associated with dense deposits in the kidney basement membrane. Kidney Int. *1,* 420-427.

13 Arieff, A.I. (1980) Rapidly progressive glomerulonephritis. *In* Stein, J.H. (ed.), Nephrology (Grune and Stratton, New York) pp. 302–305.

14 Arisz, L., Brentjens, J.R.H., Vastenburg, G., Van der Hem, G.K., Hoedemaeker, P.J., Arends, A. and Mandema, E. (1976) Neth. J. Med At the 25th Anniversary of the percutaneous renal biopsy: The state of the art. *19,* 29–40.

15 Arisz, L., Noble, B., Milgrom, M., Brentjens, J.R. and Andres, G.A. (1979) Experimental chronic sterum sickness in rats. A model of immune complex glomerulonephritis and systemic immune complex deposition. Int. Arch. Allergy *60,* 80–88.

16 Asamar, H., Dittrich, P. and Lederer, B. (1969) Die Bedeutung immunohistologischer Befunde für die nephrologische Diagnostik. Klin. Wochenschr. *47,* 759–771.

17 Baldwin, D.S. (1977) Poststreptococcal glomerulonephritis. A progressive disease? Am. J. Med. *62,* 1–1.

18 Baldwin, D.S., Levine, B.B., McCluskey, R.T. and Gallo, G.R. (1968) Renal failure and intestinal nephritis due to penicillin and methicillin. N. Engl. J. Med. *279,* 1245–1252.

19 Baldwin, D.S., Gluck, M.C., Schacht, R.G., Moussalli, A. and Gallo, G.R. (1973) Long term follow-up of poststreptococcal glomerulonephritis. *In* Kincaide-Smith, P., Mathew, T.H. and Lovell-Becker, E. (eds.), Glomerulonephritis (Wiley, New York) pp. 327–344.

20 Bannayan, G.A. (1980) Electron microscopy. *In* Stein, J.H. (ed.), Nephrology (Grune and Stratton, New York) pp. 117–123.

21 Banowsky, L.H. and Chauvenet, P.C. (1980) Renal transplantation. *In* Stein, J.H. (ed.), Nephrology (Grune and Stratton, New York) pp. 426–444.

22 Barbanel, T. and Noel, L-H. (1979) Membraneous glomerulonephritis. *In* Hamburger, J., Crosnier, J. and Grunfeld, J.-P. (eds.), Nephrology (Wiley-Flammarion, New York) pp. 489–505.

23 Barbino di Belgiojoso, G., Tarantino, A., Bazzi, C., Colosanti, G., Guerra, L. and Durante, A. (1976) Immunofluorescence patterns in chronic membranoproliferative glomerulonephritis (MPGN). Clin. Nephrol. *6,* 303.

24 Bariety, J., Druet, P., Loirat, P. and Lagrue, G. (1970) Les glomérulonéphrites pariétoprolifératives. Etude histopathologique en microscopie optique, électronique et en immunohistochimie de 49 cas. Pathol. Biol. *19,* 259–283.

25 Beirne, G.J. and Brennan, J.T. (1972) Glomerulonephritis associated with hydrocarbon solvents mediated by antiglomerular basement membrane antibody. Arch. Environ. Health *25,* 365–369.

26 Bell, E.T. (1950) Renal Diseases, 2nd ed. (Lea and Febiger, Philadelphia).

27 Beregi, E. and Varga, I. (1974) Analysis of 260 cases of membranous glomerulonephritis in renal biopsy material. Clin. Nephrol. *2,* 215–221.

28 Beregi, E., Homvas, A. and Renyi-Vamos, F. (1974) Immunohistological studies in chronic pyelonephritis. Clin. Nephrol. *2,* 113–115.

29 Berger, J. (1969) IgA glomerular deposits in renal diseases. Transplant. Proc. *1,* 939–944.

30 Berger, J. (1975) Recurrence of mesangial deposits of IgA after renal transplantation. Kidney Int. *7,* 232–241.

31 Berger, J., Yaneva, H. and Hinglais, N. (1971) Immunohistochemistry of glomerulonephritis. Adv. Nephrol. *1,* 11–30.

32 Bernard, D., Bariety, J., Druet, P., Balafrey, L., Hirbec, G. and Lagrue, G. (1974) Les glomérulonéphrites prolifératives intracapillaires. Sem. Hôp. *50,* 539–545.

33 Beutner, E.H. and Nisengard, R.J. (1973) Defined immunofluorescence and clinical immunopathology. *In* Beutner, E.N., Chorzelski, T., Bean, S.F. and Jordon, R.E. (eds.), Immunopathology of the Skin (Dowden, Hutchins and Ross, Stroudsbury) pp. 197–247.

34 Bhan, A.K., Reinherz, E.L., Poppema, S., McCluskey, R.T. and Schlossman, S.F. (1980) Location of T cell and major histocompatibility complex antigen in the human thymus. J. Exp. Med. *152,* 771–782.

35 Bohle, A. (1976) Pathologische Anatomie der Glomerulonephritiden. *In* Sarre (ed.), Nierenkrankheiten, 4th ed. (Thieme, Stuttgart) pp. 239–248.

36 Bohle, A., Gaertner, H.D., Fischbach, H., Bock, K.E., Edel, H.H., Froetscher, U., Kluthe, R., Moeninghoff, W. and Scheler, F. (1974) The morphological and clinical features of membranoproliferative glomerulonephritis in adults. Virchows Arch. *363,* 213–224.

37 Bohle, A., Eichenseher, N., Fischbach, H., Neild, G.H., Wehner, H., Edel, H.H., Losse, H., Renner, E., Reichel, W. and Schuetterle, L.E. (1976) The different forms of glomerulonephritis: morphologic and clinical aspects, analyzed in 2,500 patients. Klin. Wochenschr. *54.* 59–73.

38 Border, W.A., Lehman, D.H. Egan, J.D., Sass, H.J., Glode, J.E. and Wilson, C.B. (1974) Antitubular basement membrane antibodies in methicillin-accociated interstitial nephritis. N. Engl. J. Med. *291,* 381–384.

39 Bourgoigne, J.J. and Jacob, A.I. (1980) Chronic renal failure – classification. *In* Stein, J.H. (ed.), Nephrology (Grune and Stratton, New York) pp. 172–174.

40 Brenner, B.N. and Rector, R.C. (1976) The Kidney (Saunders, Philadelphia).

41 Brentjens, J.R., Sepulveda, M., Baliah, T., Bentzel, C., Erlanger, B.F., Elwood, C., Montes, M., Hsu, K.C. and Andres, G.A. (1975) Interstitial immune complex nephritis in patients with systemic lupus erythematosus. Kidney Int. *7,* 342–350.

42 Burkholder, P.M., Hyman, L.R. and Krueger, R.P. (1973) Classification of mixed membranous and proliferative glomerulonephritis: Recognition of three varieties. *In:* Kincaide-Smith, P., Mathew, T.H. and Lovell-Becker, E. (eds.), Glomerulonephritis (Wiley, New York) pp. 557–590.

43 Burns. J. and MacIver, A.G. (1961) Immuno-electron microscopy of the glomerular basement membrane in Goodpasture's syndrome. Rev. Eur. Etud. Clin. Biol. *16,* 48–50.

44 Cameron, J.S. (1972) A natural history of glomerulonephritis. *In* Black, D. (ed.), Renal Disease, 3rd ed. (Blackwell Scientific Publications, Oxford) pp. 295–330.

45 Cameron, J.S. (1973) A clinician's view of the classification of glomerulonephritis. *In* Kincaide-Smith, P., Mathew, T.J. and Lovell-Becker, E. (eds.), Glomerulonephritis (Wiley, New York) pp. 63-69.

46 Cameron, J.S. (1979) The nephritis of systemic lupus erythematosus. *In* Kincaide-Smith, P., D'Apice, A.J.F. and Atkins, R.C. (eds.), Progress in Glomerulonephritis (Wiley, New York) pp. 387–423.

47 Cameron, J.S. and Brown, C.B. (1970) The investigation and management of acute uremia. *In* Hamburger, J., Crosnier, J. and Grunfeld, J.P. (eds.), Nephrology (Wiley-Flammarion, New York) pp. 255–280.

48 Cammisuli, S. and Wofsy, L. (1976) Hapten-sandwich labelling. III. Bifunctional reagents for immunospecific labelling of cell surface antigens. J. Immunol. *117,* 1695–1704.

49 Christensen, T., Johansson, B.G. and Kronwall, G. (1976) Interaction of streptococci with the Fc fragment of IgG. Acta. Pathol. Microbiol. Scand. *C84,* 73–76.

50 Churg, J. and Duffy, J.L. (1973) Classification of glomerulonephritis based on morphology. *In* Kincaide-Smith, P., Mathew, T.J. and Lovell-Becker, E. (eds.), Glomerulonephritis (Wiley, New York) pp. 43–46.

51 Churg, J. and Ehrenreich, T. (1973) Membranous nephritis. *In* Kincaide-Smith, P., Mathew, T.H. and Lovell-Becker, E. (eds.), Glomerulonephritis (Wiley, New York) pp. 443–448.

52 Churg, J. and Grishman, E. (1975) Ultrastructure of glomerular disease: a review. Kidney Int. *7,* 254–261.

53 Cruickshank, B. and Hill, A.G.S. (1953) Histochemical identification of connective tissue antigens in rat. Pathol. Bacteriol. *66,* 283–289.

54 Curran, R.C. and Gregory, J. (1977) The unmasking of antigens in paraffin sections of tissue by trypsin. Experientia *33,* 1400–1401.

55 Dart, R.A., Deodhar, S.D., McCormack, L.J. and Vidt, D.J. (1972) Clinical immunopathologic studies in rapidly progressive glomerulonephritis (17 cases). Lab. Invest. *26,* 474.

56 Davies, D.R., Tighe, J.R., Wing, A.J. and Jones, N.F. (1977) Immunoglobulin deposits in membranous glomerulonephritis: immunofluorescence and immunoelectron microscopy findings. Histopathology *1,* 39–52.

57 Denk, H., Syre, G. and Weirich, E. (1977) Immunomorphologic methods in routine pathology. Application of immunofluorescence and the unlabelled antibody enzyme technique to formalin fixed paraffin embedded kidney biopsies. Beitr. Pathol. *160,* 187–194.

58 Dixon, F.J. (1968) The pathogenesis of glomerulonephritis. Am. J. Med. *44,* 493–498.

59 Dixon, F.J. (1979) Immunological renal injury produced by deposition of immune-complexes. *In* Milgrom, F. and Albini, B. (eds.), Immunopathology (Karger, Basel) pp. 117–122.

60 Dixon, F.J., Feldman, J.D. Land Vazquez, J.J. (1961) Experimental glomerulonephritis. The pathogenesis of a laboratory model resembling the spectrum of human glomerulonephritis. J. Exp. Med *113,* 899–920.

61 Dubois, E.L. (1974) Lupus erythematosus, 2nd ed. (University of California Press, Los Angeles, CA).

62 Duffy, J.L., Letteri, J., Cinque, T., Hsu, P.P., Molho, L. and Churg, J. Renal vein thrombosis and the nephrotic syndrome. Am J. Med. *54,* 663–672.

63 Earle, D.P. and Jennings, R.B. (1967) Glomerulonephritis. Prog. 3rd Int. Congr. Nephrol., Washington, 1966, *Vol. III* (Karger, Basel) p. 51.

64 Ehrenreich, T. and Churg, J. (1968) Pathology of membranous nephropathy. *In* Sommers, S.C. (ed.), Pathology Annual, *Vol. 3* (Appleton-Century-Crofts, New York) pp. 145–150.

65 Erwin, D.T., Donadio, J.V. and Holley, K.E. (1973) The clinical course of idiopathic membranous nephropathy. Mayo Clinic Proc. *48,* 697–712.

66 Fish, A.J., Sarmody, K.M. and Michael, A.F. (1979) Spatial orientation and distribution of antigens within human glomerular basement membranes. J. Lab. Clin. Med. *94,* 447–457.

67 Fish, A.J., Blau, E.D., Welstberg, N.G., Burke., Vernier, R.L. and Michael, A.F. (1977) Systemic lupus erythematosis within the first two decades of life. Am. J. Med. *62,* 99–117.
68 Forland, M. (1980) Renal biopsy. *In* Stein, J.H. (ed.), Nephrology (Grune and Stratton, New York) pp. 106–107.
69 Forland, M. (1980) Nephrotic syndrome. *In* Stein, J.H. (ed.), Nephrology (Grune and Stratton, New York) pp. 147–158.
70 Galle, P. and Mahieu, P. (1975) Electron dense alteration of kidney basement membranes. A renal lesion specific of a systemic disease. Am. J. Med. *58,* 749–764.
71 Gallo, G.R., Feiner, H.D., Katz, L.A., Feldman, G.M., Correa, E.B., Chuba, J.V. and Buxbaum, J.N. (1980) Nodular glomerulopathy associated with non-amyloidotic kappa chain deposits and excess immunoglobulin light chain synthesis. Am. J. Pathol. *99,* 621–632.
72 Ganter, P. and Berger, J. (1963) Nephropathy associating proliferative glomerulonephritis with deposits in the basal membranes. II. Histochemical studies of three cases. Nephrology *69,* 96–98.
73 Garovoy, M.R. and Strom, T.B. (1980) Poststreptococcal glomerulonephritis. *In* Stein, J.H. (ed.), Nephrology (Grune and Stratton, New York) pp. 288–292.
74 Germuth, F.G., Jr. and Rodriguez, E. (1973) Immunopathology of the Renal Glomerulus (Little, Brown and Co., Boston).
75 Germuth, F.G., Jr., Taylor, J.J., Siddiqui, S.Y. and Rodriguez, E. (1977) Immune complex disease. VI. Some determinants of the variation of glomerular lesions in the chronic bovine serum albumin-rabbit system. Lab. Invest. *37,* 162–169.
76 Gitlin, D., Craig, J.M. and Janeway, C.A. (1957) Studies on the nature of fibrinoid in the collagen diseases. Am. J. Pathol. *33,* 55–78.
77 Glassock, R.J. and Bennett, C.M. (1976) The glomerulopathies. *In* Brenner, B.M. and Rector, F.C. (eds.), The Kidney (Saunders, Philadelphia) pp. 941–1078.
78 Glassock, R.J., Abrass, C.K. and Border, W.A. (1979) Immunologic mechanism and circulating immune complexes in glomerulonephritis. *In* Kincaide-Smith, P., D'Apice, A.J.F. and Atkins, R.C. (eds.), Progress in Glomerulonephritis (Wiley, New York) pp. 27–50.
79 Gloor, F. (1966) Pathologische Anatomie der Pyelonephritis. *In* Losse, H. and Kienitz, M. (eds.), Pyelonephritis (Thieme, Stuttgart) pp. 56–61.
80 Goldwasser, R. and Shepard, C.C. (1959) Fluorescent antibody methods in the differentiation of murine and epidemic typhus sera: specificity changes resulting from previous immunization. J. Immunol. *82,* 373–380.
81 Grishman, E., Churg, J. and Parish, J.G. (1976) Glomerular morphology in nephritic heroin addicts. Lab. Invest. *35,* 415–424.
82 Grunfeld, J.-P. (1979) Chronic renal failure – general remarks . *In* Hamburger, J., Crosnier, J. and Grunfeld, J.-P. (eds.), Nephrology (Wiley-Flammarion, New York) pp. 283–288.
83 Habib, R. (1970) Classifications anatomique des néphrologies glomérulaires. Paediatr. Fortbildungskurse *28,* 327.
84 Habib, R. (1973) Classification of glomerulonephritis based on morphology. *In* Kincaide-Smith, P., Mathew, T.H. and Lovell-Becker, E. (eds.), Glomerular Nephritis (Wiley, New York) pp. 17–42.
85 Habib, R. and Levy, M. (1979) Contribution of immunofluorescence microscopy to classification of glomerular disease. *In* Kincaide-Smtih, P., D'Apice, A.J.F. and Atkins, R.C. (eds.), Progress in Glomerular Nephritis (Wiley, New York) pp. 119–144.
86 Habib, R., Kleinknecht, C. and Royer, P. (1971) Le syndrome néphrotique primitif de l'enfant. Classification et étude anatomo-clinique de 406 observations. Arch. Franc. Pédiat. 28, 277–319.
87 Habib, R., Kleinknecht, T., Gubler, M.C. and Levy, M. (1973) Idiopathic membrane proliferative glomerulonephritis in children. Report of 105 cases. Clin. Nephrol. *1,* 194–214.
88 Habib, R., Kleinknecht, T., Gubler, M.C. and Maiz, H.B. (1973) Idiopathic membranoproliferative glomerulonephritis: Morphology and natural history. *In* Kincaide-Smith, P., Mathew, T.H. and Lovell-Becker, E. (eds.), Glomerular Nephritis (Wiley, New York) pp. 491–514.

89 Habib, R., Gubler, M.C., Loirat, C., Maiz, H.B. and Levy, M. (1975) Dense deposit disease. A variant of glomerulonephritis. Kidney Int. *7,* 204–215.

90 Hadley, W.K. and Rosenau, W. (1967) Study of human renal disease by immunofluorescent methods. Arch. Pathol. *A3,* 342–351.

91 Hamburger, J. (1979) Pathogenesis. *In* Hamburger, H., Crosnier, J. and Grunfeld, J.-P. (eds.), Nephrology (Wiley-Flammarion, New York) pp. 543–552.

92 Hamburger, J., Hinglais, N. and De Montera, H. (1971) Renal biopsy in 1,000 cases of chronic glomerular disease. *In* Lovell-Becker, E., Heinemann, and Sherman (eds.), Nephrology, Cornell Seminars (Williams and Wilkins, Baltimore) pp. 63–71.

93 Hamburger, J., Crosnier, J., Dormont, J. and Bach, J.F. (1972) Renal Transplantation. (Williams and Wilkins, Baltimore).

94 Hamperl, H. (1934) Die Fluorescenzmikroskopie menschlicher Gewebe. Virchows Arch. 292, 1–51.

95 Heggeness, M.H. and Ash, J.F. (1977) Use of the avidin-biotin complex for the localization of actin and myosin with fluorescence microscopy. J. Cell Biol. *73,* 783–788.

96 Heptingstall, R.H. (1966) Pathology of the Kidney (Churchill-Livingston, London).

97 Herf, S., Pohl, S.L., Sturgill, B. and Bolton, N.K. (1979) An evaluation of diabetic and pseudodiabetic glomerulosclerosis. Am J. Med. *66,* 1040–1050.

98 Huang, F. and Kallant, N. (1968) Isolation and characterization of antigenic compounds of rat glomerular basement membrane. Can J. Biochem. *46,* 1523–1532.

99 Humair, L. (1972) Bases immunologiques des néphropathies glomérulaires. Helv. Med. Acta *36* (Suppl. 52), 1–75.

100 Jenis, E.H. and Lowenthal, D.T. (1977) Kidney Biopsy Interpretation (Davis Co., Philadelphia).

101 Jenis, E.H., Teichman, S., Briggs, W.A., Sandler, P., Hollerman, C.E., Calcagno, P.L., Knieser, M.R., Jensen, G.E. and Valeski, J.E. (1974) Fal segmental glomerulonesclerosis. Am. J. Med. *57,* 695–705.

102 Kaplan, M.H., coons, A.H. and Wendler, D.H. (1950) Localization of antigen in tissue cells; cellular distribution of pneumococcal polysaccharides types II and III in the mouse. J. Exp. Med. *91,* 15–30.

103 Kark, R.M. (1968) Renal biopsy. J. Am. Med. Assoc. *205,* 220–226.

104 Kilcoyne, M.M., Daly, J.J., Gocke, D.J., Thomson, C.E., Meltzer, J., Hsu, K.C. and Tannenbaum, M. (1972) Nephrotic syndrome in heroin addicts, Lancet *1,* 17–20.

105 Kimmelstiel, P. and Wilson, C. (1936) Inflammatory lesions in the glomeruli in pyelonephritis in relation to hypertension and renal insufficiency. Am. J. Pathol. *12,* 99–106.

106 Kincaide-Smith, P. (1975) The Kidney (Blackwell Scientific Publishers, Oxford).

107 Kincaide-Smith, P., and Hobbs, J.D. (1972) Glomerulonephritis. A classification based on morphology. Med. J. Aust. *2,* 1397–1401.

108 Klassen, J. (1979) Tubular and interstitial renal disease due to immune complexes. *In* Milgrom, F. and Albini, B. (eds.), Immunopathology (Karger, Basel) pp. 132–137.

109 Klassen, J., Elwood, C., Grossberg, A.L., Milgrom, F., Montes, M., Sepulveda, M. and Andres, G.A. (1974) Evolution of membranous nephropathy into anti-glomerular-basement membrane glomerulonephritis. N. Engl. J. Med. *290,* 1340–1344.

110 Kleinknecht, C. and Gubler, M.C. (1979) Nephrosis. *In* Hamburger, H., Crosnier, J. and Grunfeld, J.P. (eds.), Nephrology (Wiley-Flammarion, New York) pp. 433–454.

111 Kobayashi, N. (1966) An immunohistological study on renal biopsies of children. Arch. Dis. Child. *41,* 477–488.

112 Koffler, D., Agnello, V. and Kunkel, H. (1969) Variable patterns of immunoglobulin and complement dependent and the kidneys of patients with systemic lupus erythematosus. Am. J. Pathol. *56,* 305–316.

113 Koffler, D., Agnello, V. and Kunkel, H. (1974) Polynucleotide immune complexes in serum and glomerular of patients with systemic lupus erythematosus. Am. J. Pathol. *74,* 109–124.

114 Kreshnan, C. and Kaplan, M.H. (1967) Immunopathologic studies of systemic lupus erythematosus. II. Antinuclear reaction of γ-globulin eluted from homogenates and isolated

glomerular of kidneys from patients with lupun nephritis. J. Clin. Invest. *46,* 569–579.

115 Krumlowsky, F.A., Greco, F., Herdson, P.B. and Lazar, P. (1974) Renal disease associated with toxic eyidemal necrolysis (Lyell's disease). Am. J. Med. *57,* 817–825.

116 Lalli, A.F. (1969) Medullary sponge kidney disease. Radiology *92,* 92–96.

117 Lambert, P.P. (1979) Major syndromes. *In* Hamburger, J., Cromer, J. and Grunfeld, J.P. (eds.), Nephrology (Wiley-Flammarion, New York) pp. 157–183.

118 Lamîere, N. (1980) Toxic nephropathy. *In* Stein, J. (ed.), Nephrology (Grune and Stratton, New York) pp. 361–367.

119 Lamm, M.E., Koo. G.C., Stockpole, C.W. and Hammerling, V. (1972) Hapten-conjugated antibodies and visual markers used to label cell-surface antigens for electron microscopy: an approach to double labelling. Proc. Natl. Acad. Sci. U.S.A. *69,* 2732–3736.

120 Lange, K. and Treser, G. (1973) Editorial: acute poststreptococcal glomerulonephritis. Mechanisms and sequelae. Clin. Nephrol. *1,* 55–62.

121 Lehman, D.H., Wilson, C.B. and Dixon, F.J. (1975) Extraglomerular immunoglobulin deposits in human rephritis. Am J. Med. *58,* 765–786.

122. Lerner, R.A., Glassock, R.J. and Dixon, F.J. (1967) The role of anti-glomerular basement membrane antibody in the pathogenesis of human glomerulonephritis. J. Exp. Med. *126,* 989–1004.

123 Levinsky, N.G. and Alexander, E.A. (1976) Acute renal failure. *In* Brenner, B.M. and Rector, F.C. (eds.), The Kidney (Saunders, Co., Philadelphia) pp. 806–837.

124 Levy, M., Gubler, M.C. and Habib, R. (1979) New concepts on membranoproliferative glomerulonephritis. *In* Kincaide-Smith, P., d'Apice and Atkins (eds.), Progress in Glomerulonephritis (Wiley, New York) pp. 177–208.

125 Lewis, E.J., Cavallo, T., Herrington, J.T. and Cotran, R.S. (1971) An immunopathologic study of rapidly progressive glomerulonephritis in the adult. Hum. Pathol. *2,* 185–208.

126 Lindeman, R.D. (1974) Percutaneous renal biopsy. Kidney *7,* 1–5.

127 Lindemann, W. (1900) sur le mode d'action de certains poisons renaux. Ann. Inst. Pasteur *13,* 49–60.

128 MacDonald, M.K. (1973) Dense disease. *In* Kincaide-Smith, P., Malthew, T.H. and Lovell-Becker, E. (eds.), Glomerulonephritis (Wiley, New York), pp. 515–530.

129 Mahieu, P., Dardenne, M. and Bach, J.F. (1971) Isolation of glycopeptide antigenic site from kidney basement membrane. Lancet *2,* 314.

130 Mandalenakis, N., Mendoza, N., Pirani, C.L. and Pollack, V.E. (1971) Lobular glomerulonephritis and membranoproliferative glomerulonephritis. Medicine *50,* 319–355.

131 Masugi, M. (1934) Uber die experimentelle Glomerulonephritis durch das spezifische Antinierenserum. Beitr. Pathol. Anat. *92,* 429–466.

132 McCluskey, R.T. (1971) The value of immunofluorescence in the study of human renal disease. J. Exp. Med. *134,* 242–255s.

133 McCluskey, R.T. (1974) Immunologic mechanisms in renal disease. *In* Heptingstall, R.H. (ed.), Pathology of the Kidney, 2nd ed. (Little, Brown and Co., Boston) pp. 273–318.

134 McCluskey, R.T. and Andres, G.A. (eds.) (1978) Immunologically Mediated Renal Disease (Marcel Dekker, New York).

135 McIntosh, R.M. and Griswold, W.R. (1971) Antigen identification in Goodpasture's syndrome. Arch. Pathol. *92,* 329–333.

136 McIntosh, R.M., Kulvinskas, C. and Kaufman, D.B. (1971) Cryoglobulins. II. The biological and chemical properties of cryoproteins in acute post-streptococcal glomerulonephritis. Int. Arch. Allergy *41,* 700–718.

137 McIntosh, R.M., Griswold, W.R., Cheineck, W.B., Williams, G., Strauss, J., Kraufman, D.B., Koss, M.N., McIntosh, J.R., Cohen, R. and West, R. (1975) Cryoglobulins. III. Further studies on the nature, incidence, clinical, diagnostic, prognostic, and immunopathologic significance of cryoproteins in renal disease. Quart. J. Med. *44,* 285–307.

138 McLean, R.H. and Michael, A.F. (1978) Immunologic mechanisms and renal disease. *In* Pediatric Kidney Disease (Little, Brown and Co., Boston) pp. 128–150.

139 McPhaul, J.J., Jr. and Dixon, F.J. (1970) Characterization of immunoglobulin G antiglomeru-

lar basement membrane antibodies eluted from glomerulonephritis Kidney. J. Clin. Invest. *49,* 308–317.

140 Meadows, R. (1973) Renal Histopathology (Oxford University Press, London).

141 Mellors, R.C. and Ortega, L.G. (1956) Analytical pathology; new observations on pathogenesis of glomerulonephritis, lipid nephrosis, periarteritis nodosa, and secondary amyloidosis in man. Am. J. Pathol. *32,* 455–499.

142 Mellors, R.C., Siegel, M. and Pressman, D. (1955) Analytic pathology; histochemical demonstration of antibody localization in tissues, with special reference to antigenic components of Kidney and Lung. Lab. Invest. *4,* 69–89.

143 Mellors, R.C., Ortega, L.G. and Holman, H.R. (1957) Role of gamma globulins in pathogenesis of renal lesions in systemic lupus erythematosus and chronic membranous glomerulonephritis, with an observation on the lupus erythematosus cell reaction. J. Exp. Med. *106,* 191–202.

144 Michael, A.F., Westberg, N.G., Fish, A.J. and Vernier, R.L. (1971) Studies on chronic membranoproliferative glomerulonephritis with hypocomplementemia. J. Exp. Med. *134,* 208s–227s.

145 Michel, B., Milner, Y. and David, K. (1973) Preservation of tissue-fixed immunoglobulins in skin biopsies of patients with lupus erythematosus and bullous disease-preliminary report. J. Invest. Dermatol. *59,* 449–452.

146 Milgrom, F. and Witebsky, E. (1960) Rabbit antibodies against γ-globulins resembling the rheumatoid factor. Fed. Proc. *19,* 197.

147 Min, K.W., Gyorkey, F., Gyorkey, P., Yium, J.J. and Eknoyan, G. (1974) The morphogenesis of glomerular crescents in rapidly progressive glomerulonephritis. Kidney Int. *5,* 47–56.

148 Morel-Maroger, L., Leathem, A. and Richet, G. (1972) Glomerular abnormalities in nonsystemic diseases. am J. Med. *53,* 170–184.

149 Morel-Maroger, L., Adam, C. and Richet, G. (1973) The value of immunofluorescence in the diagnosis of glomerulonephritis not related to systemic diseases. *In* Kincaide-Smith, P., Mathew, T.H. and Lovell-Becker, E. (eds.), Glomerulonephritis (Wiley, New York) pp. 81–110.

150 Morel-Maroger, L., Meny, J.P., Leroux-Robert, C. and Richet, G. (1973) Mesangial IgA deposits. *In* Kincaide-Smith, P., Mathew, T.H. and Lovell-Becker, E. (eds.), Glomerulonephritis (Wiley, New York) pp. 301–304.

151 Muehrcke, R.C., Kark, R.M., Pirani, C.L. and Pollak, V.E. (1957) Lupus nephritis: a clinical and pathologic study based on renal biopsies. Medicine *36,* 2–145.

152 Murphy, W.M., Deodhar, S.D. and McCormack, L.J. (1972) Immunopathologic studies and membranous glomerulopathy (69 cases). Lab. Invest. *26,* 486.

153 Murphy, W.M., Deodhar, S.D., McCormack, L.J. and Osborne, D.G. (1973) Immunopathologic studies in glomerular desease with membranous lesions. Am. J. Clin. Pathol. *60,* 364–376.

154 Noble, B., Olson, K.A., Milgrom, M. and Albini, B. (1980) Tissue deposition of immune complexes in mice receiving daily injections of bovine serum albumin. Clin. Exp. Immunol. *42,* 255–262.

155 Noel, N.H., Draz, D., Ganeval, D. and Jugers, P. (1978) Glomerulosclerosis nodulaire du myelome. Abstract 7, Int. Congress Nephrology, p. L16.

156 Olsen, S., Petersen, V.P. and Sommer-Hansen, E. (1974) Immunofluorescence studies of extracapillary glomerulonephritis. Acta. Pathol. Microbiol. Scand. Suppl. *249,* 20–28.

157 Ooi, Y.M., Vallota, E.H. and West, C.D. (1976) Classical complement pathway activation in membranoproliferative glomerulonephritis. Kidney Int. *9,* 46–53.

158 Ortega, L.G. and Mellors, R.C. (1956) Analytical pathology; role of localized antibodies in pathogenesis of nephrotoxic nephritis in rat. J. Exp. Med. *104,* 151–170.

159 Parker, R. and Bennett, W.M. (1980) Interstitial disease. *In* Stein, J.H. (ed.), Nephrology (Grune and Stratton, New York) pp. 355–361.

160 Penner, E., Albini, B., Andres, G.A. and Milgrom, F. (1979) Dissociation of immune complexes in kidney biopsies by antigen excess. Fed. Proc. *38,* 1412.

161 Pirani, C.L. and Pollak, V.E. (1978) Systemic lupus erythematosus glomerulonephritis

nephritis. *In* McCluskey, R.T. and Andres, G.A. (eds.), Immunology Mediated Renal Diseases (Dekker, New York) pp. 19–38.

162 Pollak, V.E. and Pirani, C.L. (1974) Pathology of the kidney in systemic lupus erythematosus: Serial renal biopsy studies and the effects of therapy on kidney lesions. *In* Dubois, E.L. (ed.), Lupus Erythematosus (University of Southern California Press, Los Angeles, CA) pp. 72–89.

163 Pollak, V.E., Pirani, L. and Schwartz, F.D. (1964) The natural history of the renal manifestations of systemic lupus erythematosus. J. Lab. Clin. Med. *63,* 537–550.

164 Pollak, V.E., Mendoza, N. and Pirani, C.L. (1973) Immunohistologic observation in mesangial proliferative glomerulonephritis. *In* Kincaide-Smith, P., Mathew, T.H. and Lovell-Becker, E. (eds.), Glomerulonephritis (Wiley, New York) pp. 633–640.

165 Pollak, V.E., Pirani, C.L. and Cline, D.H. (1973) The natural history of membranous glomerulopathy. *In* incaide-Smith, P., Mathew, T.H. and Lovell-Becker, E. (eds.), Glomerulonephritis (Wiley, New York) p. 429.

166 Porch, P.A. and Williams, G. (1973) Mesangial cells in membranous glomerulonephritis. J. Pathol. *109,* XI–XII.

167 Pressman, D., Hill, R.F. and Foote, F.W. (1949) Zone of localization of anti-mouse kidney serum as determined by radioautographs, Science *109,* 65–66.

168 Randall, R.E., Williamson, W.C. Jr., Mullinex, F., Tung, M.Y. and Still, W.J.S. (1973) Manifestation of synthetic light chain deposits. Am. J. Med. *60,* 293–299.

169 Rao, T.K.S, Nicortis, A.D., Chen, C.K., Rosenthal, J., Bion, C., Delano, D.G. and Freidman, E.A. (1978) Membranoproliferative glomerulonephritis (MPGN) – an unusual manifestation of multiple myeloma. Kidney Int. *14,* 549.

170 Rees, A.J., Lockwood, C.M. and Peters, D.R. (1979) Nephritis due to antibodies to GBM. *In* Kincaide-Smith, P., D'Apice, A.J.F. and Atkins, R.C. (eds.), Progress and Glomerulonephritis (Wiley, New York) pp. 347–366.

171 Reichlin, M. (1981) Systemic lupus erythematosus. *In* Milgrom, F., Abeyounis, C.J. and Kano, K). (eds.), Principles of Immunological Diagnosis in Medicine (Lea and Febiger, Philadelphia) pp. 331–336.

172 Reinherz, E.L., Kung, P.C., Goldstein, G. and Schlossman, S.F. (1979) Separation of functional subsets of human T cells by a monoclonal antibody. Proc. Natl. Acad. Sci. U.S.A. *76,* 4061–4065.

173 Roman-Franco, A.A., Turiello, M., Albini, B., Ossi, E., Milgrom, F. and Andres, G.A. (1978) Anti-basement membrane antibodies and antigen-antibody complexes in rabbits injected with mercuric chloride. Clin. Immunol. Immunopathol. *9,* 464–481.

174 Rosen, S. (1971) Membranous glomerulonephritis: current studies. Human Pathol. *2,* 209–231.

175 Rossmann, P., Tirka, J. and Hradcova, L. (1972) Extramembranous deposits and "membranous" glomerulonephritis. Virchows Arch. *A356,* 293–306.

176 Royer, P., Habib, R. Vermeil, G., Mathieu, H. and Alizon, M. (1962) Le glomérulonéphrites prolongées de l'enfant. Am. Pediat. *38,* 173–187.

177 Sagel, I., Treser, G., Ty, A., Yshizawa. N., Kleinberger, H. Yuceoglu, M., Wesserman, E. and Lange, K. (1973) Occurrence and nature of glomerular lesions after group A streptococci injections in children. Ann. Intern. Med. *79,* 492–499.

178 Sainte-Marie, G. (1962) A paraffin embedding technique for studies employing immunofluorescence. J. Histochem. Cytochem. *10,* 250–258.

179 Scheinman, J.I., Fish, A.J. and Michael, A.F. (1974) The immunohistopathology of glomerular antigens. The glomerular basement membrane, collagen, and actomyosin antigens in normal and diseased kidneys. J. Clin. Invest. *54,* 1144–1154.

180 Scheinman, J.I. Foidart, J.M. and Michael, A.F. (1980) The immunohistology of glomerular antigens. The collagenous antigens of the glomerulus. Lab. Invest. *43,* 373–381.

181 Scheinman, J.I. Foidart, J.M., Gehson-Robey, P., Fish, A.J. and Michael, A.F. (1980) The immunohistology of glomerular antigens. IV. Laminin, a defined non-collagen basement membrane glycoprotein. Clin. Immunol. Immunopathol. *15,* 175–189.

182 Schiffer, M.S., Michael, A.F., Kim, Y. and Fish, A.J. (1981) Distribution of glomerular

basement membrane antigens in diseased human kidneys. Lab. Invest. *44,* 234–240.

183 Schoenfeld, P.Y. and Humphreys, M.H. (1976) A general description of the uremic state. *In* Brenner, B.M. and Rector, F.C. Jr. (eds.), The Kidney (Saunders, Philadelphia) pp. 1423–1477.

184 Schreiner, G.E. (1971) Renal biopsy. *In* Strauss, M.B. and Welt, L.G. (eds.), Diseases of the Kidney, 2nd ed. Vol.I (Little, Brown, and Co., Boston) pp. 197–208.

185 Seegal, B.C., Hsu, K.S., Fiaschi, E. and Andres, G. (1959) La tecnica degli anticorpi applioata allo studio della patogenesi della nefrite umana. Rass. Fis. Clin. Ter. *38,* 1–8.

186 Seymour, A.E. Spargo, B.H. and Penksa, R. (1971) Contributions of renal biopsy studies to the understanding of disease, Am. J. Pathol. *65,* 550–598.

187 Shevach, E.M., Jaffe, E.S. and Green, I. (1973) Receptors for complement and immunoglobular in human and animal lymphoid cells. Transplant. Rev. *16,* 3–27.

188 Shibata, S. (1970) Further purification of the glycoprotein that induces nephrotoxic antibody: Isolation of the active polysaccharide fraction mainly composed of glucose. J. Immunol. *104,* 215–223.

189 Sinniah, R. and Feng, P.H. (1976) Lupus nephritis: Correlation between light, electron microscopic and immunofluorescent findings and renal function. Clin. Nephrol. *6,* 340–351.

190 Smolens, P. and Lifschitz, M.D. (1980) Acute renal failure. *In* Stein, J.H. (ed.), Nephrology (Grune and Stratton, New York) pp. 159–171.

191 Spargo, B.H. and Ordoñez, N.G. (1977) Differential diagnosis of crescentic glomerulonephritis. Human Pathol. *8,* 187–204.

192 Stachura, I., Whiteside, T.L. and Kelly, R.H. (1981) Circulatory and deposited immune complexes in patients with glomerular disease. Am. J. Pathol. *103,* 21–30.

193 Steblay, R.W. (1962) Glomerulonephritis induced in sheep by injection of heterologous glomerular basement membrane. J. Exp. Med. *116,* 253–264.

194 Steblay, R.W. and Rudofsky, V.H. (1971) Renal tubular disease and auto-antibodies against tubular basement membrane induced in guinea pigs. J. Immunol. *107,* 589–594.

195 Stein, J.H. (ed.) (1980) Nephrology (Grune and Stratton, New York).

196 Striker, G.E., Cutler, R.E., Huang, T.W. and Benditt, E.P. (1973) Renal failure, glomerulonephritis and glomerular epithelial cell hyperplasma. *In* Kincaide-Smith, P., Mathew, T.H. and Lovell-Becker, E. (eds.), Glomerulonephritis (Wiley, New York,) p. 1141.

197 Strom, T.B. and Garovoy, M.R. (1980) Acute nephritis. *In* Stein, J.H. (ed.), Nephrology (Grune and Stratton, New York) pp. 144–146.

198 Szymanski, C.H. (1977) Subpopulations of Cellular Infiltrates in Interstitial Nephritis. Thesis. State University of New York at Buffalo, New York.

199 Tauber, J.W., Polley, M.J. and Zabriskie, J.B. (1976) Non-specific complement activation by streptococcal structures. II. Properdin-independent initiation of the alternate pathway. J. Exp. Med. *143,* 1352–1366.

200 Tauber, J.W., Falk, J.A. Falk, R.E. and Zabriskie, J.B. (1976) Non-specific complement activation by streptococcal structures. I. Re-evaluation of HLA cytotoxicity inhibition J. Exp. Med. *143,* 1341–1351.

201 Thoenes, W. (1973) Pathohistologische Systematik der Glomerulonephritis. Nieren- und Hochdruckkrankheiten. *5,* 199–207.

202 Tonder, O., Milgrom, F. and Witebsky, E. (1964) Mixed agglutination with tissue section. J. Exp. Med. *119,* 265–274.

203 Treser, G., Semar, M., Ty, A., Sagel, I., Franklin, M.A. and Lange, K. (1970) Partial characterization of antigenic streptococcal plasma membrane components in acute glomerulonephritis. J. Clin. Invest. *49,* 762–768.

204 Van Zieten, M.J., Leber, P.D., Bhan, A.K. and McCluskey, R.T. (1977) Experimental celmediated interstitial nephritis induced with exogenous antigen. J. Immunol. *118,* 589–593.

205 Varga, R., Thomson, K.J., Wilson, D., Cameron, J.S., Turner, D.R., Gill, D., Chantler, C. and Ogg, C.S. (1976) Mesangiocapillary glomerulonephritis with dense "deposits" in the basement membranes of the kidney. Clin. Nephrol. *5,* 73–82.

206 Vazquez, J.J. and Dixon, F.J. (1956) Studies on the immunohistochemical composition of

inflammatory and degenerative lesions. Am J. Pathol. *32,* 615–615.

207 Velosa, J., Miller, K. and Michael, A.F. (1976) Immunopathology of the end-stage kidney. Am. J. Pathol. *84,* 149–162.

208 Vernier, R.L. (1968) Glomerulonephritis. *In* Miescher, P.A. and Müller-Eberhard, H. (eds.), Textbook of Immunology, *Vol. I,* (Grune and Stratton, New York) pp. 365–373.

209 Walker, W.G. (1976) Renal diseases and disturbances in renal function. *In* Harvey, A.M., Johns, R.J., Owens, A.H. and Ross, R.S. (eds.), The Principles and Practice of Medicine, 19th ed. (Appleton-Century-Crofts, New York) pp. 129–200.

210 Wegmann, W. and Leumann, E.P. 91973) Glomerulonephritis associated with (infected) ventriculo-atrial shunt. Clinical and morphological findings. Virchows Arch. *A359,* 185–200.

211 West, C.D., mcAdams, A.J., McConville, J.M., Davis, N.C. and Holland, N.H. (1965) Hypocomplementemic and normacomplementems persistent (chronic) glomerulonephritis; clinical and pathologic characteristics. J. Pediat. *67.* 1089–1112.

212 Wick, G., Furthmayer, H. and Timpl, R. (1975) Purified antibodies to collagen: an immunofluorescence study of their reaction with tissue collagen. Int. Arch. Allergy *48,* 664–679.

213 Williams, R.C., Jr. (1980) Immune Complexes in Clinical and Experimental Medicine (Harvard Press, Cambridge).

214 Wilson, C.B. (1979) Immune reactions with antigens in or of the glomeruli. *In* Milgrom, F. and Albini, B. (eds.), Immunopathology (Karger, Basel) pp. 127–131.

215 Wilson, C.B. (1980) Immunological Considerations. *In* Stein, J.H. (ed.), Nephrology (Grune and Stratton, New York) pp. 275–286.

216 Wilson, C.B. (1980) Goodpastures Syndrome. *In* Stein, J.H. (ed.), Nephrology (Grune and Stratton, New York) pp. 306–310.

217 Wilson, C.B. and Smith, R.C. (1972) Goodpasture's syndrome associated with influenza A_2 virus infection. Ann. intern. Med. *76,* 91–94.

218 Wilson, C.B. and Dixon, F.J. (1973) anti-glomerular basement membrane antibody induced glomerulonephritis. Kidney Int. *3,* 74–89.

219 Wilson, C.B. and Dixon, F.J. (1974) Diagnosis of immunopathologic renal disease. Kidney Int. *5,* 389–401.

220 Wilson, C.B. and Dixon, F.J. (1976) The renal response to immunological injury. *In* Brenner, B.M. and Rector, F.C., Jr. (eds.), The Kidney (Saunders, Philadelphia) pp. 838–940.

221 Wofsy, L., Baker, P.C., Thompson, K., Goodman, J., Kinura, J. and Henry, C. (1974) Hapten sandwich labelling. I. A. general procedure for simultaneous labeling of multiple cell surface antigens for fluorescence and electron microscopy. J. Exp. Med. *140,* 523–537.

222 Yoshizawa, N., Treser, G., Sagel, I., Ty, A., Ahmed, U. and Lange, K. (1973) Demonstration of antigenic sites in glomeruli of patients with acute poststreptococcal glomerulonephritis by immunofluorescence and immunoferritin techniques. Am. J. Pathol. *70,* 131–150.

223 Zabriskie, J.B., Utermohlen, V., Read, S.E. and Fischetti, V.A. (1973) Streptococcus related glomerulonephritis. Kidney Int. *3,* 100–104.

224 Zollinger, H.U. (1966) Niere und ableitende Harnwege. *In* Doerr, W. and Uehlinger, E. (eds.), Spezielle pathologische Anatomie, *Vol. III.* (Springer, Berlin).

225 Zollinger, H.U. (1970) Entzundliche Glomerulomerkrankungen. Pathol Eur. *512,* 2–12.

226 Zollinger, H.U. and Mihatsch, M.J. (1978) Renal Pathology in Biopsy (Springer, Berlin).

227 Zollinger, H.U., Colombi, A. and Schiltknecht, J. (1971) New clinical and ultrastructural aspects of leptospirosis ictero-haemorrhagica (Weil's disease). Virchows Arch. *A354,* 336–342.

Wick et al. (eds) Immunofluorescence Technology. Selected Theoretical and Clinical Aspects © Elsevier Biomedical Press, 1982

CHAPTER 13

Immunofluorescence microscopy on paraffin sections

T. RADASZKIEWICZ and H. DENK

Division of Gastroenterologic Pathology and Hepatopathology (Hans Popper-Laboratory), Department of Pathology, University of Vienna School of Medicine, 1090 Vienna, Austria

13.1. INTRODUCTION

Application of immunomorphologic techniques to routine (formaldehyde-fixed, paraffin-embedded) material is a major prerequisite for their general use in diagnostic pathology. It has been shown in the last few years that several different antigens are still detectable by immunofluorescence microscopy in fixed paraffin-embedded tissue and are not destroyed by the fixation and embedding procedure. Intra- and extracytoplasmic immunoglobulins, lysozyme, hepatitis B surface antigen (HBsAg) and hepatitis B core antigen (HBcAg), α_1-antitrypsin [4, 8, 9, 14, 15, 19, 23, 24, 25, 31] and some tumor-associated antigens (for review, see Denk and Platzer, Chapter 14, this volume) have been successfully demonstrated by immunofluorescence microscopy on paraffin sections. In addition, hormones such as insulin, gastrin [1, 17, 20], glucagon, somatostatin, pancreatic polypeptide [11], actin [5], pepsinogen II [17], and alkaline phosphatase, especially in duodenal enterocytes and goblet cells [2], could also be localized in paraffin sections by immunofluorescence, thus allowing further characterization of tumors of endocrine origin. It should be kept in mind, however, that some differences in the results of the immunofluorescence test on paraffin and frozen sections of the same specimen have been reported. According to Choi and Reiner [6] IgG and IgM could be demonstrated more often in pretreated (0.1% trypsin for 2 h at 37°C) paraffin sections of kidney biopsies than in frozen sections, whereas IgA was more easily detected in frozen sections. Complement components (C3, C1q, C4) could not be visualized in paraffin-embedded material by these authors. Similar observations were also occasionally made in our laboratory with kidney biopsies (Syré, unpublished observations). With intracytoplasmic immunoglobulins, lysozyme and HBsAg we have not observed differences in immunomorphology performed on frozen sections and on formalin-fixed paraffin-embedded material. Cell surface-associated immunoglobulins and Fc receptors, however, could as yet not be detected in paraffin-embedded material.

13.2. FIXATION OF TISSUE

To detect intracytoplasmic antigens, the cells have to be treated with certain fixatives in order to allow antibodies to enter the cells and to stabilize soluble antigens in frozen sections. In tissue sections, the cells are opened at the cut surface and, consequently, cytoplasmic antigenic determinants are accessible for antibodies. Fixation preserves morphology but often destroys or alters antigenic reactivity by cross-linking proteins and carbohydrates. This may be prevented by using dehydrating substances for fixation, e.g. ethanol, methanol, ethanol-containing acetic acid, chloroform or ethyl ether, which only precipitate proteins without affecting antigenic reactivity. Although fixatives which cross-link protein and sometimes carbohydrate components of the antigens may negatively affect antigenic determinants, a series of fixatives other than precipitating ones can still be used for immunofluorescence on paraffin sections: most commonly, buffered formalin (4–10%), paraformaldehyde or Bouin's fixative (75 ml saturated aqueous picric acid, 25 ml formalin, 5 ml glacial acetic acid) are used for fixation of pathologic material. Glutaraldehyde which preferentially reacts with the ϵ-amino groups of lysine [12] destroys most of the antigenic determinants but can, in low concentrations, be mixed with formaldehyde or paraformaldehyde. It has been shown by Smit et al. [28] that 0.05% glutaraldehyde added to formalin does not decrease the number of lymphocytes stained for surface immunoglobulins in smears. Alternative fixatives are dimethylsuperimidate which specifically reacts with the ϵ-amino groups of lysine [13] and periodate–lysine–paraformaldehyde [18]. In the latter fixation procedure, periodate oxidized the membrane carbohydrates to aldehydes which are then cross-linked via the amino groups of lysine. In addition, paraformaldehyde stabilizes intracellular proteins.

13.3. EMBEDDING PROCEDURES

In order to infiltrate tissues with paraffin, it is necessary to displace the aqueous fixing fluids by dehydration, most often performed with alcohol. Since most water-miscible fluids are not paraffin solvents, it is necessary to first dehydrate with a water miscible fluid and then replace the dehydrating agent with a paraffin solvent. Usually the fixed tissues are dehydrated in 70% alcohol, then in 80%, 96% and 100% alcohol for different periods of time.

Following dehydration the tissue is transferred into paraffin solvents such as xylene, benzene, toluene, chloroform or petroleum ether. Thereafter, paraffin infiltration is achieved at a temperature a few degrees above the melting point of the paraffin. In routine embedding procedures, most commonly paraffin with a melting point of 55–56°C is used. Under these conditions good results were obtained in immunofluorescence, especially after treatment with proteases [14, 15, 24]. To prevent temperature-dependent destruction of some antigenic determinants, paraffins with a lower melting point may be used. Polyester wax as embedding medium [29], which has a low melting point (37° C) and is soluble in alcohol and acetone, has been tested in preliminary immunofluorescence studies by Sainte-Marie [27]. A different paraffin-embedding procedure for the demonstration of bovine gamma-globulin, horse ferritin, influenza A viral antigens, diphtheria and tetanus toxoids, and antibodies in the mouse spleen by immunofluorescence on paraffin sections has been described by Sainte-Marie [27]. After fixation of the specimens in 95% alcohol at 4°C, dehydration in absolute ethanol (4°C, four changes, 1–2 h duration each), passing the tissue through three consecutive baths of precooled (4°C) xylene for 1–2 h, paraffin infiltration was performed at 56°C (four times, 1–2 h each), and the tissue was finally embedded in paraffin at 56°C. The blocks were stored at 4°C and the sections floated on a water bath at 40°C only for a short duration. Slides were deparaffinized with xylene and finally washed after removal of xylene with 95% alcohol with phosphate-buffered saline at low temperature.

13.4. ENZYME TREATMENT

Fixation and embedding procedures may destroy and/or mask a certain proportion of antigenic determinants. In addition, non-specific background staining is often high in formaldehyde-fixed paraffin sections, despite the fact that formalin fixation of the tissue diminishes the net positive charge (relative to that of labeled immunoglobulins) [34] by blocking some amino groups and should, therefore, reduce background staining caused by electrostatic attraction of antibodies. Background staining of formalin-fixed paraffin-embedded material can be diminished and specific staining, at least of some antigens, eg. HBsAg and cytoplasmic immunoglobulins, can be enhanced by pretreatment of the dewaxed sections with proteases such as pronase and trypsin [3, 7–9, 14, 15, 23, 24, 26]. The favourable effect of enzyme digestion was also revealed in the unlabeled antibody enzyme (peroxidase–anti-peroxidase) technique (PAP) [24, 26] as well as in the enzyme (peroxidase)-labeled antibody technique (Radaszkiewicz, unpublished observation). The pronase effect could be substantiated quantitatively by measuring the specific and background fluorescence, as shown with HBsAg in paraffin-embedded liver biopsy material [24] (Table 13.I) Enzyme digestion is particularly important if the direct immunofluorescence method is used. Double staining of various intracytoplasmic

TABLE 13.I

SPECIFIC AND BACKGROUND FLUORESCENCE OF HBsAg IN PROTEASE-PRETREATED PARAFFIN SECTIONS OF LIVER BIOPSIES AS REVEALED BY MICROPHOTOMETRY (From Radaszkiewicz et al. [24].)

Specimen[b]	Fluorescence (photometer units)[a]			
	Specific fluorescence		Background fluorescence	
	Without protease	With protease	Without protease	With protease
1	23.2 ± 5.1	46.8 ± 15.9[c]	12.1 ± 2.3	4.5 ± 1.1[c]
2	33.9 ± 8.2	102.0 ± 20.3[c]	8.0 ± 1.1	4.0 ± 1.0[c]
3	34.9 ± 7.7	112.5 ± 17.7[c]	11.5 ± 2.0	6.4 ± 3.3[c]
4	22.1 ± 7.0	82.9 ± 25.2[c]	10.0 ± 2.3	5.9 ± 2.6[c]
5	26.1 ± 7.4	69.7 ± 15.5[c]	11.6 ± 3.8	3.6 ± 1.6[c]
6	44.9 ± 19.5	109.3 ± 18.7[c]	12.3 ± 2.3	10.8 ± 3.3[d]
7	54.3 ± 12.6	91.5 ± 22.6[c]	17.2 ± 3.8	5.4 ± 1.8[c]
8	38.5 ± 7.9	113.5 ± 19.6[c]	18.7 ± 4.7	5.5 ± 3.0[c]
9	29.5 ± 9.5	102.6 ± 23.3[c]	14.5 ± 2.1	10.2 ± 2.2[c]
10	19.8 ± 6.9	99.0 ± 24.0[c]	10.3 ± 1.5	5.9 ± 1.6[c]
11	24.4 ± 7.9	87.9 ± 29.2[c]	7.3 ± 1.2	4.7 ± 1.4[c]

[a] Mean values ± S.D.
[b] In each specimen 14–54 liver cells were evaluated.
[c] Significantly different from untreated specimens ($P<0.005$).
[d] $P<0.02$.

immunoglobulins in human malignant lymphomas with commercially available fluorescein isothiocyanate (FITC) - and tetramethylrhodamine isothiocyanate (TRITC)-labeled antisera in direct immunofluorescence was unsuccessful in untreated paraffin sections. However, after protease pretreatment double staining was rendered possible because of increased sensitivity [22] (Figs. 13.1 and 13.2). The protease effect is not limited to the immunomorphologic demonstration of immunoglobulins, lysozyme and HBsAg. Buffa et al. [3] immunohistochemically detected cholecystokinin in duodenal and jejunal mucosa on paraffin sections pretreated with trypsin. Huang et al. [15] localized fibrin, α_1-antitrypsin, HBcAg, α-fetoprotein (AFP) and carcinoembryonic antigen (CEA) in formalin-fixed paraffin sections by immunofluorescence and, with respect to some of these antigens, found enhancement of specific and reduction of background staining after treatment of the sections with trypsin for 2 h. Exceptions, however, exist. With CEA, an increase of specific staining intensity could not be achieved by trypsin digestion [15]. Protease digestion of formalin-fixed paraffin sections also did not appreciably influence the intensity of specific staining of AFP-containing cells, but was still valuable by suppressing background staining (Denk and Platzer, Chapter 14, this volume). Specific decoration of immunoglobulins after pronase pretreatment of the sections was also found in tissues fixed in 10% formaldehyde and embedded in glycol-methacrylate [32]. Contrary to the results of Dorsett and Joachim [10],

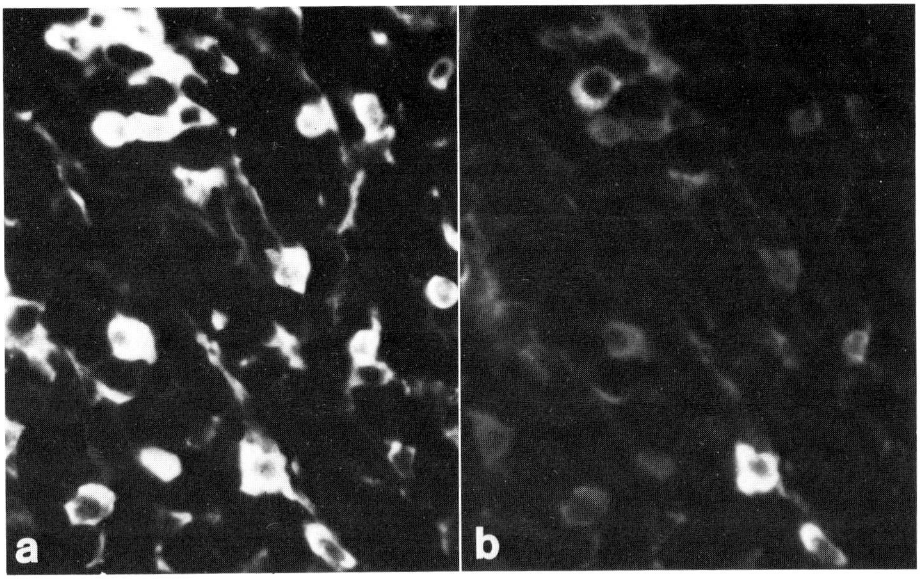

Fig. 13.1. Immunocytic malignant lymphoma of the IgM/κ type. Double immunofluorescence staining of the same paraffin section pretreated with 0.1% protease for 10 min at 37°C. a) Demonstration of intracytoplasmic κ chains in plasma cells and lymphoplasmacytoid cells with FITC-conjugated rabbit anti-human κ chain globulin (Behring-Werke, Marburg, F.R.G.). b) Application of TRITC-conjugated goat anti-human IgA globulin (Nordic Immunology, Lausanne, Switzerland) on the same section. Only two cells positively stained for κ chains (a) contain IgA. Original ×780.

complement could not be identified by immunofluorescence in trypsin-digested sections (C3, C1q, C4) by Huang et al. [15] and Choi and Reiner [6]. According to the method of Dorsett and Joachim [10] specimens were fixed in Bouin's fixative instead of formalin and not pretreated with proteases.

The mechanism by which protease pretreatment of paraffin sections exerts its beneficial effect on background staining and specific fluorescence of certain antigens is unclear. Huang et al. [15] suggested unmasking of certain immunoreactive sites. Vogt et al. [33] have shown that certain protein antigens lose their antigenicity if embedded in epoxy resins, e.g. styrene, which could be due to a binding of the monomers of epoxy resins, polyesters and other embedding compounds to free amino groups of the antigenic determinants [21]. The significance of amino groups in relation to antigenicity can be judged from the effect of carbobenzoxychloride. Carbobenzoxychloride blocks free amino groups of antigens by peptide-like bond formation [16, 33.]. In sections treated with carbobenzoxychloride, certain antigens are, therefore, not reactive in immunofluorescence [30]. The carbobenzoxychloride blockade can be reversed by treatment of the sections with non-specific proteases which seem to cleave peptide-like bonds between carbobenzoxychloride and amino groups of the antigen, thus restoring antigenicity [30]. Another possibility is that the protease randomly splits peptide bonds of the carbobenzoxychloride-modified tissue and that the cleavage leads to the formation of new antigenic

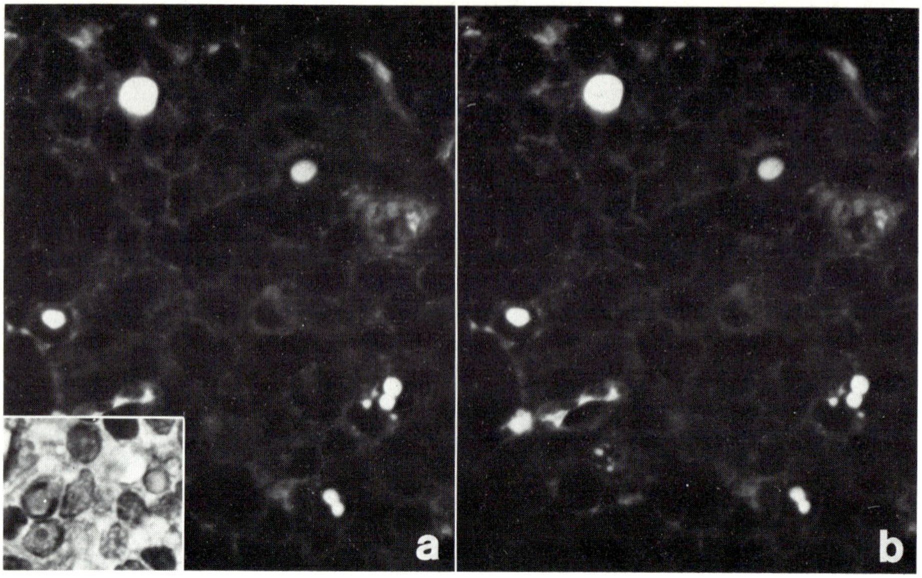

Fig. 13.2. Immunocytic malignant lymphoma of the IgM/κ type. Double immunofluorescence staining of the same paraffin section pretreated with 0.1% protease for 10 min at 37°C. a) Several intranuclear inclusions stained with FITC-labeled rabbit anti-human κ-chain globulin (Behring-Werke, Marburg, F.R.G.). b) The same intranuclear immunoglobulin inclusions are stained with TRITC-labeled goat anti-human IgM globulin (Nordic Immunology, Lausanne, Switzerland). Inset: PAS staining of a paraffin section of the same case demonstrating an intranuclear (PAS-positive) immunoglobulin inclusion. Original ×780.

determinants with which antibodies can react [30]. A similar mechanism is also possible in the case of immunohistochemical staining of protease-pretreated paraffin sections, at least with regard to certain antigens. Pilot studies, however, showed that carbobenzoxychloride did not interfere with antibody binding to HBsAg before and after protease treatment (Radaszkiewicz and Denk, unpublished observations), indicating that amino groups may not be crucially involved in HBs antigenicity and that the beneficial effect of protease may not be due to uncovering of reactive amino groups.

13.5. SUMMARY

In summary, the immunofluorescence procedure employed in our laboratory for the investigation of formaldehyde-fixed paraffin-embedded material is presented. Small pieces should be fixed to ensure proper penetration of the fixative, since otherwise background staining, especially in the center of the specimen, will be high and specificity of the staining difficult to assess. In our laboratory, phosphate-buffered 8–10% formalin, pH 7.4, is used as a fixative. Dehydration, clearing, and paraffin infiltration are automatically accomplished by a Technicon tissue processor and the specimens are embedded in paraffin in the conventional way. The sections (4 μm thick) are incubated for

2–4 h at 60°C in order to ensure adherence to the slide. The dewaxed (3 × xylene) and rehydrated sections may, in addition, be covered with 0.3% celloidine to prevent detachment (but celloidine in some instances may interfere with penetration of the antibodies). They are incubated with 0.1% protease (type V or VII, Sigma Chem. Comp., St. Louis, MO) in 0.15 M phosphate-buffered saline (PBS), pH 7.4, for 15 min (demonstration of intracytoplasmic immunoglobulins) or 60 min (demonstration of HBsAg). Protease digestion is interrupted by transferring the slides into ice-cold PBS for 60 min. Afterwards, direct or indirect immunofluorescence is performed in the usual way with antisera diluted according to the results of chessboard titrations. The same technique of fixation, embedding and protease pretreatment can also be combined with other immunohistochemical techniques, for instance the enzyme-labeled antibody technique (Radaszkiewicz, unpublished observations) or the unlabeled antibody peroxidase–anti-peroxidase (PAP) method [24].

REFERENCES

1 Arnal-Monreal, F.M., Goltzman, D., Knaack, J., Wang, N.-S. and Huang, S.-N. (1977) Immunohistologic study of thyroidal carcinoma and pancreatic insulinoma. Cancer *40,* 1060–1070.

2 Böcker, W. (1974) Use of a triple layer enzyme method as an alternative to immunofluorescence for the detection of tissue antigens. Beitr. Pathol. *153,* 410–414.

3 Buffa, R., Solcia, E. and Go, V.L.W. (1976) Immunohistochemical identification of the cholecystokinin cell in the intestinal mucosa. Gastroenterology *70,* 528–532.

4 Burns, J. (1975) Background staining and sensitivity of the unlabeled antibody-enzyme (PAP) method. Comparison with the peroxidase labeled antibody sandwich method using formalin fixed paraffin embedded material. Histochemistry *43,* 291–294.

5 Bussolati, G., Alfani, V., Weber, K. and Osborn, M. (1980) Immunocytochemical detection of actin on fixed and embedded tissues: its potential use in routine pathology. J. Histochem. Cytochem. *28,* 169–173.

6 Choi, Y.J. and Reiner, L. (1980) Immunofluorescence of renal lesions in paraffin-embedded and fresh-frozen sections. Am. J. Clin. Pathol. *73,* 116–119.

7 Curran, R.C. and Gregory, J. (1977) Unmasking of antigens in paraffin sections of tissue by trypsin. Experientia *33,* 1400–1401.

8 Denk, H., Radaszkiewicz, T. and Witting, Ch. (1976) Immunofluorescence studies on pathologic routine material: application to malignant lymphomas. Beitr. Pathol. *159,* 219–225.

9 Denk, H., Syré, G. and Weirich, E. (1977) Immunomorphologic methods in routine pathology. Application of immunofluorescence and the unlabeled antibody–enzyme (peroxidase–antiperoxidase) technique to formalin fixed paraffin embedded kidney biopsies. Beitr. Pathol. *160,* 187–194.

10 Dorsett, B.H. and Joachim, H.L. (1978) A method for the use of immunofluorescence in paraffin-embedded tissues. Am. J. Clin. Pathol. *69,* 66–73.

11 Gepts, W., DeMey, J. and Mirachal-Pipeleers, M. (1977) Hyperplasia of "pancreatic polypeptide" cells in the pancreas of juvenile diabetes. Diabetologia *13,* 27–35.

12 Hajdu, J., and Friedrich, P. (1975) Reaction of glutaraldehyde with NH compounds. A spectrophotometric method for the determination of glutaraldehyde concentration. Anal. Biochem. *65,* 273–280.

13 Hassel, J. and Hand, A.R. (1974) Tissue fixation with diimidoesters as an alternative to aldehydes. I. Comparison of cross-linking and ultrastructure obtained with dimethylsuperimi-

date and glutaraldehyde. J. Histochem. Cytochem. *22,* 223–239.
14 Huang, S.-N. (1975) Immunohistochemical demonstration of hepatitis B core and surface antigens in paraffin sections. Lab. Invest. *33,* 88–95.
15 Huang, S.-N., Minassian, H. and More, J.D. (1976) Application of immunofluorescent staining on paraffin sections improved by trypsin digestion. Lab. Invest. *35,* 383–390.
16 Kabat, E. and Mayer, H.H. (1971) Experimental Immunochemistry (Thomas, Springfield, IL).
17 Lechago, J., Sun, N.C.J. and Weinstein, W.M. (1979) Simultaneous visualization of two antigens in the same tissue section by combining immunoperoxidase with immunofluorescence techniques. J. Histochem. Cytochem. *27,* 1221–1225.
18 McLean, I.W. and Nakane, P.K. (1974) Periodate lysine-paraformaldehyde fixative. A new fixative for immunoelectron microscopy. J. Histochem. Cytochem. *22,* 1077–1083.
19 Nayak, N.C. and Sachdeva, R. (1975) Localization of hepatitis B surface antigen in conventional paraffin sections of the liver. Comparison of immunofluorescence, immunoperoxidase, and orcein staining methods with regard to their specificity and reliability as antigen marker. Am. J. Pathol. *81,* 479–493.
20 Nieuwenhuijzen-Kruseman, A.C., Knijnenburg, G., Brutel de la Riviere, G. and Bosman, F.T. (1978) Morphology and immunohistochemically defined endocrine function of pancreatic islet cell tumors. Histopathology *2,* 389–399.
21 Putnam, F.W. (1953) The chemical modification of proteins. *In* Neurath, H. and Bailey, K. (eds.), The proteins, *Vol. 1,* part B, Academic Press, New York) p. 893.
22 Radaszkiewicz, T. (1980) Maligne und benigne Lymphome: Histologische Klassifikation und immunmorphologische Untersuchungen. Wien. Klin. Wochenschr. *92,* 819–833.
23 Radaszkiewicz, T. and Denk, H. (1979) Immunohistologic detection of immunoglobulins in malignant lymphomas and its value in histopathologic diagnosis. Virchows Arch. A, Pathol. Anat. Histol. *381,* 141–158.
24 Radaszkiewicz, T., Dragosics, B., Abdelfattah-Gad, M. and Denk, H. (1979) Effect of protease pretreatment on immunomorphologic demonstration of hepatitis B surface antigen in conventional paraffin-embedded liver biopsy material: quantitative evaluation. J. Immunol. Methods *29,* 27–33.
25 Ray, M.B. and Desmet, V.J. (1975) Immunofluorescent detection of alpha I-antitrypsin in paraffin embedded liver tissue. J. Clin. Pathol. *28,* 717–721.
26 Reading, M. (1977) A digestion technique for the reduction of background staining in the immunoperoxidase method. J. Clin. Pathol. *30,* 88–90.
27 Sainte-Marie, G. (1962) A paraffin embedding technique for studies employing immunofluorescence. J. Histochem. Cytochem. *10,* 250–256.
28 Smit, J.W., Meijer, C.J.L.M. Cecary, F. and Feltkamp-Vroom, T.M. (1974) Paraformaldehyde fixation in immunofluorescence. Preservation of tissue and cell surface antigens. J. Immunol. Methods *6,* 93–98.
29 Steedman, H.F. (1957) Polyester wax. A ribboning embedding medium for histology. Nature *179,* 1345–1347.
30 Takamiya, H., Bodemer, W. and Vogt, A. (1978) Masking of protein antigen by modification of amino groups with carbobenzoxychloride (benzyl chloroformate) and demasking by treatment with nonspecific protease. J. Histochem. Cytochem. *26,* 914–920.
31 Tsuji, T., Naito, K., Tokuyama, K., Okada, T. and Kosaka, K. (1976) Detection of HBs antigen in routine paraffin embedded liver tissue by enzyme-labelled antibody technique. Acta Med. Okayama *30,* 69–73.
32 Van de Velde, S. (1980) Fluorescent microscopy of glycolmethacrylate-embedded tissue. Am. J. Clin. Pathol. *73,* 119–121.
33 Vogt, A., Takamiya, H. and Kim, W.A. (1976) Some problems involved in postembedding staining. *In* Feldmann, G., Druet, P., Bignon, J. and Avrameas, S. (eds.) Immunoenzymatic Techniques, Inserm Symp. *2.* (North-Holland, Amsterdam) pp. 109–115.
34 Von Mayersbach, H. (1966) Immunohistology. *In* Grauman, W. and Neumann, K. (eds.), Handbook of Histochemistry. I. General Methodology, part 2 (Gustav Fischer-Verlag, Stuttgart) pp. 188–268.

Wick et al. (eds) Immunofluorescence Technology. Selected Theoretical and Clinical Aspects © Elsevier Biomedical Press, 1982

CHAPTER 14

Immunofluorescence demonstration of tumor-associated antigens

H. DENK and B. PLATZER

Department of Pathology, Division of Gastroenterologic Pathology and Hepatopathology (Hans Popper-Laboratory), University of Vienna School of Medicine, Vienna, Austria

14.1. INTRODUCTION

Spontaneous and experimentally induced tumors express and eventually release substances with antigenic properties that, quantitatively and/or qualitatively, differ from products of non-neoplastic cells. Some of them may play a role in the immunological recognition of tumor cells by the host (for review, see ref. 6). These antigens can be demonstrated by immunomorphological techniques. Consequently, immunomorphology may not only be helpful in elucidating the biology of a tumor but may, at least in some instances, provide diagnostic and prognostic hints. In the present communication, tumor-associated antigens will be discussed in a broad sense, including oncofetal antigens, blood group antigens, transplantation antigens, secretion products and hormones. It is not intended, however, to discuss technical details concerning antigen and antibody preparation which are covered by numerous reviews [39, 77, 105, 114].

14.2. CARCINOEMBRYONIC ANTIGEN (CEA) OF THE DIGESTIVE SYSTEM

CEA is a glycoprotein or comprises a family of glycoproteins with a molecular weight of approximately 200,000 (for review, see ref. 114) [35, 38, 68, 69]. Slight differences in physicochemical and immunochemical properties between CEAs derived from different sources have been reported [69]. A number of substances, such as normal glycoprotein (NGP), normal cross-reacting antigen (NCA) and NCA-2, breast carcinoma glycoprotein (BCGP), fetal sulphoglycoprotein antigen (FSA), and CEA-associated antigen (CEX), share antigenic determinants with CEA and are therefore detected along with CEA if antisera to purified CEA are used without absorption with the respective antigens [14, 15, 17, 114]. In contrast to the original assumption of the tumor- and organ specificity of CEA [39, 40], CEA or CEA-like substances have been detected in malignant and benign tumors arising in different organs but also in a diversity of non-neoplastic (mostly inflammatory) conditions [14, 38, 56, 114].

14.2.1. Localization of CEA as revealed by immunofluorescence (and other immunomorphological techniques)

In adenocarcinomas of the gastrointestinal tract, including pancreatic cancers, CEA is concentrated at the luminal surface of the tumor cells, and is present to a lesser degree in the cytoplasm and within the glandular lumina, sometimes mixed with (but not identical with) mucous secretions [8, 28, 29] (Fig. 14.1a–c). An extravasation of CEA into surrounding tissue has occasionally been observed [54] (Fig. 14.2). Cytoplasmic CEA-specific staining is,

---

Fig. 14.1. a) Well-differentiated adenocarcinoma containing CEA in superficial and intraluminal position (frozen section). ×100. b) Well-differentiated colonic adenocarcinoma with concentration of CEA at the luminal cell surface (formalin-fixed, paraffin-embedded material). ×560. c) Moderately well-differentiated colonic adenocarcinoma with CEA in superficial position (frozen section). ×100.

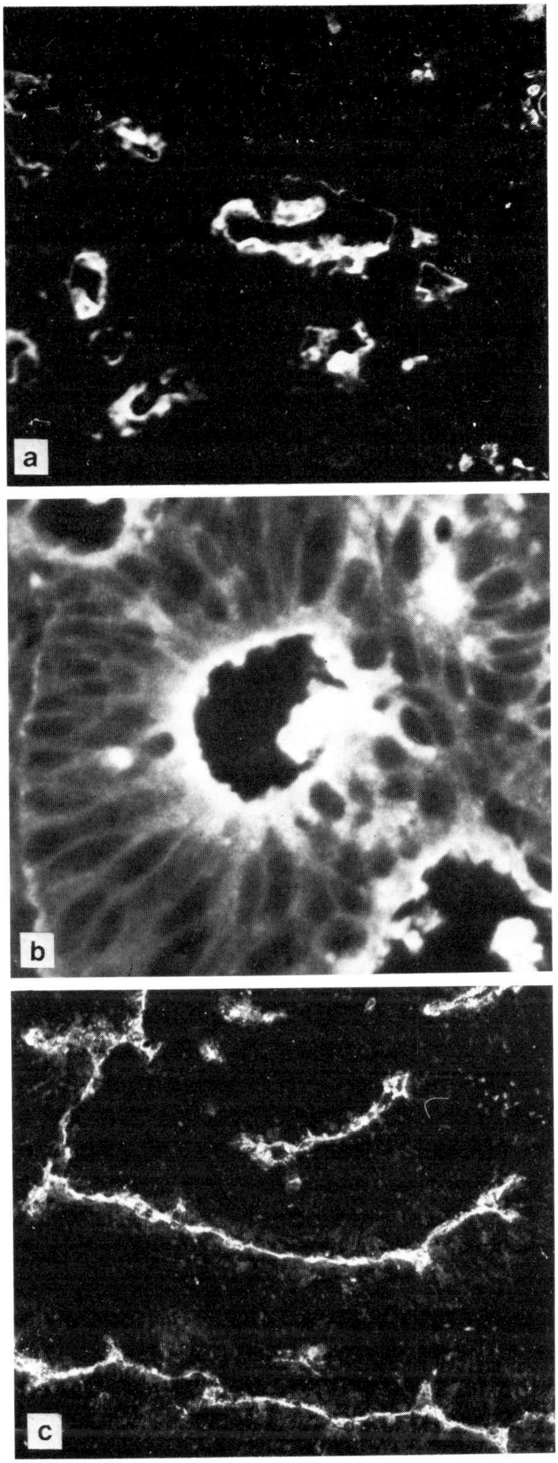
a
b
c

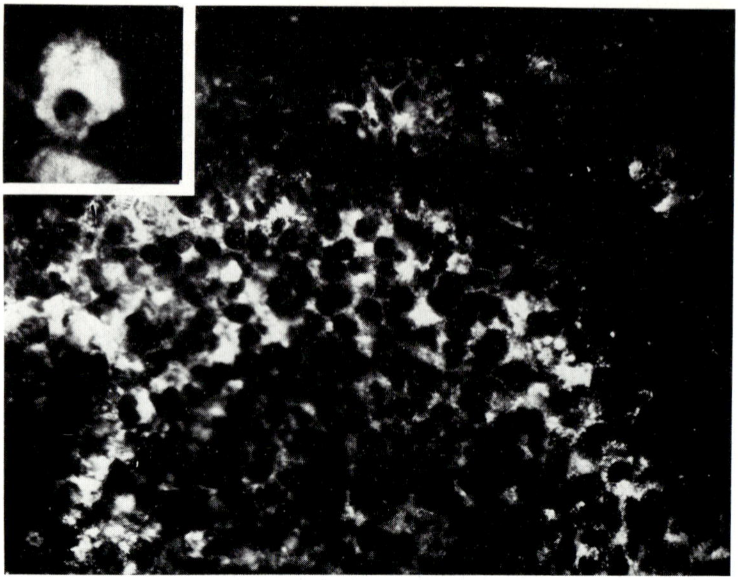

Fig. 14.2. Poorly differentiated gastric carcinoma with moderate amounts of CEA also in extracellular position. The inset shows a signet ring cell containing cytoplasmic CEA (frozen section). ×400. Inset ×800.

however, most conspicuous in tumor cells of the signet ring cell type [14, 28, 29] (Fig. 14.2, inset).

A good correlation between the expression of CEA by various tumors and the degree of differentiation has repeatedly been noted [8, 14, 28, 29, 42]. Well to moderately well differentiated neoplasms expressed CEA in higher amounts than poorly differentiated ones. In colonic adenomas, with or without severe cellular atypia, immunofluorescence revealed the concentration of the antigen at the apical pole of the cells [13, 111]. These findings are, however, in conflict with those reported by Isaacson and LeVann [56], employing an immunoperoxidase technique on formalin-fixed, paraffin-embedded material. Under these conditions CEA was only detectable in highly atypical glands indicative of malignant transformation. In colon mucosa samples derived from tumor-free patients CEA was not detectable by immunofluorescence [13]. Non-neoplastic mucosa in close proximity to the carcinoma was, however, weakly CEA-positive, probably due to passive adsorption of tumor-derived material rather than to de novo synthesis [14, 42]. In inflammatory bowel disorders, such as hemorrhoids and ulcerative colitis, CEA was detectable, indicating that CEA cannot be considered a marker of cancerous and precancerous conditions [8, 14]. In addition, CEA-specific staining has been observed in gastric mucosa with differentiated or proliferating intestinal metaplasia as well as in the glandular neck cells, particularly in the antral region [14, 29].

Hepatocellular carcinomas did not contain CEA, at least in a concentration detectable by immunomorphology [38]. In normal liver, a linear CEA-specific fluorescence was observed in bile ducts in a luminal position. Whereas CEA was confined to the cytoplasm of ductular cells in alcoholic cirrhosis, staining of these cells in non-alcoholic conditions, e.g. extrahepatic biliary obstruction, was less uniform and constant [38].

CEA has also been detected by immunomorphological techniques, including immunofluorescence, in carcinomas of various other organs. Among ovarian malignancies, a high percentage of mucinous cystadenocarcinomas was CEA-positive [43]. CEA in periluminal position was detected in about 60% of endometrial adenocarcinoma specimens. The number of positive cells varied from 1% to 20% of the total cell population. Well-differentiated tumors contained a larger number of CEA-positive cells. CEA was also found in atypical hyperplasia with wide variation in the percentages of positive cells. Specimens with cystic hyperplasia and benign endometrial polyps were consistently CEA-negative.

In cervical carcinomas the frequency of positive results increased with an increasing degree of atypia and with advanced clinical disease (70–80% in advanced disease) as shown by Lindgren et al. [72]. However, while CEA-positivity seems to reflect an aggressive potential in premalignant lesions, survival data did not disclose differences in malignancy between CEA-positive and -negative tumors.

CEA has also been found in lung, breast and laryngeal carcinomas [8, 42, 62, 89, 120]. Shousha and Lyssiotis [104] were able to demonstrate CEA by immunomorphology in 66% of breast carcinomas. In addition, 90% of metastasizing tumors were found to be CEA-positive, suggesting a relationship between the presence of CEA on the tumor cells and the propensity to metastasize. CEA-positive foci in mammary dysplasia may, under these circumstances, indicate early stages of malignant transformation. Wahren et al. [120] detected CEA only in 42% of primary mammary carcinomas by indirect immunofluorescence. In isolated cells, the cytoplasmic fluorescence was more intense at the periphery of the cell, but not all cells in a cluster were CEA-positive. A direct correlation between the morphological results and the plasma CEA level did not exist. In contrast, Goldenberg et al. [42] found only one CEA-positive breast cancer out of 64. About 25% of bronchial carcinomas were CEA-positive irrespective of whether they belonged to the adenoid or squamous variety. CEA-specific positive immunofluorescence (membrane and, occasionally, cytoplasmic staining) has been observed in medullary carcinomas of the thyroid but not in other types of thyroid cancers and benign disorders of this gland [51].

No clear-cut correlation exists between the tissue content, as revealed by immunofluorescence and other immunomorphological procedures, and the serum CEA levels, as determined by radioimmunoassay [43, 75–77, 102, 124]. In patients with colonic adenomas, plasma CEA was elevated in about one-third as compared to 100% of patients bearing malignant tumors. Plasma CEA was unrelated to the number of polyps in the patients, but apparently depended on the accessibility of the polyp to the blood stream [102]. In alcoholic liver disease a positive correlation between proliferation of CEA-containing bile ductules and plasma CEA levels has been demonstrated (see ref. 38), which did not exist in non-alcoholic liver disorders.

A variety of substances share antigenic determinants with CEA (=cross-reactive antigens; see ref. 114). NCA has a molecular weight of about 100,000. The carbohydrate content is 30% compared to 60% of CEA. NCA [125], identical with the NGP of Mach and Pusztaszeri [74] and the CEX of Darcy et al. [23], shows extensive NH_2-terminal amino acid sequence homology to CEA [37]. NCA, similar to CEA, is present at the apical pole of the cells lining the tumor glands and at the surface of non-cancerous colonic mucosa epithelial cells [14]. In addition, the lateral cell membranes were also often specifically decorated with NCA antibodies. In tumors without glandular organization NCA-specific staining identical to CEA was observed. NCA was also detected at the surface as well as in cytoplasmic position in polymorphonuclear leucocytes and monocyte–macrophage-like mononuclear cells [15]. NCA-2 is another substance cross-reacting with CEA [14, 16]. A specific antiserum, in indirect immunofluorescence, decorated intraluminal material and the luminal surface of colon tumor cells. Goblet cells of non-neoplastic mucosa derived from tumor-bearing and tumor-free patients contained cytoplasmic NCA-2. In gastric mucosa, NCA-2 antibodies did not only decorate tumor cells and intraluminal deposits but also strongly reacted with intestinal metaplastic foveolar cells; deep gastric glands (apparently of the antral type) showed irregular cytoplasmic staining with positive and negative glands [16]. Fetal intestine also contained fair amounts of NCA-2 as revealed by immunofluorescence microscopy [16]. It is noteworthy that the staining of intestinal metaplastic areas with anti-CEA serum, as previously reported by Burtin et al. [14] and Denk et al. [29], was almost abolished by absorption of the sera with NCA-2, indicating that the positive reaction might have been due to a considerable extent to NCA-2 antibodies present in these sera [16]. Kuo et al. [62] have isolated a membrane glycoprotein from human breast carcinomas (BCGP) which also shares an antigenic determinant with CEA. This substance, however, differs from CEA in its chemical composition as revealed by polyacrylamide gel- and immunoelectrophoresis [62]. It is less immunogenic in the rabbit than is CEA. In immunofluorescence, this antigen could be detected in well-differentiated breast carcinomas in higher quantities than in poorly differentiated and anaplastic ones. In addition, fibroadenomas and breasts with fibrocystic disease showed faint fluorescence, indicating that BCGP cannot be regarded as tumor-specific.

14.2.2. Methodology

Several procedures have been employed for isolation of the antigen and preparation of antibodies, and most of them are reviewed by Terry et al. [114]. An improved isolation procedure for CEA by ethanol precipitation has recently been published by Pritchard and Egan [93].

For visualization of the antigen in tissues, usually snap-frozen sections, unfixed or fixed in absolute ethanol, 95% methanol, 95% ethanol or acetone for 10–20 min, have been processed mostly for indirect and, occasionally, direct immunofluorescence [62, 86]. More recently, specimens fixed in 4–10% phosphate-buffered formalin (Denk et al., unpublished) [26, 38, 42, 54, 56, 102, 104], 95% ethanol [51], Bouin's reagent [16] or, according to Sainte-Marie [101, 16], embedded in paraffin after dehydration have been found to be equally suitable for the demonstration of CEA and cross-reacting antigens by immunofluorescence and immunoperoxidase techniques after rehydration in PBS, pH 7.2, or Tris-saline buffer, pH 7.6 [104]. Fixed and paraffin-embedded material is superior to frozen sections because of better preservation of structural details. Pretreatment of dewaxed tissue sections with proteases (pronase, trypsin) [28, 29, 33, 54, 95], which is advantageous for the demonstration of several antigens (immunoglobulins, lysozyme, hepatitis-B-surface antigen, insulin, etc.) in formalin-fixed paraffin-embedded material by decreasing background and increasing specific fluorescence, is not beneficial with respect to CEA [54] (Denk and Platzer, unpublished). Immunomorphology performed on formalin-fixed and paraffin-embedded material is slightly less sensitive than on frozen sections, if the immunoperoxidase reaction is used [42, 102]. This holds true also for immunofluorescence (Denk and Platzer, unpublished observations). Goldenberg et al. [42] have shown, using the three-step unlabelled antibody-immunoperoxidase reaction, that in frozen, ethanol-fixed specimens CEA is detectable if present in concentrations above 0.7 μg/g of tissue, whereas the threshold level is at 3–5 μg/g CEA in formalin-fixed paraffin-embedded tissue. Most benign tumors and non-malignant tissues had CEA levels below 0.7 μg/g and consequently were not stained for CEA [42]. The position of CEA in the tissue may also affect the result of the immunomorphological reaction. Negative tests have often been obtained with cyst fluid of mucinous cystadenocarcinomas known to be rich in CEA, possibly because CEA-containing material was washed out [42]. The slightly lower sensitivity of the immunomorphological test on paraffin material may be the reason for some discrepancies concerning the presence of CEA or CEA-like activity in different tissues [42]; see also the conflicting results concerning CEA in colonic adenomas as reported by Burtin et al. [13] and Tappeiner et al. [111], on the one hand, and by Isaacson and LeVann [56] on the other. An additional influence on the detection of CEA in tissue specimens may be their age [102].

14.2.3. Significance of immunomorphological CEA determinations

Because of the lack of organ and cancer specificity, the immunomorphological demonstration of CEA in tissues does not seem to have diagnostic and prognostic significance in most organs at the present time. Since the significance of CEA in cancer is still unresolved, any speculation on the meaning that the demonstration of CEA in histological specimens may have for cancer diagnosis and prognosis is still premature. In judging the results presented one should, in addition, bear in mind that "CEA" comprises a family of glycoproteins with cross-reactivity and that it is still possible that a single substance with pronounced tumor specificity may emerge on the basis of which immunomorphology could eventually gain diagnostic and prognostic importance.

In endometrium, CEA staining might be useful in delineating preneoplastic changes, since about 60% of endometrial cancer specimens and areas with atypical hyperplasia were CEA-positive [55]. In carcinomas, the positive correlation of CEA content with the histological degree of differentiation of the tumor, particularly in colonic carcinomas [28], could indicate a better prognosis of CEA-rich neoplasms. In pre-invasive dysplastic lesions of the uterine cervix the CEA content, as demonstrated by immunomorphology, seems to reflect a higher aggressive potential [72]. This, however, did not apply for invasive cancers, since survival data of patients with CEA-positive and negative tumors did not disclose any correlation between the CEA content and malignancy [72]. Immunomorphological staining of cytologic smears may eventually assist in diagnosis, particularly in breast, pancreatic, bladder and bronchial cancers.

14.3. ALPHA-1-FETOPROTEIN (AFP)

AFP is a major component of fetal serum and has been shown to reappear in association with hepatoma both in experimental animals and man (for review, see ref. 1). Fetal liver is the major site of AFP synthesis. Human AFP, similar to that found in animals bearing experimentally induced tumors, is an alpha-globulin with a molecular weight of 70,000 (see ref. 1). The physicochemical characteristics resemble those of albumin. AFP differs, however, from albumin in its carbohydrate content [99] (see also ref. 105 for review). AFP does not seem to be autoantigenic but easily evokes heteroantibodies if injected into an appropriate animal [77]. By radioimmunodiffusion, AFP can be detected in 50–80% of patients with primary hepatocellular carcinoma; by more sensitive techniques, e.g. radioimmunoassay, increased AFP levels have been found in almost all patients with hepatocellular carcinoma (for review, see refs. 20, 77, 100). Besides, hepatocellular carcinoma tumors containing yolk sac elements also express AFP [57, 88, 110, 112, 113]. Elevated serum AFP levels have also been found to be associated with other tumors, liver metastases and a variety of non-neoplastic conditions, such as viral hepatitis and liver cirrhosis, associated with liver cell regeneration [1].

14.3.1. Localization of AFP as revealed by immunofluorescence (and other immunomorphological techniques)

AFP can be demonstrated within the cytoplasm of fetal and neoplastic hepatocytes (for review, see refs. 77 and 94). In the embryo, hepatic AFP-

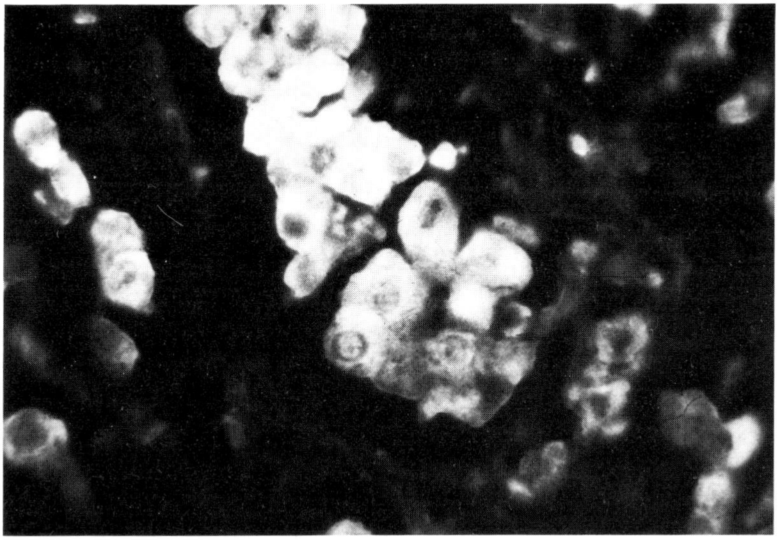

Fig. 14.3. Moderately well-differentiated hepatocellular carcinoma containing cytoplasmic AFP (formalin-fixed, paraffin-embedded material). ×500.

specific fluorescence decreases towards term. In liver tumors, the intensity of AFP staining and the number of AFP positive liver cells are highly variable (Fig. 13.3), and in many tumors, even in those with elevated serum AFP levels, only few cells are specifically stained [1, 44, 77]. AFP positivity may actually indicate a special stage of differentiation (for review, see refs. 1 and 77). AFP-positive hepatomas may be more dedifferentiated toward a fetal stage than those lacking AFP [4, 115].

In livers of rats treated with carcinogens (see, e.g., ref. 45) AFP-positive cells appear 3 weeks after commencement of carcinogen feeding, first in the periportal areas and then dispersed throughout the lobule. AFP-positive cells produced under these conditions show the morphological characteristics of less differentiated "transitional" cells.

In tumors derived from polypotential germ cells (endodermal sinus tumor, embryonal carcinoma) variable AFP-specific immunostaining can be observed in the cells lining the endodermal sinuses (for review, see ref. 1) [88, 112].

14.3.2. Methodology

The reviews by Abelev [1] and Ruoslahti et al. [99] may be consulted for details concerning the antigen and antibody preparation. An improved purification procedure for human AFP from ascitic fluid of hepatoma-bearing patients has been described by Gold et al. [41]. This technique is less time-consuming and yields large quantities of pure AFP. AFP are preserved after formalin fixation and paraffin embedding. Pronase digestion of deparaffinized tissue sections does not appreciably influence the intensity of specific staining, but suppresses background fluorescence (unpublished results). Frozen sections can be subjected to immunofluorescence staining procedures unfixed and after fixation in cold ethanol [57, 94, 112]. Purtilo and Yunis [94] compared frozen unfixed and formalin (10%)-fixed sections and did not report differences in staining intensity. Since AFP is easily washed out of cells containing it originally and can also penetrate cells with impaired permeability, proper fixation is essential to prevent erroneous results in immunofluorescence (for review, see ref. 1). Guilluozo et al. [45] have also studied the influence of different fixation conditions on the specificity of AFP staining. If liver fragments were fixed for 10 min in cold alcohol–acetic acid without prior drying, non-specific staining of all parenchymal cells was seen and the same staining pattern was obtained if fixation in the same media was performed under constant agitation for 30 min prior to paraffin embedding. Under these conditions, staining for IgG paralleled that of AFP, indicating the non-specific nature of the staining reaction due to the passive uptake of plasma constituents. If the Sainte-Marie [101] fixation and embedding procedure was used, only a fraction of hepatocytes was AFP-positive and IgG was limited to the sinusoids. Adequate fixation was also achieved in phosphate-buffered (0.1 M, pH 7.4) 10% paraformaldehyde for 6–8 h at 4°C, subsequent incubation overnight in 10% glycerol in phosphate buffer, freezing in liquid nitrogen-cooled isopentane for cryostat sectioning, or fixation in 6% paraformaldehyde–1% glutaraldehyde in sodium cacodylate buffer (0.1 M, pH 7.4) for 4 h at 4°C and further processing for cryostat sectioning as described above. These studies indicate that extensive inflow of proteins from extracellular compartments into liver cells, preventable by adequate fixation, may occur and cause erroneous immunofluorescence results.

14.3.3. Significance of immunomorphological AFP determinations

So far, no convincing evidence exists that the immunomorphological demonstration of AFP in hepatocellular carcinomas has any prognostic significance despite the notions of Alpert [4], Peyrol et al. [91], Purtilo and Yunis [94] and Thung et al. [115] that AFP-positive hepatomas are less differentiated and mimic a fetal or hepatoblastic state. In tumors of germ cell origin, the immunomorphological AFP determination may help in delineating yolk sac elements [1, 113].

14.4. FETAL SULPHOGLYCOPROTEIN ANTIGEN (FSA)

FSA has been described by Häkkinen [46] and can be detected by immunofluorescence in gastric mucosa as well as in gastric juice by double immunodiffusion (for review, see ref. 48). It is a carbohydrate-rich sulfated glycoprotein which is resistant to the acid milieu of the stomach, can be boiled for 5–10 min without apparent loss or change of antigenicity and precipitated with ethanol. It shares a common antigenic determinant with CEA. The antigen has been detected in the gastric juice of almost all patients with stomach cancer but not in that of young controls. It is not strictly cancer-specific, however, since it has been found in 3–7% of non-cancerous samples of gastric juice derived from older patients (for review, see ref. 77). The antigen cross-reacts with salivary glycoproteins and with glycoproteins from normal gastric juice. Some FSA preparations exhibit blood group reactivity. Extensive field studies conducted by Häkkinen and his coworkers [48] revealed the value of FSA determinations as a screening test for gastric cancer in the high-risk population of Finland.

14.4.1. Localization of FSA as revealed by immunofluorescence

FSA is a regular constituent of the fetal alimentary tract. In gastric cancer specimens two types of FSA-specific staining patterns have been observed: i) absence from non-neoplastic mucosal cells but presence in cancer cells, and ii) presence on both non-tumorous and cancer cells. Cytoplasmic fluorescence of tumor cells was usually less intense than that of the non-neoplastic cells. The antigen was absent from small and large bowel mucosa.

14.4.2. Methodology

Antigen and antibody are, at the present time, not commercially available and studies have, so far, only been conducted by Häkkinen and coworkers (see refs. 47 and 48 for further information). Ethanol and formalin-fixed material embedded in paraffin are suitable for the demonstration of FSA, although staining was stronger in alcohol- than in formalin-fixed material [50].

14.4.3. Significance of immunomorphological FSA determinations

FSA is clearly cancer-associated but not cancer-specific. Whereas the detection of FSA in gastric juice seems to be valuable as a screening test for gastric cancer, the significance of immunomorphological detection in tissue sections is doubtful, particularly in view of the lacking cancer specificity. Whether FSA-positive non-neoplastic cells can eventually be regarded as precancerous is unproved [50].

14.5. OTHER ONCOFETAL ANTIGENS

Oncofetal antigens different from those discussed in the preceding paragraphs have been found in association with different tumors, and the morphological distribution of some of them has been studied by immunomorphological techniques. Oncofetal antigens have been found in glial tumors [116, 117], in pancreatic cancers (for review, see ref. 97), and in kidney tumors [61]. The latter, the fetorenal antigen, is present in fetuses as well as in human and animal serum containing antibodies to the hepatitis B antigen. It seems to share an antigenic determinant (or determinants) with the hepatitis B surface antigen. The antigen can be demonstrated in frozen sections of fetal urinary system, including collecting ducts of kidneys, renal pelvis, ureter and urinary bladder, at the apical cell pole. Other organs, including the gastrointestinal tract, were negative. The clinical significance of the determination of this antigen in tissue sections is not established. The alpha-2H-globulin, an iron-containing macroglobulin immunologically related to ferritin (for review, see ref. 77), is a normal component of fetal liver and is also found in the serum of newborns up to the second postnatal month [11]. It can be detected in serum of hepatoma patients but also in a variety of gastrointestinal tumors and in inflammatory diseases. Children with hepatitis, hepatoblastomas and cholangiomas showed elevated serum levels still rising with progression of the disease. Other oncofetal antigens described in the literature are the beta-fetoprotein, described by Alpert [4] in fetal liver and hepatomas, immunologically closely related to ferritin, and the sarcoma-associated cytoplasmic antigen [119] occurring in sarcoma cells and in embryonal tissue. Antibodies to this antigen have been demonstrated by immunofluorescence with a high frequency in patients with sarcomas but also other tumors.

14.6. TUMOR-ASSOCIATED ANTIGENS WITH BLOOD GROUP REACTIVITY

14.6.1. Localization of blood group (BG) antigens

Antigens with BG reactivity exist in alcohol- and water-soluble form in epithelial cells [107–109]. The alcohol-soluble BG are associated with cell membranes, the water-soluble ones are present in intra- and extracytoplasmic secretion products. In carcinomas, at least of the gastrointestinal tract, alcohol-soluble BG prevail, at least as determined by immunomorphological procedures [31]. The membrane-bound BG reactivity can easily be demonstrated by immunofluorescence in the squamous epithelium of the oral cavity [22]. Erythrocyte adherence, another and highly sensitive method of detecting BG in tissue sections [25, 31], results in a more diffuse pattern, so it is not possible to clearly assign the antigen to specific cell structures.

14.6.2. Methodology

Commercial human BG antisera as well as rabbit antibodies have been successfully employed in indirect immunofluorescence with FITC-coupled anti-human or anti-rabbit IgG in the second layer [21, 25, 49]. In unfixed frozen tissue sections both alcohol- and water-soluble BG are preserved and easily detectable. In formalin-fixed, paraffin-embedded material, however, alcohol-soluble BG are not demonstrable by immunofluorescence, possibly due to partial extraction or modification of their antigenicity [25, 59]. This is, however, not the case with respect to the specific erythrocyte adherence reaction, which, possibly due to its superior sensitivity, is still able to uncover glycolipid-related BG reactivity in material embedded in paraffin after formalin fixation [31]. In our hands, therefore, the specific erythrocyte adherence reaction outruns immunofluorescence in detection of tissue bound BG.

14.6.3. Significance of immunomorphological BG determinations

Presence and distribution patterns of BG in non-neoplastic and neoplastic tissues were studied by using various immunomorphological techniques [30–32]. Davidsohn [24] reported loss or diminution of these antigens in a diversity of carcinomas arising from tissues which originally expressed BG and reported a positive correlation between loss of BG and the anaplasia of the tumor as well as its tendency to metastasize. In carcinomas of the oral cavity BG were also decreased in most but not all instances. BG were, in addition, diminished in peritumoral mucosa with cell atypia, suggesting that alterations of BG antigenicity are tumor-associated changes which, in some instances, may precede overt carcinomas [22]. In tumors arising from urinary bladder epithelium, antigen loss prevails in more pleomorphic, anaplastic, infiltrating and rapidly fatal tumors, but exceptions are numerous [58]. This would imply a diagnostic and prognostic significance of morphological BG determinations in tumor tissue as well as in potentially precancerous lesions [25, 103]. According to our experience, however, this does not hold true for every carcinoma. Particularly in gastric cancers we were unable to find a correlation between (alcohol-soluble) BG content and tumor differentiation or propensity to produce metastases [27]. In about 60% of carcinomas of the distal colon, BG reappear and, in this localization, may be regarded as oncofetal antigens [31]. The presence or absence of BG surface antigens in colonic carcinomas may determine the biological behaviour of the tumor via modulation of the immunological host response directed against the tumor [2]. Davidsohn and coworkers [24] have emphasized that loss of BG in tumors of the uterine cervix indicates malignancy, propensity to metastasize, and, consequently, poor prognosis. Our own experience, however, is at variance with this statement (unpublished observation). At the present stage of our knowledge, we believe that the determination of BG is of limited usefulness at least in routine diagnosis. This does not, however, restrict the importance of studies concerning the antigenicity of tumor cells which are essential for the understanding of the biology of a given tumor. In colonic adenomas, for example, the determination of BG provides an objective measure of the degree of differentiation [32].

14.7. EXOCRINE SECRETION PRODUCTS OF TUMORS

Secretion products of certain tumors may serve as markers and may be helpful in their characterization. This applies, for example, to milk (whey) proteins in mammary and uterine cancers. The main whey proteins are casein, lactalbumin, lactoferrin and secretory IgA which can be separated by gel filtration, ion-exchange chromatography and fractional salt precipitation [65]. Casein is a milk phosphoprotein which precipitates at acidic pH. Lactalbumin levels have been studied by radioimmunoassay in the blood of normal individuals, lactating mothers, and patients with breast carcinoma. Upper levels of lactalbumin in normal individuals were about 20 ng/ml. There was no significant elevation in many breast cancer patients, whereas an increased level was found during lactation. Lactoferrin with a molecular weight of 80,000 and secretory IgA (MW 390,000) are present in most external secretions of the body [78]; are found as normal plasma constituents; and are not significantly elevated in patients with malignancies. Casein or casein-like substances were detected by Bussolati et al. [19], at the surface of cells and within the lumina of lactating glands. Some intracellular fluorescence close to the apical pole of the cells was also seen. In adult non-lactating breasts, fluorescence staining was confined to some ducts and alveoli. Prepubertal breasts were casein-negative. In dysplastic mammary glands, casein was detected in ductules and acini mainly at the luminal surface of the cells. Well-differentiated mammary carcinomas were casein-positive, showing surface staining in addition to diffuse cytoplasmic fluorescence. Poorly differentiated tumors expressed less or no casein. The presence of casein in mammary Paget cells may indicate their origin from cells of intraductal carcinomas, whereas extramammary Paget cells may be derived from sweat or sebaceous glands which are also stained with casein antibodies [18]. The specificity of casein for mammary, sebaceous, and sweat gland epithelia was, however, challenged by additional studies of Bussolati and coworkers [19, 92] and Hustin [55] showing that casein or casein-like material may be produced by some adenocarcinomas of the gastrointestinal tract, endometrium and the lung. Moreover, casein-specific reactivity was observed within the glands and at the luminal surface of the cells in cystic hyperplasia but not in functioning cyclic uterine mucosa. In addition, some, but not all, endometrial polyps and carcinomas were casein-positive, possibly indicating unopposed estrogen action [55].

14.7.1. Methodology

Details concerning the preparation of antigens and antibodies have been described by Bussolati et al. [19]. The antigenicity of casein is not lost during the process of routine fixation (10% formalin, formol–alcohol–acetic acid, Bouin's solution) and (paraffin, paraplast) embedding, and the antigen can subsequently be detected by indirect immunofluorescence and peroxidase immunostaining. In contrast, the secretory piece of IgA, alpha-lactalbumin, and lactoferrin are labile, and frozen sections are required [18, 60]. The value of enzyme predigestion of the sections with respect to suppression of background staining and enhancement of specific fluorescence has not yet been explored.

14.7.2. Significance of immunomorphological detection of whey proteins

The immunomorphological demonstration of whey proteins in tissue sections may be advantageous in the characterization of tumors, as shown by Bussolati and Pich [18], with respect to Paget's disease of the nipple, and in the assessment of the functional state and differentiation of a breast tumor [19]. It should be borne in mind, however, as shown by the same authors, that casein is not specific for tumors of breast derivation. So far, there is no evidence that the presence or absence of casein can in any way be related to prognosis.

14.8. RECEPTOR PROTEINS ON TUMOR CELLS

The detection of hormone receptors, e.g. for estrogen, progesterone, and prolactin, plays an increasingly important role in predicting the response of a tumor to hormonal therapy, particularly in breast cancer [81, 96]. Immunomorphological and histochemical techniques allow a direct correlation between receptor content and histological features of the tumor.

14.8.1. Localization of receptor proteins in mammary cancer

Receptor proteins have been detected by immunomorphological and histochemical methods in the cytoplasm and/or nucleus in hyperplastic and neoplastic glands [90]. Receptor distribution was fairly uniform in non-neoplastic conditions, whereas cancer cells showed variable degrees of staining intensity, ranging from negative to strongly positive. It has been proposed, on the basis of the morphological studies, that all mammary cancers contain estrogen receptor-positive and -negative cells; consequently, breast cancers should be graded according to the ratio of positive and negative cells [66]. De Souza et al. [34] demonstrated membrane receptors for prolactin, growth hormone and placental lactogen, using immunoperoxidase techniques. Positive membrane staining for prolactin was seen in 53% of human breast cancer specimens. Similar results were obtained for growth hormone, whereas only a few tumors were positive for placental lactogen.

14.8.2. Methodology

Fixation of tissue sections containing estrogen receptor-positive cells in cold (–20°C) acetone, 3.7% buffered formaldehyde or 1% glutaraldehyde abolishes an estrogen-binding capacity [66]. Unfixed, frozen sections are, therefore, used in the indirect immunofluorescence test with anti-estradiol serum (after prior incubation with estradiol) in the first and the appropriate FITC-conjugated antiserum in the second layer [84]. In a modification of the technique [64], immunomorphology is also applicable to fixed, paraffin-embedded material. This modification rests on the fact that the receptor is protected by incubation of the tissue sections with estradiol prior to fixation (2 mm thick sections are incubated with 17-beta-estradiol at room temperature for 1 h prior to fixation in cold picric acid–formaldehyde, washed for 5 h in cold buffer and subsequently embedded in paraffin). The protective estrogen is apparently removed during fixation and embedding, and has to be resupplied prior to immunomorphological staining. Preliminary studies by the same authors revealed that the estrogen-stabilized receptor also resists formalin fixation.

14.9. HORMONES

Immunomorphology in many instances allows subclassification of tumors arising from cells with endocrine activity. Arnal-Monreal et al. [5] applied indirect immunofluorescence to medullary thyroid carcinomas and pancreatic islet cell tumors. Medullary thyroid carcinomas expressed large amounts of immunoreactive calcitonin. Detection of insulin (Fig. 14.4), glucagon and gastrin [5, 82, 85] allows for the tracing of islet cell tumors to specific progenitor cells. A variety of hormones (corticotropin, beta-lipotropin, growth hormone, prolactin, thyrotropin, gonadotropin) could be detected in pituitary adenomas [34, 53, 87]. Mostly the indirect immunoperoxidase technique was used [53, 87], but indirect immunofluorescence seems to be equally suitable [52]. Elde et al. [36] examined the cellular localization of somatostatin in central, peripheral and autonomic nervous system and in the gastroenteropancreatic tract by direct immunofluorescence. The direct immunofluorescence technique was also used to search stomach and duodenal mucosa for gastrin-producing cells [80, 82, 106]. Cholecystokinin has been detected by indirect immunofluorescence in cells in the duodenal and jejunal mucosa of dog and man [10].

14.9.1. Methodology

Most of the hormones mentioned above tolerate fixation without significant loss of antigenicity. Frozen sections or material fixed in Bouin's solution, 10% neutral formaldehyde, 4% formaldehyde and phosphate-buffered, 4% parafor-

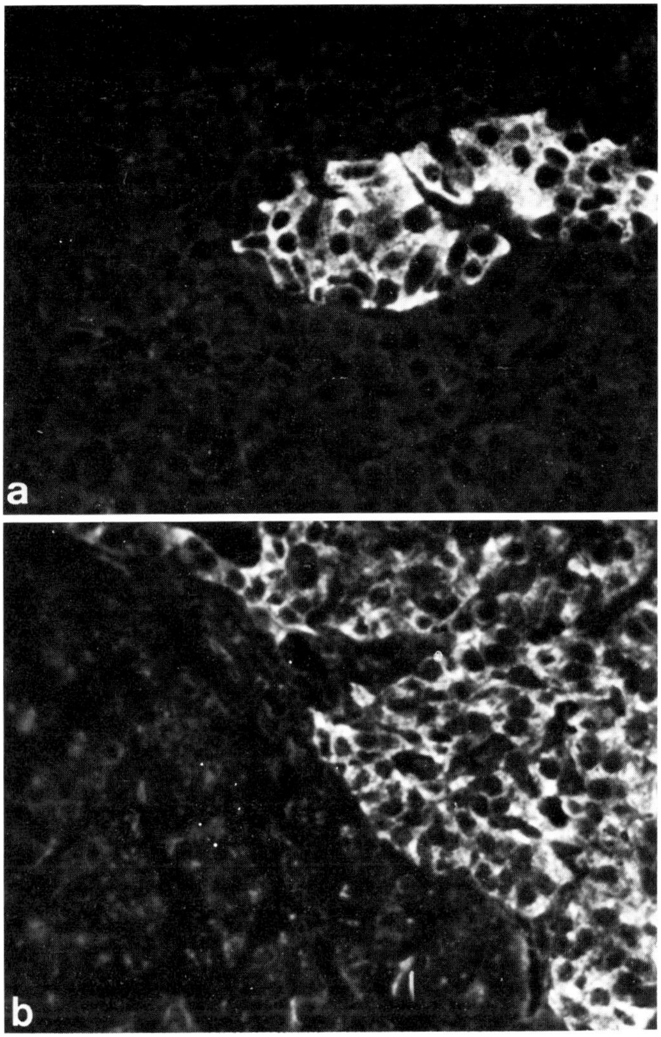

Fig. 14.4. Insulin-containing B cells. a) Pancreatic Langerhans islet. ×560. b) Islet cell tumor (insulinoma). ×320. (Both formalin-fixed, paraffin-embedded material).

maldehyde have been used after paraffin or paraplast embedding [36, 52, 53, 79, 85, 87]. In our own experience, pronase pretreatment for 10–60 min is advantageous but not critical, particularly with respect to background reduction. According to Arnal-Monreal et al. [5], trypsin pretreatment significantly improves the quality of immunofluorescence by elimination of background staining and enhancement of sensitivity. With respect to the immunomorphological detection of somatostatin, freeze-drying of the specimens at the temperature of liquid nitrogen in a propane–propylene mixture and subsequent exposure to formaldehyde or diethylpyrocarbonate vapors and embedding in paraffin proved to be the method of choice [3]. With diethylpyrocarbonate fixation the intensity of specific staining was higher than with formaldehyde.

14.10. MISCELLANEOUS TUMOR-ASSOCIATED ANTIGENS

Tumor-associated antigens have been detected in melanoma, Wilms tumor, Hodgkin's disease and bronchial carcinoma. In melanoma, common membrane and cytoplasmic antigens have been suggested by several authors on the basis of immunofluorescence staining of melanoma cell preparations grown in tissue culture with sera of melanoma patients [83], of cell suspension dispersed from fresh tumor material [70], of touch imprints fixed in acetone for 10 min at ambient temperature and then air-dried [121], or of cultured melanoma cells fixed in 96% methanol [67]. Wood and Barth [121] observed that several antibodies present in sera of patients with melanoma were directed against tumor-associated rather than tumor-specific cytoplasmic antigens. Antibodies directed against membrane antigens, however, appeared to be patient-specific [71]. The lack of cross-reactivity is similar to that seen in experimental tumors induced by carcinogens, which also show unique tumor antigens in each case [7]. The significance of antibodies directed against melanoma cell surface antigens has not yet been determined. These antibodies may be used to isolate membrane antigens in order to develop specific radio- or enzyme-immunoassays [67].

An antigen associated with Hodgkin's disease has been described by Long et al. [73]. Using acetone-fixed cells derived from cultured Hodgkin's disease tissue, the antigen could be detected on the cell surface as well as within the cytoplasm by indirect immunofluorescence.

A neoantigen (w-antigen), predominantly associated with human nephroblastomas, has been described by Burtin and Gendron [12]. The w-antigen is soluble in phytic acid and resists several enzymes, but not pronase. It is destroyed by perchloric acid and altered in its antigenicity by periodic acid. No cross-reactivities have been observed between the w-antigen and several oncofetal antigens, including CEA and AFP. By immunofluorescence using frozen sections the antigen has been detected in the cytoplasm and in intercellular deposits.

Another antigen (HLTAA) has been isolated from bronchial carcinomas and appears to be distinct from other tumor-related proteins and glycoproteins, including CEA, AFP, ferritin, lactoferrin, alpha-2H-globulin, placental alkaline phosphatase [9]. This antigen has not yet been immunolocalized.

14.11. CONCLUDING REMARKS

Immunomorphological techniques are indispensable tools in any attempt to correlate chemical composition with morphological structure. These methods not only play a major role in basic research, but also are applied with increasing frequency in pathology. In conjunction with light microscopy they are able to provide information of diagnostic and prognostic significance. Immunomorphological detection of tumor-associated antigens is of paramount importance to the understanding of tumor biology. Its practical value, however, particularly in pathology, still remains to be assessed.

REFERENCES

1 Abelev, G.I. (1974) Alpha-fetoprotein as a marker of embryospecific differentiation in normal and tumor tissue. Transplant. Rev. 20, 3–37.

2 Abdelfattah-Gad, M. and Denk, H. (1980) Epithelial blood group antigens in human carcinomas of the distal colon: further studies on their pathologic significance. J. Natl. Cancer Inst. *64,* 1025–1028.

3 Alumets, J., Sundler, F. and Häkanson, R. (1977) Distribution, ontogeny and ultrastructure of somatostatin immunoreactive cells in the pancreas and gut. Cell Tissue Res. *185,* 465–479.

4 Alpert, M. (cited by Purtilo, D.T. and Yunis, E.J., 1971, Lab. Invest. *25,* 291–294).

5 Arnal-Monreal, F.M., Goltzman, D., Knaack, J., Wang, N.-S. and Huang, S.-N. (1977) Immunohistologic study of thyroidal carcinoma and pancreatic insulinoma. Cancer *40,* 1060–1070.

6 Baldwin, R.W. (1977) Tumor-associated antigens. Z. Krebsforsch. *89,* 1–8.

7 Baldwin, R.W. and Embleton, M.J. (1971; cited by Lewis, M.G. and Philips, T.M., 1972, Int. J. Cancer, *10,* 105–111).

8 Bordes, M., Michiels, R. and Martin, F. (1973) Detection by immunofluorescence of carcinoembryonic antigen in colonic carcinoma, other malignant or benign tumors, and noncancerous tissues. Digestion *9,* 106–115.

9 Braatz, J.A., McIntire, K.R., Princler, G.L., Kortright, K.H. and Herberman, R.B. (1978) Purification and characterization of a human lung tumor-associated antigen. J. Natl. Cancer. Inst. *61,* 1035–1046.

10 Buffa, R., Solcia, E. and Go, V.L.W. (1976) Immunohistochemical identification of the cholecystokinin cell in the intestinal mucosa. Gastroenterology *70,* 528–532.

11 Buffe, D., Rimbaut, C., Fuccaro, C. and Burtin, P. (1972) Isolement et caractérisation d'une alpha-2-ferroprotéine: la globuline alpha-2-H. Ann. Inst. Pasteur *123,* 29.

12 Burtin, P. and Gendron, M.C. (1973) A tumor-associated antigen in human nephroblastomas. Proc. Natl. Acad. Sci. U.S.A. *70,* 2051–2054.

13 Burtin, P., Martin, E., Sabine, M.C. and Von Kleist, S. (1972) Immunological study of polyps of the colon. J. Natl. Cancer Inst. *48,* 25–32.

14 Burtin, P., Von Kleist, S., Sabine, M.C. and King, M. (1973) Immunological localization of carcinoembryonic antigen and nonspecific cross-reacting antigen in gastrointestinal normal and tumoral tissues. Cancer Res. *33,* 3299–3305.

15 Burtin, P., Quan, P.C. and Sabine, M.C. (1975) Nonspecific cross-reacting antigen as a marker for human polymorphs, macrophages and monocytes. Nature *255,* 714–716.

16 Burtin, P., Sabine, M.C. and Chavanel, G. (1977) A comparative study of the localization of CEA and NCA_2 in cancerous and normal gastrointestinal tissue. Int. J. Cancer *19,* 634–641.

17 Burtin, P., Calmettes, C. and Fondaneche, M.C. (1979) CEA and non-specific cross-reacting antigen (NCA) in medullary carcinomas of the thyroid. Int. J. Cancer *23,* 741–745.

18 Bussolati, G. and Pich, A. (1975) Mammary and extramammary Paget's disease. Am. J. Pathol. *80,* 117–127.

19 Bussolati, G., Pich, A. and Alfani, V. (1975) Immunofluorescence detection of casein in human mammary dysplastic and neoplastic tissues. Virchows Arch. A *365,* 15–21.

20 Chayvialle, J.A.P., Brissot, P., Pelletier, M.J., Hita de Nercy, Y., Lambert, R. and Bourel, M. (1977) Alpha-fetoprotein screening in patients with idiopathic hemochromatosis and liver cirrhosis. Digestion *16,* 118–127.

21 Dabelsteen, E. (1972) Quantitative determination of blood group substances A of oral epithelial cells by immunofluorescence and immunoperoxidase methods. Acta Pathol. Microbiol. Scand. Sect. A *80,* 847–853.

22 Dabelsteen, E. and Pindberg, J.J. (1973) Loss of epithelial blood group substance A in oral carcinomas. Acta Pathol. Microbiol. Scand. Sect. A *81,* 435–444.

23 Darcy, D.A., Turberville, C. and James, R. (1973) Immunological study of carcinoembryonic antigen (CEA) and a related glycoprotein. Br. J. Cancer *28,* 147–160.

24 Davidsohn, I. (1972) Early immunologic diagnosis and prognosis of carcinoma. Am. J. Clin. Pathol. *57,* 715–730.

25 Davidsohn, I., Kovarik, St. and Lee, Ch.L. (1966) A, B, and O substances in gastrointestinal carcinoma. Arch. Pathol. *81,* 381–390.

26 Delellis, R.A., Rule, A.H., Spiler, I., Nathanson, L., Tashjian, A.H. and Wolfe, H.J. (1978) Calcitonin and carcinoembryonic antigen as tumor markers in medullary thyroid carcinoma. Am. J. Clin. Pathol. *70,* 587–594.

27 Denk, H. (1979) Blood group antigens and CEA in stomach cancer. *In* Synopsis, G.I. and Pfeiffer, C. (eds). Gastric Cancer (Witzstrock Publishing House, New York–Baden-Baden–Cologne) pp 191–128.

28 Denk, H., Tappeiner, G., Eckerstorfer, R. and Holzner, J.H. (1972) Carcinoembryonic antigen (CEA) in gastrointestinal and extragastrointestinal tumors and its relationship to tumor-cell differentiation. Int. J. Cancer *10,* 262–272.

29 Denk, H., Tappeiner, G., Davidovits, A. and Holzner, J.H. (1973) The carcinoembryonic antigen (CEA) in carcinomata of the stomach. Virchows Arch. A *360,* 339–347.

30 Denk, H., Tappeiner, G. and Holzner, J.H. (1974) Independent behaviour of blood group A- and B-like activities in gastric carcinomata of blood group AB individuals. Nature *248,* 428–430.

31 Denk, H., Tappeiner, G., Davidovits, A., Eckerstorfer, R. and Holzner, J.H. (1974) Carcinoembryonic antigen and blood group substances in carcinomas of the stomach and colon. J. Natl. Cancer Inst. *53,* 933–942.

32 Denk, H., Holzner, J.H. and Obitisch-Mayr, I. (1975) Epithelial blood group antigens in colon polyps. I. Morphologic distribution and relationship to differentiation. J. Natl. Cancer Inst. *54,* 1313–1317.

33 Denk, H., Radaszkiewicz, T. and Weirich, E. (1977) Pronase pretreatment of tissue sections enhances sensitivity of the unlabelled antibody enzyme (PAP) technique. J. Immunol. Methods *15,* 163–167.

34 De Souza, I., Salih, H. and Hobbs, J.R. (1976) Affinity-purified antibodies enabling immunoperoxidase reactions to demonstrate membrane receptors for prolactin, growth hormone and placental lactogen. *In* Peeters, H. (ed.), Protides of the Biological Fluids, *Vol. 24,* (Pergamon Press, Oxford–New York–Toronto–Sydney–Paris–Frankfurt) pp. 803–809.

35 Edgington, T.S., Astarita, R.W. and Plow, E.F. (1975) Association of an isomeric species of carcinoembryonic antigen with neoplasia of the gastrointestinal tract. N. Engl. J. Med. *293,* 103–107.

36 Elde, R., Hökfelt, T., Johansson, O., Schultzberg, M., Efendić, S. and Luft, R. (1978) Cellular localization of somatostatin. Metabolism *27,* 1151–1159.

37 Engvall, E., Shively, J.E. and Wrann, M. (1978) Isolation and characterisation of the normal cross-reacting antigen: homology of its NH_2-terminal amino-acid sequence with that of carcinoembryonic antigen. Proc. Natl. Acad. Sci. U.S.A. *75,* 1670–1674.

38 Gerber, M.A. and Thung, S.N. (1978) Carcinoembryonic antigen in normal and diseased liver tissue. Am. J. Pathol. *92,* 671–680.

39 Gold, Ph. and Freedman, S. (1965) Demonstration of tumor-specific antigens in human colonic carcinomata by immunological tolerance and absorption techniques. J. Exp. Med. *121,* 439–462.

40 Gold, Ph. and Freedman, S.O. (1965) Specific carcinoembryonic antigens of the human digestive system. J. Exp. Med. *122,* 467–481.

41 Gold, Ph., Labitan, A., Wong, H.C.G., Freedman, S., Krupey, J. and Shuster, J. (1978) Physicochemical approach to the purification of human $alpha_1$-fetoprotein from the ascites fluid of a hepatoma-bearing patient. Cancer Res. *38,* 6–12.

42 Goldenberg, D.M., Sharkey, R.M. and Primus, F.J. (1976) Carcinoembryonic antigen in histopathology: Immunoperoxidase staining of conventional tissue sections. J. Natl. Cancer Inst. *57,* 11–22.

43 Goldenberg, D.M., Sharkey, R.M. and Primus, F.J. (1978) Immunocytochemical detection of carcinoembryonic antigen in conventional histopathology specimens. Cancer *42,* 1546–1553.

44 Goussev, A.I., Engelhardt, N.V., Masseyeff, R., Camain, R. and Basteris, B. (1971) Immunofluorescent study of alpha-fetoprotein in liver and liver tumor. Int. J. Cancer *7,* 207–217.

45 Guillouzo, A., Belanger, L., Beaumont, C., Valet, J.P., Briggs, R. and Chiu, J.F. (1978) Cellular and subcellular immunolocalization of alpha$_1$-fetoprotein and albumin in rat liver. Reevaluation of various experimental conditions. J. Histochem. Cytochem. *26,* 948–959.

46 Häkkinen, I.P.T. (1966) An immunochemical method for detecting carcinomatous secretion from human gastric juice. Scand. J. Gastroenterol. *1,* 28–32.

47 Häkkinen, I.P.T. (1974) FSA-fetal sulphoglycoprotein antigen associated with gastric cancer. Transplant. Rev. *20,* 61–76.

48 Häkkinen, I.P.T. (1978) Antigenic properties of gastric glycoproteins: *In* Piper, D.W. (ed.), UICC Technical Report Series *34* (International Union Against Cancer, Geneva) pp. 70–78.

49 Häkkinen, I.P.T. and Virtanen, S. (1970) The appearance of blood group and organ-specific antigens in human gastric glycoprotein. Int. Arch. Allergy *39,* 272–279.

50 Häkkinen, I.P.T., Järvi, O. and Grönroos, J. (1968) Sulphoglycoprotein antigens in the human alimentary canal and gastric cancer. An immunohistological study. Int. J. Cancer *3,* 572–581.

51 Hamada, S. and Hamada, S. (1977) Localization of carcinoembryonic antigen in medullary thyroid carcinoma by immunofluorescent techniques. Br. J. Cancer *36,* 572–576.

52 Hauser-Gunsbourg, N., Doerr-Schott, J. and Dubois, M.P. (1978) Identification by immunofluorescence of prolactin- and somatotropin-producing cells in the pituitary gland of the mexican axolotl (Ambystoma mexicanum, Shaw). Cell Tissue Res. *194,* 497–501.

53 Heitz, P.U. (1979) Multihormonal pituitary adenomas. Hormone Res. *10,* 1–13.

54 Huang, S.N., Minassian, H. and More, J.D. (1976) Application of immunofluorescent staining on paraffin sections improved by trypsin digestion. Lab. Invest. *35,* 383–390.

55 Hustin, J. (1978) Immunohistochemical demonstration of several tumor markers in neoplastic and preneoplastic states of the uterine mucosa. Gynecol. Obstet. Invest. *9,* 3–15.

56 Isaacson, P. and LeVann, H.P. (1976) The demonstration of carcinoembryonic antigen in colorectal carcinoma and colonic polyps using an immunoperoxidase technique. Cancer *38,* 1348–1356.

57 Itoh, T., Shirai, T., Naka, A. and Matsumoto, S. (1974) Yolk sac tumor and alpha-fetoprotein: clinicopathological study of four cases. Gann *65,* 215–226.

58 Kay, H.E.M. and Wallace, D.M. (1961) A and B antigens of tumors arising from urinary epithelium. J. Natl. Cancer Inst. *26,* 1349–1365.

59 Kent, S.P. (1954) The demonstration and distribution of watersoluble O (H) antigen in tissue sections using a fluorescein-labeled extract of *Ulex europeus* seed. J. Histochem. Cytochem. *12,* 591–599.

60 Kihm, U. (1973) Immunhistochemische Darstellung der Casein- und β-Lactoglobulinsynthese in der Rindermilchdrüse. Histochemie *35,* 273–281.

61 Kistler, G.S. and Sonnabend, W. (1974) Antikörper gegen ein fetorenales Antigen in Hepatitis-B-Patienten, Trägern von Nierentumoren und gesunden Individuen. Schweiz. Med. Wochenschr. *104,* 485–497.

62 Kuo, T.-T., Rosai, J. and Tillack, T.W. (1973) Immunological studies of membrane glycoproteins isolated from human breast carcinomas. Int. J. Cancer *12,* 532–542.

63 Kuhlmann, W. (1975) Purification of mouse alpha$_1$-fetoprotein and preparation of specific peroxidase conjugates for its cellular localization. Histochemistry *44,* 155.

64 Kurzon, R.M. and Sternberger, L.A. (1978) Estrogen receptor immunochemistry. J. Histochem. Cytochem. *26,* 803–808.

65 Laurence, D.J.R. (1978) Milk proteins and mammary cancer: a review. Invest. Cell Pathol. *1,* 5–22.

66 Lee, S.H. (1978) Cancer cell estrogen receptor of human mammary carcinoma. Cancer *44,* 1–12.

67 Leong, St. P.L., Sutherland, C.M. and Krementz, E.T. (1977) Immunofluorescent detection of common melanoma membrane antigens by sera of melanoma patients immunized against autologous or allogeneic cultured melanoma cells. Cancer Res. *37,* 4035–4042.

68 Leung, J.P., Eshdat, Y. and Marchesi, V.T. (1977) Colonic tumor membrane-associated glycoprotein: isolation of antigenically-active peptides after chemical cleavage. J. Immunol. *119,* 664–670.

69 Leung, J.P., Plow, E.F., Eshdat, Y., Marchesi, V.T. and Edgington, T.S. (1977) Delineation of three classes of CEA antigenic determinants: identification of membrane-associated CEA as an independent species of CEA. J. Immunol. *119,* 271–276.

70 Lewis, M.G. and Phillips, T.M. (1972) The specificity of surface membrane immunofluorescence in human malignant melanoma. Int. J. Cancer *10,* 105–111.

71 Lewis, M.G., Ikonopisov, R.L., Nairn, R.C., Phillips, T.M., Hamilton Fairley, G., Bodenham, D.C. and Alexander, P. (1969) Tumor specific antibodies in human malignant melanoma and their relationship to the extent of the disease. Br. Med. J. *3,* 547–552.

72 Lindgren, J., Wahlström, T. and Seppälä, M. (1979) Tissue CEA in premalignant epithelial lesions and epidermoid carcinoma of the uterine cervix: prognostic significance. Int. J. Cancer *23,* 448–453.

73 Long, J.C., Aisenberg, A.C. and Zamecnik, P.C. (1974) An antigen in Hodgkin's disease tissue cultures: fluorescent antibody studies. Proc. Natl. Acad. Sci. U.S.A. *71,* 2285–2289.

74 Mach, J.P. and Pusztaszeri, G. (1972) Carcinoembryonic antigen (CEA). Demonstration of a partial identity between CEA and a normal glycoprotein. Immunochemistry *9,* 1031–1034.

75 Martin, E.W., Kibbey, W.E., di Vecchia, L., Anderson, G., Catalano, Ph. and Minton, J.P. (1976) Carcinoembryonic antigen. Clinical and historical aspects. Cancer *37,* 62–81.

76 Martin, F. and Devant, J. (1973) Carcinoembryonic antigen in normal human saliva. J. Natl. Cancer Inst. *50,* 1375–1379.

77 Martin, F., Martin, M.S. and Bourgeaux, C. (1976) Fetal antigens in human digestive tumors. Eur. J. Cancer *12,* 165–175.

78 Masson, P., Heremans, J.F. and Prignot, J. (1967) Immunohistochemical localization of the iron binding protein lactoferrin in human bronchial glands. (Cited by Pich, A., Bussolati, G. and Carbonara, A., 1976, J. Histochem. Cytochem. *24,* 940–947).

79 McGuigan, J.E. (1968) Immunochemical studies with synthetic human gastrin. Gastroenterology *54,* 1005–1011.

80 McGuigan, J.E. (1968) Gastric mucosal intracellular localization of gastrin by immunofluorescence. Gastroenterology *55,* 315–326.

81 McGuire, W.L. (1978) Steroid receptors in human breast cancer. Cancer Res. *38,* 4289–4291.

82 Mitschke, H. (1977) Funktionelle Pathomorphologie des gastrointestinalen endokrinen Zellsystems. *In* Büngeler, W., Eder, M., Lennert, K., Peters, G., Sandritter, W. and Seifert, G. (eds.), Veröffentlichungen aus der Pathologie, *104* (Gustav Fischer Verlag, Stuttgart–New York) pp. 140–150.

83 Muna, N.M., Marcus, St. and Smart, Ch. (1969) Detection by immunofluorescence of antibodies specific for human malignant melanoma cells. Cancer *23,* 88–93.

84 Nenci, I., Beccati, M.D., Piffanelli, A. and Lanza, G. (1976) Detection and dynamic localization of estradiol–receptor complexes in intact target cells by immunofluorescence technique. J. Steroid Biochem. *7,* 505–510.

85 Nieuwenhuijzen-Kruseman, A.C., Knijnenburg, G., Brutel de la Riviere, G. and Bosman, F.T. (1978) Morphology and immunohistochemically-defined endocrine function of pancreatic islet cell tumors. Histopathology *2,* 389–399.

86 Norland, Ch. C., Maass, E.G. and Kirsner, J.B. (1969) Identification of colon carcinoma by immunofluorescent staining. Cancer *23,* 730–739.

87 Osamura, R.Y. and Watanabe, K. (1978) An immunohistochemical study of epithelial cells in the posterior lobe and pars tuberalis of the human adult pituitary gland. Cell Tissue Res. *194,* 513–524.

88 Palmer, Ph.E. and Wolfe, H.J. (1978) Immunocytochemical localization of oncodevelopmental proteins in human germ cell and hepatic tumors. J. Histochem. Cytochem. *26,* 523–531.

89 Pascal, R.R., Mesa-Tejada, R., Bennett, S.J., Garces, A. and Fenoglio, C.M. (1977) Carcinoembryonic antigen. Immunohistologic identification in invasive and intraepithelial carcinomas of the lung. Arch. Pathol. Lab. Med. *101,* 568–571.

90 Pertchuck, L.P., Tobin, E.H., Brigati, D.J., Kim, D.S., Bloom, N.D., Gaetjens, E., Berman, P.J., Carter, A.C. and Degenshein, G.A. (1978) Immunofluorescent detection of estrogen receptors in breast cancer. Comparison with dextran-coated charcoal and sucrose gradient assays. Cancer *41,* 907–911.

91 Peyrol, S., Grimaud, J.A., Chayvialle, J.A., Veyre, B., Paliard, P. and Lambert, R. (1978) Tissular immunoenzymatic detection of hepatic alpha-fetoprotein in human hepatomas. Digestion *18,* 351–370.

92 Pich, A., Bussolati, G. and Carbonara, A. (1976) Immunocytochemical detection of casein and casein-like proteins in human tissues. J. Histochem. Cytochem. *24,* 940–947.

93 Pritchard, D.G. and Egan, M.L. (1978) Isolation of carcinoembryonic antigen by an improved procedure. Immunochemistry *15,* 385–387.

94 Purtilo, D.T. and Yunis, E.J. (1971) Alpha-fetoprotein. Its immunofluorescent localization in human fetal liver and hepatoma. Lab. Invest. *25,* 291–294.

95 Radaszkiewicz, T., Dragosics, B., Abdelfattahgad, M. and Denk, H. (1979) Effect of protease pretreatment on immunomorphologic demonstration of hepatitis-B-surface antigen in conventional paraffin-embedded liver biopsy material: quantitative evaluation. J. Immunol. Methods *29,* 27–33.

96 Rich, M.A., Furmanski, P. and Brooks, S.C. and the Breast Cancer Prognostic Study Surgery and Pathology Associates (1978) Prognostic value of estrogen receptor determinations in patients with breast cancer. Cancer Res. *38,* 4296–4298.

97 Rochman, H. (1978) Tumor associated markers in clinical diagnosis. Ann. Clin. Lab. Sci. *8,* 167–175.

98 Ruoslahti, E. and Seppälä, M. (1971) Studies of carcinofetal proteins. III. Development of a radioimmunoassay for alpha-fetoprotein. Demonstration of alpha-fetoprotein in serum of healthy human adults. Int. J. Cancer *8,* 374–383.

99 Ruoslahti, E., Pihko, H. and Seppälä, M. (1974) Alpha-fetoprotein: immunochemical purification and chemical properties. Expression in normal state and in malignant and non-malignant liver disease. Transplant. Rev. *20,* 38–60.

100 Ruoslahti, E., Salaspuro, M., Pihko, H., Andersson, L. and Seppälä, M. (1974) Serum alpha-fetoprotein: diagnostic significance in liver disease. Br. Med. J. *8,* 527–529.

101 Sainte-Marie, G. (1962) A paraffin embedding technique for studies employing immunofluorescence. J. Histochem. Cytochem. *10,* 250–256.

102 Sharkey, R.M., Hagihara, P.F. and Goldenberg, D.M. (1977) Localization by immunoperoxidase and estimation by radioimmunoassay of carcinoembryonic antigen in colonic polyps. Br. J. Cancer *35,* 179–189.

103 Sheahan, D.G., Horowitz, St. A. and Zamcheck, N. (1971) Deletion of epithelial ABH isoantigens in primary gastric neoplasms and in metastatic cancer. Am. J. Dig. Dis. *16* 961–969.

104 Shousha, S. and Lyssiotis, T. (1978) Correlation of carcinoembryonic antigen in tissue sections with spread of mammary carcinoma. Histopathology (OXF) *2,* 433–447.

105 Shuster, J., Livingstone, A., Banjo, C., Silver, H.K.B., Freedman, S.O. and Gold, Ph. (1974) Immunologic diagnosis of human cancers. Am. J. Clin. Pathol. *62,* 243–257.

106 Stave, R. and Brandtzaeg, P. (1976) Immunohistochemical investigation of gastrin-producing cells (G cells). The distribution of G cells in resected human stomachs. Scand. J. Gastroenterol. *11,* 705–712.

107 Szulman, A.E. (1960) The histological distribution of blood group substances A and B in man. J. Exp. Med. 111, 785–799.
108 Szulman, A.E. (1961) The histological distribution of the blood group substances in man as disclosed by immunofluorescence. II. The H antigen and its relation to A and B antigens. J. Exp. Med. *115,* 977–1015.
109 Szulman, A.E. (1963) The histological distribution of the blood group substances in man as disclosed by immunofluorescence. III. The A, B and H antigens in embryos and fetuses from 18 mm in length. J. Exp. Med. *119,* 503–531.
110 Talerman, A., Van der Pompe, W.B., Haije, W.G., Baggerman, L. and Boekestein-Tjahjadi (1977) Alpha-fetoprotein and carcinoembryonic antigen in germ cell neoplasms. Br. J. Cancer *35,* 288–291.
111 Tappeiner, G., Denk, H., Eckerstorfer, R. (1973) Vergleichende Untersuchungen über Auftreten und Lokalisation des carcinoembryonalen Antigens (CEA) und eines normalen perchlorsäureextrahierbaren Dickdarmschleimhaut-Antigens (NC) in Carcinomen und Polypen des Dickdarms. Virchows Arch. A *360,* 129–140.
112 Teilum, G., Albrechtsen, R. and Nørgaard-Pedersen, B. (1974) Immunofluorescent localization of alpha-fetoprotein synthesis in endodermal sinus tumor (yolk sac tumor). Acta Pathol. Microbiol. Scand. Sect. A *82A,* 586–588.
113 Teilum, G., Albrechtsen, R. and Nørgaard-Pedersen, B. (1975) The histogenetic-embryologic basis for reappearance of alpha-fetoprotein in endodermal sinus tumors (yolk sac tumors) and teratomas. Acta Pathol. Microbiol. Scand. Sect. A *83,* 80–86.
114 Terry, W.D., Henkart, P.A., Coligan, J.E. and Todd, Ch. W. (1974) Carcinoembryonic antigen: characterization and clinical applications. Transplant. Rev. *20,* 100–129.
115 Thung, S.N., Gerber, M.A., Sarno, E. and Popper, H. (1979) Distribution of five antigens in hepatocellular carcinoma. Lab. Invest. *41,* 101–105.
116 Trouillas, P. (1971) Carcinofetal antigen in glial tumors. Lancet *2,* 552.
117 Trouillas, P. (1972) Immunologie des tumeurs cérébrales: l'antigène carcino-foetal glial. Ann. Inst. Pasteur *122,* 819–828.
118 Von Kleist, S. and Burtin, P. (1969) Localisation cellulaire d'un antigène embryonnaire de tumeurs coliques humaines. Int. J. Cancer *4,* 874–879.
119 Wahren, B. (1975) Fetal antigens in human tumors. Acta Med. Scand. *198,* 337–340.
120 Wahren, B., Lidbrink, E., Wallgren, A., Eneroth, P. and Zajicek, J. (1978) Carcinoembryonic antigen and other tumor markers in tissue and serum or plasma of patients with primary mammary carcinoma. Cancer *42,* 1870–1878.
121 Wood, G.W. and Barth, R.F. (1974) Immunofluorescent studies of the serologic reactivity of patients with malignant melanoma against tumor-associated cytoplasmic antigen. J. Natl. Cancer Inst. *53,* 309–316.
122 Woods, K.L. (1977) Predictive classification of human breast carcinomas based on lactalbumin synthesis. Lancet *1,* 14–16.
123 Zamcheck, N. (1975) The present status of CEA in diagnosis, prognosis and evaluation of therapy. Cancer *36,* 2460–2468.
124 Zamcheck, N., Doos, W.G., Prudente, R., Lurie, B.J. and Gottlieb, L.S. (1975) Prognostic factors in colon carcinoma. Correlation of serum carcinoembryonic antigen level and tumor histopathology. Hum. Pathol. *6,* 31–45.
125 Von Kleist, S., Chavanel, G. and Burtin, P. (1972) Identifications of a normal antigen that cross reacts with the carcinoembryonic antigen. Proc. Natl. Acad. Sci. U.S.A. *69,* 2492–2494.

Wick et al. (eds) Immunofluorescence Technology. Selected Theoretical and Clinical Aspects © *Elsevier Biomedical Press, 1982*

CHAPTER 15

Demonstration and analysis of immune complexes in tissues and in circulation with special reference to immunofluorescence techniques

EDWARD PENNER and BORIS ALBINI*

Department of Microbiology, State University of New York at Buffalo, Buffalo, NY 14214, U.S.A.

*To whom correspondence should be addressed.

15.1. INTRODUCTION

The concept of immune complex (IC)-mediated pathogenesis, although somewhat ill-defined against other antibody-mediated reactivity detrimental to the host, has proven exceptionally fruitful in the understanding of a number of human and experimental diseases [112, 113, 149, 317, 621, 684]. In a broad sense, all products of antibody–antigen reactions may be referred to as "immune complexes". A number of immunopathological entities may be distinguished with regard to the topographical site of the actual antibody–antigen reaction.

First, antigen may be an integral component of the host's tissue. Antibody present in circulation or produced locally interacts with it. Any derangement in morphology or function ensuing from this immune reaction occurs in the structure of which the antigen is an integral component or in its immediate neighborhood.

Alternatively, antibodies may bind via Fc to cell receptors. Antigen in circulation or tissue fluid may interact with the cell-bound antibody. Here, the site of immune reaction and inflammation is determined by the distribution of cells "armed" with cytophilic antibodies and by the availability of antigen. Examples of such reactivity are anaphylaxis, involving in man predominantly IgE and basophilic granulocytes or mast cells [288, 290], and antibody-dependent cell-mediated cytotoxicity (ADCC) featuring K cells or macrophages cooperating with antigen-specific immunoglobulins [308, 489].

Third, antibody may react with antigen as both reactants diffuse through tissue fluid. IC preferentially form at structures reducing the rate of diffusion: basement membranes, elastic laminae, etc. ("in situ formation of IC"). In the classical "Arthus reaction", antigen injected into the skin and diffusing through the tissue meets antibodies originating from the blood stream in the vessel lumen, vessel walls, and surrounding tissue [38, 115, 139, 280]. Some observations suggest that the formation of immune deposits at the dermoepidermal junction in systemic lupus erythematosus (SLE) of man [610] and in lupus-like syndromes of mice [448] may be analogous to this mechanism. Breakdown of epidermal DNA by UV irradiation may produce a flux of antigen towards the dermis. At the dermo-epidermal junction, antigen may meet antibody diffusing from the vasculature, and IC may form. Similarily, IC found in follicular laminae of thyroids in experimental murine thyroiditis [111], spontaneous autoimmune thyroiditis of Obese chickens [315, 324, 680], and Hashimotos thyroiditis [314] in man could form in this way. Leakage of antigen from testicular tubules and diffusion of antibodies from vessels have been implicated in the formation of IC in vasectomized rabbits [68].

Fourth, antigens may be trapped in tissue structures. Subsequently, antibody may bind to these tissue-fixed antigens [220, 299, 376]. This mechanism of in situ IC formation has been termed the "passive hemagglutination type" [411]. Thus, glomerular basement membrane (GBM) can bind DNA and concanavalin A (Con A) and circulating antibodies may react with the GBM-bound antigen [220, 299]. Recently, some experimental studies were interpreted as showing that IC may form in situ in glomeruli upon perfusion of isolated kidneys with bovine serum albumin (BSA) and antibodies to it [183]. However, it still is difficult to evaluate these findings; kidney structures may undergo rapid deterioriation upon perfusion [542] and the serum preparations used for perfusion may contain minute amounts of IC [126]. Physicochemical properties of basement membranes, e.g. high local concentration of electrically charged molecules (such as polyanionic sites) [98, 321, 322] and properties of collagen may be responsible for the interaction of antigen with tissue structures. Immune mechanisms, on the other hand, may have the same effect. In the heterologous phase of nephrotoxic serum nephritis (NSN), foreign immunoglobulin is fixed to GBM [326]. This immunoglobulin by itself is immunogenic and induces the formation of antibodies to immunoglobulin of the foreign species used to produce nephrotoxic serum [326]. IC formation presumably occurs in situ as circulating antibodies to foreign species immunoglobulin bind to the immunoglobulins of the nephrotoxic serum fixed by immunologic mechanisms to the GBM [14, 326, 684, 688].

Furthermore, antibody may be trapped in tissue structures and react with circulating antigen [162]. This hypothesis, somewhat neglected in recent years, may receive support in the results of Fleuren et al. [182]. In addition, experiments with isolated heart perfusions suggested that immune deposits occurred in vessel walls only when the heart was first perfused with antibody to BSA and then with BSA, but not vice versa (Albini, B. and Milgrom, F., unpublished observation).

Finally, antibody and antigen may interact and form IC in circulation (serum sickness type pathology). In the wake of such interactions, inflammatory mediators may be recruited in circulation and after deposition in tissues. Human and experimental serum sickness have been, and to a great extent still are, considered to be mediated by such mechanisms [112, 113, 149, 150, 206, 317, 621, 684, 688]. The results obtained in what is considered by many the crucial experiment for testing the hypothesis of the pathogenic role of circulating IC in serum sickness, namely the induction of lesions comparable to those seen in serum sickness by passive transfer of in vitro-formed IC, are subject to controversial interpretations [55, 185, 206, 237, 341, 390–392, 465]. Numerous experiments have documented deposition of passively transferred IC in glomeruli; the immune deposits, however, are found only in mesangial and subendothelial sites, whereas in the classical serum sickness model of the rabbit, IC are found predominantly in subepithelial locations. This discrepancy in location of immune deposits in actively and passively induced pathology either may indicate that IC found in tissues in serum sickness are formed in situ [125] or reflects a lack of additional factors (e.g. increased permeability of vessel walls) in the passive transfer experiments [338].

In recent years, the term IC-mediated pathology has been reserved for the three last categories discussed above: Arthus reaction-like mechanisms, "passive hemagglutination" type phenomena, and "serum sickness" pathology. One may venture, therefore, to define IC as reactants consisting of antigen and antibody linked via the epitopes on the antigen moiety and the antigen-binding site of the antibody and forming either in circulation or in tissues which do not contain the antigen as an integral component of their normal structure. Academically, this definition may not be fully satisfactory. It may be considered too wide by pathologists and too narrow by immunologists; however, it seems to be of some practical value for immunopathology. IC-mediated pathology, in most cases, offers a characteristic morphological presentation entailing characteristic functional abnormalities (see section 15.1.6.). Whereas rather narrow definitions such as that claimed here for IC-mediated reactions are useful as crystallization points in the process of understanding disease entities and in evaluating tissue samples, it should be understood that classification of immunopathological events as attempted most notably by Coombs and Gell [119] always remain rather artificial and simplified models for complex biological processes. According to their nomenclature, IC-mediated injury is labeled "type III reaction: damage by antigen–antibody complexes". The difficulty which may arise in the use of strict terminology is exemplified in interpreting recent reports on Heymann nephritis [126]. This experimental nephritis is induced in rats by immunization with brush border (BB) antigens of proximal convoluted tubules of the kidney [263]. Immunofluorescence tests revealed immune deposits in a granular pattern in the GBM of animals with Heymann nephritis, thus suggesting IC-mediated pathogenesis [215]. Deposition of circulating IC in glomeruli seemed likely after evidence for antigen [215] and IC [55] being in serum had been obtained. Recently, however, it has been shown that heterologous and homologous sera containing antibodies to BB induced formation of immune deposits in isolated perfused kidneys in patterns comparable to those seen in Heymann nephritis [126, 646]. Similarly, Sugisaki et al. [597] were able to induce Heymann nephritis by passive transfer of serum or its 7 S fractions. Again, interpretation of these results seems difficult in view of technical problems related to perfusion techniques, to ensuring total absence of IC from perfusates, and to evaluating the extent of analogy between in vitro and in vivo models. Nevertheless, the hypothesis was forwarded that in Heymann nephritis circulating antibodies bind to antigen of the podocytes or of the lamina rara externa of GBM [126, 646]. According to this interpretation, the immunopathic mechanisms are mediated by antibody reaction to integral antigens of tissues, and, according to the Coombs and Gell [119] classification, would represent a "type 2" reaction.

The sequence of serological and pathological events in serum sickness was conclusively established by experiments conducted by Germuth [205, 209] and Dixon [149–153] and their groups. In acute "one-shot" serum sickness [149, 181, 204] incipient antibody production leads to immune elimination of

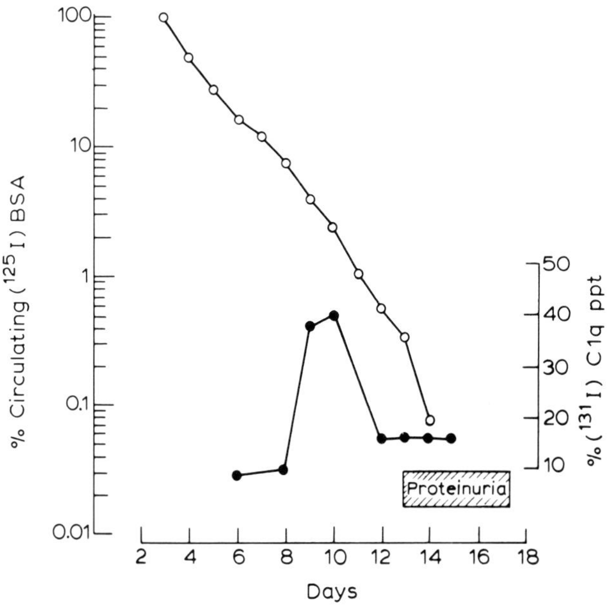

Fig. 15.1. The presence of IC in serum following immune elimination of antigen and preceding development of proteinuria in rabbits with acute serum sickness. IC were detected using a C1q binding assay. (Reproduced from ref. 460, with kind permission of the author and the publisher.)

antigen demonstrated by measuring antigen nitrogen in blood or, more specifically, measuring radiolabelled antigen. Histological lesions seen in serum sickness develop when antigen has almost disappeared and antibody concentration in serum begins to rise. With methods for the detection of circulating IC available (reviewed in ref. 706), IC have indeed been demonstrated in the sera of rabbits with one-shot serum sickness during the period of clinical symptoms (Fig. 15.1) [460]. In the wake of increasing antibody titers in serum, the histopathology and the functional derangements characteristic of serum sickness resolve. When low doses of antigen are administered daily to rabbits over long periods of time, chronic serum sickness develops [153, 208]. In this disease, the sequence of serological events is reversed if compared to acute serum sickness; after some time of continuous injection of foreign antigen the host reduces the output of antibody (Fig. 15.2) [14]. IC-mediated tissue injury occurs when antibody is no longer detectable and antigen becomes demonstrable [14]. The sequence of events in both acute and chronic serum sickness suggests that IC form in circulation and are deposited in tissues leading to structural and functional impairment and disease [152]. The development of immunofluorescent techniques [120] and their application to studies in IC-mediated diseases [121, 149, 389, 688] made it possible to convincingly link the data on immunological events to findings in tissue pathology.

In conclusion, there is general agreement that serum sickness indeed is mediated by interactions of antibody with antigen probably resulting in

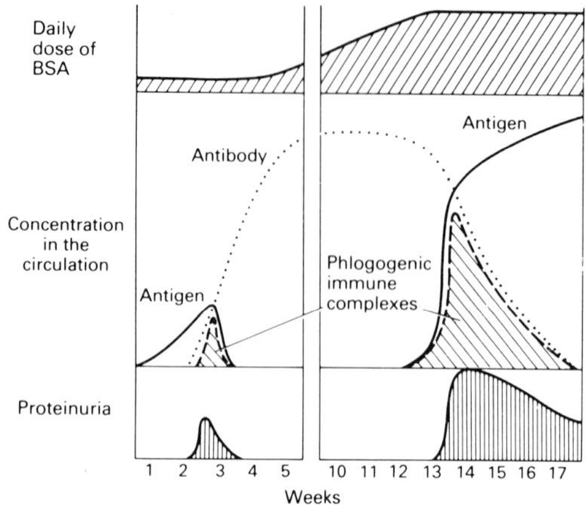

Fig. 15.2. Dose of daily injected BSA, serological data, and extent of proteinuria in a rabbit with chronic serum sickness. The early, acute-phase proteinuria and the late, chronic-phase proteinuria occur when antibody and antigen concentrations approach equivalence. (Reproduced from ref. 14, with kind permission of the authors and the publisher.)

circulating IC [152, 518]. In many other diseases, serologic, clinical, and morphologic findings strongly suggest the same pathogenic mechanisms as seen in serum sickness [150–152, 688]. The possible mechanisms by which IC may appear in tissue and cause injury (deposition of circulating IC vs. in situ formation) have been studied extensively (see above). Whereas the discussion among researchers favouring a pathogenic role of circulating IC [152] and those committed to in situ formation [125] is stimulating and fruitful, it seems yet premature to rule out either of these mechanisms in the pathogenesis of spontaneous IC-mediated diseases in man and animals.

In the following paragraphs, parameters characterizing, and phenomena associated with, IC formation will be reviewed. No exhaustive discussion can be envisaged in the framework of this chapter.

15.1.1. Properties of immune complexes (IC)

The character and pathogenic potential of IC depend, among other things, on the nature of antigen and antibody, the type of antigen–antibody interaction involved, and the molar ratio of antigen to antibody. These aspects of IC-mediated pathology have been reviewed extensively [112, 113, 149, 317, 460, 621, 684, 688, 706], and a brief outline should suffice here.

The rate of deposition of circulating IC, the turnover of its components, and the recruitment of inflammatory mediators all seem to be influenced by the structure of the "lattice" determining the architecture of IC [237, 382, 383], Christian [107–109] has distinguished several lattice types in IC. Small IC with no or only very limited lattice formation are rarely or not at all deposited in tissue, and they do not induce tissue injury. Large IC with highly complex lattice formation recruit inflammatory mediators very actively; they may readily be "solubilized" [607], taken up by phagocytotic cells, or may form intravascular precipitates. They are not likely to deposit in tissues if formed in circulation, but may be involved in anaphylactoid reactions. IC of intermediate size, with stable lattice formation, seem to be those which deposit in tissues and are capable at the same time of recruiting inflammatory mediators. Although somewhat oversimplified, this scheme still is of value in attempts to understand the structure–function relationships in IC.

The nature of the antigen obviously influences the lattice structure of IC. The variety and differential specificity of antigens first was exposed in the experiments of Obermayer and Pick [464]. The size of the antigen determines to some extent the size of the IC and its solubility [206]. Valency of antigens obviously is very important. Univalent antigens are capable of forming IC composed of Ag_1Ab_1 or Ag_2Ab_1 (possibly Ag_nAb_1). The antigen cannot bridge two or more antibody molecules; no lattice formation occurs and IC remain in circulation [554]. Interaction with cell receptors virtually is absent; thus, e.g., platelet aggregation is induced by IC with multivalent but not monovalent antigens. Multivalent antigens, in general, can form stable lattices [36, 236, 249, 252, 383, 407, 479]. The exception are "monogamous" large multivalent antigens which form Ag_1Ab_1 complexes [335]. The physicochemical properties of antigens may modulate the lattice structure and determine trapping or binding of IC in tissue. The distribution of epitopes on the antigen molecule, the number of distinct epitopes, and their local densities all may influence the extent and type of lattice structure.

Only recently, antigenic sites of myoglobin [42, 56], lysozyme [42], and BSA [41, 239] have been defined. Clarification of epitopes of BSA is of special interest, as the classical animal model for IC-mediated diseases, chronic serum sickness, most frequently is induced with this antigen. Five amino acid sequences have been implicated in the antigenic determinants. These epitopes saturate 50% of antibody reactivity [41]. The other 50% could be constituted by "discontinuous" antigenic sites [239].

The properties of antibodies also influence the lattice formation. Distinct immunoglobulin classes differ in their valence for epitopes: the valence is 2 for monomeric IgG, IgA, IgE, and IgD; 4 for dimeric secretory IgA; and 10 for IgM reacting with small haptens and 5 for the same immunoglobulin reacting with large antigens [237, 407, 578]. Avidity also may be of importance. Avidity is defined by the association constant K_0 with the dimensions $l \cdot mol^{-1}$ [311, 586]. The higher the value for K_0, the less ligands are needed to saturate all antigen-binding sites. In most systems studied, increased temperature causes decreased K_0, but in some systems, no change is seen in the range of 4–40°C. Studies on the avidity of antibodies are much more easily performed with hapten-antibody systems than with systems involving large molecules as ligands. Alpers et al. [23] showed that mice producing large amounts of high-avidity antibodies eliminate antigens much faster than mice producing low amounts of low-avidity antibodies. Soothill and Steward [577] documented a correlation between low-avidity antibody containing IC in circulation and incidence of glomerulonephritis in mice infected neonatally with lymphocyte choriomeningitis virus. Steward et al. [588] also described the presence of low-avidity antibodies to DNA in NZB/WF1 mice. Similarly, Winfield et al. [693] found low-avidity antibodies in IC of SLE patients with active nephritis. In a recent report, an inbred mouse strain selected for the production of low-avidity antibodies developed serum sickness glomerulonephritis in the wake of BSA immunization, whereas another mouse strain selected for producing high-avidity antibodies did not develop glomerulonephritis after the same schedule of immunization [587]. The avidity of antibodies found in circulating IC, however, may not be representative for that of IC deposited in tissues. Thus, Winfield et al. [693], in patients with circulating low-avidity antibodies, found high-affinity antibodies in eluates from kidney lesions. What is usually measured in serum is a mean value of avidities of various antibodies. IC deposited in tissues, however, may contain a selected population of these antibodies. Other problems also complicate studies on the avidity of antibodies present in IC. In studying eluates for antibody (see below), the elution technique was shown to influence the results significantly. Bartolotti [48] described increasing avidity of antibody preparations in eluates obtained with buffers of decreasing pH.

The size of antibodies obviously influences the size of IC and the extent of lattice formation. There have been reports indicating that IC containing IgM preferentially deposit in the glomerular mesangium, whereas smaller IC containing IgG lodge in the peripheral glomerular capillary loops [206].

Finally, the capability of antibodies participating in IC to activate inflammatory mediators and to interact with cell receptors, their half-life in circulation and in tissues, the propensity to induce antibodies to either their Fc portion (rheumatoid factors (RF)) or Fab regions (anti-antibodies (AA) and anti-idiotypic antibodies (AIA)), and their tendency to interact with each other and form aggregates all are likely to influence the fate of IC.

The role of antibodies to immunoglobulin (i.e., RF, AA, and AIA) in the pathogenesis of IC-mediated diseases, although suggested long ago [415], has been demonstrated convincingly only recently in a wide spectrum of immunopathological entities. The association of RF with the disease process of rheumatoid arthritis is well established, and reviews on this subject are readily available [109, 657, 709]. The possibility that RF may potentiate glomerular immunopathology was suggested by the experiments of McCormick and his coworkers [394]. Elegant experiments by Robinson and Schultman [524] possibly visualized antibodies to immunoglobulins in studies using electron microscopy of IC (Fig. 15.3). Chronic disease ensuing from injection of heterologous antiserum to brush border could be the consequence of host reactivity to immunoglobulin [647]. Circulating IC consisting of antibodies to DNA and RF, but lacking the antigen, DNA, have been reported in MRL/1 mice with lupus-like syndrome [298]. In human SLE, the paradigm of IC-mediated diseases, Agnello et al. [8] have shown the renal immune deposits to react with fluorescein isothiocyanate (FITC) - labeled AIA to immunoglobulins

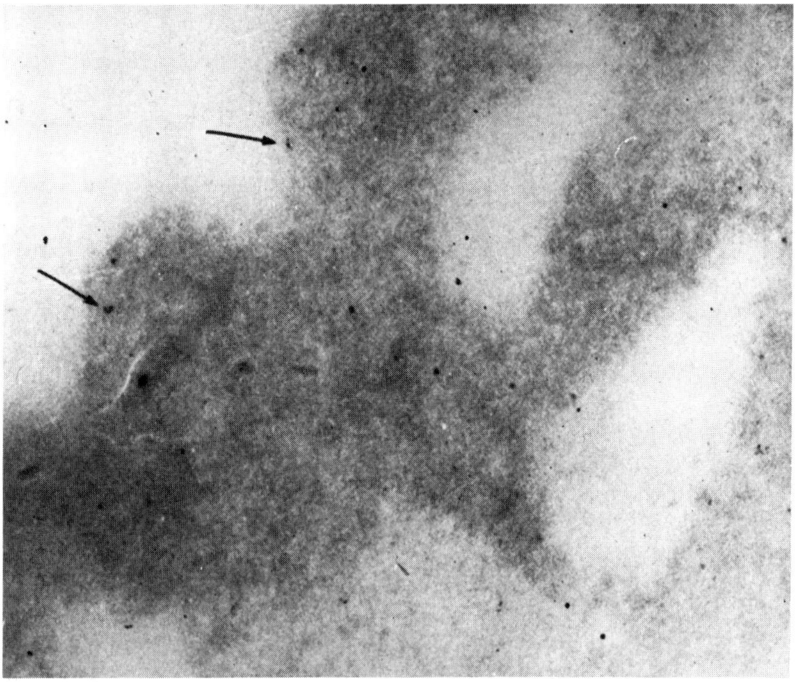

Fig. 15.3. Ferritin–anti-ferritin complexes in electron microscopy. Positive staining reveals large amounts of proteinaceous material between antigen molecules (arrows), suggesting the presence of antibodies to immunoglobulins participating in the formation of IC. (Reproduced from ref. 524, with kind permission of the authors and the publisher.)

isolated from patients with SLE. Rossen and coworkers [535] reported on glomerular binding of FITC-conjugated aggregated human IgG in patients with a variety of IC-mediated diseases. A role for antibodies to immunoglobulin was suggested by experiments of Milgrom and Witebsky in 1960 [414]. Subsequently, the work of McIntosh and his group substantiated this notion in a number of studies [397, 398]. Studies on the dissociation of IC deposited in tissue [482] showed participation of antibodies to immunoglobulins in chronic serum sickness of the rabbit and in post-streptococcal glomerulonephritis, idiopathic membranous nephropathy, and SLE in human patients. These data strongly suggest that antibodies to immunoglobulins participate in the pathogenesis of many IC-mediated diseases; they may contribute to and modify the lattice structure of IC, may perpetrate the inflammatory injury evoked by tissue-fixed IC by additional interaction with "primary" IC, or may constitute the bulk of antibodies in IC, especially late in diseases, when "primary" antigens may not be detectable any more in IC (e.g. in post-streptococcal glomerulonephritis [29, 635]). In addition to this role in IC causing tissue injury, interactions of antibodies, especially AIA, with immunoglobulins may influence immune regulation.

The antigen–antibody interactions are reversible and non-stoichiometric [165, 510]. They involve Van der Waals forces [370, 477], hydrogen bonding [478], hydrophobic interactions [165], and Coulombic forces [251]. As antigen competes with water for the binding sites on antibodies, antigens less soluble in water will form more stable bonds with antibodies than highly water-soluble ones [510]. Precipitation of antigen–antibody complexes may also be interpreted as lowering of the solubility by mutual neutralization of polar groups [76, 333], i.e. the combination of antigen and antibody reduces the number of free polar groups on IC so much that they are too few to ensure solubility in aqueous solutions. The relative role of these interactions in antibody–antigen complex formation varies among distinct IC systems. Thus, in BSA anti-BSA IC, both Coulombic and Van der Waal forces contribute effectively to the reaction [649]. In IC containing DNA, on the other hand, Coulombic interactions predominate [650]. The antigen–antibody reaction may be completed very fast in the presence of sufficient antibody [465]; over 90% or 95% of the reactants did form IC 20 s after mixing antibody with egg albumin [253], 1 min after combination of serum from a patient with syphilis and the lipoid antigen [158], and less than 3 s upon combination of pneumococcal polysaccharides and specific antibodies at 0°C [388]. Sometimes, however, antigen–antibody reactions are completed only after hours [155], especially if antibody is not present in sufficient amounts [569].

An elaborate mathematical model describing IC formation has been formulated [581]. It seems promising because it considers both the dynamic and non-stoichiometric characters of the antigen–antibody interactions. This mathematical approach makes it possible to simulate IC formation using computers. Antibodies may also be looked upon as molecules functioning in a manner somewhat analogous to allosteric enzymes [265–267].

In addition to the properties of antigen and antibody, the relative concentrations of antigen (and thus of effective epitopes) and antibody (and thus of effective binding sites) influence the lattice formation and size of IC. This is exemplified in the simple precipitation curve of IgG antibodies and antigens with a molecular weight between 50,000 and 150,000. The most insoluble IC form in the area of the antigen–antibody equivalence or in slight antigen excess. Further antigen excess leads to dissociation of IC; antibody excess, if extreme, also leads to solubilization of IC [510].

Some properties of immune reactants which influence the physicochemical and biological characteristics of IC have been confirmed in in vivo studies e.g. distinct patterns of glomerulonephritis could be distinguished in rabbits receiving the same dose of antigen but producing low, medium, or high concentrations of circulating antibodies [206]. However, it is still extremely difficult to evaluate, with any degree of certainty, the contribution of the individual parameters described above on the formation of IC or their effect on the disease process.

15.1.2. Soluble mediators of inflammation in IC-induced tissue injury

It is conceivable that IC, simply by their presence, produce derangement of tissue structure. Spacial arrangements of basement membrane components may be disturbed, the distribution of charges in tissues may be altered or cell coats may be blanketed by IC. In addition, the capacity of phagocytic cells may be over-strained by IC, inducing a deficit in phagocytic function also for other foreign particles. Most of IC-mediated injury studied up to now involves the recruitment of inflammatory mediators [436]. Complement activation and reaction with Fc and complement receptors on inflammatory cells are the best understood mechanisms. The Hageman-factor system may be activated indirectly, especially upon initial induction of tissue lesions [683].

Both classical and alternative activation pathways of complement may be induced by IC of appropriate size and lattice structure [44, 211, 227, 440, 441, 525]. Two or three antibody molecules of the IgG class in IC seem to be the minimum for efficient complement classical pathway activation [116, 380]. Nevertheless, under unusual circumstances, this requirement may be reduced to one IgG molecule and a hapten [218] or increased to a tetramer [283] of IgG moieties. A single molecule of IgM complexed to antigen binds C1, but larger IC containing more than one IgM are better activators [43, 75, 294, 375, 408, 504]. The capacity to activate complement is lower in soluble IC than in antigen–antibody interactions on cell surfaces or in contact with tissue structures [508]. In view of assays used for the detection of circulating IC, it is important to remember that uncomplexed monomeric IgG or IgM may bind to C1q [43, 375, 442]. This binding, however, is very weak and reversible. C1q reacts with C_H2 of IgG [305], and C_H4 of IgM [282, 560]. Activation occurs by IC or immunoglobulin aggregates containing IgG1, IgG2, IgG3, but not IgG4 [211, 287, 539, 578]. Binding of C1q by IgG seems to require the presence of C_H3 and is influenced by quaternary interactions with distant regions of the antibody molecule, possibly with Fab [23, 284, 558]. Two reports have been published claiming classical pathway activation by IgA fragments or IC containing IgA and IgG [83, 685].

The precise mechanism of activation is still not established. Activation after reaction with antigen or aggregation may occur by allosteric events inducing conformational changes in the Fc region of the immunoglobulin [265–267, 408]. Such conformational changes have been substantiated by findings indicating a new epitope on antibody molecules after interaction with antigen [412, 413, 416], and other experiments [39, 97, 285, 520, 584], especially measurements of circularly polarized fluorescence [214, 300, 553]. These conformational changes, however, do not suffice for activation of complement [97]. Since polyvalent antigen can, and monovalent cannot, induce, after interaction with antibodies, the classical pathway of complement activation, and since aggregated immunoglobulins very efficiently react with C1q [286, 287], the hypothesis that activation of classical pathway is mediated by increased local density of Fc portion obtained through bridging antibodies by antigen has recently gained support [439]. It seems quite possible that both mechanisms contribute to the classical pathway of complement activation.

IC may, under physiological conditions, activate complement via the alternative pathway [72, 226, 400, 579]. IC containing soluble antigens may even preferentially activate complement using this pathway [584]. Some aggregated immunoglobulins also may activate complement via the alternative pathway. Aggregates of IgA [72, 226, 579] and possibly also of IgE [291, 292] are effective in the activation process. Aggregated IgG, however, seems rather ineffective [584].

The activation of the alternative pathway is initiated by interactions of serum proteins with the Fab_2 fragment, and Fc seems not necessary for this reaction [502, 546, 557] with the exception of activation by aggregated IgE [291, 292]. C3 is activated in alternative pathway reactions via the factor B-properdin-dependent C3 convertase, which is more stable than the classical pathway C3 convertase and requires factor B and properdin but not C1, C4, or C2 for its generation. Even in soluble IC activating complement primarily via the classical pathway, the amplification loop of the alternative pathway seems essential in efficient complement activation [400]. Particulate IC, on the other hand, seem not to require complement recruitment via the amplification loop.

There is a significant difference in efficiency of complement activation by IC containing particulate or soluble antigens [400]. The former consume complement at a rate 1.5–2 times higher than the latter. This difference probably is even greater for IC containing IgM as antibody [130, 508].

C3 activated via either pathway binds to immune precipitates covalently by disulfide bonds [508] and non-covalently via hydrophobic interactions [349, 607]. The whole sequence of assembly of complement components in the course of activation is much better understood for IC containing particulate antigens than it is for IC containing soluble antigens.

In vitro-formed IC or immune aggregates vary in their capability to bind or activate complement, and the factors influencing their behaviour are not yet well understood [196]. Thus, in vitro-formed immune aggregates or IC may bind complement without initiating activation; they may activate complement without much demonstrable binding of complement components; or they may bind and activate complement. This seemingly erratic behaviour of in vitro-formed IC poses serious problems for establishing control preparations and standard curves to be used in tests for the detection of circulating IC.

Binding of complement components influences the size of IC (the molecular weight of C1q is 400,000, that of C3b is 171,000–195,000). In addition, intercalation of complement components obviously has an impact on the lattice structure. Therefore, complement activation changes the solubility of IC. Both increases and decreases of solubility of IC upon interaction with complement have been described ("biphasic" interaction). This biphasic interaction was first suggested in experiments performed by Heidelberger in 1941 [250]. Increasing complement activation first led to increased binding of complement to antibody in IC; after reaching a maximum, however, the amount of bound complement decreased with increasing available complement. This type of reactivity is reflected in two opposite effects on the solubility of IC. Maurer and Talmage [387] and Förster and Weigle [188] showed that binding of complement by IC decreases solubility. On the other hand, Miller and Nussenzweig

[420], in 1975, reported data indicating that excess of complement leads to detachment of IC bound to cell surfaces via cell receptors. Through work of the group of Nussenzweig, the mechanism involved in this process of "partial solubilization" has been elucidated [607]. The solubilization of IC is mediated by the alternative pathway of complement activation, requiring the presence of factors B and D, properdin, C3 and Mg^{2+} ions [604]. Classical pathway activation, although enhancing the solubilization process [606], does not suffice by itself to efficiently solubilize IC. The solubilization mechanism is envisioned as the effect of intercalation of excess C3b in the lattice structure of IC, ultimately breaking up the lattice structure [607]. The requirement of the alternative pathway may find its explanation in the higher efficiency and stability of factor B-properdin-dependent C3 convertase over classical pathway-C3 convertase [607]. It is obvious that IC (which, under physiological conditions, preferentially activate complement via the alternate pathway) will be solubilized more efficiently than immune aggregates containing IgG (which preferentially activate the classical pathway). This may be of importance in evaluating tests for the detection of circulating IC, in which standards of aggregated immunoglobulins are used. The solubilization of IC renders, as end product, a macromolecular IC with almost all of the antigen still present, some of the antibody lost, and with molecular weights smaller than the original "active" IC [607]. Complement to antibody ratios found in solubilized IC are close to 1, and the IC are shifted towards antigen excess [607]. Solubilized complexes have been found in fractions ranging in molecular weight from 11S to larger than 19S [607]. The distribution of molecular weights of solubilized IC is comparable for solubilized IC derived from all IC without influence of original Ab to Ag ratios. The solubilization of IC may also be achieved by interaction of monovalent Fab fragments of antibodies to immunoglobulin involved in IC, but not by divalent fragments of the same antibodies or by staphylococcal protein A; therefore, monovalent proteins seem to be required to achieve solubilization by intercalation into lattices formed by antigens and antibodies [607]. Solubilization requires *nascent* C3b, probably involving a short-lived binding site on antibody molecules [131]. Purified C3b, therefore, does not lead to solubilization of IC upon incubation [605]. The C3 interaction with antibodies decreases the affinity for antigens, an effect essential in the release of antibodies from IC during solubilization [607]. Solubilization is more effective with IC containing low-avidity antibodies than in IC containing high-avidity antibodies [607]. The specific location of the receptor site for C3-determining solubilization is not known, and both Fab and Fc portions may be involved [607]. Solubilized IC are not degraded any further by incubation with fresh serum. Solubilization of IC also changes the biological activity of IC [607]. Solubilized IC do not bind to mouse lymph node cells in vitro [420] or to circulating blood cells in vivo [419]. IC bound to lymph node cells detach from these cells upon incubation in excess complement (i.e. fresh serum) [419]. Interestingly, the binding of IC to Fc receptors on cells [607] and that to staphylococcal protein A [547] are also inhibited after solubilization. Thus,

phagocytosis of soluble IC is impaired by solubilization of the IC [667], and there is suggestive evidence that solubilized IC are incapable of efficiently binding C1q or activating the complement cascade [607]; they are "dead end" IC with impressively reduced biological activity. Experiments by Bartolotti and Peters [49] strongly indicate that resolution of experimental acute serum sickness nephritis may depend on the solubilization of IC via complement activation.

Activation of complement components, in addition to changing solubility and biological activity of IC, has profound effects on immune reactivity [377, 564] and inflammatory mediators [174, 666]. A number of excellent reviews are available on these aspects of complement activation [191, 422, 541]. In the following, the discussion will be limited to the interaction of activated complement components with cell surface receptors [66, 156, 159, 473]. These interactions may be essential to the outcome of IC-mediated pathology and have been widely used in assays for the detection of IC in circulation (reviewed in refs. 621 and 706).

15.1.3. Interaction of IC with cell receptors

IC interact with cells predominantly via three groups of cell surface receptors: antigen receptors [6, 232, 241, 515, 669], receptors for Fc of immunoglobulins [274, 276, 474, 703], or complement receptors [157, 275, 277]. Thus, B cells possibly may bind IC via specific surface immunoglobulins interacting with the antigen in IC, and T cells may do so via their antigen-binding unit. Cell receptors for complement components and for the Fc portion of immunoglobulins have been demonstrated on a variety of inflammatory, lymphoid, and other cells. With which of these receptors a given IC interacts may depend on the characteristics of the Ag–Ab complex (it could be envisioned that, e.g., IC in antigen excess be favoured in interactions with antigen receptors on cell surfaces), the immunoglobulin class of the antibody involved in IC, local density of receptors (e.g. Fc receptors on different cells vary in their binding capability), and the ability of IC to fix complement (IC effectively fixing complement do not react with Fc receptors [543] and "solubilized" IC do not react with C3 receptors of cells [607]). Interactions of IC with cell receptors are involved in phagocytosis [594] and in immunoregulation. Finally, IC may interact with cells, e.g. bacteria, via moieties activating complement; endotoxin of *Salmonella* [434] and components of *Streptococcus* [106, 342]; or molecules binding to immunoglobulins: *Staphylococcus* [187] and *Streptococcus* [106, 342]. IC containing excess antibodies to cell surface epitopes could bind to such cells via antigen receptors.

15.1.3.1. Complement-mediated interactions

Erythrocytes from man and other primates have receptors for C3b [212] and C4b [122]. The same receptor reacts with both complement components [533]. The interaction of IC with cells via complement components is less stable, i.e.

more dynamic in vivo than it is in vitro. In vivo, IC are released continuously from cells by C3b inactivator and beta H which convert C3b and C4b in C3d and C4d [105, 123, 350, 540, 676], and by excess C3 [607]. Since erythrocytes do not possess receptors for these latter components (i.e. C3d, C4d), IC are released from these cells. Nevertheless, IC attached to erythrocytes via complement components enhance significantly in vivo phagocytosis by neutrophilic granulocytes [450, 522]. It is conceivable that elimination of circulating IC may be influenced indirectly by interaction of C3b and C4b with erythrocytes.

Immune adherence does not occur with platelets in primates and man [52, 254, 255, 259, 443]. Moreover, binding of complement components to IC does inhibit attachment of IC to platelets via Fc receptor (see below) and subsequent platelet aggregation [260, 499]. C1q, however, may interact with C1s present on platelet surface membranes [99, 594, 671]. This reaction indeed may promote platelet aggregation [672].

Neutrophilic granulocytes possess a vast array of receptors for various complement components [33, 160, 212, 459, 512, 513, 533, 620]. Receptors for C3a [216] and C5a [103] are present, but only the interaction with C5a seems to be essential in chemotaxis [279]. Mature human neutrophilic granulocytes have C3b and C4b receptors [534]. Immature forms of these cells (which make up to 20% or more of the bloods neutrophilic granulocyte population), contain C3d or C3bi receptors [532]. C3b, C4b receptors sometimes are referred to as "CR1", C3d receptors as "CR2", and C3bi receptors as "CR3". In mice, also mature neutrophilic granulocytes carry C3d receptors [513]. The degradation [532] of C3b may be circumvented by interaction with properdin and factor B of the alternative pathway [172, 556]. Inactivation of C4b is inhibited by interaction with C2 and with C4b-binding protein [123, 180, 547]. Intact C3b may bind to both CR1 (via its C3c portion) and to CR2 (via its C3d portion); in contrast, C4b binds only to CR1 [261]. C4c and C4d do not interact with cell receptors on neutrophilic granulocytes [73], but C3bi interacts with CR3 [532]. As shown recently, the lack of interaction of C3bi with mature neutrophilic granulocytes may be caused by rapid conversion of C3bi to C3d by surface elastase rather than by loss of CR3 [112, 301]. Interactions of neutrophilic granulocytes with complement components seem essential for the efficient adherence of the cells to IC. Furthermore, they mediate secretion of lysosomal enzymes, enhanced glucose oxidation and metabolism in general, and the release of H_2O_2 and prostaglandins [261, 708]. Large IC are better suited to induce enhanced phagocytosis and secretion than small ones [256, 257]. It is interesting that IC which cannot be taken up by neutrophilic granulocytes are more efficient in inducing secretion of lysosomal enzymes than soluble, phagocytosable IC [261]. Thus, surface-bound IC are 500 times more efficient in stimulating secretion than soluble IC in vitro. This may explain the savage impact of neutrophilic granulocytes on tissues containing IC firmly deposited in basement membranes.

C3a and C5a interact with receptors on basophilic granulocytes and mast cells [216, 279]. Binding induces degranulation and release of heparin, histamine, and other vasoactive amines, eosinophil-chemotactic factor, and factors affecting platelets (PAF and PLF) [57–60, 89, 323, 645]. Recently, C3b receptors have also been described on platelets. Complement components may, therefore, mediate much of the anaphylactoid reactions presumably contributing to the deposition of IC in tissues by changes of permeability of vessel walls [58].

Human, but not murine, eosinophils display C3b, C4b, and C3d receptors on their surface [33, 234, 254, 511, 603]. C3b receptors may increase in density after interaction of eosinophils with chemotactic factors [33, 34]. These cells also possess C3a and C5a surface receptors. Eosinophilic granulocytes are considered to have a regulatory role on the impact of mediator release by basophilic granulocytes and mast cells [325, 704]. This regulatory role is accomplished by inactivation of inflammatory mediators, induction of resynthesis of mediators in those cells, modulation of mediator release, and phagocytosis, preferentially of IC containing homocytotropic antibodies [675]. In addition, eosinophils may participate in the elimination of helminthic parasites [84–87].

IC may bind to macrophages via receptors for C3b and C4b [275, 356]. In contrast to previous reports, it now seems proven that macrophages do not have "CR2" binding C3d but bear "CR3" reacting with C3b IC. Complement receptor interactions, in the macrophage as in the neutrophilic granulocyte, mediate attachment of IC to the cells but not phagocytosis [161, 224, 230, 386]. Engulfment requires simultaneous reaction with both Fc and complement receptors. This, however, may be true only for particles and not for soluble IC [331, 653]. Upon ingestion of IC, macrophages may release lysosomal enzymes which participate in the inflammatory process [92, 674]. In addition, activated macrophages have been shown to release plasminogen-activating factor upon interaction with soluble IC in vitro [225]. This reaction links interaction of complement with cell receptors to the fibrinolytic coagulation systems of serum and tissue fluid [542]. Interaction of factor Bb of the alternative pathway with macrophages leads to activation, immobilization, and spreading of these cells [228]. This reaction seems to depend on C5 synthesis by macrophages [599]. Soluble C3b induces the release of hydrolases, which cleave C3, providing thus another amplification mechanism for complement activation. Some reports suggest enzyme release from macrophages induced by C3a [555]. This reaction entails the death of the cell. C5a may be chemotactic for guinea pig macrophages [572]. The dendritic Langerhans cells of the skin have C3b receptors [589].

B cells have been shown to possess high-affinity receptors for C4b, C3b, C3d, and C1q [617]. Alpha-antitrypsin may be the receptor of B cells for C3 components [345]. IC bind preferentially via these complement receptors to B cells, and binding of IC to B cells via Fc receptors is impaired or abolished by reaction of IC with complement [316]. Binding of IC to B cells and release of IC from them via activation of the alternative pathway may influence the immune response and thus the outcome of the IC-mediated disease [607, 621]. The presence of complement receptors on T cells has been suggested only in very few studies. Clq receptors may be found on human T cells [575] and some results indicate C3b receptors to be present on activated or neoplastic T cells [47, 104, 565, 633].

Receptors for C3 have also been described on cells not involved in immune response or inflammation. Human and rabbit hepatocytes can bind IC via C3 receptors [271, 272]. The podocytes and mesangium of human kidney glomeruli [201, 202, 424, 573], but not of other species, and human choroid plexus cells [40] have C3b receptors. It is possible that these receptors interact with IC in vivo and determine the site of deposition of IC formed in circulation or secure "anchorage" for IC formed in situ.

15.1.3.2. Interactions of IC with cells via Fc portions of immunoglobulins

Various cell types bear receptors for the Fc portion of immunoglobulins. Only in few cases (prominently the receptors for IgE on basophilic granulocytes and mast cells, and the IgG receptors on macrophages), the affinity of the receptors for the immunoglobulin is high enough to warrant binding of monomeric immunoglobulin. In most instances, Fc receptors preferentially or exclusively bind complexed or aggregated immunoglobulins. This preferential binding of IC (over monomeric immunoglobulins) by most Fc receptors may either be caused by a configurational change in the Fc portion of immunoglobulin after reaction with the antigen or be induced by increased local density of Fc fragments after aggregation by binding to polyvalent antigens. The nature of Fc receptors, although studied extensively in recent years, is still not well characterized. It is of interest that cells bearing Fc receptors kept in culture shed the Fc receptor into the culture supernatant [611]. The binding site of immunoglobulins to Fc receptors seems to be localized in a decapeptide sequence of the CH3 disulfide loop [110].

Whereas erythrocytes do not have Fc receptors, Fc receptors interacting with all subclasses of human IgG are found on human platelets [258, 297, 498]. IC containing polyvalent but not monovalent antigens [329] of a size greater than 19 S readily induce aggregation of platelets and release of inflammatory mediators, and nucleotides [329, 437, 471, 488, 498]. As mentioned before, complement activation by IC inhibits binding to the Fc receptors [316].

Neutrophilic granulocytes bear Fc receptors binding to all subclasses of IgG [355, 406]. The affinity is somewhat greater for IgG1 and IgG3 than for the other subclasses. Aggregated myeloma proteins of the IgA class have also been shown to bind to neutrophilic granulocytes via Fc receptors [689]. It is not known whether IgA and IgG Fc receptors are the same molecular entities. Together with complement receptors, Fc receptors of neutrophilic granulocytes modulate many of the functions of the cell. Interactions with the Fc receptor seem essential in the enhancement of phagocytosis of particulate antigens in mice and man. Fc receptors on these cells are neither sensitive to trypsin nor to neuraminidase [356].

The IgE Fc receptors on basophilic granulocytes and mast cells show high affinities (10^8–10^9 M^{-1}) and therefore react readily with monomeric immunoglobulin [293]. They are extremely specific for IgE of their own species, and cross-reactivities are found only with IgE of the most closely related species. These cells also carry Fc receptors for IgG [295].

IgE receptors have not been found consistently on human eosinophils, although some data do indicate that 25–30% of these cells may possess such Fc receptors [278]. Murine and human eosinophils, however, have Fc receptors reacting with IgG. These IgG receptors have a much lower affinity than Fc receptors for IgE of mast cells. Fc receptors for IgG may mediate the ADCC-like reaction seen in defense to helminthic infestations [84–86]. It has been suggested that the defective defense mechanism in *Schistosoma* infestation may be caused by binding of circulating IC to eosinophil Fc receptors [331].

Macrophages bear Fc receptors which interact with monomeric IgG1 and IgG3, aggregated IgG2, and possibly also IgG4 [578]. It is striking that the IgG subclasses binding to macrophages most avidly also are the ones activating most efficiently the classical sequence of complement. The density of receptors and their affinity for immunoglobulins may increase after activation of the cell [517]. Binding of monomeric immunoglobulins occurs spontaneously, whereas binding of IC containing particulate antigens requires active cell metabolism, appropriate temperature, and concentration of Mg^{2+} and Ca^{2+} [476]. In mice, two distinct Fc receptors for IgG2a and IgG2b have been demonstrated [259, 642]. Whether in humans two distinct Fc receptors for IgG1 and IgG3 exist on macrophages, and whether there are separate receptors for monomeric and aggregated immunoglobulins (i.e. also IC), is not yet resolved [25, 262, 664]. In the mouse macrophage, one of the receptors (FcR1) is trypsin-sensitive, whereas FcR2 is not [262, 642, 643, 664]. These two receptors may mediate different effector functions, with FcR1 primarily being involved in phagocytosis and FcR2 in ADCC [665]. It has been shown that Fc receptors on macrophages redistribute and cap in the surface membrane after interaction with a particulate antigen [529, 631]. Fc receptors contribute to both the binding and the phagocytosis of particulate complexes, whereas complement receptors facilitate only the binding [161, 386]. In opsonization, complement and Fc receptors, if simultaneously saturated, show an impressive synergistic effect on phagocytosis [161]. However, evidence is accumulating that phagocytosis of IC and of non-opsonized particles may be two distinct processes [410, 451, 514]. This is of special interest for the study of the function of the reticuloendothelial system (RES) in IC-mediated diseases (see section 15.1.4).

B, T, and K cells have Fc receptors [670]. B-cell receptors for IgG do not bind monomeric immunoglobulins but react with aggregated IgG and IC [144]. Fc receptors on murine B cells show a close association with surface immunoglobulins [1, 186]. This association induced by ligand binding of surface immunoglobulins, however, may be lost after activation of B cells, possibly releasing such cells from regulatory signals conveyed via Fc receptors [559]. There is also strong evidence for a close relation of Ia and Fc receptors [143,

145]. Nevertheless, the Fc receptor seems distinct from both surface immunoglobulins and Ia. Subpopulations of B cells have also been reported to carry Fc receptors for IgE [221, 222], IgA [235], and IgM [179, 527]. Interestingly, there is no association between IgM Fc receptors and Ia-like antigens. T cells may bind IC via Fc receptors for IgG, IgM, IgA, and IgE, [24, 50, 353, 354, 372, 425, 593, 702, 703]. The expression of Fc receptors on T cells may reflect the states of reactivity of these cells [703]. Most of the T cells bear IgM Fc receptors (75%) [425, 426]. From more recent studies it seems that the same T-cell population may express both IgM and IgG Fc receptors [501]. A shift from IgG Fc receptor to IgM Fc receptor on T cells has been described by Pichler et al. [500, 501] following interaction with IC. This phenomenon, documented in vitro, could mediate changes induced by IC on the immune response. The quality of Fc receptors seems also to be associated with distinct locomotive behaviours of T cells. Parrot et al. [475] described that T cells with IgM Fc receptors but not those with IgG Fc receptors respond to chemoattractants. K cells carry high-affinity receptors for IgG, especially for IgG1 and IgG3 [124, 143, 490, 580, 694]. The interaction of Fc receptors for IgG on lymphocytes and IC depends on the degree of aggregation (or possibly lattice structure) and subclasses of immunoglobulins involved [262]. Highly aggregated IgG bind with higher affinity than monomeric IgG, and IgG1 and IgG3 bind better than IgG2 and IgG4 to human lymphocytes; IgG1 and IgG2a bind better than IgG2b in mice [143, 154, 355, 696].

15.1.4. The reticuloendothelial system (RES) and IC

Since long it has been suspected that the status of the RES may influence the persistence of IC in circulation. Impaired phagocytosis in IC-mediated diseases had been suggested by the studies of Menabuoni as early as 1908 [190]. Wilson and Dixon [687] postulated in 1971 that an alteration of the function of mononuclear phagocytes may occur in chronic serum sickness of rabbits. They found depressed phagocytosis of autologous, aggregated serum albumin 10 min (but not 24 h) after administration of the immunizing antigen, BSA. Already in 1953, Biozzi et al. [69] had obtained convincing evidence that the clearance of carbon particles followed saturation kinetics. Haakenstad and Mannik [236] showed in 1974 that the same phenomenon occurred with large-lattice IC (larger than Ag_2Ab_2). In mice, the hepatic uptake of IC reached a maximum at 300 μg of antibodies complexed to antigen. They [236] obtained evidence that saturation of Kupffer cells in the liver resulted in prolonged circulation and enhanced deposition of IC in glomeruli of kidneys. Non-immune phagocytosis of various distinct particles showed competitive inhibition. Benaceraff et al. [54] demonstrated inhibition of uptake of carbon particles following administration of IC. This concept of "tiring out" of the RES, however, seems not to tell the whole story [99, 410]. Results obtained by radiolabeled marker studies in chronic serum sickness of rabbits have shown that non-immune phagocytosis of technetium-labeled sulfur colloid is enhanced during the initial stage of chronic serum sickness, whereas the uptake of specific BSA–anti-BSA IC is significantly reduced or does not occur at all at the same time [451]. The same studies have shown that during the period preceding late-phase proteinuria in chronic serum sickness, antigen and presumably IC localize in the first 5–60 min in phagocytic cells of the RES and in neutrophilic granulocytes [452]. There is no deposition in basement membranes. During the period of avid deposition of IC in basement membranes, early uptake by cells of the RES and other phagocytes is diminished or absent, and localization of antigen in basement membranes presumably in the form of IC occurs only after 6–24 h of injection of the antigen.

Phagocytosis of colloid particles seems not to be affected in the same way as phagocytosis mediated by immune reactions during chronic serum sickness. The short-lived inhibition of phagocytosis seen immediately after injection of antigen may reflect the immediate uptake of IC. Changes in Fc or C receptors of phagocytic cells may be involved in the prolonged saturation of RES in late stages of chronic IC-mediated diseases. Frank and his associates [192] indeed have obtained evidence for defective Fc-receptor function on cells of patients with SLE. Recently, correction of RES blockade has been described by Lockwood et al. [369] after plasmapheresis. This finding may indicate interaction of serum factors with IC and/or phagocytic cells in the RES blockade. It has been suggested that the therapeutical effect of plasmapheresis in IC-mediated disease, rather than resulting from the removal of antibodies to DNA or of IC, could be corrected by the supply of fresh serum and thus complement to the patient, thus altering the complement to IC ratio. The results obtained in radiolabeled marker studies in chronic serum sickness of the rabbit (discussed above) also could be interpreted as caused by decreased reactivity of circulating IC (e.g. by solubilization) with complement receptors on phagocytic cells. In addition to cells of the RES, neutrophilic granulocytes (NG) participate in the early uptake of IC. Early after injection of antigen in the chronic serum sickness of rabbit, NG are gorged with IC (Fig. 15.4). These

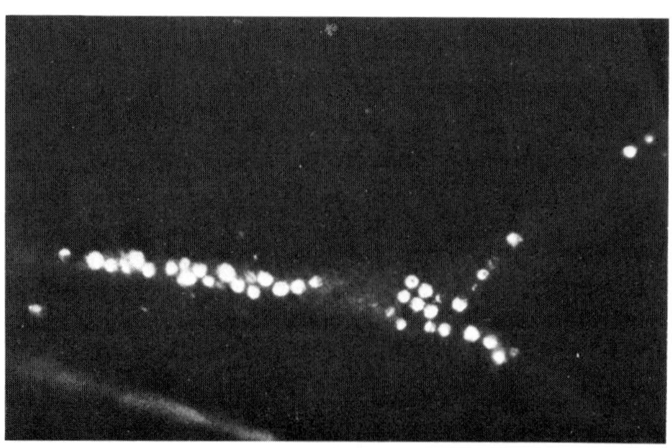

Fig. 15.4. Granulocytes with phagocytized BSA–anti-BSA IC in a vessel of the peritoneum of a rabbit with chronic serum sickness. Staining for BSA. ×250.

cells preferentially migrate to the lungs where they abound within a few minutes of antigen injection. It is somewhat surprising that this phenomenon had been suggested already in 1907 by Bianca Bienenfeld [67], who described the decrease in the number of circulating neutrophilic granulocytes immediately after antigen injection in serum sickness and suggested that these cells "may migrate... to visceral organs".

15.1.5. Inflammatory manifestations of IC-mediated diseases

Activation of the complement cascade and interaction of IC with inflammatory and tissue cells leads to acute or chronic inflammatory processes. As expected, changes of permeability of vascular and other basement membranes, induction of the coagulation and plasmin systems, phagocytosis and secretion or spill-over of hydrolytic enzymes and other lysosomal components contribute in varying degrees to the shaping of the IC-mediated disease. The degree to which specific mediators are recruited is influenced by the nature and components of IC, by the environment, in which IC are formed or deposited, and by the general status of the host. The morphological aspects of IC-mediated tissue lesions are discussed in section 15.2.

15.1.6. IC and immune response

Obviously, IC formation depends on the quality and quantity of antibodies produced. Thus the immune response in IC-mediated diseases is of great interest. There are two perspectives of the immune response to be studied in IC-mediated pathology: 1) possible derangements of the lymphoid system and regulatory mechanisms predisposing for IC formation; and 2) the changes of the immune response induced by prolonged presence of IC in circulation and in lymphoid organs.

Both in human SLE and in lupus-like syndromes of inbred mice, B-cell hyperreactivity manifests as hypergammaglobulinemia, autoantibody production and spontaneous polyclonal activity [352, 435]. In mice, a derangement of "regulatory" T cells has been suggested by Cantor et al. [91]. Con A-induced suppressor T cells, however, seem to be normal [629]. Lupus-prone mice have increases numbers of mature B cells in the spleen, especially those secreting IgG antibodies [629]. T-cell deficiencies have been suggested in human SLE [3, 4, 70, 71, 80, 240, 368, 531, 596, 654]. Interestingly, infiltrating lymphocytes in lesions of SLE do not react with T-cell rosettes, nor form complement or Fc rosettes [602]. This suggests lack or reduction in surface moieties making up the normal inventory of B, T, or K cells. All these derangements may contribute either to the enhanced propensity to manifest autoimmunity or to development of IC-mediated lesions, or to both. Studies on the influence of derangements of the immune system on IC formation seem more promising in experimentally induced diseases, where autoimmunity is not of primary importance and the antigens involved in IC are known. In chronic serum sickness of chickens induced by daily injection with BSA [19], thymectomy significantly increases the incidence of glomerulonephritis (20% of "intact" white Leghorn chickens develop glomerulonephritis; 65% of thymectomized chickens do so).

From extensive in vitro and in vivo studies it is well established that IC may influence the immune response [2, 26, 38, 55, 90, 101, 148, 176–178, 248, 268, 348, 359, 427–430, 463, 470, 567, 571, 590, 641, 673, 701]. Recently, it was shown that in rabbits with chronic serum sickness induced by high doses of BSA, the B-cell response to this antigen is "shut-off" at a time when phlogogenic IC are present in the circulation and tissue lesions occur. This induction of humoral unresponsiveness is specific and coincides with a switch back from IgG to IgM antigen receptors on lymphoid cells of the spleen [12, 19, 20]. Concomitantly, the relative number of cells carrying IC on their surface increases in spleen from less than 0.2% to 4%, and preliminary studies do indicate the reappearance of T-cell sensitivity by BSA.

The importance of a better understanding of the immune response in IC-mediated diseases has only recently been realized (e.g. refs. 12, 19, 149, 684), and new knowledge in this field may be instrumental in devising effective therapy.

15.2. DEMONSTRATION OF IMMUNE COMPLEXES IN TISSUES

Suggestive evidence for the presence of IC in tissues may be obtained in conventional histology. Convincing evidence relies on immunohistology and electron microscopy. Definitive demonstration of IC in tissues rests on integration of data obtained with several methods.

15.2.1. Conventional light microscope histology

Conventional histology may indirectly suggest the presence of IC in tissues by visualization of inflammatory, degenerative, and/or proliferative lesions compatible with IC-mediated pathology and, more convincingly, by demonstration of deposits of foreign material in tissue.

15.2.1.1. Features of tissue lesions in IC-mediated pathology

Formation of IC in the vessel walls, as exemplified in the Arthus reaction [38, 114, 280] leads to acute localized necrotizing vasculitis with impressive infiltration of the vessel wall and surrounding tissue with polymorphonuclear, mainly neutrophilic granulocytes. These cells phagocytize and catabolize IC and seem instrumental in the ensuing necrosis of the vessel [38, 68, 111, 113, 138, 139, 246, 280, 305, 314, 324, 374, 448, 610]. Tissue deposition of IC which are progressing from antigen excess towards equivalence, as seen, e.g., in one-shot serum sickness, leads to endothelial proliferation, infiltration of variable extent with polymorphonuclear granulocytes, and increased vascular permea-

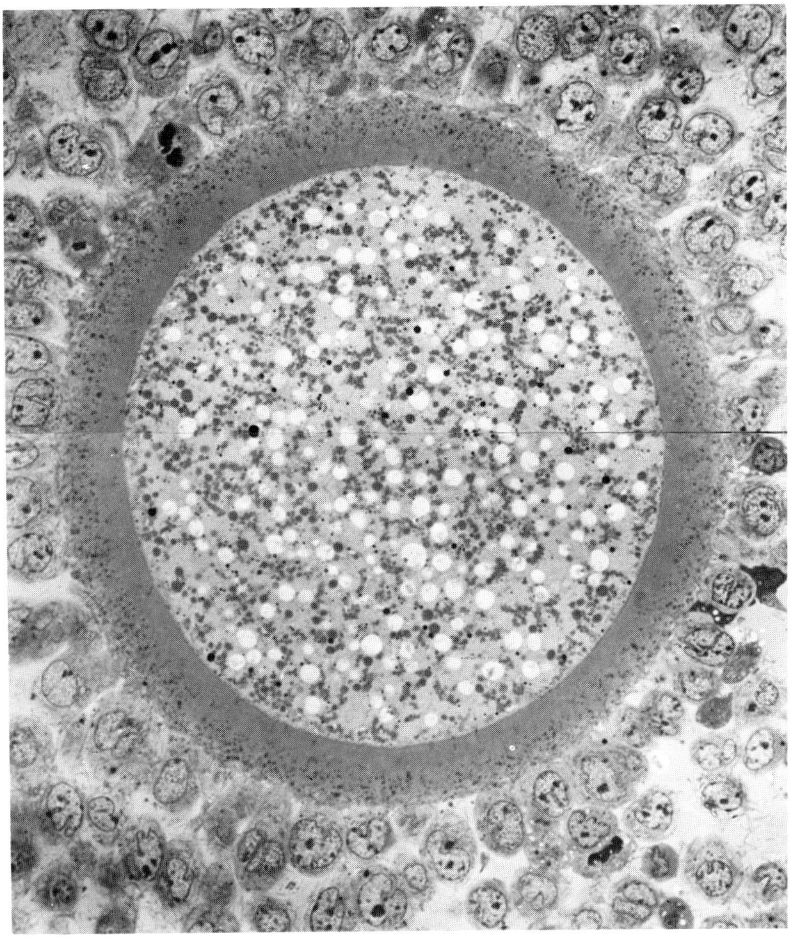

Fig. 15.5. A follicle of the ovary of a rabbit with chronic serum sickness. In this plastic-embedded toluidine-stained section IC deposits are seen as dark granules predominantly in the outer portion of the zona pellucida. (Unpublished micrograph by Albini, Ossi, and Andres.)

bility [112, 115, 339]. Deposition of IC progressing from antibody towards antigen excess, as seen in chronic serum sickness, may induce a broad spectrum of lesions. Most commonly, degenerative rather than inflammatory features predominate [390]. Membranous lesions with thickening and transformation of basement membranes are accompanied by no or only negligible endothelial proliferation. In such tissue lesions, proliferative and ultimately scarring reactions become predominant with progression of the disease. Hyaline degeneration and fibrosis are the tombstones of severe chronic IC-mediated pathology (Fig. 15.5). Polymorphonuclear granulocytes participate in such tissue lesions to a varying degree. In some cases, they add a significant exudative aspect to the chronic IC-mediated tissue lesion. In summary, IC-mediated tissue injury presents as thickening or transformation of basement membranes, the presence of polymorphonuclear leucocytes, predominantly endothelial proliferation, with increased vascular permeability, and ultimately ends in degeneration, necrosis, fibrosis, and obsolescence of the normal tissue structure. IC, especially those containing antibodies lacking the ability to activate complement, may induce tissue lesions without participation of complement and polymorphonuclear leucocytes [257].

15.2.1.2. Histological presentation of IC deposits

In some instances, IC may be seen with conventional light microscope. Haematoxylin–eosin and periodic acid-Schiff staining may suggest deposits in basement membranes by uniform increase in thickness or by granularity (deposits stain reddish). Sections stained with toluidine blue or methylene blue may show large dark-blue IC deposits as seen in IC-oophoritis or as "humps" in post-streptococcal glomerulonephritis. The use of thin sections [684] of plastic-embedded material [17] makes interpretation of granular, toluidine-stained material more reliable. The impressive subendothelial deposits of IC in some cases of lupus nephritis may be seen as wire-loop lesions in conventional light microscopy [399, 509]. Trichrome stain and van Gieson may reveal orange granules of IC in basement membranes [705], and silver stain may show spikes originating from the basement membrane surrounding the IC deposits (silver staining thus functions somewhat as a "cast" of IC deposits) [309]. These abnormal deposits in tissue seen by light microscopy may suggest, by granularity, size, and location the IC character. Light microscopy, however, can never be accepted as definitive proof for the presence of IC in tissues, because other derangements of tissue structures not related to IC may evoke similar morphological changes.

15.2.2. Conventional electron microscopy

In conventional electron microscopy, IC in tissues manifest as electron-dense (opaque osmophilic) deposits (Fig. 15.6) [705]. The demonstration that electron-dense deposits indeed are accumulations of IC came from studies in immunoelectron microscopy. Andres and co-authors [28] demonstrated the presence of the antigen, BSA, in electron-dense deposits on the GBM of rabbits with chronic serum sickness using ferritin-labelled antibody to BSA (Fig. 15.7). Electron-dense deposits of IC, although quite characteristic in shape and texture, have to be distinguished from collagen, reticulin bundles, and cytoplastic processes.

The electron-dense deposits may be finely granular or lanceolar; they may be present as large individual deposits (as seen, e.g., in the zona pellucida of ovaries or as humps in post-streptococcal disease), as tightly packed, continuous, ribbon-like deposits, or rather diffuse thickening and increase of electron density of basement membranes. Ultrastructural studies allow for precise distinction of the site of IC deposition or formation,e.g. subendothelial, intramembranous or subepithelial deposits in GBM (see Chapter 12, this volume). With progressive disease, the characteristics of dense deposits may

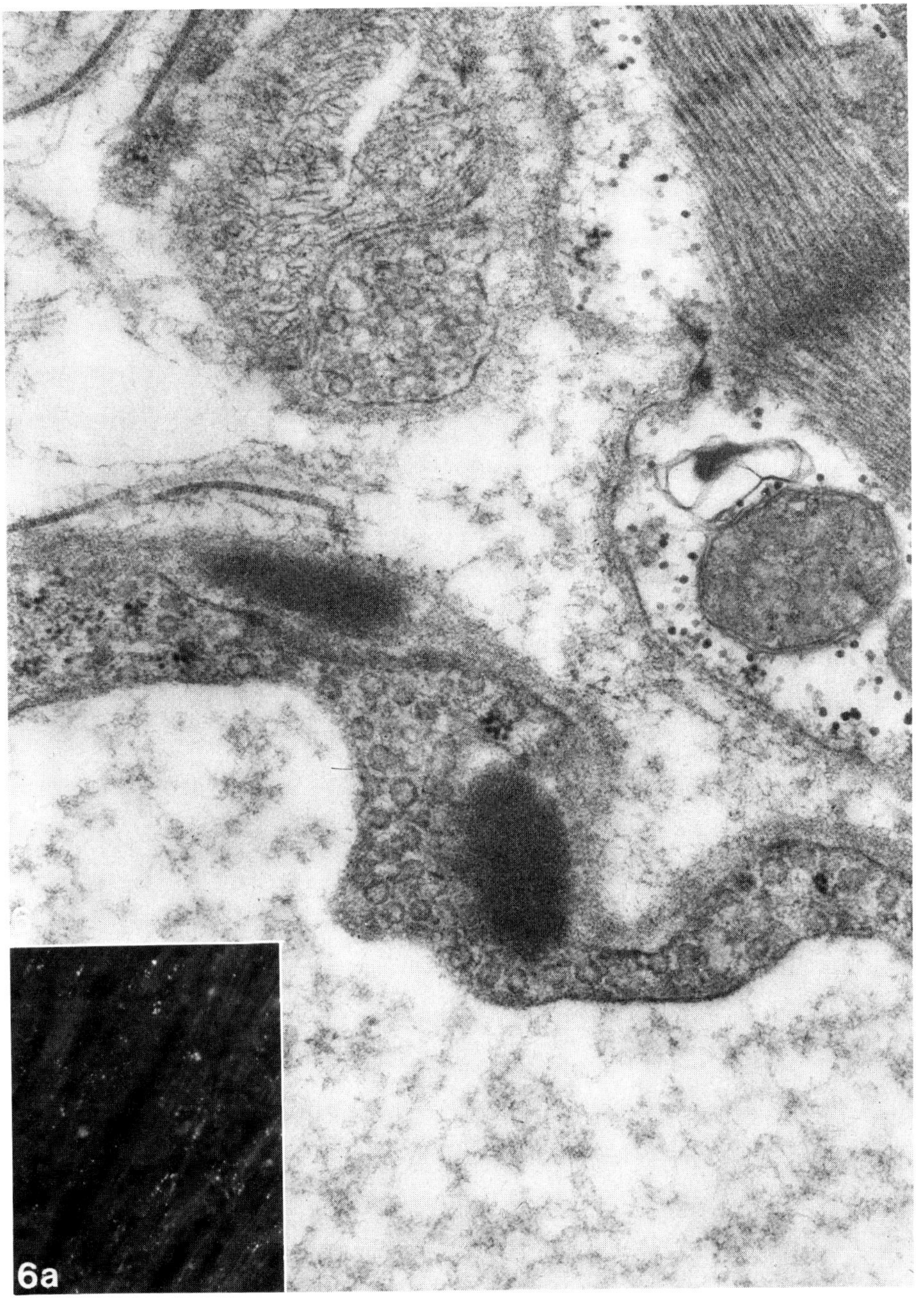

Fig. 15.6. Discrete electron-dense deposits in a heart capillary of a rabbit with chronic serum sickness. ×45,600. a) Immunofluorescent staining of the same heart tissue for BSA ×190.

change, with areas of electron lucency appearing in and around deposits, finally changing the electron-dense deposit into the empty, electron-lucent remnant often seen in late stages of membranous glomerulonephritis (see Chapter 12). Sometimes, no electron dense deposits are seen in tissues with

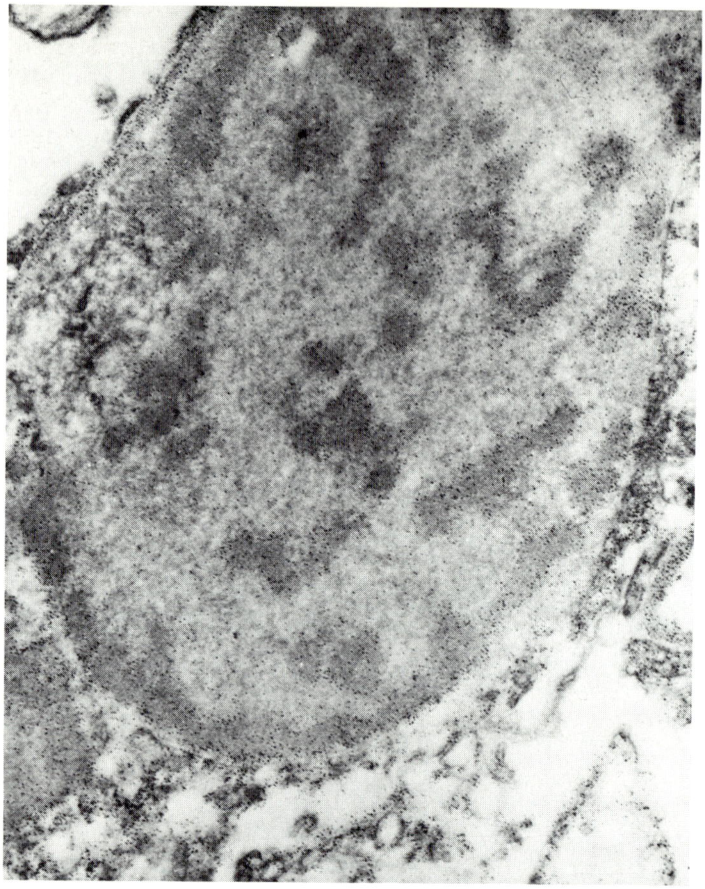

Fig. 15.7. Immunoferritin-labelled antibody to BSA is found in electron-dense deposits in the glomerular capillary wall of a rabbit with chronic serum sickness (courtesy of Dr. G.A. Andres). Microphotograph reproduced with kind permission of the author and publisher [28].

extensive immune deposits seen in immunofluorescence. Thus, e.g., in the space of Dissé in liver sinusoids, BSA and IgG are detectable by immunofluorescent staining in chronic serum sickness of rabbits [79]. No electron-dense deposits were seen in the same tissue. Similar results were obtained with livers from rabbits injected with mercury chloride developing systemic IC disease [528]. It seems possible that electron-dense deposits are washed out in some tissues during processing for electron microscopy; alternatively, electron-dense deposits may only form in media with certain viscosity and characteristics (e.g. basement membranes).

15.2.3. Immunohistology

Immunohistology at the light microscopy level of resolution probably is the most useful technique in the study and diagnosis of IC-mediated diseases. The methodology most widely used in immunohistology is immunofluorescence.

Among 250 kidney biopsies with IC deposition demonstrable by immunofluorescence, Zollinger and Mihatsch [705] reported on 45% giving negative results in electron microscopy; on the other hand, electron-dense deposits were seen in only 0.6% of patients with negative immunofluorescence results.

15.2.3.1. Immunofluorescence

This technique has been greatly improved in the last two decades by defining and standardizing the optics, light sources, and, most importantly, the fluorochrome-antibody conjugates. The WHO has contributed significantly to achieving the goal of making immunofluorescence reproducible and results obtained in different laboratories comparable (see chapter 1, this volume).

Immunohistological methods not only allow for identification of IC in tissues, but also for analysis of their constituents. Reviews of immunofluorescence procedures and their standardization [62, 269, 270, 337, 447, 682] are available, and constant improvements make their use increasingly productive both in research and in clinical laboratories. The importance of well-defined techniques, reagents, and instruments for meaningful immunopathological analyses cannot be overstressed [6, 62, 269, 270, 337, 447].

The immunofluorescent staining procedure for the detection of IC deposited in tissues is the direct staining technique [447]. Tissues from patients or experimental animals are obtained either by biopsy or autopsy and are incubated with FITC- or TRITC-labelled antisera to immunoglobulins, antigens, or complement components. The preservation of antigenicity and structure of the tissue determines the outcome of the test. Post-mortem autolysis destroys tissue structure, changes antigenic make-up, prevents accurate localization of immune reactants, and increases non-specific staining. Therefore, tissues should be processed as soon as possible after performing a biopsy or at the earliest time feasible after death. Tissues are best snap-frozen in liquid nitrogen and kept until use at –70°C (e.g. refs. 270, 447, 682). To prevent drying, tissue should be embedded in OCT, a fluid guaranteeing optimal freezing and preservation of the frozen tissue. Drying increases non-specific staining (especially at the edges of the cracked tissue portions) and may significantly diminish antigenicity of tissue components. Alternatively, the tissue may be frozen in an acetone–dry ice mixture, or in the cryotome (most instruments have a quick-freeze device). Both of these methods give acceptable results but are inferior to freezing in liquid nitrogen.

Some organs have to be kept in expanded condition in order to assure unequivocal interpretation. Eyes and lungs may be injected with 5% solution of albumin from any species [418]. Sometimes better results in immunofluorescence are obtained by isolation of specific organ structures. Thus, demonstration of IC in choroid plexus is easier after preparation of the plexus and orientation in OCT on the bolt. Small tissue fragments, as obtained frequently with biopsy procedures, may float away from the slide, especially during prolonged incubations. This may effectively be prevented either by using gelatine or agarose-coated slides or by placing a drop of agarose on the tissue section [483]. The latter procedures also have the advantage of slowing down (and hence preventing) large precipitates of FITC conjugated antibodies from reaching the tissue section, without interfering with penetration of immunoglobulin [483]. Demonstration of immune reactants in IC may require partial elution. In particular, elution of antibody from IC may "unearth" epitopes on antigens formerly "blanketed" by the antibodies (see below).

Strong background staining may pose a great difficulty in interpreting results. The background staining may have various causes: autofluorescence and reaction of FITC-labeled antibody with connective tissue components, basement membranes, and charged groups, etc. [270, 447, 682]. Some tissues are more prone to background staining than others. Thus the epidermis and dermis of skin and lymph nodes often show intense fluorescence. Dried and decaying tissue and tissue margins and cracks abound with background staining. On the other hand, characterization of immune reactants and optimization by selection of purified monospecific conjugates at defined working dilutions are essential in keeping undesired staining low. Many conjugates, especially to mouse and rat immunoglobulin, react with nuclei. Recently, it was found that antiglobulin sera may contain specificities reacting with serum enzymes [363]. The use of affinity chromatography-purified or monoclonal antibodies for the preparation of conjugates should allow for improved specificity. Where optimal conditions cannot be achieved, the use of counterstains may be helpful. Evans blue and diamond black have been used. Rhodamine-conjugated BSA has been proposed for covering reactive groups of the tissue prior to incubation with specific FITC-coupled antisera. In addition, the old concept [544] of using formalin-fixed and paraffin-embedded tissue for immunofluorescence tests has been revived recently (see Chapter 13, this volume). Deparaffinized tissue sections are treated with pronase or trypsin prior to routine immunofluorescent staining [129, 140, 273]. The feasibility of using paraffinized tissue in immunofluorescence makes old material accessible to re-evaluation with this method. Furthermore, transport of biopsy and autopsy material is possible without continuous cooling. It seems, however, that not all antigens can be demonstrated in fixed and paraffin-embedded tissues. The time of fixation of tissue in formalin is crucial in determining the preservation of antigenicity. Finally, tissues may be fixed in a medium developed by Michel et al. [409] and kept in it for several weeks without loss of antigenicity. This medium has been used extensively and successfully as "transport medium" for specimens of the skin [409]. Preliminary evidence suggests that it can be used in some types of IC-mediated kidney diseases as well.

In our experience, tissues in which IC are suspected are used best for immunofluorescent staining procedures without any fixation [13, 30]. Some authors, however, do recommend fixation in acetone as a routine procedure (see for review, ref. 447).

FITC- or TRITC-labelled antisera ("conjugates") to all human immunoglobulin classes (and most subclasses) are commercially available. Also, reagents for the detection of C3 (in most cases, for C3c) and C4 are manufactured. Conjugates are now available for the detection of immunoglobulins of most animal species used in experimental research. A number of manufacturers provide the customer with a data sheet on the characteristics of their products. In most cases, additional information can be obtained upon request. Nevertheless, it is important to conduct the appropriate tests with each new batch of conjugates purchased. The characteristics to be defined are the specificity, the amount of antibody present, and the F/P ratio [64]. The conjugate should have a high antibody content and a F/P ratio of roughly 2.0–2.4. This makes it possible to use a reasonably high dilution of the conjugate without non-specific staining of tissues caused by immunologically non-specific interactions of FITC with tissue components. Simple titration on known positive tissue should make it possible to establish optimal working dilutions. In addition to demonstration of immunoglobulin present in IC deposits, immunofluorescent staining may also be used to document the antibody specificity of the immunoglobulin by fluorochrome conjugated to the "presumed" antigen. This method was used with success in studies on kidneys of rabbits with chronic serum sickness. It was not successful with IC in the thyroids of Obese strain chickens. Alternatively, a "sandwich"method may be employed: tissue speci-

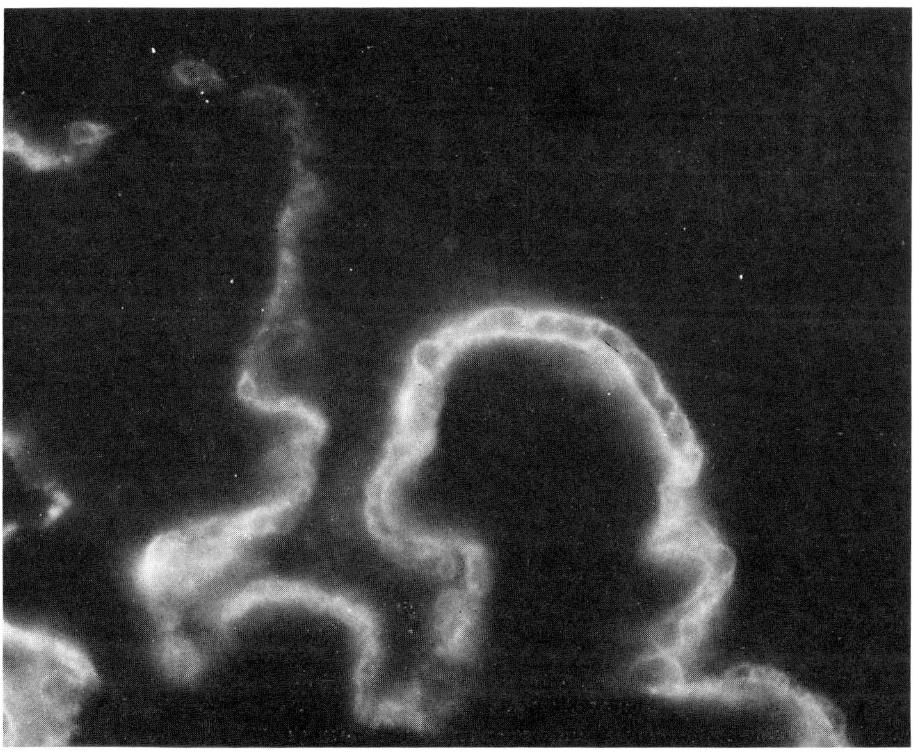

Fig. 15.8. Immunofluorescent staining of kidney of a rabbit with chronic serum sickness with fluorochrome- conjugated antiserum to rabbit IgG. Staining on a thin section (1.5 μm). ×1720.

mens containing the antibody are incubated with antigen and subsequently with the specific antibody. The concentrations of the reagents have to be determined very carefully to ensure optimal results.

Tissues for routine immunofluorescence staining procedures should be cut in a cryostat at a thickness of 3–4 μm. Thicker sections do not allow for optimal localization and extent of staining and are more liable to show non-specific staining when microscopes with transmitted light are employed. Recently, thin sections (1–1.5 μm) have been used for immunofluorescence [551, 552]. In combination with phase contrast microscopy, such preparations allow for exact localization of immune reactants, thereby rivalling the precision of electron microscopy (Fig. 15.8). Some tissue samples may be investigated without

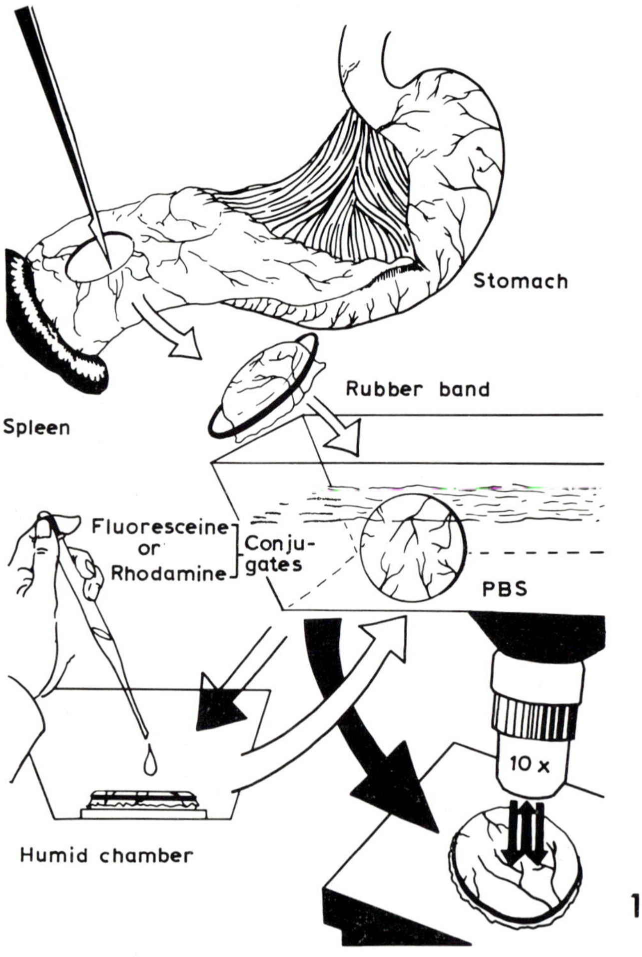

Fig. 15.9. Preparation of synovial or serosal tissue for immunofluorescent staining. The thin tissue is placed over a petri dish (or microscopic slide) and washed in PBS. Fluorochrome-conjugated antisera to immunoglobulins, complement components or the antigen are placed on the tissue and incubated for 45–60 min. The preparation is examined in an immunofluorescence microscope equipped with epi-illumination optics. (Reproduced with kind permission of the authors and the publisher from ref. 13).

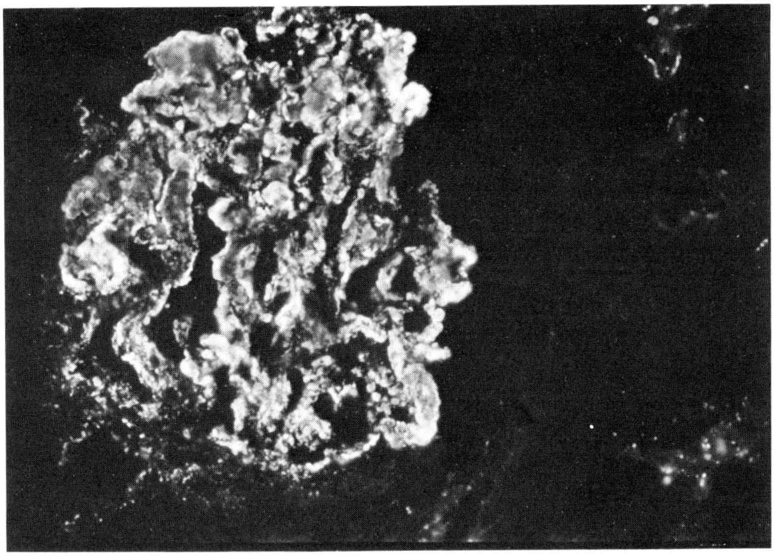

Fig. 15.10. Glomerulus of a rat with mercury-induced glomerulonephritis. Granular to ribbon-like immune deposits (rat IgG) are seen in the glomerular capillary walls. ×400.

sectioning, e.g. specimens of the serosae or synovia (Fig. 15.9). More time has to be allowed for the penetration of these thick tissue specimens (e.g. 45 instead of 30 min incubation) and incident light is preferably used in microscopy [13].

Testing tissue samples for the presence of IC does not require sophisticated microscopic equipment; the smaller and cheaper immunofluorescence microscopes of a number of manufacturers give satisfactory results. These microscopes should be equipped with an excitation-barrier filter combination, using blue light for excitation and a high energy yield. If available, an additional set of filters for UV light excitation may be of advantage improving the localization in tissue by autofluorescence [437]. Transmitted light illumination in general is sufficient, and focusing on the specimen on the slide is much easier than with incident illumination. With thick section or very high magnifications (800× or more), however, epi-illumination should be used.

The immunofluorescence of a preparation soon deteriorates, even when slides are kept in the dark and in the refrigerator. In general, slides should be read during the first week after staining, preferably in the first 48 h. Methods have been proposed recently to decrease quenching of immunofluorescent staining [357]. Under certain circumstances they may be of great help but cannot substitute prompt reading of preparations.

In immunofluorescence tests, IC have been associated most often with granular staining (Fig. 15.10) [389]. This general axiom is very helpful and has the merit of differentiating IC-mediated from antibody-mediated diseases (e.g. disease mediated by antibodies to basement membranes). Uptake of IC by phagocytic cells (Fig. 15.11) also renders a characteristic granular pattern of immunofluorescence staining easily differentiated from localization of IC in

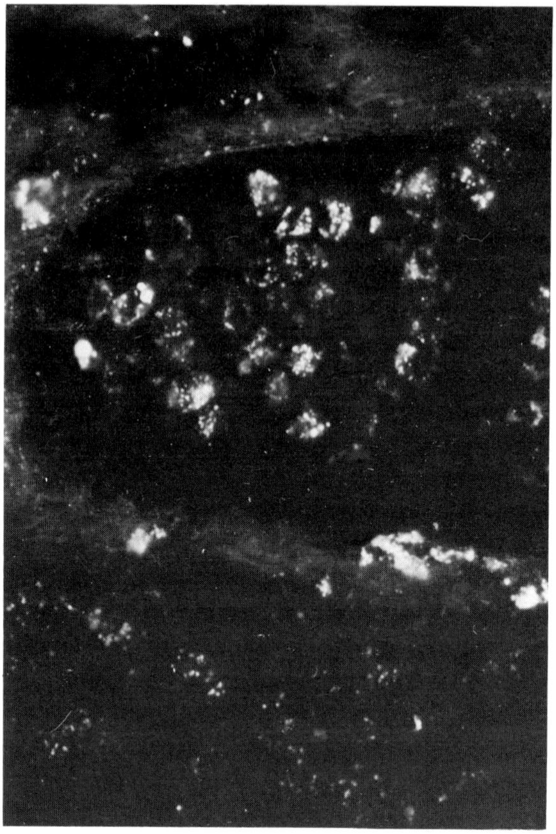

Fig. 15.11. Immunofluorescent staining of a large vessel and surrounding tissue of the omentum of a rabbit with chronic serum sickness. Antigen (BSA) is seen in granular deposits in phagocytic cells in the vessel lumen and in the surrounding tissue. ×400.

basement membranes (Fig. 15.10) [452]. It has to be kept in mind, however, that distinct granular staining is only one of the staining patterns seen with IC in tissue sections; both the structure, in which IC localize, and the amount and character of IC contribute to the pattern of staining. Table 15.I summarizes the major tissue structures, in which IC are detected by immunofluorescent staining procedures most frequently. In Table 15.II, a number of morphological patterns are presented which may be found with IC localization in vessel walls and some other tissues. Immunofluorescence staining procedures give suggestive evidence for the site of immune deposits (Table 15.III). Precise localization in tissue sometimes is possible only with the help of electron microscopy.

One component of an immune reactant may be detected in immunofluorescence with a pattern distinct from other components. Thus, in anti-GBM nephritis, granular deposition of C3 has been described together with linear deposits of immunoglobulin in the glomeruli [210]. In some conditions, combined linear staining of antibodies directed to basement membranes and granular or ribbon-like staining of IC occurs and in these conditions IC easily may be overlooked. This was seen, e.g. in mercury chloride-induced disease of

TABLE 15.I

TISSUE STRUCTURES FREQUENTLY INVOLVED IN IC DEPOSITION

Eye	vessels of iris
	uvea
	ciliary body
Heart	vessels
Intestine	vessels
	basal lamina
Kidney	vessels
	mesangium
	glomerular basement membrane
	tubular basement membrane
	Bowman's capsule
Liver	vessels
	sinusoids (Disse's space)
Lung	vessels
	alveolar basement membrane
Ovary	vessels
	zona pellucida
	basement membrane between granulosa and theca
Plexus chorioideus	vessels
Serosae	vessels
Skin	vessels
	dermo-epidermal junction
Spleen	vessels
	basement membrane of red pulp
Synovia	vessels
Testis	vessels
	basal lamina of tubules
Thyroidea	vessels
	basal lamina of follicles
Uterus	vessels
	basal lamina of glands

TABLE 15.II

PATTERNS OF IMMUNOFLUORESCENT STAINING CONSISTENT WITH IC DEPOSITION OR FORMATION

Morphology	finely granular
	coarsely granular
	lanceolar (interrupted-linear)
	ribbon-like
Site	subendothelial
	along elasticae
	intramembranous
	mesangial (in kidney)
	subepithelial
	along connective tissue fibers
	intracellular
	on cell membranes

TABLE 15.III

APPROACH TO DIAGNOSIS OF IC-MEDIATED DISEASES (SEROLOGY AND IMMUNOPATHOLOGY)

Suggestive evidence	Antibody and antigen present in serum (simultaneously or consecutively) Complement concentrations in serum decreased Light microscopy: inflammation characterized by predominantly granulocytic infiltrate; granular deposits (toluidine blue PAS, or Masson's trichrome); thickening and irregularities of basement membranes
Corroborative evidence	Immune deposits (Table 15. II) in immunofluorescence or immunoenzyme staining (immunoglobulins, C3, C4) Electron microscopy: electron-dense (opaque) deposits; tissue derangements (e.g., fusion of podocytes, thickening of basement membranes) Demonstration of functional changes: increased permeability, abnormal EKG, ascites, etc. Immune complexes in circulation and in body fluids
Conclusive evidence	Antigen deposition (immunofluorescence, immunoenzyme techniques; immunoferritin) Elution of immune deposits and assay by serological procedures Dispersion of tissue-bound immune complexes by antigen excess Positive anti-antibody absorption test with tissue sections Demonstration of the same antigen in IC in tissue and in circulation.

rabbits, in which antibodies first react with basement membranes and ultimately IC are formed which deposit in these membranes. When IC just start to be found in basement membranes, they are easy to miss (Fig. 15.12). Similarly, in some rabbits with chronic serum sickness induced by BSA injections, a seemingly double linear pattern of staining for IgG may be seen in glomeruli (Fig. 15.8) of which one line probably is caused by antibodies to GBM-associated antigens (possibly similar or identical to those described by Wilson, C.B., et al., personal communication); the other seemingly linear staining probably represent ribbon-like deposits of IC. Finally, it should be expected that tissue antigens distributed in a discrete pattern may give granular staining when reacted with FITC-labeled antisera.

In IC-mediated pathology, double staining with antisera conjugated to distinct fluorochromes may be used to show beyond doubt that the immune reactants containing antigen, antibody, and complement indeed are at the same site. Thus, Clagett et al. [111] convincingly showed antigen and antibody in IC deposited in the follicular basal lamina of thyroids by double staining. Double staining may be performed in several modifications, and the selection of a method has to be done for every individual approach [437, 682]. The availability of a new fluorochrome giving blue staining (SITS) [536] may, despite some discouraging experience with this agent, make it possible to use a

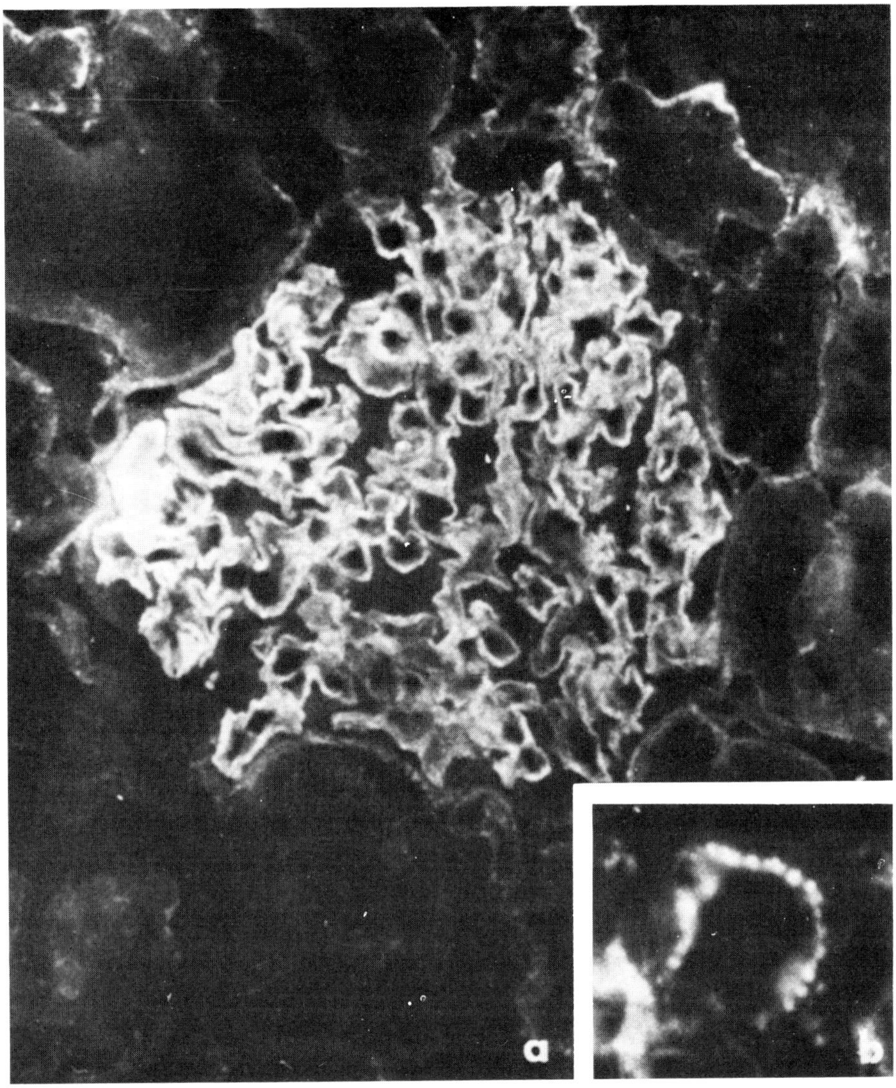

Fig. 15 12. Immunofluorescent staining of kidney tissue from a rabbit with mercury chloride-induced glomerulonephritis. Initial IC deposition superimposed on antibody depostition in the GBM. The granularity is barely visible on the main figure but is obvious in the inset. ×400 (inset: ×1000). (Reproduced with kind permission of the authors and publisher, from ref. 528.)

triple stain to demonstrate immunoglobulin, antigen, and complement simultaneously in immune deposits.

Although direct immunofluorescent staining procedures are usually used for detection of IC components in tissues, indirect immunofluorescent staining procedures may increase the sensitivity of the test [437, 682]. Unfortunately, these indirect procedures also decrease specificity. Similarly, complement-mediated immunofluorescence procedures increase sensitivity and the danger for non-specific staining [437, 682]. Immunofluorescence tests have recently been used also in the evaluation of tissue injury. Morphological derangements and increased or decreased production of tissue elements can be made visible. Thus, i.e. collagen [632, 681] and other connective tissue components [184, 551, 552] have been evaluated in pathological tissues. In addition, immunofluorescence may be used to examine functional derangements. Permeability changes of the vasculature can be followed by using macromolecules (e.g. dextrans) conjugated to fluorochromes [13].

Many "small" improvements in immunofluorescence technique are made as a result of everyday confrontation with preparation and microscopy (e.g. ref. 683). The publication of such seemingly trivial but valuable observations is essential in ensuring improved interpretation of biopsy and autopsy specimens in both diagnostic routine and research.

15.2.3.2. Immunoenzyme techniques

Immunoenzyme techniques are useful both in light microscopy and in ultrastructural studies [45, 229, 445, 446]. The principle of these immunohistological assays is analogous to that of immunofluorescence. A marker – an enzyme – is bound to an immunologically reactive molecule, e.g. antibodies or antigen [445]. The presence of the marker at sites of immune reactivity (i.e. the presence of antigen or antibodies) is visualized by the transformation of a leucobase into a dye [229]. Thus, in assays using horseradish peroxidase as the marker enzyme, diaminobenzidine undergoes polymerization and cyclization in the presence of peroxidase-oxidative [563]. This large molecular end-product containing conjugated double bonds precipitates at the site of immune reactions as a dark-brown dye. Treatment with osmium-tetroxide aids precipitation and further darkens the colour of the dye. Immunoenzyme techniques have several advantages over immunofluorescence; the preparations do not fade and may be stored over long periods of time for documentation; conventional light microscopes are sufficient to read the slides; and the test tissue may be analysed in light and electron microscopy using the same immunohistological reagents. Unfortunately, immunoenzyme techniques have not been as well defined as immunofluorescence. Still, attempts to compare some parameters of horseradish peroxidase and FITC-conjugated antisera in light microscopy suggest a high sensitivity for immunoenzyme techniques [45, 496, 561, 562]. In tissues with much autofluorescence, e.g. skin sections, immunoenzyme techniques may have the additional advantage of diminished background staining. For detection of IC, immunoenzyme techniques may be used in lieu of immunofluorescence in light microscopy. They are often indispensable for localization of IC in the ultrastructure of tissues. As with immunofluorescence tests, techniques are available allowing for use of paraffin embedded, formalin-fixed material; the results are comparable to those obtained with immunofluorescence.

The problems encountered in immunoelectron microscopy in general all come to bear on work with tissue-deposited IC. These problems encompass the achievement of a balance between good tissue preservation and penetration by the marker-antibody conjugate, the preservation of enzyme and antibody activity during conjugation, and the ability to have an electron-dense product as the end result of the reaction which does not diffuse too much but has enough contrast to the environment to allow for definitive identification and localization. In immunoenzyme techniques the possibility of endogenous enzymes (e.g. peroxidase in polymorphonuclear granulocytes) should be kept in mind. All these aspects have been reviewed extensively [10, 16, 32, 65, 585]. The reader is referred to these reviews. The introduction of triple-layer technique [384] and PAP [431] techniques has enhanced significantly sensitivity and technical feasibility of immunoenzyme techniques. Immunoelectron microscopy will undoubtedly remain reserved primarily for research and will not be used for specific problems of evaluation of patients' tissues. Studies in immunoelectron microscopy render the best results when preceded by immunofluorescence and/or immunoenzyme assays in light microscopy.

15.2.3.3. Immunoferritin techniques

Ferritin coupled to antiserum is a powerful tool for the detection and localization of immune reactants, especially those easily accessible, i.e. cell surface components [32, 568]. It is more difficult to use in studies on immune reactants lodged deep in tissues because of the large size of ferritin-antibody conjugates and poor penetration of tissues. Important insights into the

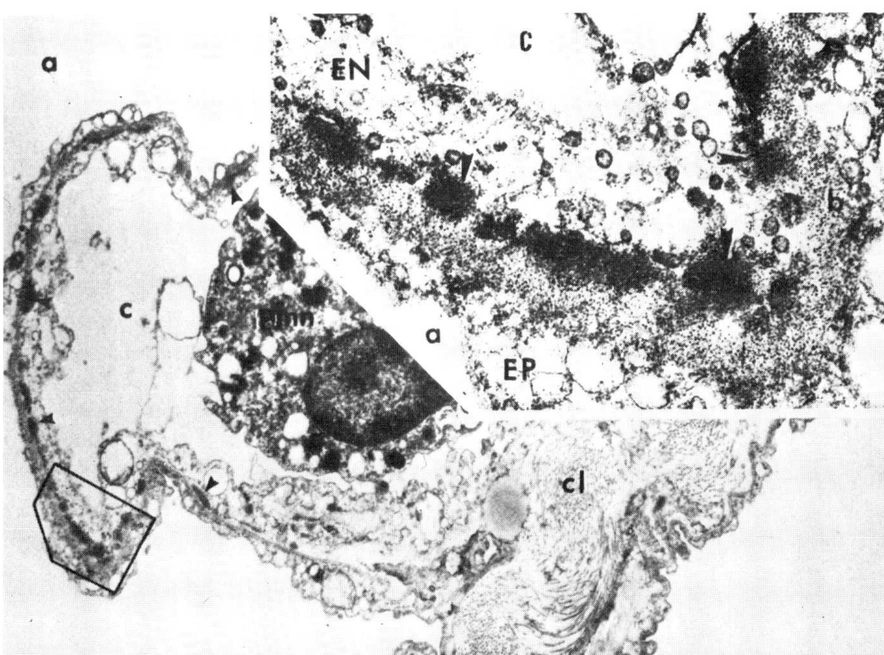

Fig. 15.13. Immunoelectron microscopy of the lung from a rabbit with chronic serum sickness. Complement deposits (arrows) are detectable in the electron-dense areas and in the basement membrane. a, alveolar space; c, capillary; pmn, polymorphonuclear cell; cl, collagen fibres; EN, endothelial cell; EP, epithelial cell; b, basement membrane. (Reprinted with the permission of the authors and publisher, from ref. 477.)

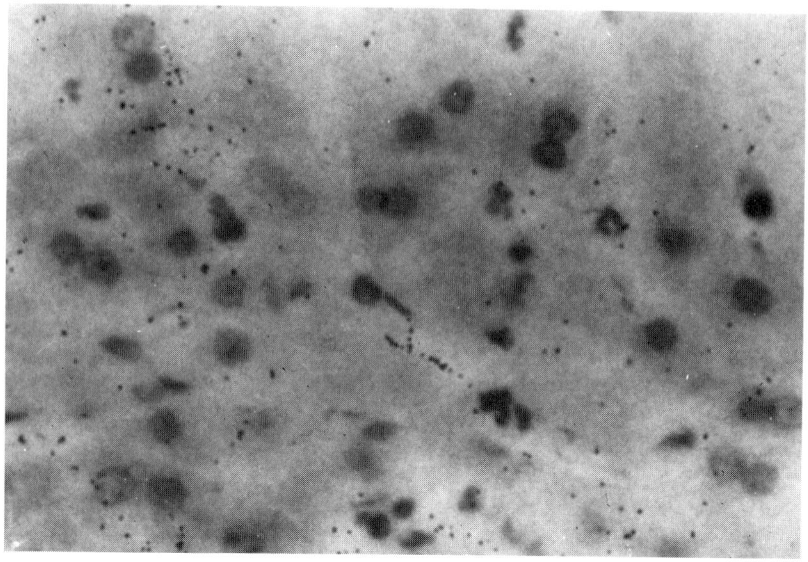

Fig. 15.14. Autoradiography (or radioautography) of the liver of a rabbit with chronic serum sickness injected 24 h earlier with radioactive BSA (^{125}I-BSA). Silver granules marking the site of the deposition of BSA presumably forming part of IC are seen in Disse's space. ×400. (Unpubl. micrograph by Neuland, Albini and Andres.)

ultrastructure of Masugi nephritis [27] and chronic serum sickness in rabbits [30] have been gained by this method. Recently, it was shown that cationized ferritin indeed may penetrate basement membranes in vivo [660], thus overcoming the major hurdle posed previously to the use of this marker in in vivo studies [661]. Immunoferritin techniques, in a few cases, may detect immune reactants not demonstrable in immunofluorescence. In the lung disease of systemic chronic serum sickness in rabbits, complement components could not be demonstrated by immunofluorescent staining but became detectable in immunoferritin reactions [77] (Fig. 15.13).

15.2.3.4. Autoradiography

Autoradiography [526] of tissues of animals injected with radiolabeled antigen has been used to document the pattern and extent of tissue deposition of IC (Fig. 15.14) [452]. Autoradiography in light microscopy allows for only rough localization, as the irradiation emanating from the antigen molecule reaches an area on the photosensitive emulsion much larger than occupied by the antigen itself. It may, however, also be used in electron microscopy.

15.2.4. Additional techniques

IC deposition in tissue may be tested for by the anti-antibody consumption test [319]. In this test, a "novel" antigenic site on antibody molecules of the IgG class is detected, which appears only upon IC formation with specific antigen [412, 413, 416]. The test itself is an agglutination inhibition test [318, 319].

Anti-antibody (AA) first is reacted with 4–10μm thick sections of the tissue to be tested. IC present in the tissue will "consume" the AA present in the preparation. Subsequent incubation of the preparation with Rh antibody-sensitized red cells will not lead to agglutination, i.e. the test is positive. Alternatively, if no IC are present in the tissue, AA remains free and reactive in the preparation. Upon incubation with sensitized erythrocytes it bridges the incomplete antibodies and induces agglutination, i.e. the test is negative. With this method, IC in tissues have been demonstrated in patients with renal allograft rejection [319] and leprosy [320]. This test, up to now the only one to evaluate immune deposits in tissues directly for being IC, promises to be of help in differentiating immunoglobulin aggregates from IC deposited in tissues.

Circumstantial evidence for the presence of IC in some tissues may be obtained by demonstrating saturation of IC receptors; that is, receptors for C [201] in tissues. The feasibility of this approach has been shown for IC deposition in SLE glomerulonephritis by Gelfand et al. [203]. The lack of reactivity of kidney sections from SLE patients with EAC in contrast to kidney tissue from normal individuals has been convincingly interpreted as representing saturation of normally present C receptors on podocytes of the glomerulus by IC. Whereas this method is not suitable for the detection of tissue-deposited IC, it may furnish additional evidence.

An attempt to establish a flow chart for screening tissue for the presence of IC in tissue specimens was made in Table 15.III. Whereas it is desirable to obtain all possible evidence for the presence of IC in a specimen, positive results in 1a and c together with evidence for IC obtained in 2 will be considered sufficient to assume deposition of IC (Table 15.III). On the other hand, isolated evaluation of biopsy or autopsy tissue in either light, electron, or immunofluorescent microscopy alone often will not satisfy the requirement for sufficient evidence for reliable diagnostic work.

15.3 DEMONSTRATION OF IMMUNE COMPLEXES IN CIRCULATION

Until recently, evidence for circulating IC could be obtained only indirectly. Decreased concentrations of complement [190, 233, 281, 347, 655, 658], detection of both antigen and antibody in the same or in consecutive serum samples [149, 503, 684], increased amounts of heavy molecular fractions in serum, and demonstration of mixed cryoglobulinemia [397, 398] were interpreted as suggestive evidence for circulating IC. After some attempts to use increased precipitability and other physicochemical properties of IC for their demonstration, assays were developed detecting IC on the basis of their biological properties. A wide variety of such methods have been and are continuously described. The overwhelming number of assays developed is a sure sign for both the need of a reliable method for the detection of IC and the rather discouraging results obtained with all the methods proposed until now.

The most widely used test procedures avail themselves of changes occurring in the Fc portion of immunoglobulins upon interaction with antigen: activation of the complement cascade, reactivity or enhanced reactivity with rheumatoid factors and other antibodies to immunoglobulins, and interaction with Fc receptors on cells. Some assays detect complement activation irrelevant to the pathway, be it classical or alternative, by detecting reactivities which reside in the "common components" of both pathways, notably C3. Recently, the appearance of a "new" antigenic site on the Fab fragment of complexed immunoglobulins has been used successfully for screening sera for circulating IC. This "anti-antibody agglutination inhibition test" has the great advantage of probably detecting only IC and not aggregated immunoglobulins. These antigen-independent methods of demonstration of circulating IC are much more promising than antigen-dependent assays. In most human IC-mediated diseases, the antigens involved are not known. Unfortunately, the clinical use of tests designed to detect circulating IC in most instances is not yet satisfactory. In many tests there is interference by the presence of aggregated immunoglobulins. In some tests, even monomeric immunoglobulins may interact with the markers used and thus give false-positive results. Often it is not precisely known which type of IC is detected by a given test procedure. Thus, even when IC are convincingly demonstrated in serum, it is difficult to determine whether these IC are disease-specific and/or pathogenic or merely "non-specific bystander" IC which could be expected to occur in the course of intermittent infections or other trivial events. Therefore, further analysis of IC demonstrated in circulation is of paramount importance in the effort to understand better their pathogenic role.

The various procedures used to demonstrate circulating IC detect distinct IC populations, or at least detect various IC populations with variable sensitivity. Serious attempts to define the IC detected in individual tests as to their physicochemical nature and the components involved have been made only recently. This insight seems essential for any serious attempt of interpretation of data on circulating IC.

The availability of assays for the detection of circulating IC has undoubtedly opened a whole new perspective in the understanding of IC-mediated diseases. However, it seems equally true that these tests are in their very infancy, and that experimental work combined with experience gained in testing clinical samples is necessary to make routine clinical use of these tests satisfactory. We readily concur with those questioning the general clinical value of tests for IC demonstration for individual patients. But the academic gain and the potentials of assays detecting circulating IC are great, and benefit undoubtedly is gained for future patients. In addition, testing of human samples seems essential in making detection of circulating IC reliable, well-defined, and useful in clinical routines. Furthermore, there are a few clinical conditions in which assays for the detection of circulating IC have been shown to be of great benefit for the individual patients. Obtaining complement and anti-DNA concentrations in serum of SLE patients does not always supply satisfactory

TABLE 15.IV. PHYSICOCHEMICAL AND ANTIGEN-DEPENDENT METHODS USED FOR THE DETECTION OF CIRCULATING IC

Assays	Size of IC	Sensitivity	Major causes for	
			False-positive results	False-negative results
I. Based on physicochemical characteristics				
A. Size				
1. Sucrose density gradient	L.M.	+ +	High MW macromolecules	Small IC (Ag_2Ab_1)
2. Sedimentation in isokinetic gradients	L.M.	+ +	idem	idem
3. Polyacrylamide gel electrophoresis (PAGE)	L.M.	+ +	idem	idem
4. Sephadex chromatography	L.M.	+ + +	idem	idem
5. BioGel A 1.5 M agarose chromatography	L.M.	+ + +	idem	idem
6. Analytical ultracentrifugation	L.M.	+	idem	idem
B. Solubility				
1. Ammonium sulfate precipitation	L.M.	(+)	idem	idem
2. Polyethylene glycol (PEG) precipitation	L.M.	(+)	idem	idem
3. Cryoprecipitation	L.M.(S)	+ +	Cryofibrinemia, monoclonal globulins	Inadequate harvesting technique
C. Net surface charge	L.M.S.	+ + (?)	?	?
D. Morphology: electron microscopy	L.M.S.	+ +	Aggregates other than Ag–Ab	No characteristic shape of Ag or lack of label
II. Based on the demonstration of antigen				
A. Use of IC-antigen specific antisera	(L)M.S.	?	Aggregated antigen	Antigen not accessible
B. Use of radiolabelled antigens[a]				
C. Infectivity of serum prior and after dissociation of IC[b]				

[a] Limited by radioactivity hazards and necessity to inject antigen into host. [b] Limited to IC-containing microbial and parasitic antigens. L, large; M, medium; S, small.

TABLE 15.V

ASSAYS FOR THE DETECTION OF CIRCULATING IC BASED ON BIOLOGICAL REACTIVITY OF ANTIGEN-COMPLEXED IMMUNOGLOBULINS

	Immunoglobulin class (and subclass) of IC detected	Size of IC	Sensitivity	Major cause for	
				False-positive results	False-negative results
A. ACTIVATION OF COMPLEMENT					
1. Via classical pathway only: interaction with Clq					
a.) agarose precipitation test	IgG1, IgG3, IgG2	L.M.(S.)	+ + +	Presence of DNA, endotoxin, C-reactive protein, β_2-microglobulin, virus, C1s, aggregated or monomeric IgG	IC not activating C via classical pathway, Rf or AA bound to IC; endogenous C1q
b.) radiolabeled C1q + precipitation with PEG		L.(M.)	+ +	idem	idem
c.) precipitation + double immunodiffusion		L.(M.)	+ +	idem	idem
d.) C1q deviation test		L.(M.)	5–10 μg	idem	idem
e.) C1q solid-phase radioimmunoassays		L.(M.)	5–10 μg	Aggregated or monomeric IgG	idem
2. Via classical or alternative pathways					
a.) microcomplement test	IgG1, IgG3, IgG2, (IgG4)? IgM, IgA, (IgE)?	L.M.S.	+ +	Heating of serum required which may lead to aggregation of IG	IC not activating C3

b.) activation of C3 – precipitation by antibody to C3					
i.) solid-phase radioimmunoassy		?	+ +	Monomeric and aggregated IC	idem
ii.) EAC-rosette inhibition test		?	?	?	idem
iii.) conglutinin binding (solid-phase radioimmunoassay)		?	?	Monomeric or aggregated Ig	IC not activating C3 catabolism of C3 (short life time of C3bi)
iv.) erythrocyte receptor assay		L.(M.)	?	Aggregated Ig, antibodies to erythrocytes	IC not reacting with C3 IC with C3d alone
v.) Raji cell receptor assays:					
immunofluorescence		M.S.	3–5 μg	Aggregated Ig antibodies to lymphocytes	IC not activating C3
radioimmunoassay		M.S.	1–5 μg		
B. INTERACTION WITH NEW EPITOPES ON COMPLEXED IMMUNOGLOBULIN					
1. Assays using rheumatoid factors					
a.) immunoprecipitation	IgG	?	100 μg	Aggregated and monomeric IgG	RF in serum
b.) agglutination-inhibition	IgG	(L).M.S.	1–25 μg	idem	idem (antibodies to erythrocyte)
c.) competitive inhibition assays with radiolabeled markers	IgG	idem	idem	idem	idem
2. Assay using immune antiglobulin sera: agglutination inhibition	IgG, IgA, IgM	L.M.S.	+ + +	idem	RF-containing IC not detectable

TABLE 15.V (continued)

	Immunoglobulin class (and subclass) of IC detected	Size of IC	Sensitivity	Major cause for	
				False-positive results	False-negative results
3. Assays using anti-antibodies: agglutination inhibition	IgG	M.(S.)	1–5 μg	(?)	RF in test serum (IC binding C?; antibodies to erythrocytes)(?)
4. Assays using cellular Fc receptors					
a.) platelet aggregation test	IgG	L.(M.)	(1)5–10 μg	Aggregated IgG; myxovirus, enzymes, antibodies to platelets	IC binding C
b.) L1210 murine leukemia cell assay	IgG(IgM)	?	+ +	Aggregated or monomeric IgG	idem
c.) inhibition of ADCC	IgG(IgM)	?	5–10 μg	idem	idem; antilymphocytic antibodies; complement-induced lysis
d.) inhibition of EA rosettes	IgG?	?	?	Aggregated and monomeric IgG antilymphocytic antibodies	?
e.) degranulation of eosinophilis granulocytes or mast cells	IgE(IgG)	?	?	Macromolecules inducing degranulation	
f.) interaction with staphylococcal protein A[b]	IgG1, IgG2, IgG4, IgM(?)	varies with test[b]	?	?	RF or AA bound to IC

C. PHAGOCYTOSIS OF IC					
1. By polymorphonuclear granulocytes	Ig	L.M.	?	Aggregated IgG, non-specific IF staining	Catabolites of IC in lysosomes (soluble IC)
2. By guinea pig peritoneal macrophages	Ig	?	?	?	?
3. By polymorphonuclear-granulocytes: killing of *E. coli*	Ig	?	?	?	?

[a] Even IC.
[b] Used as a modification in A1e, A2bv.

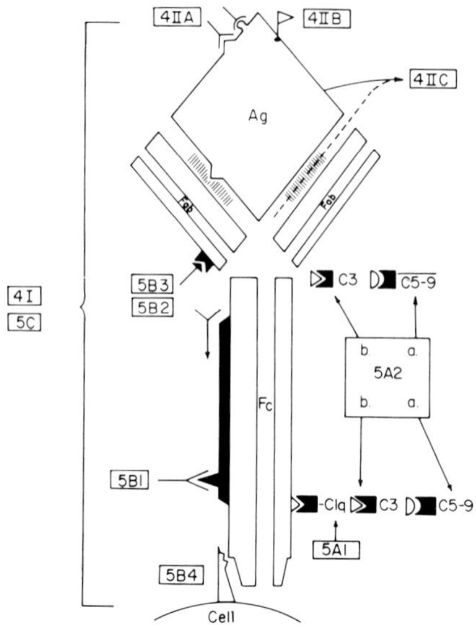

Fig. 15.15. Diagrammatic representation of an IC. The framed numbers refer to Tables 15.IV and 15.V, indicating the component of the IC involved in the various methods used in assays for the detection of circulating IC.

clinical information to monitor disease activity or development of kidney disease [88]. Testing for circulating IC allows for more precise evaluation of the course of SLE [493]. Detectable IC in serum have been shown to parallel closely disease activity in a number of patients with rheumatoid arthritis [462]. Especially neurological complications and development of nodules seem to correlate with circulating IC [118]. Levinsky et al. [365] reported on a female patient with diffuse proliferative glomerulonephritis in which IC concentrations assayed in serum paralleled disease activity and rendered important data to aid management of the disease.

A brief overview of the available tests is given in Tables 15.IV, 15.V and Fig. 15.15. More detailed accounts are available in a number of reviews [460, 621, 684, 706]. The discussion focusses on the microassay modification for the detection of IC using Raji cells and immunofluorescence. The anti-antibody agglutination assay will be described to some extent, as it has been used for comparative studies in our laboratory and is still not described extensively in most reviews.

15.3.1. The Raji cell assay

The density of C3 receptors varies on peripheral human blood lymphocytes. Such cells also carry surface immunoglobulins. A human lymphoblastoid cell line derived from a patient with Burkitt's lymphoma, however, displays high densities of C3b (and possible C3d) receptors, Fc receptors of low avidity or low density (reacting with human immunoglobulins only), but no surface immunoglobulins [146, 622–624]. This Raji cell line has been used by Theofilo-

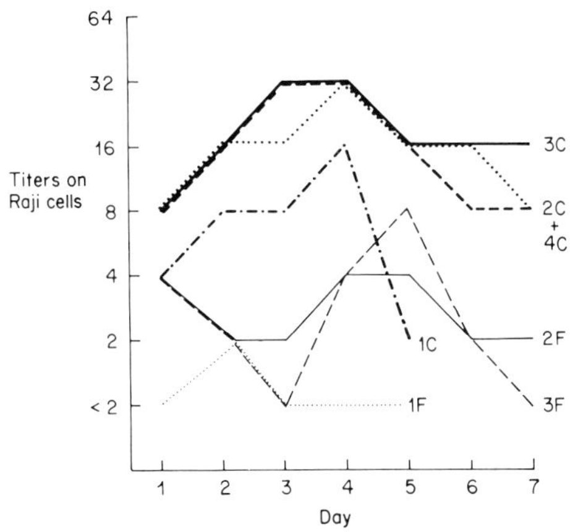

Fig. 15.16. Titers of in vitro-formed IC (BSA and rabbit anti-BSA) with (C) or without (F) complement on Raji cells harvested at different times after initiation of culture. The IC were detected with a fluorescein-conjugated antiserum to rabbit IgG.

TABLE 15.VI

BLOCKING OF COMPLEMENT RECEPTOR–COMPLEMENT INTERACTION BY PREINCUBATION OF IC–COMPLEMENT–CONTAINING PREPARATIONS WITH SUPERNATANT[a] OF 72 h CULTURES OF RAJI CELLS

No preincubation		Supernatant					
		1:80	1:40	1:20	1:10	1:5	1:1
1:1	+ +	+ +	+ +	+ +	+ +	+	±
1:2	+ +	+ +	+ +	+	+	−	−
1:4	+	+ +	+ +	+	+		
1:8	+	+	+ +	+	±		
1:16	+	+	+	+	−	−	−
1:32	+	+	+	±	−	−	−
1:64	+	±	+	±	−	−	−
1:128	±	−	−	−	−	−	−

[a] Supernatant concentrated 50:1. Blocking could be demonstrated only with soluble IC but not with EAC.

poulous and associates [146, 622–624] to develop an assay for the detection of circulating IC. The reactivity of receptors for C3 and Fc of IgG varies over time of culture (Fig. 15.16). This variation of reactivity probably reflects changes in density and/or avidity of surface receptors. The interaction of IC with the Fc receptors is always weak. This interaction is stronger for large aggregates of immunoglobulin, especially when complement is not activated. To completely avoid interactions with Fc receptors it is best to harvest Raji cells 72 h after initiation of culture, when the expression of C3 receptors is maximal and that of Fc receptors negligible (Fig. 15.16). Complement receptors seem to be shed into the culture fluid (Albini and Glurich, unpublished observation). This has been suggested by blocking the interaction of IC with Raji cells after incubation of IC with concentrated culture fluid (Table 15.VI). Shedding of Fc receptors and their transfer to primarily Fc-negative cells have been described earlier [611] with other cell types. To obtain optimal results in Raji cell assays, undisturbed and controlled growth of the cells is required. A steady growth is

TABLE 15.VII

THE RAJI CELL ASSAY: IMMUNOFLUORESCENCE TEST AND RADIOIMMUNOASSAY (RIA)

1. Harvest 72 h Raji cells Wash thoroughly in RPMI 1640. Count cells. Adjust suspension to	immunofluorescence (IF) test: 3×10^6/ml	RIA: 2×10^6/200 lambda
2. Add test serum	25 lambda of 1:2, 1:4, 1:8, etc. dilution + 20 lambda of cell suspension	25 lambda of a 1:4 dilution + 50 lambda of cell suspension
3. Incubate for	45 min at 4°C	45 min at 37°C
4. Wash with	50 lambda of RPMI 1640 medium containing NaN_3 (3×)	1 ml Spinners medium (3×)
5. Add	25 lambda of fluorescein (or rhodamine) conjugated anti-serum to immunoglobulin or antigen	"optimal amount" of radiolabelled antiserum to immunoglobulin (or staphylococcal protein A)
6. Incubate for	45 min at 4°C	30 min at 4°C
7. Wash with	50 lambda of RPMI containing NaN_3 (2×) and with 50 lambda PBS containing NaN_3 (2×)	1 ml Spinners medium (3×) containing 1% HSA
8. Decant supernatant	Place cells on slide. Dry under a fan. Coverslip with glycerol	
9. Read results	under an immunofluorescence microscope (5–10 dilutions)	in a gammacounter (duplicates or triplicates).
10. Express results	Highest serum dilution giving detectable cell surface immunofluorescence is the titer of immune complexes in serum (semiquantitative)	The counts obtained are compared to values obtained with known amounts of aggr. gamma globulin. Results are given as "amount of aggregated gammaglobulin-equivalent": (quantitative).

seen usually for a period of 6–18 months; then the number of cells in culture increases (e.g. from 12–16 × 10^6 to 20–32 × 10^6 per culture). This should be taken as an indication to discard the culture and initiate a new inoculum. With high cell counts, the results of the assay become erratic, and false-negative and false-positive results can be seen in consecutive experiments. To assure optimal conditions for the evaluation of IC in Raji cell assays, the following precautions should be taken: 1) cells should be harvested 72 h after feeding culture medium; 2) cells should be used only if the cell count of the culture does not exceed 18 × 10^6 cells/culture; 3) each test should be run with a positive and negative control serum; 4) cells should be washed well (3–5 times) prior to use in the assay; 5) the final preparations should be evaluated as soon as possible after the incubation and washes have been performed; and 6) cells should always be tested for viability prior and after incubation with test serum. The principles of the Raji cell assay are depicted in Table 15.VII. The detection of molecules bound to Raji cells may be accomplished by FITC or TRITC-conjugated or radiolabeled antisera to immunoglobulins [622] or antigen [625, 626] or by staphylococcal protein A coupled to FITC or ^{125}I.

15.3.1.1. The Raji cell radioimmunoassay [620, 625]

The procedure is outlined in Table 15.VII. The "marker" reagent is radiolabeled anti-immunoglobulin or staphylococcal protein A. The results are expressed as equivalent of aggregated gammaglobulin. With every test, a series of preparations of Raji cells, sera containing serial dilutions of aggregated gamma globulin, and the radiolabeled antiserum to immunoglobulin are run. By plotting measured radioactivity (c.p.m.) against the dilutions of aggregated gammaglobulin used in a test it is possible to establish a "standard curve" from which the values for "aggregated gamma globulin equivalent" may be determined after amounts of radioactivity in test sera have been established [620, 625]. Only one dilution of test serum is used (usually 1 : 2 or 1 : 4) but the preparations are done in triplicate. This method has been widely used for the detection of IC of human and animal origin [621, 684]. The sensitivity of the method is very good (minimum IC detected 6–12 μg/ml). Use of staphylococcal protein A is widely advocated for this assay and seems to give values very well comparable to those obtained by using antisera to immunoglobulins. If serum samples are diluted serially, the various dilutions often do not give the same value for the amount of IC in undiluted serum. As aggregated immunoglobulins (which are used to establish the standard curve) behave in many ways differently from IC and as IC of various distinct classes and sizes vary in ability to activate C3 (see section 15.1.2), the expression of results as aggregated gammaglobulin equivalent at best allows for semiquantitative interpretation (despite evoking the impression of strictly quantitative data). The presence of lymphocytotoxic antibodies in the test serum [690] or deterioration of cell viability during the test may lead to false-positive results. Balancing these disadvantages, however, are the advantages of this test: it is

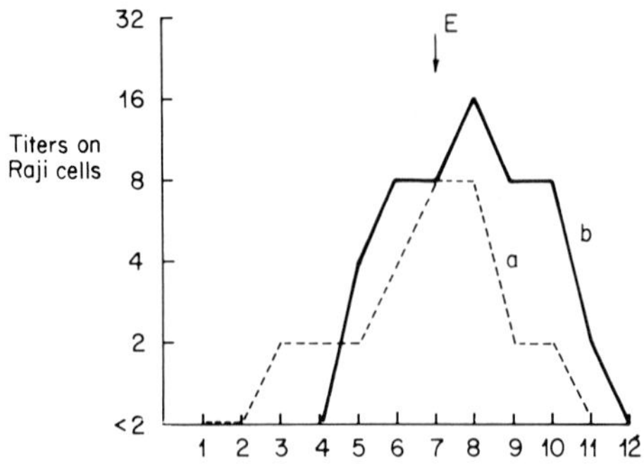

Fig. 15.17. Titers of in vitro-formed IC (horse IgG–human anti-horse IgG) on Raji cells harvested 72 h after initiation of culture. The IC were detected by fluorescein-conjugated antiserum to human IgG (b) and by rhodamine-conjugated antiserum to horse IgG (a). The antigen concentration was diluted serially from 1 to 12, with the concentration of antbodies remaining constant.

simple and easy to perform, is evaluated in a gammacounter (i.e. no active reading or microscopy is required) and the presentation of data as "micrograms equivalent" satisfies the modern passion for quantitation.

15.3.1.2. The Raji cell immunofluorescence procedure.
Immunofluorescent staining was used in the original report by Theofilopoulos et al. [622]. The sera were either not diluted at all or were used at only one low dilution; the intensity of staining was recorded. This rather crude technique obviously did not render satisfactory results. However, using defined immunofluorescent staining [64] and the procedure described by Schauenstein et al. [549] (and Chapter 4, this volume), large numbers of patient sera can be tested in a short time allowing for semiquantitative results, namely the determination of end-titers. In our laboratory, up to 30 patients' sera have been tested in a single run. The assay follows the flow chart given in Table 15.VII. To work up large numbers of sera, it is essential to set the tests as described by Schauenstein et al. [549]. The washing fluids (RPMI 1640 and PBS) should contain 0.7 nM NaN_3 to prevent capping [491]. Experiments with in vitro-formed IC containing human or rabbit antibodies suggest that the maximum sensitivity of the test is obtained with IC at antigen–antibody equivalence or in slight antigen excess (Fig. 15.17). As expected, antigen can be detected more easily in antigen-excess IC, whereas immunoglobulin is better demonstrable in antibody-excess IC.

Sera to be used in the Raji cell test obviously should not be decomplemented. Very old sera containing IC (stored for 18 months or more) often have a decreased reactivity with Raji cells, and normal sera stored over prolonged periods of time may show false-positive results.

If reasonably fresh sera (less than 18 months) are used, a titer of 1 : 4 is considered "positive". The highest titers observed by us were 1 : 512. Normal blood donor populations gave a positive result of 6%, and among 22 healthy laboratory personnel, one had IC in circulation (also found by AA inhibition assay).

Decomplemented sera may be used after addition of guinea pig complement.

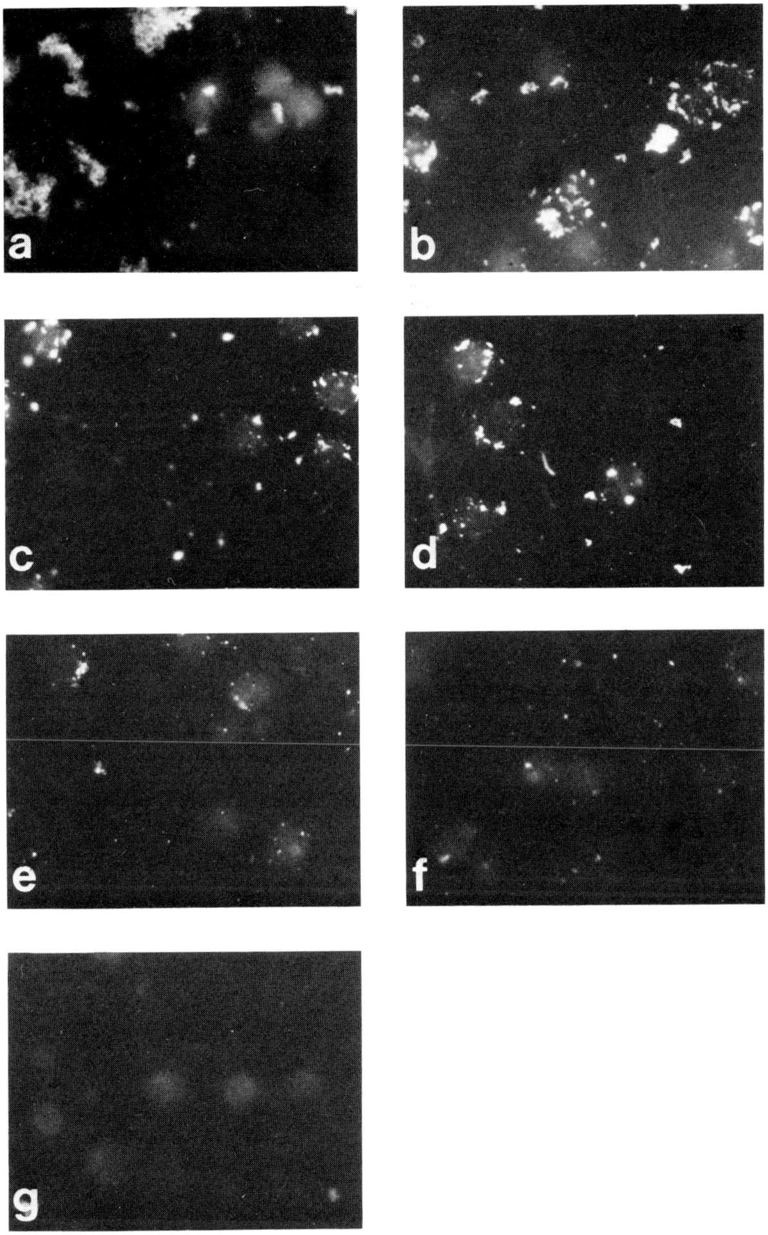

Fig. 15.18. Titration of a test serum containing IC (patient with SLE) on Raji cells. Dilutions: a), 1:2; b), 1:4; c), 1:8; d), 1:16; e), 1:32; f), 1:64; and g), 1:128. The lowest dilution (1:2) only shows precipitates between the cells. The higher dilutions show decreased amounts of immune precipitates and definitive staining of cell membranes. The dilution of 1:64 gives only a ± staining. The next dilution is negative. ×250.

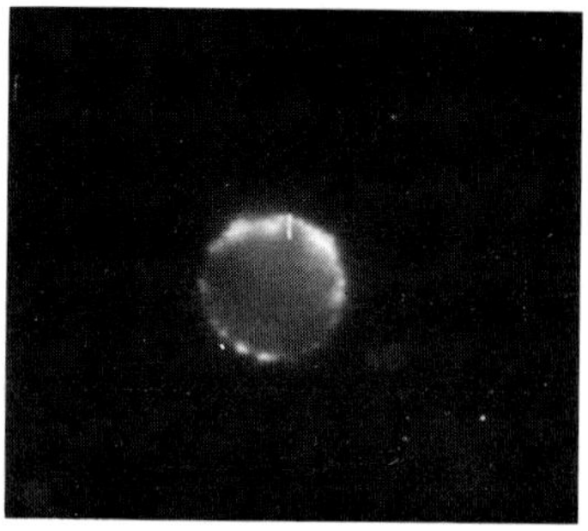

Fig. 15.19. Immunofluorescent staining for human immunoglobulin on the surface of a Raji cell incubated with a serum from a patient with allograft rejection. Serum dilution 1:8. ×400.

The optimal complement concentration has to be established by titration. Excess of complement may lead to "solubilization" of IC [607], and thus to false-negative results. Still, the titers obtained for IC in sera after decomplementation and reconstitution of complement are lower for IC-containing preparations and higer for IC-free sera than found in fresh preparations. Under these conditions, only titers higher than 1 : 8 can be considered positive. Therefore, addition of complement to sera prior to Raji cell assay should only be resorted to as a last measure.

As Raji cells are grown in the presence of fetal calf serum, antibodies to calf and bovine serum may interact with fetal calf serum proteins adsorbed to Raji cells, and thus render false-positive results. This complication can be avoided by thorough washing of Raji cell suspensions in large volumes of medium prior to the tests. With many patients' sera, prozone-like phenomena may be observed at serum dilutions of 1 : 2 and 1 : 4. In addition, heavy immune precipitates may blurr the reading of preparations at these low dilutions (Fig. 15.18).

The typical appearence of immunofluorescent staining of IC on Raji cells is shown in Fig. 15.19. The titration of a patient's serum (SLE) on Raji cells is shown in Fig. 15.18. The presence of antibodies to lymphoid cell surface antigens in sera may lead to the presence of linear to granular immunoglobulin deposits on the cell. With most antilymphocytic antibodies, Raji cells show intracellular uptake of the FITC conjugate used: a high percentage of the cells shows cloudy staining of the cytoplasm. Despite convincing reports on the rather insignificant role of lymphocytotoxic antibodies for the Raji cell assay [625, 628, 639, 690], we have observed these antibodies in sera from three patients with SLE in a series of 13, and in sera of four patients with SLE out of a series of 23; four of the sera did have lymphocytotoxic antibodies with a titer of 8, one with a titer of 4, and two were positive when tested without dilution.

Results with sera of patients with SLE, rheumatoid arthritis, alcoholic liver diseases, primary biliary cirrhosis, membranous nephropathy, and leprosy are summarized in Table 15.VIII.

IC involving antibodies of various immunoglobulin classes can be distinguished in Raji cell assays. IC containing IgA have first been described in the

TABLE 15.VIII

RAJI CELL ASSAY: RESULTS WITH SERA FROM PATIENTS WITH SLE, KIDNEY ALLOGRAFTS (KA), LEPROSY (L), MEMBRANOUS NEPHROPATHY (MN) AND WITH SERA FROM NORMAL INDIVIDUALS (N)

	Test groups				
Serum dilution	N	SLE	KA	L	MN[a]
<1:2 (= neg.)	21	0	10	26	4
1:2	0	2	0	7	2
1:4	0	0	9	8	0
1:8	1	5	8	5	1
1:16	0	3	3	2	0
1:32	0	5	0	7	0
1:64	0	1	0	0	0
1:128	0	2	0	1	0
1:256	0	1	0	0	0
N	22	19	30	56	7
% pos.	5%	100%	67%	54%	43%

[a] In membranous nephropathy, consecutive sera were tested over prolonged periods of time (3 months to 2 years). The four patients listed as negative never showed positive results; one of the patients listed as positive had positive tests on two occasions, the others only on one occasion during the observation period.

immunofluorescence micromethod [481] and then with the use of radiolabeled antisera [241]. IC containing IgM were detected in sera of patients with leprosy and primary biliary cirrhosis [320, 484]. Antigens may be detected in IC using Raji cells and fluorochrome-conjugated antigen-specific antisera. In studies with preformed IC, the antibody and the antigen may be labeled with fluorochromes prior to reaction. Thus, both antigen and antibody may be seen in the same IC. Complement components cannot (or can only inconsistently) be detected in IC after reaction with C receptors on Raji cells. Thus, the use of fluorochrome or radiolabelled antisera to complement components seems infeasible.

15.3.2. The anti-antibody inhibition assay

Anti-antibodies (AA) were first described in 1956 by Milgrom et al. [416]. These antibodies occur in the sera of some humans and rabbits. They are, in humans, of the IgM class. They occur in relatively low frequency in the populations of healthy or hospitalized individuals tested thus far (~ 1 out of 2000). AA react with other antibodies after these have interacted with antigen. Aggregated gammaglobulin reportedly does not react with AA [195]. The anti-antibody combines with an antigenic determinant in the $F(ab)_2$ fragment of antibodies.

AA are used in an agglutination–inhibition test for the detection of circulating IC [319]. The anti-antibody is incubated first with the test serum; IC of the IgG class present in the serum will combine with AA. The indicator reaction in this consumption test is agglutination of human erythrocytes sensitized with "incomplete" antibodies to Rh blood group antigens. Agglutination occurs only when the antibodies reacted with erythrocyte antigens are "bridged" by AA. Therefore, the absence of agglutination indicated the presence of IC in a test serum, and positive agglutination indicated the absence of IC. The degree of inhibition is expressed as titer (i.e. the highest dilution of test serum still giving a negative reaction in the agglutination indicator system).

The antigenic specificities responsible for reaction with high-titered AA seem not to be allotypic determinants [317], despite some suggestive evidence that low-titered AA indeed may show allotypic specificities [449].

The AA inhibition assay is highly sensitive in the detection of IC in antibody–antigen equivalence or in slight antigen excess. This test is unique among all assays described up to now in not detecting aggregated IgG [317, 621].

RF present in test sera may aggregate sensitized erythrocytes. This may lead to false-negative results in this assay [317, 621]. Pretreatment of test sera with 2-mercaptoethanol destroys RF. IC consisting of IgM-class RF and IgG (now in the role of antigen) are not detected by the AA inhibition assay; IgG has to react as antibody in IC to be detected in this assay. The assay is easy to perform and has a high specificity for IC. The necessity for elaborate and extensive screening procedures for detecting sera containing high-titered AA limits, at least at present, the usefulness of this procedure for general clinical laboratories.

15.4. FURTHER ANALYSIS OF IMMUNE COMPLEXES

Immunohistological techniques described in section 15.2 of this chapter allow for detection of IC in tissues and for some definition of the constituents of IC. Immunoglobulin class and subclass, nature of antigen, and complement components recruited by the IC may be determined. To accomplish further analysis, however, IC or their components must be solubilized and eluted from the tissue. Circulating IC may be detected by the variety of assays outlined in Tables 15.IV and 15.V. Some insight into their composition may be gained by considering the type of IC detected by individual test methods (e.g. complement binding or not) and by selecting the reagents used (e.g. marker-antisera conjugates specific for IgG, IgA and IgM in Raji cell assay). Detailed analysis usually requires enrichment of IC and separation from other serum components. In the following, elution techniques and enrichment methods for IC will be described. These are the two basic procedures in the course of any detailed characterization of IC. Finally, selected specialized techniques useful in characterization will be discussed briefly.

TABLE 15.IX

METHODS USED MOST FREQUENTLY FOR ELUTION OF TISSUE-BOUND IC

	Efficiency in eluting	
	Ag[a]	Ab[a]
1 M Propionic acid, pH 2.7	+ + +	(+)
0.02 M Citrate buffer, pH 3.2	+	+ +
Glycine buffer, pH 2.6/2.8/3.0	(+)	+ +
0.1 M Borate buffer, pH 11.5	+ +	(+)
0.1 M Glycine buffer, pH 1.5/11.0/ 11.5/12.0	+	+ +
8 M Urea	+	+ +
3 M KBr at pH 9	+ +	+ +
3 M KI at pH 7.2	+ +	+ +
2–3 M NaSCN, KSCN, at pH 5.8 or 9.0–10.5	+ +	+ +
2–3 M NaCl at pH 7.3	+	+ +
2.5 M $MgCl_2$ at pH 7.3	+	+ +
2–4% Propanol at acid or alkaline pH	+ +	+(+)
50–60% Ethylene glycol at acid or alkaline pH	+ +	+(+)
50% DMSO at acid or alkaline pH	+ +	+(+)

[a] As tested with BSA/anti-BSA IC deposited anti-BSA in rabbit kidney.

15.4.1. Elution techniques

Antibody, antigen and, to a very limited extent, intact IC deposited in tissues may be brought into solution by a number of techniques [48, 362, 699]. This solubilization may be accomplished by agents capable of dissolving immune precipitates [313, 616], dissociating antibodies or antigen from immunoadsorbents [132, 698], or breaking down basement membranes [327, 381]. Even though distilled water and buffered saline may elute more or less effectively IC or their components from tissues, two main approaches have been used for elution: 1) acid buffers at low or high salt concentrations and chaotropic ions; or 2) excess of the immunologically active components of IC, especially of antigen.

The reagents used most commonly for elution are listed in Table 15.IX. The efficiency of various elution techniques in view of relative amounts of immune reactants solubilized and biological activity of the immune reactants after solubilization vary among different elution techniques. Detailed analyses of elution techniques have been published by Bartolotti [48] and by Woodroffe and Wilson [699]. Woodroffe and Wilson [699] reported that 1 M propionic acid at pH 2.7 eluted 86%, and 0.1 M borate buffer at pH 11.25 80% of ^{125}I-BSA from IC deposits. These buffers, however, reduced the antibody reactivity. In their hands, the best preservation of antibody reactivity was obtained by incubation of kidney homogenates with 0.02 M citrate buffer at pH 3.2. The antibody reacted well in immunodiffusion, immunofluorescence, and radioimmunoassays, but showed impaired complement fixation. On the other hand, elution with chaotropic agents yielded antibodies capable of complement activation. In the study by Bartolotti [48], a chaotropic agent, namely 3 M KBr at pH 9, gave the best results in elution of antigens from IC. In this study, repeated extractions with the chaotropic agent were performed. The same author suggests a stepwise alkaline gradient of pH 10.5–11.1 using 0.1 M glycine-NaOH. Also 8 M urea gave satisfactory elution of IC. Elution in the cold seems better than at higher temperatures. According to Bartolotti [48], acid buffers seem effective in eluting antibodies present in IC but not in solubilizing antigens. Only 5–23% of BSA was eluted with glycine-HCl buffers at pH 3.0–2.6. On the other hand, Woodroffe and Wilson [699] found significant elution of antigen with citrate buffer at pH 3.2 (over 50%) and with propionic acid (86%). Woodroffe and Wilson [699] reported that 75% of BSA eluted reassembles with antibodies under neutral pH conditions; this may have accounted for the low percentages obtained by Bartolotti [48]. Decreasing pH of acid buffers allows for elution of increasingly avid antibodies [48]. Optimal elution conditions, however, probably vary with the population of IC studied. Table 15.X gives a comparison of elution studies with BSA–anti-BSA IC, thyroglobulin–antithyroglobulin IC, and IC found in mercury chloride-induced glomerulonephritis of rabbits. Recombination of antibody and antigen in eluates may be prevented by separation in acid sucrose density gradient [699].

The same elution techniques may also be applied to tissue sections [174]. With appropriate sensitive methods, antibody and antigen content of such eluates may be tested [174, 699]. In addition, elution predominantly of antibody may increase the reactivity of conjugates with antigen in immunohistological tests. Reconstitution of IC after elution of antibodies using antibodies of the specificity expected to be involved in IC has been accomplished [31]. The use of specific immune reactants for elution of IC or their components is useful in corroborating or establishing the specificity of reactant (antigen or antibody) and could be used, at least in experimental animals injected with radiolabeled antigen, for quantitative studies.

First evidence for "solubilization" of IC in antigen excess was obtained by Pedersen [480] and Heidelberger and Pedersen [252] and then summarized in Goldberg's theory of antigen–antibody interactions. Dissolution of IC has been accomplished in vivo by injection of excess antigen into rabbits with chronic serum sickness [644, 687] and into mice with IC deposits in kidneys [379]. This method can be used to establish the identity of antigens involved in specific IC. Dissociation and elution of IC occur only in the presence of the specific antigen. Thus, inspection of, e.g., kidney biopsies taken prior and after administration of antigen excess will allow for detection of partial or complete dissociation of IC using immunohistological techniques. Recently, elution of IC by antigen excess was performed on tissue sections [483]. In chronic serum sickness of

TABLE 15.X

COMPARISON OF VARIOUS ELUTION METHODS ON TISSUE SECTIONS FROM CHICKENS WITH SPONTANEOUS AUTOIMMUNE THYROIDITIS, RABBITS WITH CHRONIC SERUM SICKNESS, AND RABBITS WITH MERCURY CHLORIDE-INDUCED SYSTEMIC IC DISEASE

Tissues for elution procedure	Thyroids of 7 week[a] old OS chickens	Kidneys from[b] rabbits with SCSS	Kidneys from rabbits with MISICD[c]
Citrate buffer, pH 3.2	+ + + +[d]	−	±
Glycine buffer, pH 2.8/3.0	+ + +	−	NT
Glycine buffer, pH 9.0/11.5	+ + + +	−	NT
KI	−	−	+ + +
KSCN	+ + +	±	+ + +
Phosphate-buffered saline, pH 7.2	+ + +	+ +	±
Glycine buffer, pH 9.5/DMSO	+	−	NT
(Staining prior to elution:	+ + +	+ +	+ + +)

[a] IC in follicular basal lamina. OS, obese strain.
[b] IC in GBM. SCSS, Systemic chronic serum sickness.
[c] IC in GBM and TBM. MISICD, mercury-induced systemic IC disease.
[d] Staining after elution.

rabbits, at the onset of the late proteinuric phase [453], elution of IC could be accomplished by incubation of tissue with excess of antigen. In human idiopathic membraneous glomerulonephritis, aggregated human immunoglobulins did dissociate glomerular IC deposits [483, 598].

Prolonged incubation with antigen is necessary, and small biopsy specimens tend to float off the slides during washing procedures. Application of one drop of 0.5% agarose on top of the tissue plazed on the slide prevents such complications [483]. Antibody excess could also be used; as shown in precipitation curves, extremely large excess of antibodies usually is necessary [312].

Antibody obtained by elution techniques should be tested for specificity in indirect immunofluorescence tests, double immunodiffusion, passive hemagglutination tests, and radioimmunoassays. Any antigenic specificity detected should be confirmed by absorption with pure antigenic preparation. The setbacks of the elution technique are the preferential elution of low-avidity antibodies, possible changes induced during the procedure in the structure of immunoglobulins (sometimes entailing partial or total abolishment of immune reactivity), and interaction of eluted antibodies with eluted antigens. Eluted IC usually are a minimal fraction of the eluate and probably undergo structural changes during the procedure, prohibiting the use of eluates for gathering information on the precise characteristic of tissue-deposited IC themselves.

15.4.2. Enrichment and purification of circulating IC

The use of cryoglobulins and methods enriching IC based on physicochemical properties have been discussed earlier. Other purification methods select IC by biological properties of the immune reactants involved. Some of the latter procedures are discussed in the following paragraphs.

Isolation of circulating IC (or IC from other body fluids) first was accomplished by physicochemical procedures [93, 120, 358, 692]. The isolated material sometimes contains immunoglobulin or complement components, but it is doubtful if it represents IC. Subsequently, interaction of IC with C1q attached to Sepharose has been used by Svehag and Burger [601] to isolate IC by affinity chromatography and desorption with diaminoalkyl compound. This basic procedure has been improved more recently by Casali and Lambert [94]. They used lipid-free serum precipitated with 2.5% polyethylene glycol (PEG) prior to passage through a column with polymethylene metacrylate beads coated with C1q. This method was used to enrich IC from serum of patients with Kala Azar which were analyzed subsequently by acid pH dissociation of antigen and antibody, immunoelectrophoresis, SDS-PAGE, and ultracentrifugation [94]. The same authors developed a procedure using conglutinin for the isolution of IC [94]. IC activating C3 may also be purified using Raji cells as described by Theofilopoulos et al. [627]. IC bound to Raji cells were labelled with lactoperoxidase. These moieties then were eluted from the cell surface with isotonic citrate buffer at pH 3.2 or were isolated by precipitation with antibodies from cell homogenates. Antigen and antibody present in IC were analysed by sucrose density gradient and SDS-PAGE. IC not activating complement have been purified using affinity chromatography with staphylococcal protein A coupled to Sepharose [637]. Double diffusion in agar, immunoelectrophoresis, and counterimmunoelectrophoresis were used for analysis of enriched IC fractions. Similar to other methods of enrichment of IC, Chenais et al. [102] precipitated the IC first with ammonium sulfate and further fractionated the preparation by filtration in Ultrogel AcA 34 (LKB Instruments); one serum was precipitated also in 5% PEG. The combination of physicochemical methods and biological reactions seems the most promising approach in attempts to purify IC from body fluids.

15.4.3. Characterization of IC: size, lattice structure, kinetics of deposition in tissues and of disappearance from serum

The size of IC in fluids (eluates or enriched fractions from body fluids) has been estimated using gel chromatography columns, SDS-PAGE procedures, or sucrose density gradients. These methodologies, although extensively used, have many pitfalls and deficiencies. It is extremely difficult to preserve the original IC structure, and it should be kept in mind that during the procedures to determine the IC size the composition of IC may change. The reviews of Haakenstad and Mannik [237] and the thesis of Fagundus [169] give a good synopsis of available methodology and an evaluation of various techniques. Indirect evidence for the composition of IC, i.e. Ag_nAb_m, may be obtained from studies on the size of IC and quantitation of antigen and antibody. Radiolabeled immune reactants forming part of IC make such quantitation easier, and studies on in vitro-formed IC paved the way for approaching the problem of characterizing IC formed in vivo.

The disappearance of IC from blood, plasma, or serum has been studied using various methods [151, 208]. The most extensively used approach is monitoring concentrations of radiolabeled antigen [151, 206, 451, 609, 686]. In concert with determination of molecular size and demonstration of antibody in the same molecular weight fraction where antigen is found, as well as demonstration of IC by specific assays from body fluids, some insight into the kinetics of the disappearance of IC may be gained by this approach [151, 206, 451, 609, 686].

Estimates on the kinetics of deposition of IC may be obtained by a method based on the approach of Wilson and Dixon [686], allowing for continuous measurement of radioactivity in tissue over prolonged periods of time [451]. In this approach, antigen concentrations are measured in tissues and the presence of IC has to be inferred from other analyses [451]. This methodology has clearly established differences in uptake of IC by cells and deposition in basement membranes of tissues. Similarly, the time of maximum deposition has been shown to vary with progression and character of chronic serum sickness in rabbits. Earlier studies have indicated that IC are detectable in tissues only up to 18 h after IC formation [117]. This seems to be the case in chronic serum sickness of rabbits injected with a low dose of antigen [451]. In rabbits with high doses of antigen high concentrations of IC are still found in tissues 24 and 48 h after injection of radiolabeled antigen [451].

15.4.4. Additional characterization of IC components

The components of IC can be defined to some extent as they present in IC. Thus, immunohistological techniques allow for the detection of antibody class and subclass and nature of antigen as well as activated complement components (see section 15.2). Such characterization may also be carried out with purified circulating IC using labeled antisera or radioimmunoassays and ELISA. In most cases, however, dissociation of IC is a prerequisite for detailed and reliable characterization of its components. Thus, IC in antigen or antibody excess may not be suitable for assays detecting the relatively deficient component and useful data and estimates on the avidity of antibodies require availability of uncomplexed immune reactants.

Tissue-bound IC recovered by elution techniques are usually dissociated, at least in part [621]. The antibody and antigen tend to reassemble under appropriate conditions (e.g. neutral pH after acid elution [699]). The "secondary" IC thus formed may be expected to differ from the ones present in tissue prior to elution. Separation of antibody and antigen in eluates may be accomplished effectively by sucrose gradient centrifugation in acid buffer [699]. IC purified from body fluids and IC in tissue homogenates or unsatisfactorily separated IC in eluates can be dissociated by low or high pH, high salt solutions, or chaotropic ions by affecting ionic bonds [199, 200, 340, 362], inducation of repulsive Van der Waals forces [648, 649, 651], or electrophoresis at 56°C [417]. Dissociation of ionic bonds in IC has been used widely, although often with only partial success because of the other bonds remaining intact. Repulsive Van der Waals forces of the London variety have been recruited only recently for dissociation experiments [648, 652]. Hamaker [244] was the first to mention the possibility that Van der Waals forces may be repulsive. Formulating the combining rule for two different materials in a liquid, Hamaker [244] made the prediction on the effect of Van der Waals forces which has been summarized by Van Oss et al. [651] as follows: "when the sum of the interactions of two different materials with a liquid medium is larger than the sum of the interactions between the two materials and those between the molecules of the liquid medium themselves, the net Van der Waals interaction between the two materials, immersed in that liquid medium, will be repulsive". Fowkes [189], Visser [659], Israelachvili [296] and Nir [454] showed these repulsive forces in experiments. Recently, both theoretical analysis and experimental data have corroborated this hypothesis [651]. Dissociation of IC by lowering the surface tension of the liquid medium to a value between that of antibody and antigen has been achieved studying both IC constituted by Van der Waals forces alone and IC with both ionic and Van der Waals interactions [649]. The lowering of surface tension of liquids was accomplished by addition of ethylene glycol or dimethyl sulfoxide (DMSO). In the case of IC with antigen–antibody bonds to which both ionic and Van der Waals forces did contribute, the dissociation was carried out at low or high pH [649]. Protein antigens always bind to antibodies by both ionic and Van der Waals forces, and the method of IC dissociation described by Van Oss et al. [651] seems to offer the possibility to improve significantly the prospects for reliable analysis of IC components. Some IC, however, may display only ionic forces, and thus the "conventional" splitting procedures may suffice (e.g. DNA anti-DNA) [650].

Electrophoresis at 56°C has been used for splitting of IC [417]. Usually, antigen and antibody may be demonstrated by precipitation in gel. Thus the procedure used is immunoelectrophoresis. At 56°C, antigen–antibody reactants are dissociated at a high velocity [346]. This method has been applied to the study of BSA anti-BSA and to DNA anti-DNA IC [417].

The immune reactants obtained by separating antigen, antibody, and possibly complement components from IC may be studied in conventional serological and biochemical assays. Not only can the immunoreactants be defined (e.g. the nature of the antigen) but also qualitative (e.g. avidity of antibodies) and quantitative aspects can be analysed. The reader should be reminded of the elegant studies on antibody avidity performed by Soothill, Steward, and others [23, 311, 577, 586–588, 693], and referred to the discussion given previously on this subject (see Section 15.1).

Dissociation of IC in circulation may be achieved by antigen or, more difficult, antibody excess in analogy to the procedures discussed for elution techniques [137, 535]. This method has been successfully used to define or corroborate the nature of antigens in circulating IC.

15.4.5. Detection of antibodies to immunoglobulin in IC

Recently, a role for antibodies to immunoglobulins in circulating and tissue-bound IC has been suggested in a number of IC-mediated diseases [415] and documented by a variety of analytical approaches [8, 109, 298, 394, 397, 398, 414, 482, 523, 524, 634, 647, 657, 709]. After the possibility of an involvement of RF in immunopathology had been formulated by Milgrom and Witebsky [415], it is to the great merit of McIntosh and his group [397, 398] that they paved the way for acceptance of this concept. Evidence for the participation of RF in IC found in various diseases is mounting. The techniques used to demonstrate the involvement of RF in IC encompass immunoelectron microscopy, immunohistology using anti-idiotypic antisera specific for isolated RF [8] or FITC-conjugated aggregated human IgG [659], and serological techniques applied to isolated cryoglobulins [397, 398]. Most recently, dissociation of tissue-bound IC by incubation with aggregated human IgG was taken as evidence for the presence of anti-immunoglobulin specificities, possibly including RF and anti-isotype antibodies [482, 483, 598]. In these experiments it was shown that in idiopathic membranous nephropathy and post-streptococcal glomerulonephritis, and, to a lesser degree, in SLE, IC found in glomerular capillaries may be dissolved by aggregated human IgG. It seems of special interest that IC deposited in kidney glomeruli of rabbits with systemic chronic serum sickness also require aggregated rabbit IgG to dissolve completely the IC seen late in the disease. Thus, even in a model of IC-mediated diseases clearly induced by heteroimmunization (i.e. by injection with BSA), antibodies to rabbit immunoglobulins seem to participate in IC deposited in tissues.

15.4.6. Preparation of aggregated gamma globulin (IgG) and IC in vitro

Aggregated gammaglobulin (AGG) most often is prepared by heating (e.g. ref. 620) but may be obtained also by other procedures. It was used in experiments designed to study the clearance from body fluid and deposition kinetics in tissues. AGG is considered roughly analogous to IC. This, however, is valid only to a very limited extent. Characteristics of aggregated gammaglobulins differ in many aspects from those of "true" IC [607]. The use of AGG as reference standard for some tests developed to detect circulating IC seems somewhat precarious because of the variability of characteristics of IC detected in various test sera and the differences between characteristics of IC and AGG.

In vitro-formed IC may be of great use in establishing properties and kinetics of "model" IC and in experiments on clearance and tissue deposition of

IC [237]. IC injected into a host, however, must be expected to undergo changes in composition. Recent work with covalently linked IC may help to overcome these problems [101].

15.4.7. Additional comments

The study of clinical material containing IC (body fluids and tissues) must be complemented by investigations on experimental animal models. Fortunately, a vast array of spontaneous and experimentally induced IC-mediated diseases in animals is available [18].

Isolated kidney perfusions or perfusions of kidneys in situ have been used in recent years, opening many interesting and exciting perspectives [126, 183, 543]. These methods have to be evaluated in each individual experimental setting; extensive controls are necessary to make interpretation of results obtained with these methods conclusive.

15.5. CONCLUSIONS

In this chapter, it was attempted to give a short overview of the development of the concept of IC-mediated diseases; subsequently, we have focussed on the rather large number of methods available for demonstration and analysis of tissue-bound and circulating IC, with special emphasis on immunofluorescence techniques, which have contributed so much to the understanding of IC-mediated diseases and still are the backbone of research and diagnosis in IC-mediated immunopathology. The basic concepts on the pathogenesis of IC-mediated diseases had emerged in studies pioneered by Von Pirquet, Schick, and Francioni, and were brought to a first conclusion by the endeavours of Germuth, Dixon, Christian, Kunkel, Andres, and many others. A second stage of research in IC-mediated pathology seems just to have started; the description of more and more human diseases and experimental models of IC-mediated diseases involving a host of tissues and organ systems indicates the widespread occurrence of the immunopathological entity. In addition, the focus of research has shifted: the study of the immune response in IC-mediated diseases; the role of genetic and endocrine factors in susceptibility to IC-mediated tissue injury; the definition of antigens involved in IC of human diseases; the revival of the question on whether deposits of IC in tissues represent a "common waste basket" containing a broad spectrum of microbial and other heterologous and autologous antigens or whether there are some preferred antigens involved in IC (e.g. autologous immunoglobulins); the establishment of reliable, well-defined assays for the clinical use in detection of circulating IC, and the new approaches in determining whether IC-mediated pathology is induced by deposition of circulating IC or by in situ formation; all these approaches have set, we believe, much of the ground work for a new take-off. Only application of all of the available methods in concerted efforts seems promising in studies on the properties of IC, their deposition in tissue in human diseases, and the development of a satisfactory therapy.

ACKNOWLEDGEMENTS

We would like to thank those who have introduced us to the fascinating world of immunofluorescence and immune complexes: Professors G.A. Andres, E.H. Beutner, F. Milgrom, C.J. van Oss, and G. Wick. Many thanks also go to our colleagues Drs. A. Fagundus, K. Kano, C. Neuland, B. Noble, K. Olson, E. Ossi, and A.A. Roman-Franco for helpful discussions. Miss I. Glurich's help was essential in proofreading and assembling the references and Miss P. George had the patience to type and retype this manuscript.

REFERENCES

1 Abbas, A.K. and Unanue, E.R. (1975) J. Immunol *115,* 1665.
2 Abbas, A.K. and Klaus, G.G.B. (1978) Eur. J. Immunol. *8,* 217.
3 Abdou, N.I., Sagawa, A., Pascual, E., Hebert, J. and Sadeghee, S (1976) Clin. Immunol. Immunopathol. *6,* 192.
4 Abe, T. and Homma, M. Acta Rheum. Scand. *17,* 35.
5 Abrass, C.K., Border, W.A. and Glassock, R.J. Kidney Int. *12,* 508.
6 Ada, G.L. Transpl. Rev. *5,* 105.
7 Agnello, V., Winchester, R.J. and Kunkel, H.G. (1970) Immunology *19,* 909.
8 Agnello, V., Koffler, D., Eisenberg, J.W., Winchester, R.J. and Kunkel, H.G. (1971) J. Exp. Med. *134,* 228.
9 Ahlstadt, S., Hanson, L.A. and Wadsworth, C. (1976) Scand. J. Immunol. *5,* 293.
10 Albini, B. and Andres, G.A. (1979) *In* Rose N.R., Milgrom and Van Oss, C.J. (eds.), Principles of Immunology, 2nd ed. (Macmillan, New York) p. 494.
11 Albini, B., Herzog, F. and Wick, G. (1972) Immunology *23,* 343.
12 Albini, B., Brentjens, J., O'Connell, D. and Andres, G.A. (1976) Fed. Proc. *35,* 2587.
13 Albini, B., Ossi, E. and Andres, G. (1977) Lab. Invest. *37,* 64.
14 Albini, B., Brentjens, J.R. and Andres, G.A. (1979) Immunopathology of the Kidney (Arnold, London).
15 Albini, B., Brentjens, J., Olson, K., Ossi, E. and Andres, G.A. (1979) *In* Milgrom, F. and Albini, B. (eds.), Immunopathology (Karger, Basel) p. 207.
16 Albini, B., Holubar, K., Shu, S. and Wolf, K (1979) *In* Beutner, E.H. (ed.), Immunopathology of the Skin, 2nd ed. (J. Wiley & Sons, New York), p. 93.
17 Albini, B., Ossi, E., Neuland, C., Noble, B. and Andres, G (1979) Lab. Invest. *41,* 446.
18 Albini, B., Fagundus, A., Glurich, I., Kerjaschky, D., Neuland, C, Noble, B., Olson, K., Ossi, E. and Penner, E. (1981) *In* Steffen, C. and Ludwig, H. (eds), Clinical Immunology and Allergology (Elsevier, Amsterdam) p. 177.
19 Albini, B., Glurich, I. and Andres, G.A. (1981) Acute and chronic serum sickness glomerulonephritis in intact, thymectomized and bursectomized chickens (in press).
20 Albini, B., Olson, K., Ossi, E. and Andres, G.A. (1981) in preparation.
21 Allen, R. and Isliker, H. (1974) Immunochemistry *11,* 175 and 243.
22 Almeida, J.D. and Waterson, A.P. (1969) Lancet *2,* 983.
23 Alpers, J.H., Steward, M.W. and Soothill, J.F. (1971) Clin. Exp. Immunol. *121.*
24 Anderson, C.L. and Grey, H.M. (1974) J. Exp. Med. *139,* 1175.
25 Anderson, C.L. and Grey, H.M. (1978) J. Immunol. *121,* 648.

26 Andre, C., Heremans, J.F., Vaerman, J.P. and Cambiaso, C.L. (1975) J. Exp. Med. *142,* 1509.
27 Andres, G.A., Morgan, C., Hsu, K.C., Rifkind, R.A. and Seegal, B.C. (1962) Nature *194,* 590.
28 Andres, G.A., Seegal, B.C., Hsu, K.C., Rothenberg, M.S. and Chapeau, M.L. (1963) J. Exp. Med. *117,* 691.
29 Andres, G.A., Accini, L., Hsu, K.C., Zabriskie, J.B. and Seegal, B.C. (1966) J. Exp. Med. *123,* 399.
30 Andres, G.A., Accini, L., Beiser, S.M., Christian, C.L., Cinotti, G.A., Erlanger, B.F., Hsu, K.C. and Seegal, B.C. (1970) J. Clin. Invest. *42,* 2106.
31 Andres, G.A., Kano, K., Elwood, C., Prezyne, A., Sepulveska, M. and Milgrom, F. (1976) Int. Arch. Allergy *52,* 136.
32 Andres, G.A., Hsu, K.G. and Seegal, B.C. (1978) *In* Weir, D.M. (ed.), Handbook of Experimental Immunology, Ch. 37 (Blackwell Sci. Publ., Oxford).
33 Anwar, A.R.E. and Kay, A.B. (1977) J. Immunol. *119,* 976.
34 Anwar, A.R.E. and Kay, A.B. (1978) J. Immunol. *121,* 1245.
35 Arend, W.P. and Mannik, M (1973) J. Immunol. *110,* 1455.
36 Arend, W.P., Teller, D.C. and Mannik, M (1972) Biochemistry *11,* 4063.
37 Arizs, L., Noble, B., Milgrom, M., Brentjens, J.R. and Andres, G.A. (1979) Int. Arch. Allergy *60,* 80.
38 Arthus, M.C.R. (1903) Seanc. Soc. Biol. *55,* 817.
39 Ashman, R.F., Kaplan, A. and Metzger, H. (1971) Immunochemistry *8,* 627.
40 Athen, L.R.B., Forre, O.T., Husby, G. and Williams, R.C., Jr (1979) Clin. Immunol. Immunopathol. *14,* 284.
41 Attasi, M.Z. (1978) Immunochemistry *15,* 909.
42 Attasi, M.Z. and Saplin, B.J. (1968) Biochemistry *7,* 688.
43 Augner, W., Gray, H.M., Cooper, N.R. and Muller-Eberhard, H.J. (1971) Immunochemistry *8,* 1011.
44 Austen, K.F. (1974) Transplant. Proc. *6,* 1.
45 Avrameas, S. (1970) Int. Rev. Cytol. *27,* 349.
46 Barkas, T., Al-Khateeb, S.F., Irvine, W.J., Davidson, H. and Roscoe, P. (1976) Clin. Exp. Immunol. *25,* 270.
47 Barrett, S. (1978) Clin. Immunol. Immunopathol. *11,* 190.
48 Bartolotti, S.R. (1977) Clin. Exp. Immunol. *29,* 334.
49 Bartolotti, S.R. and Peters, D.K. (1978) Clin. Exp. Immunol. *32,* 199.
50 Basten, A., Miller, J.F.A.P., Warner, N.L., Abraham, R., Chia, E. and Bamble, J. (1975) J. Immunol. *115,* 1159.
51 Baumal, R. and Broder, I. (1968) Clin. Exp. Immunol. *3,* 525.
52 Becker, E.L. and Henson, P.M. (1973) Adv. Immunol. *17,* 94.
53 Becker, E.L. Henson, P.M., Showell, H.J. and Huse, L.S. (1974) J. Immunol. *112,* 2047.
54 Benacerraf, B., Sebestyen, M. and Cooper, N.S. (1959) J. Immunol. *82,* 131.
55 Benacerraf, B., Potter, J.M., McCluskey, R.T. and Miller, F. (1960) J. Exp. Med. *111,* 195.
56 Benjamin, D.C. and Tede, J.M. (1978) J. Biol. Chem. *253,* 8087.
57 Benveniste, J. (1974) Nature *249,* 581.
58 Benveniste, J., Henson, P.M. and Cochrane, C.G. (1972) J. Exp. Med. *136,* 1356.
59 Benveniste, J., LeCouedic, J.P. and Kamoun, P. (1975) Lancet *1,* 344.
60 Benveniste, J., LeCouedic, J.P., Polansky, J. and Tence, M. (1977) Nature *269,* 170.
61 Benveniste, J., Mencine-Huerta, J.M. and Camussi, G. (1979) Adv. Infl. Res. *1,* 353.
62 Beutner, E.H. (1971) Ann. N.Y. Acad. Sci. *177.*
63 Beutner, E.H., Holborow, E.J. and Johnson, G.D. (1967) Immunology *12,* 327.
64 Beutner, E.H., Sepulveda, R. and Barnett, E.V. (1968) Bull. W.H.O. *39,* 587.
65 Beutner, E.H., Nisengard, R.J. and Albini, B. (1979) *In* Rose, N.R., Milgrom, F. and Van Oss, C.-J. (eds.) Principles of Immunology, (MacMillan, New York) p. 476.
66 Bianco, C., Patrick, R. and Nussenzweig, V. (1970) J. Exp. Med. *132,* 702.
67 Bienenfeld, B. (1907) Jahrb. Kinderheilkd. *65,* 174.
68 Bigazzi, P.E., Kosuda, L.L., Hsu, K.C. and Andres, G.A. (1976) J. Exp. Med. *143,* 382.

69 Biozzi, G., Benacerraf, B. and Halpern, B.N. (1953) Br. J. Exp. Pathol. *34,* 441.
70 Bitter, T., Bitter, F., Silberschmidt, R. and Dubois, E.L (1971) Arthritis Rheum. *14,* 152.
71 Block, S.R., Gibbs, C.B., Stevens, M.B. and Shulman, L.E. (1968) Ann. Rheum. Dis. *27,* 311.
72 Boackle, R.J., Pruitt, K.M. and Mestecky, J. (1974) Immunochemistry *11,* 543.
73 Bokisch, V.A. and Sobel, A.T. (1974) J. Exp. Med. *140,* 1336.
74 Bombardieri, S., Lightfoot, R.W. and Christian, C.L. (1973) Proc. Soc. Exp. Biol. Med. *144,* 148.
75 Borsos, T. and Rapp, W.J. (1965) Science *150,* 505.
76 Boyd, W.C. (1942) J. Exp. Med. *75,* 407.
77 Brentjens, J.R., O'Connell, D.W., Pawlowski, I.B., Hsu, K.C. and Andres, G.A. (1977) J. Exp. Med. *140,* 105.
78 Brentjens, J., Ossi, E., Albini, B., Sepulveda, M., Kano, K., Sheffer, J., Vasilion, P., Marine, E., Baliah, T., Jockin, H., and Andres, G.A. (1978) Arthritis Rheum. *21,* 868.
79 Brentjens, J., Albini, B., Mendrick, D., Neuland, C., O'Connell, D., Ossi, E., Accini, L. and Andres, G.A. (1979) *In* Milgrom, F. and Albini, B. (eds.), Immunopathology (Karger, Basel) p. 202.
80 Bresnihan, B. and Jasin, H.E. (1977) J. Clin. Invest. *59,* 106.
81 Broder, I., Baumal, R. and Keystone, E. (1968) Clin. Exp. Immunol. *3,* 537.
82 Brouet, J.C., Clavel, J.P., Danon, F., Klein, M. and Seligmann, M. (1975) Am. J. Med. *57,* 775.
83 Burritt, M.F., Calvanico, N.J., Menta, S. and Tomasi, T.B., Jr. (1977) J. Immunol. *118,* 723.
84 Butterworth, A.E., Sturrock, R.F., Houba, V. and Rees, P.H. (1974) Nature *252,* 503.
85 Butterworth, A.E., Sturrock, R.F., Houba, V., Mahmoud, A.A.F., Sher, A. and Rees, P.H. (1975) Nature *256,* 727.
86 Butterworth, A.E., David, J.R., Franks, D., Mahoud, A.A.F., David, P.H., Sturrock, R.F. and Houba, V. (1977) J. Exp. Med. *145,* 136.
87 Butterworth, A.E., Remold, H.G., Houba, V., David, J.R., David, F., David, P. and Sturrock, R.F. (1977) J. Immunol. *118,* 2230.
88 Cameron, J.S., Lessof, M.H., Ogg, C.S., Williams, B.D. and Williams, D.G. (1976) Clin. Exp. Immunol. *25,* 418.
89 Camussi, G., Mencia-Huerta, J.M. and Benveniste, J. (1977) J. Immunol. *33,* 523.
90 Cantor, H.M. and Dumont, A.E. (1967) Nature *215,* 744.
91 Cantor, H., McVay-Boudreau, L., Hugenberger, J., Naidorf, K., Shen, F.W. and Gershon, R.K. (1978) J. Exp. Med. *147,* 1116.
92 Cardella, C.J., Davies, P. and Allison, A.C. (1974) Nature *247,* 46.
93 Carella, G., Digeon, M., Feldmann, G., Jungers, P., Drovet, J. and Bach, J.F. (1977) Scand. J. Immunol. *6,* 1297.
94 Casali, P. and Lambert, P.-H. (1979) Clin. Exp. Immunol. *37,* 295.
95 Casali, P., Bossus, A., Carpentier, N.A. and Lambert, P.-H (1977) Clin. Exp. Immunol. *29,* 342.
96 Cat, A., Lafeber, G.J.M. and Klein, F. (1975) Ann. Rheum. Dis. *34,* 146.
97 Cathou, R.E., Kulczycki, A. and Haber E. (1968) Biochemistry *7,* 3958.
98 Caulfield, J.P. and Farquhar, M.G. (1976) Proc. Natl. Acad. Sci. USA *73,* 1646.
99 Cazenave, J.P., Assimek, S., Painter, R.H., Packham, M.A. and Mustard, J.F. (1976) J. Immunol. *116,* 162.
100 Chan, P.L. and Sinclair, N.R. St. C. (1971) Immunology *21,* 967.
101 Chan, E.K.L. and Boyd, N.D. (1980) J. Immunol. Methods *33,* 55.
102 Chenais, F., Virella, G., Patrick, C.C. and Fudenberg, H.H. (1977) J. Immunol. Methods *18,* 183.
103 Chenoweth, D.E. and Hugli, T.E. (1978) Proc. Natl. Acad. Sci. U.S.A. *75,* 3943.
104 Chiao, J.W., Pantic, V.S. and Good, R.A. (1974) Clin. Exp. Immunol. *18,* 483.
105 Chiraishi, S. and Stround, R.M. (1975) Immunochemistry *12,* 935.
106 Christensen, P., Johansson, B.G. and Kronvall, G. (1976) Acta Pathol. Microbiol. Scand. *C84,* 73.
107 Christian, C.L. (1969) N. Engl. J. Med. *280,* 878.

108 Christian, C.L. and Lightfoot, R.W., Jr. (1970) *In* Bonomo, L. and Turk, J.L. (eds.), Immune Complex Diseases (Carlo Erba, Milano) p. 3.
109 Christian, C.L. and Paget, A.A. (1978) *In* Samter, X.X. (ed.), Immunological Diseases (Little, Brown, & Co., Boston) p. 1061.
110 Ciccimarra, F., Rosen, F.S. and Merler, E. (1975) Proc. Natl. Acad. Sci. U.S.A. *72,* 2081.
111 Clagett, J.A., Wilson, C.B. and Weigle, W.O. (1974) J. Exp. Med. *140,* 1439.
112 Cochrane, C.G. and Koffler, D. (1973) Adv. Immunol. *16,* 185.
113 Cochrane, C.G. and Janoff, A. (1974) *In* Zweifach, B.W., Grant, L. and McCluskey, R.I. (eds.), The Inflammatory Process (Academic Press, New York) p. 85.
114 Cochrane, C.G. and Dixon, F.J. (1978) *In* Samter, M.D. (ed.), Immunological Diseases (Little, Brown & Co., Boston) p. 210.
115 Cochrane, C.G., Unanue, E.R. and Dixon, F.J. (1965) J. Exp. Med. *122,* 99.
116 Cohen, S. (1968) J. Immunol. *100,* 409.
117 Combes, B., Stastny, P., Shory, J., Eigenbrodt, E.H., Barrera, A, Hull, A.R. Carter, N.W. (1971) Lancet *2,* 234.
118 Conn, D.L., Schroeter, A.L. and McDuffie, F.C. (1976) Arthritis Rheum. *19,* 15.
119 Coombs, R.R.A. and Gell, P.G.H. (1975) *In* Gell, P.G.H., Coombs, R.R.A. and Lachmann, P.J. (eds.), Clinical Aspects of Immunology, 3rd ed. (Blackwell Sci. Publ., Oxford) p. 761.
120 Coons, A.H. and Kaplan, M.M. (1950) J. Exp. Med. *91,* 1.
121 Coons, A.H., LeDuc, E.H. and Connelly, J.M. (1955) J. Exp. Med. *102,* 49.
122 Cooper, N.R. (1969) Science *165,* 396.
123 Cooper, N.R. (1975) J. Exp. Med. *141,* 890.
124 Cordier, G., Samarut, C., Brocier, J. and Revillard, J.P. (1976) Scand J. Immunol. *15,* 233.
125 Couser, W.G. and Salant, D.J. (1980) Kidney Int. *17,* 1.
126 Couser, W.G., Steinmuller, D.R., Stilmant, M.M., Salant, D.J. and Loewenstein, L.M. (1978) J. Clin. Invest. *62,* 1275.
127 Cream, J.J., Bryceson, A.D.M. and Ryder, G. (1971) Br. J. Dermatol. *84,* 106.
128 Creighton, D.W., Lambert, P.H. and Miescher, P.A. (1971) J. Immunol. *111,* 1219.
129 Curran, R.C. and Gregory, J. (1977) Experientia *33,* 1400.
130 Czop, J.K. (1981) J. Immunol. (in press).
131 Dalmasso, A.P. and Muller-Eberhard, H.J. (1967) Immunology *13,* 293.
132 Dandliker, W.B. and Saussure, V.A. (1968) Immunochemistry *5,* 357.
133 Davey, M.P. and Korngold, L. (1981) J. Immunol. Methods (in press).
134 Davis, B.D., Dulbecco, R., Eisen, H.N., Ginsberg, H.S., Wood, W.B., and McCarty, M. (eds.) (1973) *In* Microbiology, 2nd ed. (Harper and Row, New York).
135 Davis, P., Cumming, R.H. and Vernier-Jones, (1977) J. Clin. Exp. Immunol. *28,* 226.
136 De Groot, E.R., Lamers, M.C., Aarden, L.A., Smeenk, R.J.T. and Van Oss, C.J. (1980) Immunol. Commun. *9,* 515.
137 Deliere, M., Cambiaso, C.L. and Masson, P.L. (1978) Nature *272,* 632.
138 Denk, H. Forster, O., Kovac, W. and Kraft, D. (1968) Zbl Bakt. I. Abt. Orig. *208,* 277.
139 Denk, H., Forster, O. and Kraft, D. (1969) Z. Immunitätsforsch *138,* 169.
140 Denk, H., Syre, G. and Weirich, E. (1977) Beitr. Pathol. *160,* 187.
141 Diamond, B., Bloom, B.R. and Scharff, M.D. (1978) J. Immunol. *121,* 1329.
142 Dias da Silva, W., Eisele, J.W. and Lepow, I.H. (1967) J. Exp. Med. *126,* 1027.
143 Dickler, H.B. Adv. Immunol. (1976) *24,* 167.
144 Dickler, H.B. and Kunkel, H.G. (1972) J. Exp. Med. *136,* 191.
145 Dickler, H.B. and Sachs, D.H. (1974) J. Exp. Med. *140,* 779.
146 Dietrich, M.P. and Landen, B. (1977) J. Exp. Med. *146,* 1484.
147 Digeon, M., Laner, M., Riza, J. and Bach, J.F. (1977) J. Immunol. Methods *16,* 165.
148 Dive, C.H., Nadalini, R.A., Vaerman, J.P. and Heremans, T.F. (1974) Eur. J. Clin. Invest. *4,* 241.
149 Dixon, F.J. (1963) Harvey Lect. *58,* 21.
150 Dixon, F.J. and Andres, G.A. (1971) *In* Amos, D.B. (ed.), Progress in Immunology, 1st Int. Congr. Immunol. (Academic Press, New York).

151 Dixon, F.J., Bukantz, S.C., Dammin, G.J. and Talmage, D.W. (1951) Proc. Soc. Exp. Biol. Med. *78,* 123.
152 Dixon, F.J., Vazquez, J.J., Wengle, W.O. and Cochrane, C.G. (1958) Arch Pathol. *65,* 18.
153 Dixon, F.J., Feldman, J.D. and Vazquez, J.J. (1961) J. Exp. Med. *113,* 899.
154 Dorrington, K.J. (1976) Immunol. Commun. *5,* 263.
155 Dreyer, G. and Douglas, J.S.C. (1910) Proc. Soc. (London) *B82,* 185.
156 Dukor, P. and Hartmann, K.U. (1973) Cell. Immunol. *7,* 349.
157 Dukor, P., Bianco, C. and Nussenzweig, V. (1970) Eur. J. Immunol. *1,* 491.
158 Eagle, M. (1932) J. Phys. Chem. *36,* 259.
159 Eden, A., Bianco, C. and Nussenzweig, V. (1971) Cell. Immunol. *2,* 658.
160 Eden, A., Miller, G.W. and Nussenzweig, V. (1973) J. Clin. Invest. *52,* 3239.
161 Ehlenberg, A.G. and Nussenzweig, V. (1977) J. Exp. Med. *145,* 357.
162 Ehrich, W.E. Seifter, J. and Forman, C. (1949) J. Exp. Med. *89,* 23.
163 Ehrnst, A. (1977) J. Immunol. *118,* 533.
164 Ehrnst, A. (1978) J. Immunol. *121,* 1206.
165 Eisen, H,N. (1973) *In* Davis, B.D., Dulbecco, R., Eisen, H.N., Ginsberg, H.S., Wood, W.B. and McCarthy, M. (eds.), Microbiology (Harper, New York) p. 359.
166 Eisenberg, R.A., Theofilopoulos, A.N. and Dixon, F.J. (1977) J. Immunol. *118,* 1428.
167 Ellerson, J.R., Yasmeen, D., Painter, R.H. and Dorrington, K.H. (1972) FEBS Lett. *24,* 318.
168 Engelhardt, A.V. (1940) Behringwerke-Mitteilungen 10.
169 Fagundus, A. (1981) Physicochemical and immunochemical studies on immune complexes in systemic chronic serum sickness of the rabbit. Thesis.
170 Farr, R.S. (1960) J. Infect. Dis. *103,* 542.
171 Farrell, C., Cogaard, H. and Svehag, S.-E. (1975) Scand. J. Immunol. *4,* 673.
172 Fearon, D.Y. and Austen, K.T. (1975) J. Exp. Med. *142,* 856.
173 Feizi, T. and Gitlin, N. (1969) Lancet *2,* 873.
174 Feltkamp, T.E.W. and Boode, J.H. (1970) J. Clin. Pathol. *23,* 629.
175 Feldmann, J.L., Becher, M.J., Moutsopoulos, H., Fey, K., Blackman, M., Epstein, W. and Talal, N. (1976) J. Clin. Invest. *58,* 173.
176 Feldmann, M. and Diener, E. (1970) J. Exp. Med. *131,* 247.
177 Feldmann, M. and Diener, E. (1971) Immunology *21,* 387.
178 Feldmann, M. and Diener, E. (1972) J. Immunol. *108,* 93.
179 Ferrarini, M., Hoffman, T., Fu, S.M., Winchester, R.J. and Kunkel, H.G., Jr. (1977) J. Immunol. *6,* 1525.
180 Ferreira, A., Takahashi, M. and Nussenzweig, V. (1977) J. Exp. Med. *146,* 1001.
181 Fish, A.J., Michael, A.J., Verner, R.L. and Good, R.A. (1966) Am. J. Pathol. *49,* 997.
182 Fleuren, G.J. and Hoedemaeker, P.J. (1978) Abstr. VII Int. Congr. Nephrol. p. K3.
183 Fleuren, G.J., Grond, J. and Hoedemaeker, P.J. (1980) Kidney Int. *17,* 631.
184 Foidart J.M., Bene, S.W., Yaar, M., Renard, S.I., Guilio, M., Martin, G.R. and Katz, S.D. (1980) Lab. Invest. *42,* 336.
185 Ford, P.M. (1975) Br. J. Exp. Pathol. *56,* 199.
186 Forni, L. and Pernis, B. (1975) *In* Seligmann, M., Preudhomme, J.L. and Kourilsky, T.M. (eds.) Membrane Receptors on Lymphocytes (North-Holland, Amsterdam) p. 193.
187 Forsgen, A. and Sjoqvist, J. (1966) J. Immunol. *97,* 822.
188 Forster, O. and Weigle, W.O. (1963) J. Immunol. *90,* 935.
189 Fowkes, F.M. (1967) *In* Burke, J.J. (ed.), Surfaces and Interfaces (Plenum Press, New York) p. 167.
190 Francioni, C. (1908) Rev. Clin. Ped. 321.
191 Frank, M.M. (1975) Complement (Upjohn, Kalamazoo)
192 Frank, M.M., Hamberger, M.I. and Lawley, T.J. (1979). N. Engl. J. Med. *300,* 518.
193 Franklin, E.C., Holman, H.R., Mueller-Eberhard, H.J. and Kunkel, H.C. (1957) J. Exp. Med. *105,* 425.
194 Freedman, P. and Markowitz, A.S. (1959) Lancet *2,* 45.
195 Fudenberg, H.H., Goodman, J.W. and Milgrom, F. (1964) J. Immunol. *92,* 227.

196 Furst, G., Medgyesi, G.A. Rajnavolgyi, E., Grecsinagy, M., Czikora, K. and Gergely, J. (1978) Immunology *35,* 873.

197 Fye, K.H., Becker, M.J., Theofilopoulos, A.N., Moutsopoulos, H., Feldman, J.L. and Talal, N. (1977) Am. J. Med. *62,* 783.

198 Gabriel, A. and Agnello V. (1977) J. Clin. Invest. *59,* 990.

199 Gallo, G.R. (1970) Am. J. Pathol *61,* 377.

200 Gamble, C.N. and Reardan, J.B. (1975) Engl. J. Med. *292,* 449.

201 Gelfand, M.C., Frank, M.M. and Green, I. (1975) J. Exp. Med. *142,* 1029.

202 Gelfand, J.A., Fauci, A.S. and Green, I. (1976) J. Immunol. *116,* 595.

203 Gelfand, M.C., Frank, M.M., Green, J. and Shin, M.L. (1979) Clin. Immunol. Immunopathol *13,* 19.

204 Germuth, F.G., Jr. (1953) J. Exp. Med. *97,* 257.

205 Germuth, F.G., Jr. and McKinnon, G.E. (1953) Johns Hopkins Med. J. *101,* 13.

206 Germuth, F.G., Jr. and Rodriguez, E. (1973) *In* Immunopathology of the Renal Glomerulus (Little, Brown & Co., Boston).

207 Germuth, F.G., Jr., Pace, M.G. and Tippe, M.J.C. (1955) J. Exp. Immunol. *101,* 146.

208 Germuth, F.G., Jr., Flanagan, C. and Montenegro, M.R. (1957) Bull. Johns Hopkins Hosp. *101,* 149.

209 Germuth, F.G., Jr., Senterfit, L.B. and Pollack, A.D. (1967) Johns Hopkins Med. J. *120,* 225.

210 Germuth, F.G., Jr. Choi, I., Taylor, J.J. and Rodriguez, E. (1972) Johns Hopkins Med. J. *131,* 367.

211 Gigli, I.J. (1976) Invest. Dermatol. *67,* 346.

212 Gigli, I. and Nelson, R.A. (1968) Exp. Cell. Res. *51,* 45.

213 Gitlin, J.D., Rosen, F.S. and Lachmann, P.J. (1975) J. Exp. Med. *141,* 1221.

214 Givol, D., Pecht, I., Hochmann, J., Schlessinger, J. and Steinberg, I.Z. (1974) *In* Brent, L. and Hollborow, E.J. (eds.), Progress in Immunology, II (North-Holland, Amsterdam) p. 39.

215 Glassock, R.J., Edgington, T.S., Watson, J.I. and Dixon, F.J. (1968) J. Exp. Med. *127,* 573.

216 Glovsky, M.M., Hugli, T.E., Ishizaka, T., Lichtenstein, L.M. and Erickson, B.W. (1979) J. Clin. Invest. *64,* 804.

217 Gocke, D.J., Hsu, K., Morgan, C., Bombardieri, S., Lockshin, M., Christian, C.L. (1970) Lancet *2,* 1149.

218 Goers, J.W., Ziccardi, R.J., Schumaker, V.N. and Glovsky, M.M. (1977) J. Immunol. *118,* 2182.

219 Goetzl. E.J. and Austen, F.J. (1974) J. Clin. Invest. *53,* 591.

220 Golbus, S. and Wilson, C.B. (1979) Kidney Int. *16,* 1489.

221 Gonzales-Molina, A. and Spiegelberg, H.L. (1976) J. Immunol. *117,* 1838.

222 Gonzales-Molina, A. and Spiegelberg, H.L. (1977) J. Clin. Invest. *59,* 616.

223 Gordis, E. (1960) Proc. Soc. Exp. Biol. Med. *103,* 542.

224 Gordon, S. and Cohn, Z.A. (1973) Int. Rev. Cytol. *36,* 171.

225 Gordon, S., Unkeless, J. and Cohn, Z.A. (1974) J. Exp. Med. *140,* 995.

226 Gotze, O. and Muller-Eberhard, H.J. (1971) J. Exp. Med. *134,* 90s

227 Gotze, O. and Muller-Eberhard, H.J. (1976) Adv. Immunol. *24,* 1.

228 Gotze, O., Bianco, C. and Cohn, Z.A. (1979) J. Exp. Med. *149,* 372.

229 Graham, R.C., Jr. and Karnovsky, M.J. (1966) J. Histochem. Cytochem. *14,* 291.

230 Griffin, F.M., Jr., Bianco, V. and Silverstein, S.C. (1974) J. Cell. Biol. *63,* 123a.

231 Grangeot-Keros, L., Segoud, P., Capel, F., Israki, S. and Pillot, J. (1978) J. Immunol. Methods *23,* 349.

232 Greaves, M.F. (1970) Transplant. Rev. *5,* 45.

233 Gunn, W.C. (1914/15) J. Pathol. Bacteriol. *19,* 155.

234 Gupta, R.C., Laforce, F.M. and Mills, D.M. (1976) Lab. Clin. Med. *88,* 183.

235 Gupta, S., Platsoucas, C.D. and Good, R.A. (1979) Proc. Natl. Acad. Sci. U.S.A. *76,* 4025.

236 Haakenstad, A.O. and Mannik, M. (1974) J. Immunol. *112,* 1939.

237 Haakenstad, A.O. and Mannik, M. (1977) *In* Talal, N. (ed.), Autoimmunity (Academic Press, New York). p. 278.

238 Haakenstad, A.O., Striker, G.E. and Mannik, M. (1976) Lab. Invest. *35,* 293.
239 Habeeb, A.F.S.A. and Attasi, M.Z. (1976) J. Biol. chem. *251,* 4616.
240 Hahn, B.H., Bagby, M.K. and Osterland, C.K. (1973) Am. J. Med. *55,* 25.
241 Hall, R.P., Lawley, T.J., Heck, J. Ai and Katz, S.I. (1980) Clin. Exp. Immunol. *40,* 431.
242 Hallberg, T. (1974) Scand. J. Immunol. *3,* 117.
243 Hallgren, S.B. and Wide, L. (1976) Ann. Rheum. Dis. *35,* 306.
244 Hamaker, H.C. (1968) Physica *4,* 1058.
245 Harbeck, R.J., Bardana, E.J., Kohler, P.F. and Carr, R.I. (1973) J. Clin. Invest. *52,* 789.
246 Hawn, C.V. and Janeway, C.A. (1947) J. Exp. Med. *85,* 571.
247 Hay, F.C., Nineham, L.J. and Roitt, I.M. (1976) Clin. Exp. Immunol. *24,* 396.
248 Hayward, A.R., Hayward, L., Hydyard, P.M., Moretta, L., Dagg, M. and Lawton, A.R. (1978) J. Immunol. *121,* 1.
249 Heidelberger, M. (1939) Bacteriol. Res. *3,* 49.
250 Heidelberger, M. (1941) J. Exp. Med. *73,* 681.
251 Heidelberger, M. and Kendall, F.E. (1929) J. Exp. Med. *50,* 809.
252 Heidelberger, M. and Pedersen, K.O. (1937) J. Exp. Med. *65,* 393.
253 Heidelberger, M., Treffers, H.P. and Mayer, M.M. (1940) J. Exp. Med. *71,* 271.
254 Henson, P.M. (1969) Immunology *16,* 107.
255 Henson, P.M. (1970) J. Immunol. *105,* 476.
256 Henson, P.M. (1971) J. Immunol. *107,* 1535.
257 Henson, P.M. (1971) J. Exp. Med. *134,* 114S.
258 Henson, P.M. (1976) Immunol. Communications *5,* 757.
259 Henson, P.M. and Cochrane, C.G. (1969) J. Exp. Med. *129,* 167.
260 Henson, P.M. and Spiegelberg, H.L. (1973) J. Clin. Invest. *52,* 1282.
261 Henson, P.M. and Oades, Z.G. (1975) J. Clin. Invest. *56,* 1059.
262 Heusser, C.H., Anderson, C.L. and Grey, H.M. (1977) J. Exp. Med. *145,* 1316.
263 Heymann, W., Hackel, D.B., Harwood, J., Wilson, S.G.F. and Hunter, J.L.P. (1959) Proc. Soc. Exp. Biol. Med. *100,* 660.
264 Hijmans, W. (ed) (1975) Ann. New York Acad. Sci. 254.
265 Hoffmann, L.G. (1976) Immunochemistry *13,* 725.
266 Hoffmann, L.G. (1976) Immunochemistry *13,* 731.
267 Hoffmann, L.G. (1976) Immunochemistry *13,* 737.
268 Hoffmann, M.K. and Kappler, J.W. (1978) Nature *272,* 64.
269 Holborow, E.J. (ed) (1970) Standardization of Immunofluorescence (Blackwell Sci. Publ., Oxford).
270 Holubar, K., Stingl, H. and Albini, B. (1976) Hautarzt *27,* 78.
271 Hopf, U., Meyer zum Buschenfelde, K.H. and Dirich, M.P. (1976) J. Immunol. *117,* 639.
272 Hopf, U., Brandtzaeg, P., Hutteroth, T.H. and Meyer-Buschenfelde, K.H. (1978) Scand. J. Immunol. *8,* 543.
273 Huang, S., Minassiah, H. and More, J.D. (1976) Lab. Invest. *35,* 383.
274 Huber, H. and Fudenberg, H.H. (1968) Int. Arch. Allergy *34,* 18.
275 Huber, H. and Fudenberg, H.H. (1970) Semin. Haematol. *111,* 160.
276 Huber, H., Douglas, S.D. and Fudenberg, H.H. (1969) Immunology *17,* 7.
277 Huber, H., Polley, M.J., Linscott,W.D. and Muller-Eberhard, H.J. (1968) Science *162,* 1281.
278 Hubscher, T. (1975) J. Immunol. *114,* 1379.
279 Hugli, T.E. and Muller-Eberhard, H.J. (1978) Adv. Immunol. *26,* 1
280 Humphrey, J.H. (1955) Br. J. Exp. Pathol. *36,* 268.
281 Hunsicker, L.G. (1974) Transplant. Proc. *6,* 77.
282 Hurst, M.M., Volanakin, J., Bennett, J.C. and Strout, R.M. (1974) Fed. Proc. *33,* 759.
283 Hyslop. N.E., Dourmashkin, R.R., Green, N.M. and Porter, R.R. (1970) J. Exp. Med. *131,* 783.
284 Isenman, D.E., Dorrington, R.J. and Painter, R.J. (1975) J. Immunol. *114,* 1726.
285 Ishizaka, K. and Campbell, D.H. (1959) J. Immunol. *83,* 318.
286 Ishizaka, T. and Ishizaka, K. (1959) Proc. Soc. Exp. Biol. Med. *101,* 845.
287 Ishizaka, K. and Ishizaka, T. (1960) J. Immunol. *85,* 163.

288 Ishizaka, K. and Ishizaka, T. (1971) Clin. Allergy *1,* 9.
289 Ishizaka, K., Ishizaka, T. and Sugahara, T. (1962) J. Immunol. *88,* 690.
290 Ishizaka, K., Ishizaka, T. and Hornbrook, M.M. (1966) J. Immunol. *97,* 75.
291 Ishizaka, T., Sian, C.M. and Ishizaka, K. (1972) J. Immunol. *108,* 848.
292 Ishizaka, T., Soto, C.S. and Ishizaka, K. (1972) J. Immunol. *109,* 1290.
293 Ishizaka, T., Soto, C. and Ishizaka, K. (1973) J. Immunol. *111,* 500.
294 Ishizaka, T., Tada, T. and Ishizaka, K. (1968) J. Immunol. *100,* 1145.
295 Ishizaka, T., Sterk, A. and Ishizaka, K. (1979) Fed. Proc. *38,* 1087.
296 Israelachvili, J.N.Q. (1974) Rev. Biophys. *6,* 341.
297 Israels, E.D., Nisli, G., Paraskevas, F. and Israels, L.G. (1973) Thromb. Diath. Haemorrh. *29,* 434.
298 Izui, S. and Eisenberg, R.A. (1980) Clin. Immunol. Immunopathol. *15,* 536.
299 Izui, S., Lambert, P.H. and Miecher, P.A. (1976) J. Exp. Med. *144,* 428.
300 Jaton, J.C., Huser, H., Brown, D.G., Schlessinger, J., Pecht, I. and Givol, D. (1975) Biochem. *14,* 5212.
301 Jaton, J.C., Huser, H., Riesen, W.F., Schlessinger, J. and Givol, D.J. (1976) Immunology, *116,* 1363.
302 Jewell, D.P. and MacLennan, I.C.M. (1973) Clin. Exp. Immunol. *14,* 219.
303 Johns, P. and Stanworth, D.R. (1973) J. Immunol. Methods *10,* 231.
304 Johnson, A.R., Hugli, T.E. and Muller-Eberhard, H.J. (1975) Immunology *28,* 1067.
305 Johnson, B. and Thames, K.E. (1976) J. Immunol. *117,* 1481.
306 Johnson, G.D. (1970) Cited in ref. (Moretta et al., 1975) p, 12,
307 Johnson, G.D., Holborow, E.J. and Dorling, J. (1978) *In* Weir, D.W. (ed.), Handbook of Experimental Immunology, Ch. 15 (Blackwell Sci. Publ. Oxford).
308 Jonas, W.E., Gurner, B.W., Nelson, D.S. and Coombs, R.R.A. (1965) Int. Arch. Allergy *28,* 86.
309 Jones, D.V. (1957) Am. J. Pathol. *33,* 313.
310 Joseph, B.S., Cooper, N.R. and Oldstone, M.B.A. (1975) J. Exp. Med. *141,* 761.
311 Kabat, E.A. (1981) *In* Structural Concepts in Immunology and Immunochemistry (Holt, Rinehart and Winston, Inc., New York).
312 Kabat, E.A. and Heidelberger, M. (1937) J. Exp. Med. *66,* 229.
313 Kabat, E.A. and Mayer, M.M. (1961) Experimental Immunolochemistry, 2nd ed. (C.C. Thomas, Springfield, IL) p. 781.
314 Kalderon, A.E., Bogaars, H.A. and Diamond, I. (1973) Am. J. Med. *55,* 485.
315 Kalderon, A.E., Bogaars, H.A., Holly, G. and Diamond, I. (1977) Lab. Invest. *37,* 487.
316 Kammer, G.M. and Schur, P.H. (1978) Clin. Immunol. Immunopathol. *10,* 202.
317 Kano, K. and Milgrom, F. (1980) Vox Sang. *38,* 121.
318 Kano, K., Nishimaki, T., Palosuo, T., Loza, U. and Milgrom, F. (1978) Clin. Immunol. Immunopathol. *9,* 425.
319 Kano, K., Nishimaki, T. and Milgrom, F. (1979) *In* Peeters, H. (ed.), Protides of Biological Fluids, (Pergamon Press, Oxford) p. 51.
320 Kano, K., Aranzazu, N., Nishimaki, T., Convit, J., Albini, B. and Milgrom, F. (1981) Int. Arch. Allergy *64,* 19.
321 Kanwar, Y.S. and Farquhar, M.G. (1978) J. Cell Biol. *79,* 150a.
322 Kanwar, Y.S. and Farquhar, M.G. (1979) Proc. Natl. Acad. Sci. U.S.A. *76,* 1303.
323 Kater, L.A., Austen, K.F. and Goetzl, E.J. (1975) Fed. Proc. *34,* 985.
324 Katz, D., Kite, J.H., Jr. and Albini, B. (1981) J. Immunol. *126,* XXXX.
325 Kay, A.B. (1976) Br. J. Haematol. *33,* 313.
326 Kay, C.F. (1940) J. Exp. Med. *72,* 559.
327 Kefalides, N.A. and Winler, R.J. (1966) Biochemistry *5,* 702.
328 Kehoe, J.M., Bougois, A., Capra, D.J. and Fougereau, M. (1974) Biochemistry *13,* 2499.
329 Kekomaki, R., Kauppinen, H.L., Pentinen, K. and Myllyla, G. (1977) Acta. Pathol. Microbiol. Scand. *C85,* 207.
330 Kerjaschki, D., Förster, O., Bolz, G., Scheiner, W. and Albini, (1978) *In* Sturgens (ed.), Electron Microscopy (Microscop. Soc., Toronto) p. 462.

331 Kijlstra, A., Van Es, L.A. and Haha, M.R. (1979) Immunology *37,* 673.
332 Kinsella, T.D., Baum, J. and Ziff, M. (1969) Clin. Exp. Immunol. 4, 265.
333 Kleczkowski, A. (1945) Br. J. Exp. Pathol. *26,* 41.
334 Klein, F., Van Rood, J.J., Van Furth, R. and Rosema, H. (1968) Clin. Exp. Immunol *3,* 703.
335 Klinman, N.R. and Karush, F. (1967) Immunochemistry *4,* 387.
336 Knapp, W. and Ploem, J.S. (1974) J. Immunol. Methods *5,* 259.
337 Knapp, W., Holuber, K. and Wick, G. (1978) Immunofluorescence and Related Staining Techniques (Elsevier, Amsterdam).
338 Kniker, W.T. and Cochrane, C.G. (1958) J. Exp. Med. *127,* 119.
339 Kniker, W.T. and Cochrane, C.G. (1965) J. Exp. Med. *122,* 83.
340 Koffler, D., Agnello, V., Thoburn, R. and Kunkel, H.G. (1971) J. Expl. Med. *134,* 169.
341 Koyama, A., Niwa, Y., Shigematsu, H., Taniguchi, M. and Tada, T. (1978) Lab. Invest. *38,* 253.
342 Kronvall, G. (1973) J. Immunol. *111,* 1401.
343 Kunkel, H.G., Simon, H.J. and Fudenberg, H.H. (1958) Arthritis Rheum. *1,* 289.
344 Kunkel, H.G., Mueller-Eberhard, H.J., Fudenberg, H.H. and Tomasi, T.B. (1961) J. Clin. Invest. *40,* 117.
345 Kammer, G.M. and Schur, P.H. (1978) Clin. Immunol. Immunopathol. *10,* 202.
346 Landsteiner, K. and Miller, C.P., Jr. (1925) J. Exp. Med. *42,* 853.
347 Lange, K., Wasserman, E. and Slobody, L.B. (1960) Ann. Intern. Med. *53,* 636.
348 LaVia, M.F. and LaVia, D.S. (1978) Cell. Immunol. *39,* 297.
349 Law, S.K. and Levine, R.P. (1977) Proc. Natl. Acad. Sci. U.S.A. *74,* 2701.
350 Lachmann, P.J. and Muller-Eberhard, H.J. (1971) J. Immunol. *100,* 691.
351 Lambert, P.H., Dixon, F.J., Zubler, R.H., Agnello, V., Cambiaso, C., Casali, P., Clark, J., Cowdery, J.S., McDuffie, F.C., Hay, F.C., MacLennan, I.C.M., Masson, P., Muller-Eberhard, H.J., Penttinen, K., Smith, M., Tappeiner, G., Theofilopoulos, A.N. and Verroust, P. (1978) J. Clin. Lab. Immunol. *1,* 1.
352 Lambert, P.H., Louis, J.A., Izui, S. and Kobayakawa, T. (1979) In Milgrom, F. and Albini, B. (eds.) Immunopathology, (Karger, Basel) p. 191.
353 Lamon, E.W., Skurak, H.M., Anderson, B., Whitten, H.P. and Klein, E. (1975) J. Immunol. *115,* 1288.
354 Lamon, E.W., Whitten, H.D., Skurrak, H.M., Anderson, B. and Lidin, B. (1975) J. Immunol. *15,* 1288.
355 Lawrence, D.A., Weigle, W.O. and Spiegelberg, H.L. (1975) J. Clin. Invest. *55,* 368.
356 Lay, W.H. and Nussenzweig, V. (1968) J. Exp. Med. *128,* 991.
357 Lea, D.J. and Ward, D.J. (1979) J. Immunol. Methods *31,* 191.
358 Lee, S.L. and Rivero, I. (1964) Arthritis Rheum. *7,* 321.
359 Lees, R.K. and Sinclair, N.R. St. C. (1973) Immunology *24,* 735.
360 Leon, M.D. and Yokohari, R. (1964) Science *143,* 1327.
361 Lerner, A.B. and Watson, C.J. (1947) Am. J. Med. Sci. *214,* 410.
362 Lerner, R.A., Glassock, R.J. and Dixon, F.J. (1967) J. Exp. Med. *126,* 989.
363 Leroux-Reels, G.G., Wilme, R.J. and Broe, M. (eds.) (1981) J. Lab. Clin. Med. *97,* 316.
364 Levinsky, R.J. and Soothill, J.F. (1977) Clin. Exp. Immunol. *29,* 428.
365 Levinsky, R.J., Cameron, J.S. and Soothill, J.F. (1977) Lancet *1,* 564.
366 Levinsky, R.J., Mellerson, P.N., Barratt, T.M. and Soothill, J.F. (1978) N. Engl. J. Med. *298,* 1126.
367 Levo, Y., Gorevic, P.D., Kassab, H.J., Zucker-Franklin, D. and Franklin, E.C. (1977) N. Engl. J. Med. *296,* 1501.
368 Lockshin, M.D., Eisenhauer, A.C., Kohn, R., Weksler, M., Block, S. and Mushlin, S.B. (1975) Arthritis Rheum. *18,* 245.
369 Lockwood, C.M., Worlledge, S. and Nicholas, A. (1979) N. Engl. J. Med. *300,* 524.
370 London, F.Z. (1930) Physik *63,* 245.
371 LoSpalluto, J., Dorward, B., Miller, W. and Ziff, M. (1962) Am. J. Med. *32,* 142.
372 Lum, L.G., Muchmore, A.V., Keren, D., Decker, J., Koshi, I., Strober, W. and Blaese, R.M.

(1979) J. Immunol. *122,* 65.
373 Lurhuma, A.Z., Cambiaso, S.L., Masson, P.L. and Heremans, (1977) Immunology *28,* 40.
374 Mackenzie, G.M. and Leake, W.H. (1971) J. Exp. Med. *33,* 601.
375 MacKenzie, M.R., Creevy, N. and Heh, M. (1971) J. Immunol. *106,* 65.
376 MacKenzie, M.R., Warner, N.L. and Mitchell, G.F. (1978) J. Immunol. *120,* 1493.
377 Mackler, B.F., Altman, L.C., Rosenstreich, D.L. and Oppenheim, J.J. (1974) Nature *249,* 834.
378 MacLennan, I.C.H. (1972) Clin. Exp. Immunol. *10,* 275.
379 Mannik, M. and Striker, G.E. (1980) Lab. Invest. *42,* 483.
380 Mannik, M., Arend, W.P., Hall, A.P. and Gilliland, B.C. (1971) J. Exp. Med. *133,* 713.
381 Marquart, H., Wilson, C.B. and Dixon, F.J. (1973) Kidney Int. *3,* 57.
382 Marrack, J.R. (1934) The Chemistry of Antigens and Antibodies. H.M. Stationary Office, London.
383 Marrack, J.R. (1938) Med. Res. Counc. (BG) Spec. Rep. Ser. SRS-230.
384 Mason, T.E., Phifer, R.F., Spicer, S.S., Swallow, R.A. and Dreskin, R.E. (1969) J. Histochem. Cytochem. *17,* 563.
385 Masuda, T., Miyama, K., Kuzibayashi, K., Yodoi, J., Takabayshi, A. and Kyoizumi, S. (1978) Cell. Immunol. *39,* 238.
386 Mantovani, B., Rbinovitch, M. and Nussenzweig, V. (1972) J. Exp. Med. *135,* 780.
387 Maurer, P.H. and Talmage, D.W. (1953) J. Immunol. *70,* 435.
388 Mayer, M.M. and Heidelberger, M. (1942) J. Biol. Chem. *143,* 567.
389 McCluskey, R.T. (1971) J. Exp. Med. *134,* 242s.
390 McCluskey, R.T. (1974) *In* Heptinstall, (ed.), Pathology of the Kidney, 2nd ed. (Little, Brown, & Co., Boston) p. 273.
391 McCluskey, R.T. and Benacerraf, B. (1959) Am J. Pathol. *35,* 275.
392 McCluskey, R.T., Benacerraf, B., Potter, J.L. and Miller, F. (1960) J. Exp. Med. *111,* 181.
393 McCluskey, R.T., Benacerraf, B. and Miller, F. (1960) Proc. Soc. Exp. Biol. Med. *111,* 195.
394 McCormick, J.N., Day, J., Morris, C.J. and Hill, A.G.S. (1969) Clin. Exp. Immunol *4,* 17.
395 McDougal, J.S., Redecha, P.B., Inman, R.D. and Christian, C.L. (1979) J. Clin. Invest. *63,* 627.
396 McIntosh, R.M., Kaufman, D.B., Kulvinskas, C. and Grossman, B.J. (1970) J. Lab. Clin. Med. *75,* 566.
397 McIntosh, R.M., Kulvinskas, C. and Kaufman, D.B. (1971) Int. Arch. Allergy *41,* 700.
398 McIntosh, R.M., Griswold, W.R., Chernack, W.B., Williams, G., Strauss, J., Kaufman, D.B., Koss, M.N., McIntosh, J.R., Cohen, R. and Weil, R.Q. (1975) J. Med. *44,* 285.
399 Meadows, R. (1973) Renal Histopathology (Oxford University Press, London).
400 Medicus, R.G. (1978) Fed. Proc. *37,* 1377
401 Medof, M.E. and Sukhupunyarakas, S. (1975) Fed Proc. *36,* 670.
402 Mellors, R.C. and Brzosko, W.J. (1962) J. Exp. Med. *115,* 891.
403 Mellors, R.C., Arias-Stella, J., Seigel, M., Pressman, D. (1955) Am. J. Pathol. *31,* 687.
404 Meltzer, M., Franklin, E.C. (1966) Am. J. Med. *40,* 828.
405 Meltzer, M. and Franklin, E.C. (1967) Arthritis Rheum. *40,* 489.
406 Messner, R.P. and Jelinek, J. (1970) J. Clin. Invest. *49,* 2165.
407 Metzger, H. (1970) Adv. Immunol. *12,* 57.
408 Metzger, H. (1974) Adv. Immunol. *18,* 169.
409 Michel, B., Milner, Y. and David, K. (1973) J. Invest. Dermatol. *59,* 449.
410 Michl, J., Ohlbaum, D.J. and Silverstein, S.C. (1976) J. Exp. Med. *144,* 148.
411 Miescher, P.A. *In* Milgrom, F. and Albini, B. (eds.), Immunopathology (Karger Basel) p. 173.
412 Milgrom, F. (1959) Proc. 7th Congr. Int. Soc. Blood Transfusion (Karger, Basel) p. 512.
413 Milgrom, F. (1964) Proc. 9th Congr. Int. Soc. Blood Transfusion (Karger, Basel) p.335.
414 Milgrom, F. and Witebsky, E. (1960) Fed. Proc. *19,* 197.
415 Milgrom, F. and Witebsky, E (1962) Second Int. Symp. Immunopathology (Schmid & Co., Basel) p. 337.
416 Milgrom, F., Dubiski, S. and Woznickzko, G. (1956) Vox Sang. *1,* 172,
417 Milgrom, F., Campbell, W.A. and Andres, G.A. (1976) Immunology *30,* 277.
418 Milgrom, M., Albini, B., Noble, B., O'Connell, D., Brentjens, J. and Andres, G.A. (1979) Clin.

Exp. Immunol. *38,* 249.
419 Miller, G.W. and Nussenzweig, V. (1974) J. Immunol. *113,* 464..
420 Miller, G.W. and Nussenzweig, V. (1975) Proc. Natl. Acad. Sci. U.S.A. *72,* 418.
421 Miller, G.W., Saluk, P.H. and Nussenzweig, V. (1973) J. Exp. Med. *138,* 495.
422 Minta, J.O. and Movat, H.Z. Curr. Top. Pathol. *68,* 135.
423 Moake, J.L., Kageler, W.V., Cimo, P.L., Blakely, R.W., Rossen, R.D. and Haesse, W. (1977) Ann. Intern. Med. *86,* 516.
424 Moran, J., Colasanti, G., Amos, N. and Peters, D.K. (1977) Clin. Exp. Immunol. *28,* 212.
425 Moretta, L., Ferrarini, M., Durante, M.L. and Mingari, M.C. (1975) Eur. J. Immunol. *5,* 565.
426 Moretta, L., Webb, S.R., Grossi, C.E., Lydyard, P.M. and Cooper, M.D. (1977) J. Exp. Med. *146,* 184.
427 Moretta, L., Mingari, M.C. and Romanzi, C.A. (1978) Nature *272,* 618.
428 Moretta, L., Mingari, M.C., Moretta, A. and Cooper, M.D. (1979) J. Immunol. *122,* 984.
429 Morgan, E.L. and Tempelis, C.J. (1977) J. Immunol. *119,* 1293.
430 Morgan, E.L. and Tempelis, C.J. (1978) J. Immunol. *120,* 1669.
431 Moriarty, G.C., Moriarty, C.M. and Sternberger, L.A. (1973) J. Histochem. Cytochem. *21,* 825.
432 Morito, T., Tanimoto, K., Hashimoto, Y., Hoziuchi, Y. and Fugi, T. (1976) Ann. Rheum. Dis. *35,* 415.
433 Moroz, L.A. and Rose, B. (1978) *In* Samter, M.D. (ed.), Immunological Diseases, 3rd ed. (Little, Brown, & Co., Boston) p. 570.
434 Morrison, D.C. and Ulevitch, R.J. (1978) Am. J. Pathol. *93,* 527.
435 Moutsopoulos, H.M., Boehm-Truitt, M., Kassan, S.S. and Chused, T.M. (1977) J. Immunol. *119,* 1639.
436 Movat, H.Z. (1976) Fed. Proc. 2435.
437 Movat, H.Z., Mustard, J.F., Taichman, H.S. and Uriuhara, T. (1965) Proc. Soc. Exp. Biol. Med. *120,* 232.
438 Mowbray, J.F., Holborow, E.J., Hoffbrand, A.V., Seah, P.O. and Fry, L. (1973) Lancet *1,* 400.
439 Muller-Eberhard, H.J. (1968) Adv. Immunol. *8,* 1.
440 Muller-Eberhard, H.J. (1969) Ann. Rev. Biochem. *38,* 389.
441 Muller-Eberhard, H.J. (1975) Ann. Rev. Biochem. *44,* 697.
442 Muller-Eberhard, H.J. and Calcott, M.A. (1966) Immunochemistry *3,* 500.
443 Muller-Eberhard, H.J. and Luscher, E.F. (1968) Thomb. Diath. Hemorrh. 20, 155.
444 Myllyla, G. (1973) Scand. J. Haematol., Suppl. *19,* 1.
445 Nakane, P.K. and Pierce, G.B., Jr. (1966) J. Histochem. Cytochem. *14,* 929.
446 Nakane, P.K. and Pierce, G.B., Jr. (1967) J. Cell. Biol. *33,* 307.
447 Nairn, R.C. (1976) Fluorescent Protein Tracing, 4th ed. (Churchill-Livingston, Edinburgh).
448 Natali, P.G. and Tan, E.M. (1973) Arthritis Rheum. *16,* 579.
449 Natvig, J.B. (1965) Acta Pathol Microbiol. Scand. *65,* 559.
450 Nelson, R.A. (1956) Proc. R. Soc. Med. *49,* 55.
451 Neuland, C. (1978) Kinetic studies on antigen deposition in rabbits with systemic serum sickness. Thesis, Buffalo.
452 Neuland, C., Albini, B., Andres, G., Brentjens, J., Ossi, E., Steinbach, J. and Blau, M. (1977) Kidney Int. *12,* 516.
453 Neuland, C., Albini, B., Brentjens, J., Grossberg, A.I. and Andres, G.A. (1981) Int. Arch. Allergy (in press).
454 Nir, S (1976) Prog. Surf. Sci. *8,* 1.
455 Nishimaki, T., Kano, K. and Milgrom, F. (1978) Arthritis Rheum. *21,* 639.
456 Nisonoff, A. and Pressman, D. (1958) Science *128,* 659.
457 Notkins, A.L., Hahar, S., Scheele, C. and Goffman, J. (1966) J. Exp. Med. *124,* 81.
458 Nowack, H., Gay, S., Wick, G., Becker, U. and Timpl, R. (1977) J. Immunol. Methods *12,* 117.
459 Nussenzweig, V. (1974) Adv. Immunol. *19,* 217
460 Nydegger, U.E. (1979) Rev. Physiol. Biochem. Pharmacol. *85,* 63.
461 Nydegger, U.E., Lambert, P.H., Gerber, H. and Menber, P.A. (1974) J. Clin Invest. 54, 297.

462 Nydegger, U.E., Zubler, R.H., Gabay, R., Joliat, G., Karagevrekis, C.H., Lambert, P.H. and Miescher, P.A. (1977) J. Clin. Invest. *59,* 862.
463 Oberbarenscheidt, J. and Kolsch. E. (1978) Immunology *35,* 151.
464 Obermayer, F. and Pick, E.P. (1904) Wien. Klin. Wochenschr. *17,* 265.
465 Okamura, K., Kondo, Y. and Tada, T. (1976) Lab. Invest. *35,* 293.
466 Oldstone, M.B.A. and Dixon, F.J. (1969) J. Exp. Med. *129,* 483.
467 Oldstone, M.B.A. Copper, N.R. and Larson, D.L. (1974) J. Exp. Med. *140,* 549.
468 Onyewotu, I.I., Holborrow, E.J. and Johnson, G.D. (1974) Nature *248,* 156.
469 Onyewotu, I.I., Johnson, P.M., Johnson, G.D. and Holborow, E.J. (1975) Clin. Exp. Immunol. *19,* 267.
470 Oppenheim, J.J. (1972) Cell. Immunol. *3,* 341.
471 Osler, A.G. and Siraganian, R.P. (1972) Prog. Allergy *16,* 450.
472 Palosuo, T., Kano, K., Anthone, S., Gerbasi, J.R. and Milgrom, F. (1976) Transplantation *21,* 312.
473 Parish, C.R. and Hayward, J.A. (1974) Proc. R. Soc. London B *187,* 47.
474 Paraskevas, F., Lee, S.Y., Orr, K.B. and Israelo, L.C. (1972) J. Immunol. *108,* 1319.
475 Parrot, D.M.V., Good, R.A., O'Neil, G.J. and Gupta, S. (1978) Proc. Natl. Acad. Sci. U.S.A. 75, 2392.
476 Passwell, J.H., Schneeberger, E. and Merler, E. (1978) Immunology *35,* 863.
477 Pauling, L. (1945) *In* Landsteiner. K. (ed.), The Specificity of Serological Reactions, (Harvard University Press, Cambridge).
478 Pauling, L. (1960) The Nature of the Chemical Bond, 3rd ed. (Cornell Univ. Press, Ithaca).
479 Pauling, L., Pressman, D. and Campbell, D.H. (1944) J. Am. Chem. Soc. *66,* 330.
480 Pedersen, K.O. (1936) Nature *138,* 363.
481 Penner, E., Albini, B. and Milgrom, F. (1978) Clin. Exp. Immunol. *34,* 28.
482 Penner, E., Albini, B., Andres, G.A. and Milgrom, F. (1979) Fed. Proc. *38,* 6241.
483 Penner, E., Albini, B., Glurich, I.,Andres, G.A. and Milgrom, F. (1981) (In press.)
484 Penner, E., Goldenberg, H., Albini, B., Weiser, M.M. and Milgrom, F. (1981) (In press).
485 Pentinnen, K. (1977) Ann. Rheum. Dis. 36, Suppl. *1,* 55.
486 Pentinnen, K. and Myllyla, G. (1970) Bull. W.H.O. *42,* 980.
487 Pentinnen, K., Vakeri, A. and Myllyla, G. (1971) Clin. Exp. Immunol. *8,* 389.
488 Penttinen, K., Myllyla, G., Makela, O. and Vaheri, A. (1969) Acta Pathol. Microbiol. Scand. *77,* 309.
489 Perlmann, P., Perlmann, H. and Biberfeld, P. (1972) J. Immunol. *108,* 558.
490 Perlmann, P., Perlmann, H., Wihlin, B. and Hammerstron, S. (1977) *In* Miescher, P.A. (ed.), Immunopathology (Schwabe, Basel) p. 321.
491 Pernis, B., Forni, L. and Amante, L. (1970) J. Exp. Med. *132,* 1001.
492 Pernis, B., Forni, L. and Amente, L. (1971) Ann. N.Y. Acad. Sci. *190,* 420.
493 Perrin, L.H., Lambert, P.H. and Miescher, P.A. (1975) J. Clin. Invest *56,* 165.
494 Perrin, L.H., Joseph, B.S., Cooper, N.R. and Oldstone, M.B.A. (1976) J. Exp. Med. *143,* 1027.
495 Petersson, B.A., Nilsson, A. and Stelenheim, G. (1975) J. Immunol. *114,* 1581.
496 Petts, V. and Roitt, I.M. (1971) Clin. Exp. Immunol. *9,* 407.
497 Pfeiffer, R. and Moreschi, C. (1906) Berl. Klin. Wochenschr. *43,* 33.
498 Pfueller, S.L. and Luscher, E.F. (1972) Immunochemistry *9,* 1151.
499 Pfueller, S.L. and Luscher, E.F. (1974) J. Immunol. *112,* 1201.
500 Pichler, W.J. and Broder, S. (1978) J. Immunol. *121,* 887.
501 Pichler, W.J., Lum, L. and Broder, S. (1978) J. Immunol. *121,* 1540.
502 Pillemer, L., Blum, L. and Lepow, I.H. (1954) Science *120,* 279.
503 Pirquet, C.V. (1911) Arch. Internal Med. *7,* 259.
504 Plaut, A.C., Cohen, S. and Tomasi, T.B. Jr. (1972) Science *176,* 55.
505 Ploem, J.S. (1967) Z. Wiss. Mikroskop. *68,* 129.
506 Polson, A., Potgieter, G.M., Largier, J.F., Mears, C.E.F. and Jombert, F.J. (1964) Biochim. Biophys. Acta *82,* 463.
507 Pope, R.M., Teller, D.I. and Mannick, M. (1974) Proc. Natl. Acad. Sci. *71,* 517.

508 Porter, R.R. and Reid, K.B.M. (1978) Nature *275,* 699.
509 Poskitt, T.R. and Poskitt, P.K.F. (1978) Immunol. Commun. *7,* 543.
510 Pressman, D. and Grossberg, A.L. (1973) The Structural Basis of Antibody Specificity (Benjamin, Reading).
511 Rabellino, E.M. and Metcalf, D. (1975) J. Immunol. *115,* 688.
512 Rabellino, E.M., Ross, G.D. and Polley, M.J. (1978) J. Immunol. *120,* 879.
513 Rabellino, E.M. Ross, G.D., Trang, H.Y.K., Williams, N. and Metcalf, D. (1978) J. Exp. Med. *147,* 434.
514 Rabinovitch, M., Manejias, R.E. and Nussenzweig, V. (1975) J. Exp. Med. *142,* 827.
515 Raff, M.C., Sternberg, M. and Taylor, R.B. (1970) Nature *255,* 553.
516 Reaman, G.M., Poplock, D.G., Broder, S. and Pichler, W.J. (1980) J. Immunol. *125,* 2215.
517 Rhodes, J. (1975) J. Immunol. *114,* 976.
518 Rich, A.R. (1956) Bull. Johns Hopkins Hosp. *98,* 120.
519 Riethmueller, G., Meltzer, M., Franklin, E. and Miescher, P.A. (1966) Clin. Exp. Immunol. *1,* 337.
520 Robert, B. and Grabar, P. (1957) Ann. Inst. Pasteur *92,* 56.
521 Roberts-Thompson, P.J., Hazlemen, B.L., Barnett, I.G., MacLennan, I.C.N. and Mowat, A.Z. (1976) Ann. Rheum. Dis. *35,* 314.
522 Robineaux, R. and Pinet, J. (1960) *In* Wolsterholme, G.E.W. and O'Connor, M (eds.), Cellular Aspects of Immunity (Little, Brown & Co., Boston) p. 5.
523 Robinson, J.P. (1966) J. Mol. Biol. *17,* 456.
524 Robinson, J.P. and Schultman, S.S. (1970) Immunology *20,* 883.
525 Rodrick, M., Allan, R. and Islikerty, (1978) J. Immunol. Methods *22,* 211.
526 Rogers, A.W. (1967) Techniques of Autoradiography (Elsevier, New York).
527 Romagnani, S., Maggi, E., Biagiotti, R., Giudizi, G.M., Amador, A. and Risci, M. (1978) Clin. Exp. Immunol. *32,* 324.
528 Roman-Franco, A.A., Turiello, M., Albini, B., Ossi, E., Milgrom, F. and Andres, G.A. (1978) Clin. Immunol. Immunopathol. *9,* 464.
529 Romans, D.G., Pinteric, L., Falk, R.E. and Dorrington, K.H. (1976) Immunology *116,* 1473.
530 Root, R.K., Metcalf, J., Oshino, N. and Chance, B. (1975) J. Clin. Invest. *55,* 945.
531 Rosenthal, C.J. and Franklin, E.C. (1975) Arthritis Rheum. *18,* 207.
532 Ross, G.D. and Rabellino, E.M. (1979) Fed. Proc. *38,* 1467.
533 Ross, G.D., Polley, M.J., Rabellino, E.M. and Grey, H.J. (1973) J. Exp. Med. *138,* 798.
534 Ross, G.D., Jarowski, C.I., Rabellino, E.M. and Winchester, R.J. (1978) J. Exp. Med. *147,* 730.
535 Rossen, R.D., Reisberg, M.A., Sharp, T., Suki, W.N., Schloeder, F.X., Hill, L. and Ekroyer, G. (1975) J. Clin, Invest. *56,* 427.
536 Rothbarth, P.H., Tanke, H.J., Mul, A.J., Ploem, J.S., Vliegenthart, J.F.G. and Ballieuz, R.E. (1978) J. Immunol. Methods *19,* 101.
537 Rother, K. (1972) Eur. J. Immunol. *2,* 550.
538 Rowley, D.A., Fitch, F.W., Stuart, F.P., Kohler, H. and Cosenza, H. (1973) Science *181,* 1133.
539 Ruddy, S. (1974) *In* Weissmann, G. (ed.), Mediators of Inflammation (Plenum, New York) p. 113.
540 Ruddy, S. and Austen, R.F. (1971) J. Immunol. *107,* 742.
541 Ruddy, S., Gigli, I. and Austen, K.F. (1979) N. Engl. J. Med. *287,* 489.
542 Ryan, G.B. and Majno, G. (1977) Am. J. Pathol. *86,* 183.
543 Ryan, G.B., Hein, S.J. and Karnovsky, M.J. (1976) Lab. Invest. *24,* 415.
544 Sainte-Marie, G. (1962) J. Histochem. Cytochem. *10,* 250.
545 Samarut, C., Cordier, G. and Revillard, J.P. (1979) Cell. Immunol. *42,* 18.
546 Sandberg, A.L., Oliveira, B. and Osler, A.G. (1971) J. Immunol. *106,* 282.
547 Scharfstein, J., Correa, E.B., Gallo, G.R. and Nussenzweig, V. (1974) J. Clin. Invest. *63,* 437.
548 Schauenstein, K., Wick, G., Herzog, F. and Steinbatz, A. (1975) J. Immunol. Methods *8,* 9.
549 Schauenstein, K., Wick, G. and Kink, H. (1976) J. Immunol. Methods *10,* 143.
550 Scheinberg, M.A. and Cathcart, E.S. (1976) Clin. Exp. Immunol. *24,* 317.
551 Scheinman, J.I., Foidart, J.M., Gehron-Robey, P., Fish, A.J. and Michael, A.F. (1980) Clin.

Immunol. Immunopathol. *15,* 175.
552 Scheinman, J.I., Foidart, J.M. and Michael, A.F. (1980) Lab. Invest. *43,* 373.
553 Schlessinger, J., Steinberg, I.L., Givol, D., Hahmann, J. and Pecht, I. (1975) Proc. Natl. Acad. Sci. U.S.A. *72,* 2775.
554 Schmidt, D.H., Kaufman, B.M. and Butler, V.D., Jr. (1974) J. Exp. Med. *139,* 278.
555 Schorlemmer, H.U. and Allison, A.C. (1976) Immunology *31,* 781.
556 Schreiber, R.D., Medicus, R.G., Gotze, O. and Muller-Eberhard, H.J. (1975) J. Exp. Med. *142,* 760.
557 Schur, P.H., and Becker, E.L. (1963) J. Exp. Med. *118,* 891.
558 Schur, P.H. and Christian, G.D. (1964) J. Exp. Med. *120,* 531.
559 Scribner, D.J., Weiner, H.L. and Moorhead, J.W. (1977) J. Immunol. *119,* 2084.
560 Shimizu, A., Paul, C., Kohler, H., Chinoda, T. and Putman, F.W. (1971) Science *182,* 287.
561 Shu, S. and Albini, B. (1976) J. Immunol. Methods *13,* 341.
562 Shu, S., Deng, J.S., Vetter, S. and Beutner, E.H. (1975) Cited in ref. 424 (Moran et al., 1977) p. 559.
563 Seligman, A.M., Karnovsky, M.J., Wasserkrug, H.L. and Hanker, J.S. (1968) J. Cell Biol. *38.* 1.
564 Shearer, W.T., Atkinson, J.P., Frank, M.M. and Parker, C.W. (1974) Clin. Res. *22,* 612a.
565 Shevach, E., Edelson, R., Frank, M., Lutzner, M. and Green, I. (1974) Proc. Natl. Acad. Sci. U.S.A. *71,* 863.
566 Shulman, N.R. and Barker, L.F. (1969) Science *165,* 304.
567 Sinclair, N.R. St. C. (1969) J. Exp. Med. *129,* 1183.
568 Singer, S.J. (1959) Nature *183,* 1523.
569 Smith, E.L. (1952) J. Biol. Chem. *199,* 789.
570 Smith, M.D., Veroust, P.J., Marcel-Maroger, L.M., Pesticier, A. and Couland, J.P. (1975) Br. Med. J. *2,* 274.
571 Smith, T. (1909) J. Exp. Med. *11,* 241.
572 Snyderman, R., Phillips, J.K. and Mergenbegger, S.E. (1971) J. Exp. Med. *134,* 1131.
573 Sobel, A.T. and Bokisch, V.A. (1975) Fed. Proc. *34,* 965.
574 Sobel, A.T., Gabay, Y.E. and Lagrue, G. (1976) Clin. Immunol. Immunopathol. *6,* 94.
575 Sobel, A.T., Bokisch, V.A. and Muller-Eberhard, H.J. (1975) J. Exp. Med. *142,* 139.
576 Soothill, J.F. and Hendrickse, R.J. (1967) Lancet *2,* 629.
577 Soothill, J.F. and Steward, M.W. (1971) Clin. Exp. Immunol. *9,* 193.
578 Spiegelberg, H.L. (1974) Adv. Immunol. *19,* 259.
579 Spiegelberg, H.L. and Gotze, O. (1972) Fed. Proc. *31,* 655.
580 Spiegelberg, H.L., Perlman, H. and Perlmann, P. (1976) J. Immunol. *116,* 1464.
581 Steensgaard, J., Liu, B.M., Cline, G.B. and Moller, N.P. (1977) Immunology *32,* 445.
582 Steffelaar, J.W., De-Graaff-Reitsma, C.B. and Feltkamp-Vroom, T.H.M. (1976) Clin. Exp. Immunol. *23,* 272.
583 Steffelaar, J.W., Tenkate, F.J.W., Nap, M., Swaak, A.J.G., DeGraaff-Reitsma, C.B., Elven, V.E.H. and Feltkamp-Vroom, T.H.M. (1977) Clin. Exp. Immunol. *27,* 391.
584 Steiner, L.A. and Lowey, S. (1972) J. Cell. Biol. *55,* 616.
585 Sternberger, L.A. (1979) Immunocytochemistry, 2nd ed. (Wiley & Sons, New York).
586 Steward, M.W. (1978) *In* Weir, D.W. (ed.), Handbook of Experimental Immunology, 3rd ed., Ch. 16 (Blackwell Sci. Publ., Oxford).
587 Steward, M.W. (1979) Clin. Exp. Immunol. *38,* 414.
588 Steward, M.W., Katz, F.E. and West, N.J. (1975) Clin. Exp. Immunol. *21,* 121.
589 Stingl, G., Wolff-Schreiner, E.C., Pichler, W.J., Schnait, F., Kanpp, W. and Wolff, K. (1977) Nature *268,* 245.
590 Stockinger, B. and Lemmel, E.M. (1978) Cell. Immunol. *40,* 395.
591 Stout, R.D. and Herzenberg, L.A. (1975) J. Exp. Med. *142,* 611.
592 Strauss, J., Pardo, V., Koss, M., Griswold, W. and McIntosh, R.M. (1975) Am. J. Med. *58,* 382.
593 Strober, W., Hague, N.E., Lum, L.G. and Henkart, P.A. (1978) J. Immunol. *121,* 2440.
594 Stuart, A.E. *In* Gell, P.G.H., Coombs, R.R.A. and Lachmann, P.J. (eds.), Clinical Aspects of

Immunology (Blackwell Sci. Publ., Oxford) p. 365.
595 Suba, E.A. and Csako, G. (1976) J. Immunol. *117,* 304.
596 Suciu-Foca, N., Buda, J.A., Thiem, T. and Reemtsma, K. (1974) Clin. Exp. Immunol. *18,* 295.
597 Sugisaki, T., Klassen, J. and McCluskey, R.T. Cited in ref. 413 (Milgrom, 1964)
598 Sugisaki, T., Kano, K., Brentjens, J., Anthone, S., Anthone, R., Andres, G.A. and Milgrom, F. (1982) Submitted for publication.
599 Sundsmo, J.S. and Gotze, O. (1979) Fed. Proc. *38,* 1467.
600 Svehag, S.E. (1975) Scand. J. Immunol. *4,* 687.
601 Svehag, S.E. and Burger, D. (1976) Acta Pathol. Microbiol. Scand. Sect. *C* 84, 45.
602 Szymanski, C.H. (1977) Sub-populations of cellular infiltrates in interstitial nephritis. Thesis, State University of New York, Buffalo.
603 Tai, P.C. and Spry, C.J.F. (1976) Clin. Exp. Immunol. *24,* 423.
604 Takahashi, M., Czop, J., Ferreira, A. and Nussenzweig, V. (1976) Transplant. Rev. *32,* 121.
605 Takahashi, M., Tack, B.F. and Nussenzweig, V. (1977) J. Exp. Med. *145,* 86.
606 Takahashi, M., Takahashi, S., Brade, V. and Nussenzweig, V. (1978) J. Clin. Invest. *62,* 349.
607 Takahashi, M., Takahashi, S. and Hirose (1980) Prog. Allergy *27,* 134.
608 Takenaka, T., Okuda, M., Kawabori, S. and Kubo, K. (1977) Clin. Exp. Immunol. *28,* 56.
609 Talmage, D.W., Dixon, F.J., Bukantz, S.C. and Dammin, G.J. (1951) J. Immunol. *67,* 243.
610 Tan, E.M. and Kunkel, H.G. (1966) Arthritis Rheum. *9,* 37.
611 Targowski, S.P. and Milgrom, F. (1979) Cell. Immunol. *42,* 405.
612 Targowski, S.P. and Milgrom, F. (1979) Fed. Proc. *38,* 920.
613 Tauber, J.W., Falk, J.A., Falk, R.E. and Zabriskie, J.B. (1976) J. Exp. Med. *143,* 1341.
614 Tauber, J.W., Polley, M.J. and Zabriskie, J.B. (1976) J. Exp. Med. *143,* 1352.
615 Taylor, R.B. and Basten, A. (1976) Br. Med. Bull. *32,* 152.
616 Ternynck, T. and Avrameas, S. (1900) Biochem. J. *125,* 297.
617 Tenner, A.J. and Cooper, N.R. (1979) Fed. Proc. *38,* 1467.
618 Ter Laan, B., Molenaar, J.L., Feltkamp-Vroom, T.H.M. and Pondman, K.W. (1974) J. Immunol. *4,* 393.
619 Teshima, H., Wanebo, H., Pinsky, C. and Day, N.K. (1974) J. Clin. Invest. *59,* 1134.
620 Theofilopoulos, A.N. and Dixon, F.J. (1976) *In* Bloom, B.R. and David, J.R. (eds.), In Vitro Methods in Cell-Mediated and Tumor Immunity (Academic Press, New York) p. 555.
621 Theofilopoulos, A.N. and Dixon, F.J. (1979) Adv. Immunol. *28,* 89.
622 Theofilopoulos, A.N., Bokisch, V.A. and Dixon, F.J. (1974) J Exp. Med. *139,* 696.
623 Theofilopoulos, A.N., Dixon, F.J. and Bokisch, V.A.(1974) J. Exp. Med. *140,* 877.
624 Theofilopoulos, A.N., Wilson, C.B., Bokisch, F.A. and Dixon, F.J. (1974) J. Exp. Med. *140,* 1234.
625 Theofilopoulos, A.N., Wilson, C.B. and Dixon, F.J. (1976) J. Clin. Invest. *57,* 169.
626 Theofilopoulos, A.N., Andrews, B.S., Urist, M.M., Morton, D.L. and Dixon, F.J. (1977) J. Immunol. *119,* 657.
627 Theofilopoulos, A.N., Eisenberg, R.A. and Dixon, F.J. (1978) J. Clin. Invest. *61,* 1570.
628 Theofilopoulos, A.N., Eisenberg, R.A. and Dixon, F.J. (1978) *In* Natelson, Pesce and Dietz (eds.), Clinical Immunochemistry (Assoc. Clin. Chem., Washington) p. 151.
629 Theofilopoulos, A.N., McConakey, P.J., Izui, S., Eisenberg, R.A. Pereira, A.B. and Creighton, W.D. (1980) Clin. Immunol. Immunopathol. *15,* 258.
630 Thomas, H.C. and Ferin, J. (1968) J. Clin. Endocrinol. Metabol. *28,* 1
631 Thrasher, S., Bigazzi, P.E., Yoshida, T. and Cohen, S. (1975) Immunol. Commun. *4,* 219.
632 Timpl. R., Wich, G. Furthmayer, H. and Kuhn, K. (1975) Eur. J. Biochem. *32,* 584.
633 Toben, H.R. and Smith, R.G. (1977) Clin. Exp. Immunol. *27,* 292.
634 Rossen, R.D., Reisberg, M.A., Sharp, T., Suki, W.N., Schloeder, F.X., Hill, L. and Ekroyer, G. (1975) J. Clin. Invest. *56,* 427.
635 Treser, G., Sermar, M., Ty, A., Sagel, I., Franklin, M.A. and Lange, K. (1970) J. Clin. Invest. *49,* 762.
636 Tsuda, F., Miyakawa, Y. and Mayumi, M. (1979) Immunology *37,* 681.
637 Tucker, D.F., Begent, R.H.J., and Hogg, N.M. (1978) J. Immunol. *121,* 1644.

638 Tung, K.S.K. (1977) J. Immunol. Methods *18,* 391.
639 Tung, K.S.K., Woodruffe, A.J., Ahlin, T.D., Williams, R.C. and Wilson, C.B. (1978) J. Clin. Invest. *62,* 61.
640 Uhr, J.W. (1965) Proc. Natl. Acad. Sci. U.S.A. *54,* 1599.
641 Uhr, J.W. and Moller, G. (1968) Adv. Immunol. *8,* 81.
642 Unkeless, J.C. (1977) J. Exp. Med. *145,* 931.
643 Unkeless, J.C., Kaplan, G., Plutner, H. and Cohn, Z.A. (1979) Proc. Natl. Acad. Sci. U.S.A. *76,* 1400.
644 Valdes, A.J., Senterfit, L.B., Pollack, A.D. and Germuth, F.G., Jr. (1969) Johns Hopkins Med. J. *124,* 9.
645 Valone, F.H., Witmer, D.I., Picke, H.W.C., Austen, K.F. and Goetzl, E.J. (1979) Immunology *37,* 841.
646 Van Damme, B.J.C., Fleuren, G.J. Bakker, W.W., Vernier, R.L. and Hoedemaeker, P.J. (1978) Lab. Invest. *38,* 502.
647 Van Es, L.A., Blok, A.P.R., Achoenfeld, L. and Glassock, R.J. (1977) Kidney Int. *11,* 106.
648 Van Oss, C.J., Neumann, A.W., Omenyi, S.N. and Absolom, K.R. (1978) Sep. Purif. Methods *7,* 245.
649 Van Oss, C.J., Absolom, D.R., Gorssberg, A.L. and Neumann, A.W. (1979) Immunol. Commun. *8,* 11.
650 Van Oss, C.J., Absolom, D.R. and Neumann, A.W. (1979) Sep. Sci. Technol. *14,* 305.
651 Van Oss, C.J., Absolom, D.R. and Neumann, A.W. (1980) Colloids Surfaces *1,* 45.
652 Van Oss, C.J., Absolom, D.R. and Neumann, A.W. (1980) Coll. Polym. Science *258,* 424.
653 Van Snick, J.L. and Masson, P.L. (1978) J. Exp. Med. *148,* 903.
654 Vazquez, J.J. and Dixon, F.J. (1957) Lab. Invest. *6,* 205.
655 Vaughan, J.H., Bayles, T.B. and Favour, C.B. (1951) J. Lab. Clin. Med. *37,* 698.
656 Vaughan, J.H., Barnett, E.V., Sobel, M.V. and Jacox, R.F. (1968) Arthritis Rheum. *11,* 125.
657 Vaughan, J.H., Carson, D.A., Kaplan, R.A. and Slaughter, L.S. (1979) *In* Milgrom, F. and Albini, B. (eds.), Immunopathology (1951) (Karger, Basel) p. 224.
658 Verroust, P.J., Wilson, C.J., Cooper, N.R., Edgington, T.S. and Dixon, F.J. (1974) J. Clin. Invest. *53,* 77.
659 Visser, J. (1972) Adv. Colloid Interface Sci. *3,* 331.
660 Vogt, A. (1965) Ein Beitrag zur Immunologie der Masugi-Nephritis. Thesis, Freiburg.
661 Vogt, A. (1982) Lab. Invest (in press).
662 Walwich, E.R., Inami, Y.H. and Nakamura, R.M. (1975) Am. J. Clin. Pathol. *63,* 219.
663 Wager, O., Penttinen, K., Rasanen, J.A. and Myllyla, G. (1973) Clin. Exp. Immunol. *15,* 393.
664 Walker, W.S. (1976) J. Immunol. *116,* 911.
665 Walker, W.S. (1977) J. Immunol. *119,* 367.
666 Ward, P.A. (1967) J. Exp. Med. *126,* 189.
667 Ward, P.A. and Zvaifler, N.J. (1973) J. Immunol. *111,* 1771.
668 Ward, P.A., Cochrane, C.G. and Muller-Eberhard, H.J. (1965) J. Exp. Med. *122,* 327.
669 Warner, N.L. (1974) Adv. Immunol. *19,* 67.
670 Warner, N.L. and McKenzie, I.F.C. (1977) *In* Marchalonis, J.J. (ed.), The Lymphocyte, Part II, p. 433.
671 Wautier, J.L., Tobelem, G.M., Pelteir, A.P. and Caen, J.P. (1976) Immunology *30,* 459.
672 Wautier, J.L., Souchon, H., Reid, K.B.M., Peltier, A.P. and Caen, J.P. (1977) Immunochemistry *14,* 763.
673 Weigle, W.O. (1975) Adv. Immunol. *21,* 87.
674 Weissmann, G., Dukor, P. and Zurier, R.B. (1971) Nature New Biol. *231,* 131.
675 Weller, P.F. and Goetzl, E. (1979) J. Adv. Immunol. *27,* 339.
676 Whaley, K. and Ruddy, S. (1976) J. Exp. Med. *144,* 1147.
677 Whaley, K. and Thompson, R.A. (1978) Immunology *35,* 1045.
678 Wick, G. and Beutner, E.H. (1969) Immunology *16,* 149.
679 Wick, G. and Beutner, E.H. (1970) *In* Holborow, E. J. (ed.), Standardization of Immunofluorescence (Blackwell, Oxford) p. 185.

680 Wick, G. and Graf, J. (1972) Lab. Invest. *27,* 400.
681 Wick, G., Furthmayer, H. and Timpl, R. (1975) Int. Arch. Allergy *48,* 664.
682 Wick, G., Baudner, S. and Herzog, F. (1976) Immunfluoreszenz (Mediz. Verlagsanstalt, Marburg).
683 Wiggins, R.C. and Cochrane, C. (1981) N. Engl. J. Med. *304,* 518.
684 Williams, R.C., Jr. (1980) Immune Complexes in Clinical and Experimental Medicine (Harvard Press, Cambridge).
685 Williams, D.C., Slaney, J.M., Price, J.F. and Challacombe, S.J. (1976) Nature *259,* 52.
686 Wilson, C.B. and Dixon, F.J. (1970) J. Immunol. *105,* 279.
687 Wilson, C.B. and Dixon, F.J. (1971) J. Exp. Med. *134;* 7s.
688 Wilson, C.B. and Dixon, F.J. (1976) *In* Brenner, B.M. and Rector, F.C., Jr. (eds.), The Kidney (Saunders, Philadelphia) p. 838.
689 Wilton, J.M.A. (1978) Clin. Exp. Immunol. *34,* 423.
690 Winchester, R.J., Winfield, J.B., Siegal, F., Wernet, P., Bentwich, Z. and Kunkel, H.G. (1974) J. Clin. Invest. *54,* 1082.
691 Winchester, R.J., Kunkel, H.G. and Agnello, V. (1971) J. Exp. Med. *134,* 286s.
692 Winfield, J.B., Koffler, D. and Kunkel, H.G. (1975) J. Clin. Invest. *56,* 563.
693 Winfield, J.B., Faiferman, I. and Koffler, D. (1977) J. Clin. Invest. *59,* 90.
694 Winfield, J.B., Lobe, P.I. and Hamilton, M.E. (1977) J. Immunol. *119,* 1778.
695 Wintrobe, M.M. and Buell, M.V. (1933) Bull. Johns Hopkins Hosp. *52,* 156.
696 Wisloff, F., Michaelsen, T.E. and Froland, S.S. (1974) Scand. J. Immunol. *3,* 29.
697 Wolff, K. and Schreiner, E. (1970) Arch. Klin. Expl. Dermatol. *238,* 38.
698 Wood, K.R., Stephen, J. and Smith, H. (1968) J. Gen. Virol. *2,* 313.
699 Woodroffe, A.J. and Wilson, C.B. (1977) J. Immunol. *118,* 1788.
700 Yasmeen, D., Ellerson, J.R., Dorrington, K.J. and Painter, R.H. (1976) J. Immunol. *116,* 185.
701 Yodoi, J., Takabayashi, A. and Masuda, T. (1978) Cell. Immunol. *39,* 225.
702 Yodoi, J., Ishizaka, T. and Ishizaka, K. (1979) Fed. Proc. *38,* 1088.
703 Yoshida, T.O. and Anderson, B. (1972) Scand. J. Immunol. *1,* 401.
704 Zieger, R.A. and Colten, H.R. (1977) J. Immunol. *118,* 540.
705 Zollinger, H.U. and Mihatsch, M.J. (1978) Renal Pathology in Biopsy (Springer, Berlin).
706 Zubler, R.H. and Lambert, P.-H. (1978) Prog. Allergy *24,* 1.
707 Zubler, R.H., Lange, G., Lambert, P.H. and Miescher, P.A. (1976) J. Immunol. *116,* 232.
708 Zurier, R.B. and Sayadoff, D.M. (1975) Inflammation *1,* 93.
709 Zwaifler, N.J. (1979) *In* Milgrom, F. and Albini B. (eds.) Immunopathology (Karger, Basel) p. 217.
710 Zwaifler, N.J. and Bluestein, H.G. (1976) Arthritis rheum. *19,* 844.

Subject index